Review of

PGI Chandigarh

Review of

PGI Chandigarh

Second Edition

Nov 2017
May 2017–Nov 2016

Mukhmohit Singh MBBS MD PG Dip. Diab, mRSSDI mIAPSM mIPHA
Faculty—Preventive Medicine, Public Health and Ethics
Ex. Assistant Professor, Department of Community Medicine
Ex. Epidemiologist, IDSP, Chandigarh Administration
Ex. Research Officer, PGIMER, Chandigarh
Gold SP Awardee, ERS-2012

Shveta Saini MBBS MD mIAPSM mIPHA
Faculty—Preventive Medicine and Public Health, Preventive Obstetrics and Gynecology
Ex. Assistant Professor, Department of Community Medicine

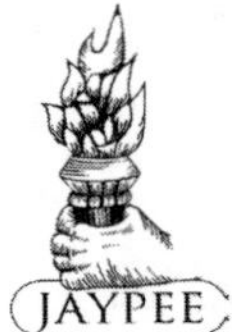

JAYPEE The Health Sciences Publisher
New Delhi | London | Panama

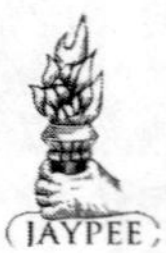

Jaypee Brothers Medical Publishers (P) Ltd

Headquarters
Jaypee Brothers Medical Publishers (P) Ltd.
4838/24, Ansari Road, Daryaganj
New Delhi 110 002, India
Phone: +91-11-43574357
Fax: +91-11-43574314
E-mail: jaypee@jaypeebrothers.com

Overseas Offices

JP Medical Ltd.
83, Victoria Street, London
SW1H 0HW (UK)
Phone: +44-20 3170 8910
Fax: +44(0)20 3008 6180
E-mail: info@jpmedpub.com

Jaypee-Highlights Medical Publishers Inc.
City of Knowledge, Bld. 235, 2nd Floor, Clayton
Panama City, Panama
Phone: +1 507-301-0496
Fax: +1 507-301-0499
E-mail: cservice@jphmedical.com

Jaypee Brothers Medical Publishers (P) Ltd.
17/1-B, Babar Road, Block-B, Shyamoli
Mohammadpur, Dhaka-1207
Bangladesh
Mobile: +08801912003485
E-mail: jaypeedhaka@gmail.com

Jaypee Brothers Medical Publishers (P) Ltd.
Bhotahity, Kathmandu, Nepal
Phone: +977-9741283608
E-mail: kathmandu@jaypeebrothers.com

Website: www.jaypeebrothers.com
Website: www.jaypeedigital.com

Inquiries for bulk sales may be solicited at: jaypee@jaypeebrothers.com

Review of PGI Chandigarh

First Edition: **2017**

Second Edition: **2018**

ISBN: 978-93-5270-221-3

Printed at: Sanat Printers

Dedicated to

Our Teachers
and
Students

PGI Review 2016–2017

Preface

Hello friends,

It does not matter what others say...

The sweat, time, hardwork, dedication...WILL pay off!

As we approach to reading of this manuscript, I would like to say that for any student aspiring for PGIMER Chandigarh, the race is for the best.

The race (or competition—as we may say) is for the best student of medicine and surgery and the one with excellent skills for time management.

The PGI examination, as we know, is composed of 250 MCQs with multiple options correct, making it imperative for the student to study and prepare to such an extent that he/she has the capacity to read, assess and mark the whole 1250 (250 × 5) options within the same stipulated time period of three hours.

As we go deeper into analysis of the PGI recall MCQs from the previous years, it comes out that the maximum MCQs in the examination are from a set of core areas as Medicine, Surgery, Obstetrics and Gynecology and Pediatrics. Now to be strong in these areas, one needs to have in-depth understanding of the concepts of the basic subjects as Pathology, Physiology, Pharmacology, Preventive Medicine, Biochemistry and Microbiology. So, one may classify these subjects as one part (approximately 50–70% of paper) and the remaining subjects as another part of the examination. Hence, you should be able to split your time accordingly for the preparation, revision and re-revision.

Overall, over the examinations, which the students have appeared, it seems that the more exposure you take for the MCQs, the better your chances are for clearing the examination with a good percentile score.

The most crucial aspect for a PG aspirant while preparing and writing the PGI entrance exam is time management. The art of solving 1250 options in limited time frame is not to be underestimated.

The chapters in this book have been strategically presented in order to provide an insight into the subject, giving you an extra edge for your preparation.

The explanations for various MCQs have been drafted in a manner to provide a complete review of the topic. The chapters on PSM include the recent changes and updates on Immunization, Tuberculosis and RNTCP, Leprosy and NLEP and Rabies updates.

The chapter on Orthopedics has been designed to contain illustrations for better understanding by the reader.

Emphasis has been put on cervical cancer, staging and management protocols, HIV and prevention of HIV from mother to child transmission, anti-phospholipid syndrome and pregnancy. The MCQs from valvular heart disease and cardiology, H1N1 and zika virus and other viral diseases have been discussed in detail. Various scoring systems for assessment of the clinical cases have been given due importance in the manuscript, which is one of the high yield areas of the PGI entrance examination.

We would like to thank all our faculty members and the review board for expediting the work on MCQs and providing the expert review of the subject matter. Our heartfelt thanks to our student contributors Dr Sajja Sai, Dr Narayan Prasad, Dr Musunuri Sai Sudha, Dr Somnath Sengupta, Dr Anshuman and others from the batch 2016-2017.

We also extend our very special thanks to Mr Harpreet Singh and Mr Rakinder Singh (operations manager NIME Institute) for providing constant support and motivation for compilation of the project.

All said and done, this project could not have been accomplished without the relentless support of our parents (Wg Cdr MS Bawa, Smt Gursharan Kaur, Dr RS Saini, and Mrs SB Saini) and daughters (Guntas and Mirajita).

We can never give them back the time we have used for writing this book. However, we do hope that the time consumed for this book is reflected by the time gained by our dear students preparing for the PGI entrance examination.

We would also extend immense gratitude to Mr Jitendar P Vij (Group Chairman), Ms Chetna Vohra (Associate Director, Content Strategies) and Ms Payal Bharti (Sr Manager, Publishing) for their valuable comments, editing, formatting and shaping the manuscript.

Keep your heads up...
God gives its "hardest" battles to His "strongest" soldiers
Realize the fire within... for only then is yours the sky and earth within...!
Humble greetings and best wishes for a splendid future...!

Mukhmohit Singh MBBS MD
Shveta Saini MBBS MD

Contents

Anatomy

1. All of the following are true about cervical lymphadenectomy except:
   a. The spinal accessory nerve, internal jugular vein, and sternocleidomastoid muscle are removed in radical neck dissection
   b. Modified radical neck dissection includes preservation of spinal accessory nerve and internal jugular vein
   c. Modified radical neck dissection includes preservation of spinal accessory nerve and sternocleidomastoid muscle.
   d. Anterior neck dissection includes removal of level V group of cervical lymph nodes

Ans. d (its level VI not V)

Option a	True	Yes, correct
Option b	True	Yes, correct
Option c	True	Yes, correct
Option d	False	No, anterior compartment lymph nodes are level 6 (not level V)
Option e	Not Available	---

2. LN removal level, correct match is:
   a. Submental nodes is level IB
   b. Posterior triangle group V
   c. Radical neck dissection: Removal of internal jugular vein
   d. Radical neck dissection: Removal of hypoglossal nerve
   e. Selective neck dissection: Removal of accessory nerve

Ans. b, c

Option a	False	No, it is level IA
Option b	True	Yes, correct
Option c	True	Yes, correct
Option d	False	No, not correct (refer to explanation)
Option e	False	No, not correct (refer to explanation)

Surgically, cervical lymph nodes are divided into 6-7 levels (only 6 according to many authors who exclude the level VII nodes) for staging of carcinoma which would also be the basis for selective neck dissection. There are 5 levels in the lateral compartment and 2 in the central compartment. Nodes not included in these system of levels are retropharyngeal group, periparotid group, buccinator group, post auricular group and suboccipital group of nodes.

Level		Lymph nodes	Boundaries
	A	Submental nodes	Bilaterally: Anterior belly of digastrics Inferiorly: Hyoid bone
I	B	Submandibular nodes	Superiorly: Mandible Posteroinferiorly: Posterior belly of digastrics Anteroinferiorly: Anterior belly of digastrics

Contd...

Contd…

Level		Lymph nodes	Boundaries
II	A (Anterior to the vertical line in relation to spinal accessory nerve) B (Posterior to the vertical line in relation to spinal accessory nerve)	Upper internal jugular (deep cervical) nodes	Superiorly: Skull base Inferiorly: Inferior border of hyoid bone and carotid bifurcation Posteriorly: Posterior border of Sternocleidomastoid (SCM) Anteriorly: Lateral border of Sternohyoid and Stylohyoid
III		Mid internal jugular (deep cervical) nodes	Superiorly: Inferior border of hyoid bone and carotid bifurcation Inferiorly: Inferior border of cricoid cartilage and junction of omohyoid muscle and IJV Posteriorly: Posterior border of SCM Anteriorly: Lateral border of sternohyoid
IV		Lower internal jugular (deep cervical nodes)	Superiorly: Inferior border of cricoids cartilage and Junction of omohyoid and IJV Inferiorly: Clavicle Posteriorly: Posterior border of SCM Anteriorly: Lateral border of sternohyoid
V	A (Above the horizontal plane marking the inferior border of arch of cricoids cartilage) B (Below the horizontal plane marking the inferior border of arch of cricoids cartilage)	Posterior triangle (spinal accessory) nodes	Superiorly: Convergence of SCM and trapezius Inferiorly: Clavicle Posteriorly: Anterior border of trapezius Anteriorly: Posterior border of SCM
VI	(Prelaryngeal or Delphian, Pretracheal, Paratracheal, Prethyroidal)	Anterior compartment (midline) nodes	Superiorly: Hyoid bone Inferiorly: Suprasternal notch Bilaterally: Carotid arteries
VII		Upper mediastinal nodes	Below suprasternal notch

Note

The highest jugular digastric node near the angle of the mandible is called the 'sentinel' node. The 'signal' node is the lowest along the internal jugular chain called the virchow nodes.

- Level 1: Oral cavity, submandibular gland
- Level 2: Nasopharynx, oropharynx, parotid, supraglottic larynx
- Level 3: Oropharynx, hypopharynx, supraglottic larynx
- Level 4: Subglottic larynx, hypopharynx, esophagus, thyroid
- Level 5: Nasopharynx, oropharynx
- Level 6 and 7: Thyroid, larynx, lung

Classical Neck Dissection

Level I-V nodes + sternocleidomastoid muscle + internal jugular vein + accessory nerve.

Modified radical neck dissection: Preserves some of the latter three structures.

Selective neck dissection: Removes some, but not all lymph nodes I-V.

Selective Neck Dissection Involves

- Supraomohyoid/Anterolateral: Level I to III
- Extended supraomohyoid: Level I to IV
- Lateral: Level II to IV
- Posterolateral: Level II to V
- Anterior or Central: Level VI
- Superior mediastinal: Level VII

3. All of the following structures traverse parotid gland except:

a. External carotid artery b. Facial nerve
c. Retromandibular vein d. Facial artery
e. External Jugular vein

Ans. d, e *Ref: Gray's anatomy, 40th/ed p879*

Option a	True	Yes, it crosses the parotid gland
Option b	True	Yes, it crosses the parotid gland
Option c	True	Yes, it crosses the parotid gland
Option d	False	No, it does not cross
Option e	False	No, it does not cross

There is no specific developmentally determined plane in which the facial nerve branches pass between superficial and deep lobes of the gland.

The parotid is an integral gland, not divided into lobes. Within the gland, the nerve branches communicate with each other, forming a plexiform arrangement that lies superficial to the retromandibular vein, which in turn is superficial to the external carotid artery. The retromandibular vein is formed within the parotid by the confluence of the superficial temporal and maxillary veins. The retromandibular vein emerges from the lower part (pole) of the gland and divides into an anterior branch which joins the facial vein and a posterior branch which joins the posterior auricular vein to form the external jugular vein; however, the division may occur within the gland and the two branches emerge from the lower pole. Lymph nodes of the preauricular (parotid) group lie on or deep to the fascial capsule of the parotid, as well as within the gland.

The retromandibular vein formed by the union of the maxillary and superficial temporal veins (which enter near the points of exit of the corresponding arteries) is superficial to the external carotid artery. It descends in the parotid gland and emerges behind the apex of the gland where it usually divides into an anterior branch which passes forwards to join the facial vein, and a posterior branch which joins the posterior auricular vein to form the external jugular vein. Occasionally, it is not connected to the external jugular vein which is then small, and the anterior jugular vein is enlarged.

4. All of the following statements are true for thyroid gland and its capsule except:
a. Pretracheal fascia is derived from deep layer of cervical fascia
b. Condensed layer of capsule forms berry ligament
c. Parathyroid glands are usually related to posterior border
d. Thyroid gland extends from sixth cervical to third thoracic vertebra
e. Recurrent laryngeal nerve course is identical in most cases on both sides of neck

Ans. d, e

Option a	True	Yes, correct
Option b	True	Yes, correct
Option c	True	Yes, correct
Option d	False	No, the gland extends from 5th cervical to 1st thoracic
Option e	False	No, the RLN has different course on both sides of the neck

Thyroid gland – anatomy:
- Extends from 5th cervical to the 1st thoracic vertebra consists of two lobes connected by median isthmus.
- Covered by pretracheal layer of deep cervical fascia.

The pretracheal facia encloses the thyroid gland and forms the false capsule.
The posterior layer of the capsule is thick.
- On the either side it forms a suspensory ligament for the thyroid gland known as '*ligament of berry*' the ligaments are attached to the cricoid cartilage and support the thyroid gland
- The fascia provides a smooth friction free surface for movement of trachea over the cartilages and thyroid gland.

Note: The recurrent laryngeal nerve course on either side is different [FAQ]

The right RLN leaves the right vagus nerve as it crosses the right subclavian artery and loops posteriorly under the artery. The right RLN initially traverses at an angle towards the tracheoesophageal groove and then runs parallel to it.

The left RLN originates from the left vagus nerve as it crosses the aortic arch. It then passes posteriorly under the arch and the ligamentum arteriosum. The left RNL travels in a course that is parallel and close to the tracheoesophageal groove. The lower origin and consequently, a longer course of the left RLN makes it more vulnerable to injury than the right RLN.

5. Fusion of bones in 22–25 years of age:
a. XiphiSternum
b. Manubriosternal joint
c. Lower end of radius and ulna
d. Shoulder
e. Coracoid process, scapula

Ans. c,d

Option a	False	No, sternum fuses after 4th decade of life
Option b	False	No, it fuses at very late age (~ > 60 years)
Option c	True	Yes, correct
Option d	True	Yes, correct
Option e	False	No, it fuses at an early age usually < 17 years of age

- Between 18–25 years: By this age long bones epiphysis unites with their shaft.
- Lower end of radius and ulna unite with their respective shafts at 18–19 years.
- Iliac crest unites with the ilium and ischial tuberosity unites with the ischium of hip bone by 20 years.
- The sternal end of clavicle unites with the sternum by 21 years.
- Secondary centers in articular facet of the rib is complete by 20–25 years.
- The bony replacement of cartilage between basi-occiput and basi-sphenoid is complete by 20–25 years.

The median age for ossification centers and their fusion is:

Table 1: The important ossification centers and their fusion

Centers of bones	Appearance	Fusion
Clavicle—medial end	15–19 years	20–22 years
Sternum	5 month IUL	60–70 years
Manubrium body (1st segment)	5 month IUL	14–25 years from below upwards
IInd segment	7 month IUL	3rd and 4th—15 years
IIIrd segment	7 month IUL	2nd and 3rd—25 years
IVth segment	10 month IUL	1st and 2nd—25 years
Xiphoid process	3 years	> 40 years with the body
Humeus (Upper end)		
• Head	1 year, all 3 units at 6 years	16 years
• Greater tubercle	3 years	4–5 years with head
• Lesser tubercle	5 years	5-7 years with greater tubercle
Humeus (Lower end)		
• Medial epicondyle	5–6 years	Capitulum, trochlea and lateral epicondyle
• Capitulum	1 year	Form conjoint tendon at 14 years
• Trochlea	9–10 years	Unites with shaft at 15 years
• Lateral epicondyle	10–12 (11) years	Medial, epicondyle unites at 16 years
Radius		
Upper end	5–6 years	15–16 years
Lower end	1–2 years	18–19 years
Ulna		
• Upper end	8–9 years	16–17 years
• Lower end	5–6 years	18–19 years

Contd...

Contd...

Centers of bones	Appearance	Fusion
• Head 1st metacarpal	2 years	15–17 years
• Head other metacarpals	1 1/2 to 2 1/2 years	15–19 years
Hip bone		
• Triradiate cartilage	11–13 years	14–15 years
• Iliac crest	14–15 years	18–20 years
• Ishchial tuberosity	15–16 years	20–22 years
• Sarcum	8 months IUL	25 years
Femur (Upper end)		
• Head	1 year	17–18 years
• Greater trochanter	4 years	17 years
• Lesser trochanter	14 years	15–17 years
Femur (Lower end)	9 months IUL	17–18 years
Tibia		
• Upper end	9 months IUL	16–17 years
• Lower end	1 year	16 years
Scapula		
• Coracoid base	10–11 years	14–15 years
• Acromion process	14–15 years	17–18 years

6. All of the following is true about central retinal artery except:

a. The central retinal artery enters into optic nerve about 5 cm behind the eyeball.

b. The central retinal artery supplies the outer 5 layers of the retina

c. It divides into equal superior and inferior branches.

d. They mainly run within the nerve fiber and ganglion cell layer of retina.

e. Arteries are easily distinguished from the veins ophthalmoscopically

Ans. a, b *Ref: Gray's anatomy 40 ed, page 1256*

Option a	False	No, it enters just 1.2 cm near to the eyeball
Option b	False	No it supplies the inner layers of the retina
Option c	True	Yes, correct
Option d	True	Yes, correct
Option e	True	Yes, correct because of the bright red color

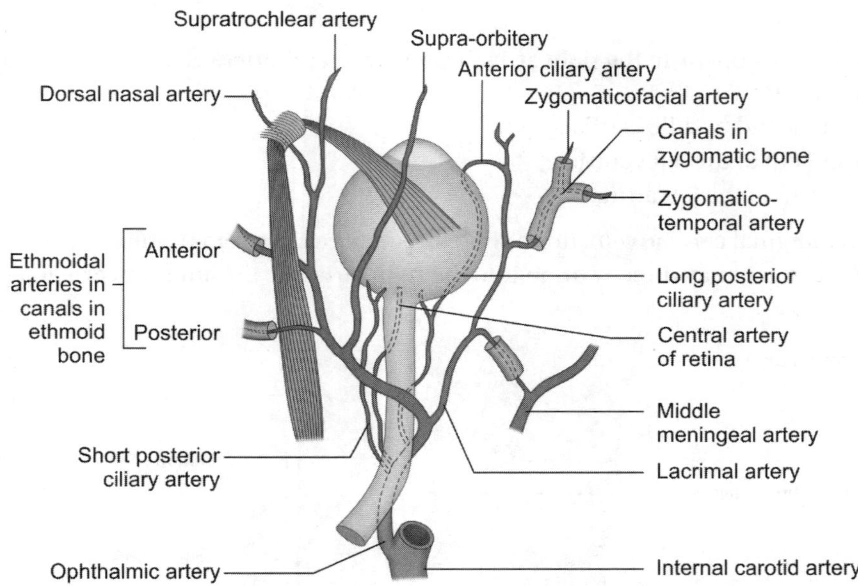

The retina has a dual blood supply. The outer five layers of retina are avascular and inner retina receives the blood supply from the branches of the central retinal artery and vein.

- The central retinal artery (CRA) enters the optic nerve as branch of the ophthalmic artery approx 1.2 cm behind the eyeball and travels within the optic nerve to cross the lamina cribrosa.
- It divides into superior and inferior branches which further divide into nasal and temporal branches - each supply the FOUR quadrants of retina (superior/inferior nasal; superior/ inferior temporal)
- The vessels run within the nerve fiber and the ganglion layer of retina
- In chronic severe HTN - the arteries may impinge upon the veins causing visible dilations at the crossings (AV Kinks).

7. All are tributaries of coronary sinus except:

a. Great cardiac vein
b. Middle cardiac vein
c. Small cardiac vein
d. Anterior cardiac vein
e. Right marginal cardiac vein

Ans. d,e *Ref: Last anatomy 12 ed, pg 323 and Gray's anatomy, 40, pg 1797*

Option a	True	Yes, correct
Option b	True	Yes, correct
Option c	True	Yes, correct
Option d	False	No, it drains directly into right atria
Option e	False	No, it drains into the small cardiac vein or directly into right atria

Coronary sinus:

The coronary sinus opens in the right atria through the semilunar valve of the coronary sinus. The tributaries are:

- ❑ Great, small and middle cardiac veins
- ❑ Posterior vein of the left ventricle
- ❑ Oblique vein of the left atrium

Note: Right marginal cardiac vein: drains into the small cardiac veins (which further join in the coronary sinus) or it may directly drain into the right atria like the anterior cardiac vein.

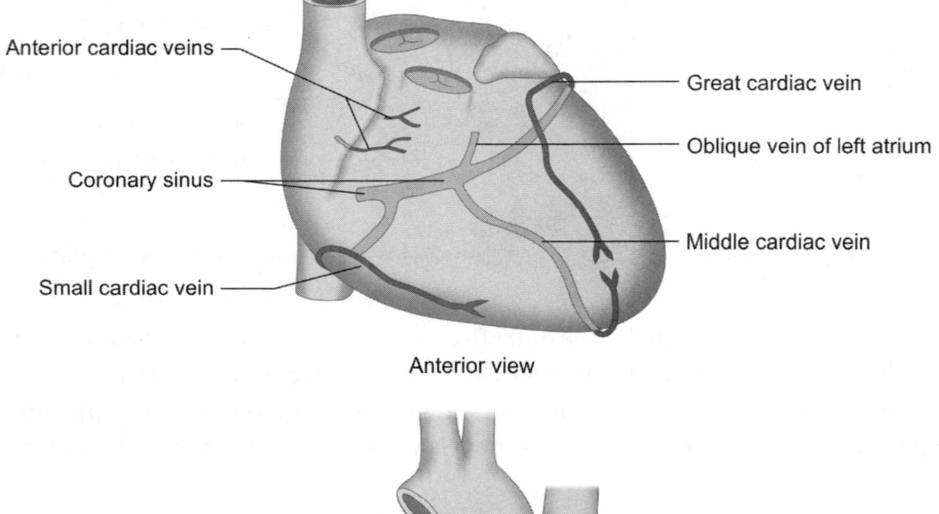

Anterior view

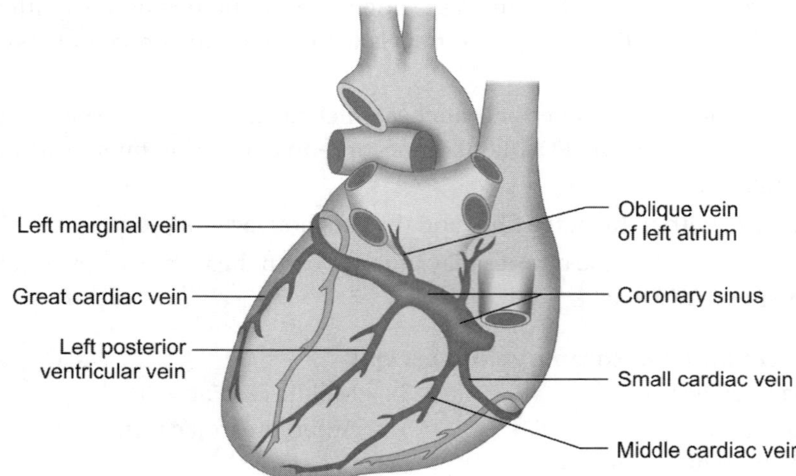

8. All are true about hangman's fracture except:

a. Also known as traumatic spondylolisthesis of the axis
b. Neurological injuries are very common
c. The pedicles of axis break symmetrically and fracture may extend to posterior part of body
d. Dens of axis mostly remain intact
e. It is bilateral fracture involving the interarticular area

Ans. b, e

Option a	True	Yes, correct
Option b	False	No, neurological deficit is very rare because spinal canal is very wide at this level
Option c	True	Yes, correct
Option d	True	Yes, correct
Option e	False	No, it is bilateral traumatic spondylolithesis of the axis (C2) with interarticular area fracture

- Hangman's fracture is a bilateral fracture of the pars interarticularis of the C2
- Motor vehicle accident/RTA is most common cause
- Mechanism of injury – sudden hyperextension followed by sudden forceful flexion.

Levine and Edwards classification (based on mechanism of injury)			
Type I	Axial compression and hyperextension	• < 3 mm horizontal displacement C2/3 • No angulation • C2/3 disc remains intact	• Rigid collar × 4–6 weeks
Type II	Hyperextension and axial load followed by rebound flexion	• > 3 mm of horizontal displacement • Significant angulation • Vertical fracture line • C2/3 disc and PLL are disrupted • Unstable fracture pattern	• If < 5 mm displacement reduction with traction then halo immobilization × 6–12 weeks • If > 5 mm displacement, surgery or prolonged traction • Usually heal despite displacement (autofuse C2 on C3)
Type IIA	Flexion distraction	• No horizontal displacement • Horizontal fracture line • Significant angulation	• Avoid traction type IIA • Reduction with gentle axial load + hyperextension, then compression halo immobilization for 6-12 weeks.
Type III	Flexion distraction followed by hyperextension	• Type I fracture with associated bilateral C2-3 facet dislocation • Rare injury pattern	• Surgical reduction of facet dislocation followed by stabilization required

9. Ureter blood supply is from:

a. Renal artery
b. Gonadal artery
c. Vesical artery
d. External iliac artery
e. Superior rectal artery

Ans. a,b,c

Option a	True	Yes, correct
Option b	True	Yes, correct
Option c	True	Yes, correct
Option d	False	No, it is by common and internal iliac artery
Option e	False	No, it is by middle rectal artery

The ureter is supplied from the:
- ❑ Renal artery
- ❑ Gonadal artery
- ❑ Common iliac artery
- ❑ Vesical artery
- ❑ Uterine arteries
- ❑ Internal iliac artery

Note:
- ❑ The abdominal part of the ureter is supplied from the medial side of the arteries
- ❑ The pelvic ureter is supplied by the vessels lateral to the ureter.

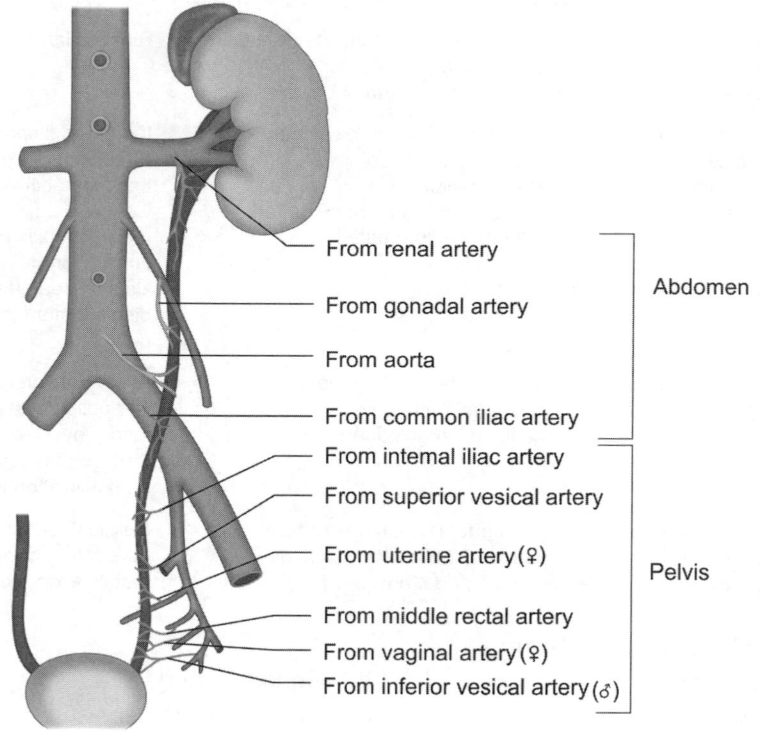

10. All are true about trochlear nerve except:
- a. It crosses midline within the midbrain
- b. Exits from brainstem anteriorly below inferior colliculus
- c. Passes between posterior cerebral and inferior cerebellar artery
- d. Runs forward in the lateral wall of cavernous sinus
- e. Has longest intracranial route

Ans. b,c

Option a	True	Yes, correct statement
Option b	False	No, it is the only nerve which emerges from the brainstem dorsally (or posteriorly) and not anterior
Option c	False	No, it passes between the posterior cerebral and superior (not inferior) cerebellar artery
Option d	True	Yes, correct statement
Option e	True	Yes, correct statement

- Trochlear nerve nucleus is located in the dorsal midbrain. The trochlear nerve fibers decussate in the brainstem to exit dorsally.

Note: It is the only cranial nerve to exit posteriorly.

- It runs along the III cranial nerve between the superior cerebellar and posterior cerebral artery.
- Courses through the cavernous sinus to emerge through the superior orbital fissure.

High Yield

- The long course of the fourth cranial nerve renders it particularly prone to injury from blunt head trauma or compression from changes in intracranial pressure, brain tumors, or swelling anywhere along its course.
- Nerves passing through the superior orbital fissure: **LFTS Nasally In Abdomen**
  - **L:** Lacrimal nerve (branch of CN VI)
  - **F:** Frontal nerve (branch of CN VI)
  - **T:** Trochlear nerve (CN IV)
  - **S:** Superior division of the oculomotor nerve (CN III)
  - **N:** Nasociliary nerve (branch of CN V1)
  - **I:** Inferior division of the oculomotor nerve (CN III)
  - **A:** Abducens nerve (CN VI)

11. Urogenital diaphragm, the correct statement is:

a. Formed by the deep transverse perinei muscle
b. Sphincter urethrae constitutes the urogenital diaphragm
c. Triangular shape
d. The bulbourethral gland is inserted into the deep perineal pouch
e. It supports the rectum

Ans. b, e

Option a	True	Yes Correct
Option b	False	No, deep transverse perinei, sphincter urethra, perineal membrane form the urogenital membrane
Option c	True	Yes Correct
Option d	True	Yes Correct
Option e	False	No, it supports the penis, prostate

The sphincter urethra l layers and deep transverse perineal muscles, superior and inferior fascia- constitute the urogenital diaphragm. The inferior fascia l layers is termed as perineal membrane, and the enclosed space between the superior and inferior fascia l layers is known as the deep perineal pouch.

Perineal membrane: Above the perineal membrane lies the membranous urethra surrounded by urethral sphincter below the apex of prostate. The membrane is pierced by the urethra, the ducts of bulbourethral glands and by nerves and vessels.

Sphincter urethrae:

- Known as external urethral sphincter
- Pear shaped
- Innervation: Perineal branch of pudendal nerve

Superficial perineal fascia:

- Known as colles fascia
- Continuation into perineum of membranous fascia (of scarpa) from the anterior abdominal wall. It is attached to the ischiopubic rami and the posterior margin of the perineal membrane and forms the **superficial perineal pouch**.

Anatomy

1. Branches of internal carotid artery are:

a. Superior hypophyseal artery
b. Inferior hypophyseal artery
c. Ophthalmic artery
d. Post cerebral artery
e. Post communicating artery

Ans. a, b, c, e *Ref: Snell's Anatomy, 9th/ed*

Option a	True	Branch of cerebral part of ICA
Option b	True	Branch of cavernous part of ICA
Option c	True	First branch of ICA distal to the cavernous sinus
Option d	False	Terminal branches of the basilar artery
Option e	True	Branch of cerebral part of ICA

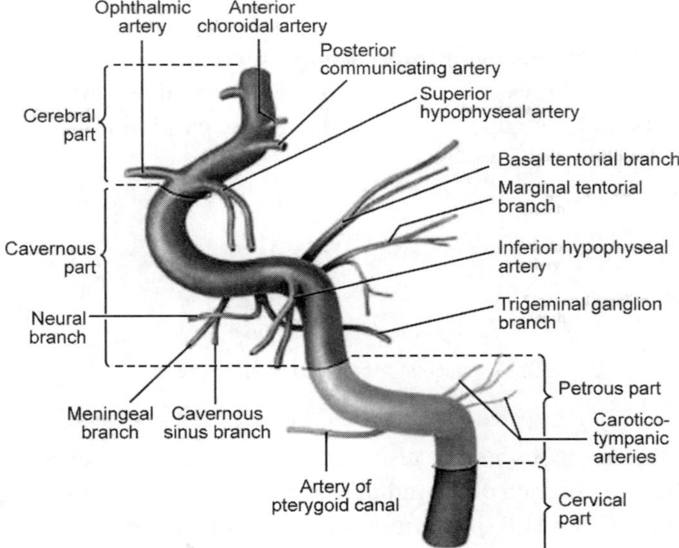

Fig. 1: Branches of internal carotid artery.

Mnemonic:

- *1st supplies the parts of head – nose and ear.*
- *Then supplies the covering of brain and pituitary.*
- *Then supplies the eyes.*
- *At last supplies the brain.*

Mnemonic to remember branches of Internal carotid artery:

A VIP'S COMMA

A: Anterior choroidal artery (C7)

V: Vidian artery (C2)
I: Inferolateral trunk (C4)
P: Posterior communicating artery (C7)
S: Superior hypophyseal artery (C6)
C: Caroticotympanic artery (C2)
O: Ophthalmic artery (C6)
M: Meningohypophyseal trunk (C4)
M: Middle cerebral artery (C7)
A: Anterior cerebral artery (C7)

Brain structures supplied by Internal carotid artery:

1. Cerebral hemispheres.
2. Eye, optic nerve, optic chiasma and optic tract.
3. Midbrain through anterior choroidal artery.
4. Thalamus and internal capsule through posterior communicating artery.
5. Pituitary gland and hypothalamus.
6. Meninges of the skull base.

2. Muscles supplied by posterior interosseous nerve are:

a. Extensor pollicis brevis
b. Extensor digitorum
c. Adductor pollicis longus
d. Flexor carpi ulnaris
e. Extensor carpi radialis brevis

Ans. a, b, e *Ref: Snell's Anatomy, 9th/ed*

Option a	True	
Option b	True	
Option c	False	Supplied by deep branch of ulnar nerve
Option d	False	Supplied by muscular branches of ulnar nerve
Option e	True	

The posterior interosseous nerve, also known as the dorsal interosseous nerve, is the continuation of the deep branch of the radial nerve after it penetrates the supinator muscle. It carries fibers from the C7 and C8 spinal nerves, and supplies the majority of the muscles in the posterior compartment of the forearm.

The posterior interosseous nerve supplies four superficial extensors and five deep extensors in the posterior compartment of the forearm.

Superficial extensor	Deep extensor
Extensor carpi radialis brevis	Supinator
Extensor digiti minimi	Extensor indicis
Extensor carpi ulnaris	Abductor pollicis longus
Extensor digitorum	Extensor pollicis longus
	Extensor pollicis brevis

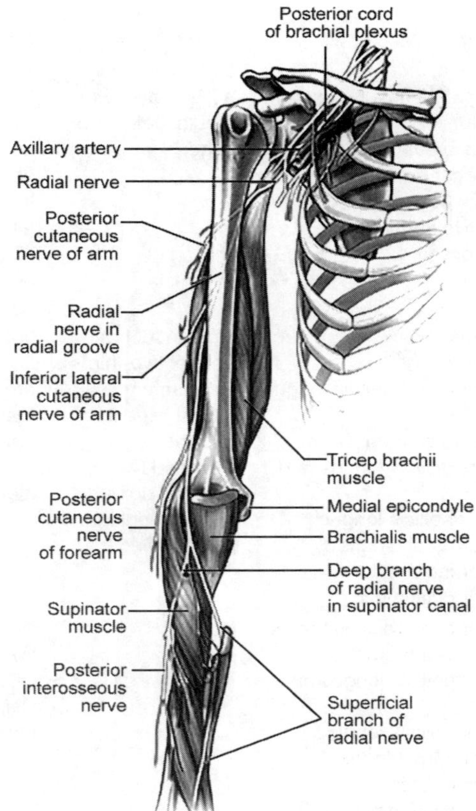

Fig. 2: Nerve supply of elbow and forearm.

Motor, sensory and functional loss in the Upper limb			
Nerve	***Motor loss***	***Sensory loss***	***Functional loss***
Median nerve (C6 to C8, T1)	Pronator teres Flexor carpi radialis Palmaris longus Flexor digitorum superficialis Flexor pollicis longus Lateral half of flexor digitorum profundus Pronator quadratus Thenar eminence Lateral two lumbricals	Palmar aspect of hand with thumb, index, middle, and lateral half of ring finger Dorsal aspect of distal third of index, middle, and lateral half of ring finger	Pronation weak or lost Weak wrist flexion and abduction Radial deviation at wrist lost Inability to oppose or flex thumb Weak thumb abduction Weak grip Weak or no pinch (ape hand deformity)
Anterior interosseous nerve (branch of median nerve)	Flexor pollicis longus Lateral half of flexor digitorum profundus Pronator quadratus Thenar eminence Lateral two lumbricals	None	Pronation weak especially at 90° elbow flexion Weak opposition and flexion of thumb Weak finger flexion Weak pinch (no tip-to-tip)

Contd…

Contd…

Nerve	Motor loss	Sensory loss	Functional loss
Ulnar nerve (C5 to C8, T1)	Flexor carpi ulnaris Medial half of flexor digitorum profundus Palmaris brevis Hypothenar eminence Adductor pollicis Medial two lumbricals All interossei	Dorsal and palmar aspect of little and medial half of ring finger	Weak wrist flexion Loss of ulnar deviation at wrist Loss of distal flexion of little finger Loss of abduction and adduction of fingers Inability to extend second and third phalanges of little and ring fingers (benediction hand deformity) Loss of thumb adduction
Radial nerve (C5 to C8, T1)	Anconeus Brachioradialis Extensor carpi radialis longus and brevis Extensor digitorum Extensor pollicis longus and brevis Abductor pollicis longus Extensor carpi ulnaris Extensor indices Extensor digiti minimi	Dorsum of hand (lateral two-thirds) Dorsum and lateral aspect of thumb Proximal two-thirds of dorsum of index, middle, and half ring finger	Loss of supination Loss of wrist extension (wrist drop) Inability to grasp Inability to stabilize wrist Loss of finger extension Inability to abduct thumb
Posterior interosseous nerve (branch of radial nerve)	Extensor carpi radialis brevis Extensor digitorum Extensor pollicis longus and brevis Abductor pollicis longus Extensor carpi ulnaris Extensor indices Extensor digiti minimi	None	Weak wrist extension Weak finger extension Difficulty stabilizing wrist Difficulty with grasp Inability to abduct thumb

3. True about homeotic genes:

a. Anatomical location of organs
b. Early organ development
c. Contain homeobox
d. Mutations are generally not lethal
e. Important for segmentation

Ans. a, b, c, e *Ref: Developmental biology—molecular biology of cell determination and differentiation—Vol 5*

Option a	True	
Option b	True	Control the pattern of body formation during early embryonic development
Option c	True	Homeobox is a sequence of DNA
Option d	False	Mutations are lethal
Option e	True	

Homeotic gene:

- Group of genes that control the pattern of body formation *during early embryonic development of organisms.*
- These genes encode proteins called transcription factors that direct cells to form various parts of the body.
- There are several subsets of homeotic genes. They include many of the *Hox* and *ParaHox* genes that are important for *segmentation.*

- ❑ A homeotic protein can activate one gene but repress another, producing effects that are complementary and necessary for the ordered development of an organism.
- ❑ Mutations in homeotic genes *cause displaced body parts,* such as antennae growing at the posterior of the fly instead of at the head. Mutations that lead to such ectopic placements are usually *lethal.*
- ❑ Homeotic genes contain a sequence of DNA known as a ***homeobox***, which encodes a segment of 60 amino acids within the homeotic transcription factor protein.
- ❑ If a mutation occurs in the homeobox of any of the homeotic genes, an organism will not develop correctly.

4. Correct statement(s) about meiosis:

a. Somatic cells not divide by meiosis because number of chromosomes reduces to half
b. Occur in germ cell which result in haploid cells
c. There is production of single ovum and single sperm from a single oocyte and spermatocyte respectively
d. Germ cells undergo meiosis
e. Meiosis is required to produce large number of eggs and sperms

Ans. a, d, e *Ref: Langman's Medical Embryology, 13th/ed*

Option a	True	
Option b	False	Meiosis occurs in gametes to produce the germ cells
Option c	False	One primary oocyte and one primary spermatocyte give rise to 4 daughter cells
Option d	True	
Option e	True	

- ❑ Meiosis, also referred to as "reduction division", is the form of division of the cell nucleus by which a cell divides into four "daughter cells" each of which has half of the number of chromosomes of the original cell.
- ❑ Meiosis only occurs in the "gametes"—prior to the formation of sperm (in males) and ova (in females).
- ❑ Meiosis occur in gametes (i.e. reproductive cells): in the ovary and testis to produce the germ cells: ova and spermatozoa.
- ❑ It consists of two successive divisions: meiosis I and meiosis II, to reduce the number of chromosomes to haploid number of 23.
- ❑ At the beginning of meiosis—I, spermatocyte and primary oocyte replicate their DNA so that each of 46 chromosomes gets duplicated into sister chromatids.
- ❑ The homologous chromosomes then align themselves in pairs ***(synapsis).***
- ❑ The pairing is exact and point for point except for the XY combination.
- ❑ Homologous pairs then separate into two daughter cells, thereby reducing the chromosome number from diploid to haploid.
- ❑ Shortly, meiosis II separates sister chromatids. Each gamete then contains 23 chromosomes.
- ❑ During meiosis, one primary oocyte gives rise to four daughter calls each with 22 plus 1 X chromosome. Only one develops into mature gamete and others degenerate subsequently.
- ❑ Similarly, one primary spermatocyte gives rise to 4 daughter cells, 2 with 22 plus 1 X chromosome and 2 with 22 plus 1 Y chromosome. In contrast to oocyte, all four develop into mature gametes.

Crossover:

- ❑ Interchange of chromatid segments between paired homologous chromosomes.

- Segments of chromatids break and are exchanged as homologous chromosomes separate.
- Genetic variability is enhanced through crossover by redistribution of genetic material and random distribution of homologous chromosomes to daughter calls.

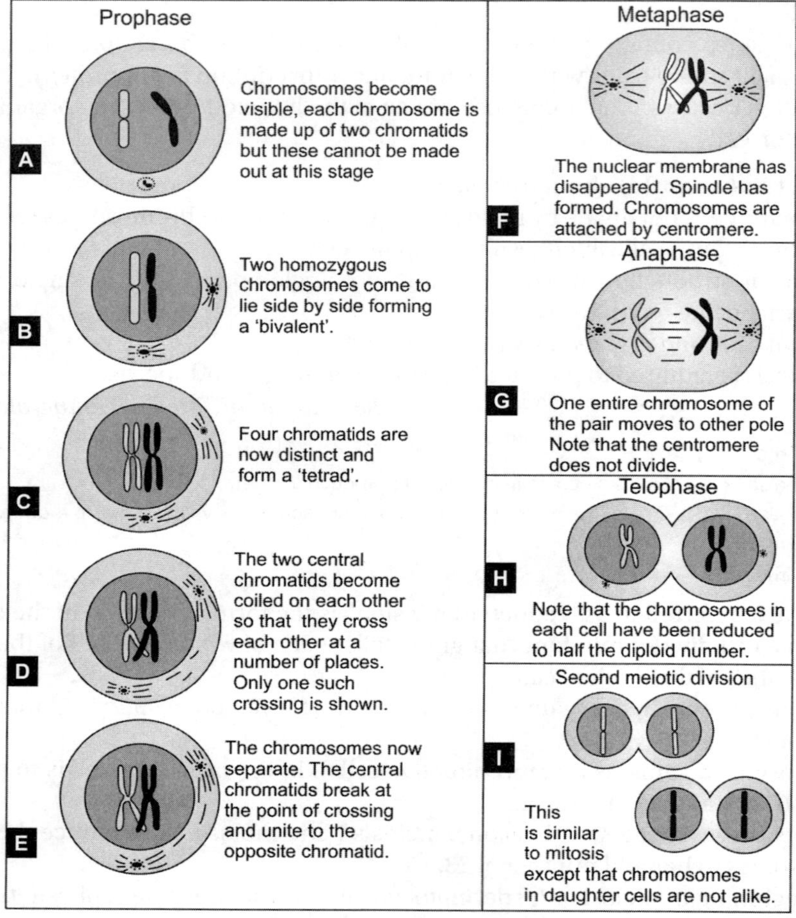

Fig. 3: Scheme to show the main steps of meiosis. Only the telophase of the second division is shown.

5. Anterior compartment of leg muscle are all *except*:

a. Extensor hallucis longus
b. Extensor digitorum longus
c. Peroneus brevis
d. Peroneus longus
e. Fibularis tertius

Ans. c, d *Ref: Snell's Anatomy, 9th/ed*

Option a	False	Anterior compartment of leg muscle
Option b	False	Lie within the peroneal compartment located at the lateral fibular region
Option c	True	
Option d	True	
Option e	False	Anterior compartment of leg muscle

Fibularis longus muscle/Peroneus longus muscle: originates at the head and the upper body of the fibula and the intermuscular septa. It inserts at the plantar side of the medial cuneiform and first metatarsal bone.

***Fibularis brevis muscle/Peroneus brevis muscle*:** has its origin more distal at the fibula and is covered by the fibularis longus muscle to its most part. Its tendon inserts at the tuberosity of the fifth metatarsal bone.

The leg is separated into anterior, lateral, superficial posterior and deep posterior compartments by intermuscular septa and surrounded by the deep fascia of the leg.

The anterior compartment of the leg is one of the four compartments in the leg between the knee and foot. These are:

- ❑ Tibialis anterior muscle
- ❑ Extensor hallucis longus muscle
- ❑ Extensor digitorum longus muscle
- ❑ Peroneus tertius muscle

These muscles primarily produce *ankle dorsiflexion* and *toe extension.*

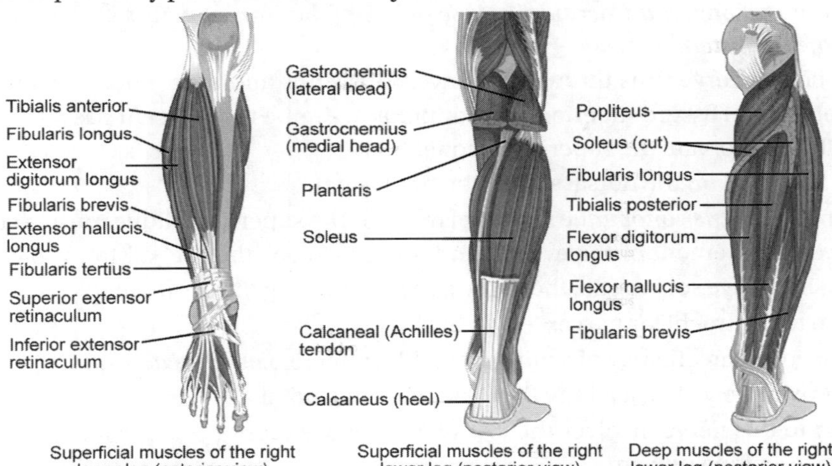

Fig. 4: Superficial and deep muscles of lower leg.

6. True about Trochlear nerve is/are:

a. Damage cause ipsilateral palsy of superior oblique muscle
b. Midbrain has the nucleus of trochlear nerve
c. Arise from ventral aspect of brainstem
d. Enters orbit via annulus of Zinn
e. Lesion may cause diplopia

Ans. b, e *Ref: Snell's Anatomy, 9th/ed*

Option a	False	Damage will result in dysfunction of the contralateral superior oblique muscle
Option b	True	The nucleus of CN IV lies at the level of the inferior colliculus in the tegmentum of the midbrain
Option c	False	Emerges from the dorsal aspect of the brainstem at the level of the caudal mesencephalon, just below the inferior colliculus
Option d	False	Enters the orbit through superior orbital fissure superior to the annulus of Zinn
Option e	True	The diplopia is typically worse in down gaze (consequently, they will often complain of difficulty reading) and lateral gaze toward the contralateral side

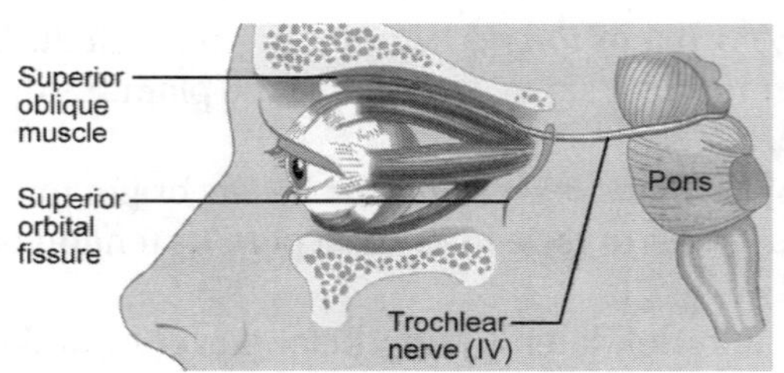

- The trochlear nerve is also known as the fourth cranial nerve, motor nerve and is the most slender of the cranial nerves.
- Its fibers course dorsally and decussate dorsal to the periaqueductal grey matter before exiting the brainstem immediately below the inferior colliculus.
- The nucleus of CN IV lies at the level of the inferior colliculus in the tegmentum of the midbrain.
- *CN IV has the longest intracranial course of any of the cranial nerves and is the only nerve to exit the brainstem dorsally.*
- The trochlear nerve runs through the cavernous sinus and then enters the orbit through the supraorbital fissure superior to the annulus of Zinn. From there, it passes ventrally and medially to innervate the superior oblique.
- It exits the brain on the dorsal side of the brain stem.
- It controls *the superior oblique muscle* of the eye. The superior oblique muscle controls the downward movement of the eyeball and, in part, keeps the eyeball from rolling upward into the orbit (eye socket). So, the nerve assists in turning the eye *downwards and laterally.*
- Damage to the trochlear nerve:
  - Most common etiology of acquired trochlear nerve palsy is *head trauma.*
  - Approximately 75% of all CN IV palsies are congenital.
  - Palsy to this nerve involves the loss of control of superior oblique muscle, resulting in the eye drifting upward.
  - Lesions will result in dysfunction of the *contralateral* superior oblique muscle.
  - Acute palsy is usually temporary (lasting from a week up to two months) and often results from head trauma. Initially, patients may complain of blurry vision, but more severe damage can cause diplopia.
  - Chronic palsy is normally congenital and results from the malformation or incomplete formation of the trochlear nerve. Chronic palsy can be noticed in childhood, but sometimes minor congenital defects of the trochlear nerve are not always noticed until adulthood. In some cases, congenital palsy can be repaired surgically.

7. No man's land in hand is:

a. Zone I
b. Zone II
c. Zone III
d. Zone IV
e. Zone V

Ans. b

Ref: Snell's Anatomy 9th/ed; http://boneandspine.com/flexor-tendon-zones-of-hand accessed on 10 June 2017.

Option a	False	
Option b	True	No man's land
Option c	False	
Option d	False	
Option e	False	

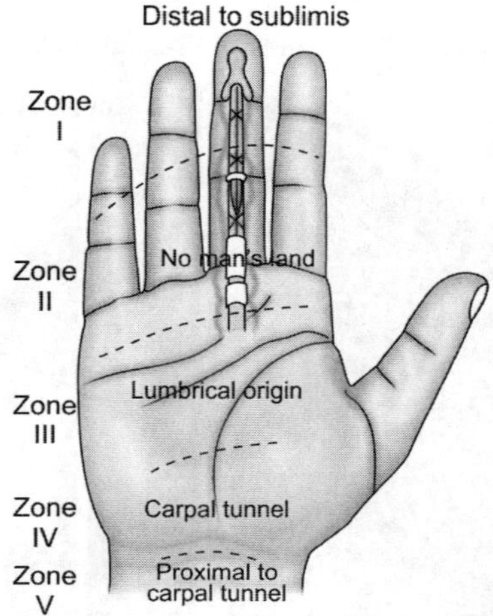

Fig. 5: Flexor tendon zones of hand.

- There are five flexor tendon zones in hand. Flexor tendon zones influence prognosis following flexor tendon repair.
- **Zone I** extends from the tip of the finger to the middle of middle phalanx. This zone consists of the profundus tendon only and is bounded proximally by the insertion of the superficialis tendons and distally by the insertion of the flexor digitorum profundus tendon into the distal phalanx.
- **Zone II** extends from the middle of the middle phalanx to distal palmar crease. It contains both flexor tendon superficialis and flexor tendon profundus. Proximal to zone II, the flexor digitorum superficialis tendons lie superficial to the flexor digitorum profundus (PDP) tendons. Within zone II and at the level of the proximal third of the proximal phalanx, the Flexor digitorum superficialis (FDS) tendons split into 2 slips, collectively known as ***Camper chiasma***. These slips then divide around the FDP tendon and reunite on the dorsal aspect of the FDP, inserting into the distal end of the middle phalanx. It has been called "***No Man's Land" or "No Man's Zone***" because repair in this zone is very difficult.
- Zone III extends from distal palmar crease to the distal edge of flexor carpal ligament. It is also called ***lumbrical zone*** because of the presence of lumbricals in this zone.
- Zone IV is the zone covered by the transverse carpal ligament.
- Zone V is the zone proximal to the transverse carpal ligament and includes the forearm.

8. Contents of aortic hiatus include:

a. Aorta
b. Thoracic duct
c. Azygos vein
d. Vagus nerve
e. Inferior vena cava

Ans. a, b, c *Ref: Snell's Anatomy, 9th/ed*

Option a	True	
Option b	True	
Option c	True	
Option d	False	Passes through esophageal hiatus
Option e	False	The caval opening passes through the central tendon of the diaphragm

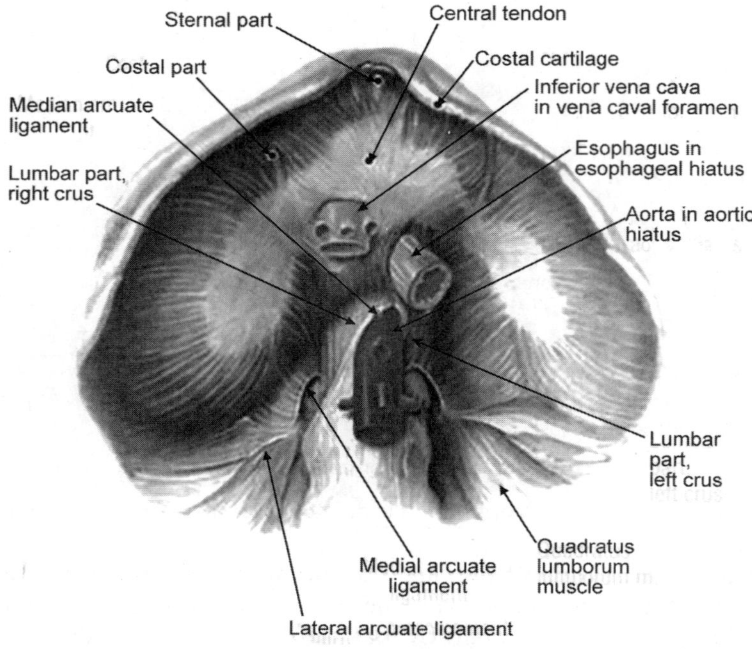

Fig. 6: Openings in diaphragm.

The aortic aperture is the route that the aorta takes on passing through the diaphragm. It is not a real aperture in the diaphragm, but an osseoaponeurotic opening between it and the vertebral column. It is characterized by:

- Lies at the level of the T12 thoracic vertebra in expiration
- Formed by the median arcuate ligaments of the diaphragm
- Passes behind the diaphragm as the arcuate ligaments only carry the aorta anteriorly
- Consequently, diaphragmatic contractions do not directly influence aortic diameter
- Lies slightly to the left of the median plane.

Relations:

- *Anteriorly*: Esophagus
- *Posteriorly*:
  - T12 vertebral body
  - Hemiazygos vein
- *Right*: Inferior vena cava

Structures passing through **the aortic hiatus include:**

- Aorta

- ❑ Thoracic duct, to the right
- ❑ Azygos vein, situated more laterally on the right
- ❑ Minor lymphatics

9. All are true about vestibulocochlear nerve *except*:

a. It has two divisions—superior and inferior vestibular
b. Vestibular nuclei situated at junction of pons and medulla
c. Nerve fibers relay at scarpa's ganglion
d. Vestibular nucleus lie in midbrain near aqueduct
e. The nerve exits at the cerebellopontine angle

Ans. d *Ref: Snell's Anatomy, 9th/ed*

Option a	True	True about vestibulocochlear nerve
Option b	True	True about vestibulocochlear nerve
Option c	True	True about vestibulocochlear nerve
Option d	False	Vestibular nuclei complex lies in the pons and medulla
Option e	True	The nerve emerges from the brain at the cerebellopontine angle and exits the cranium via the internal acoustic meatus of the temporal bone

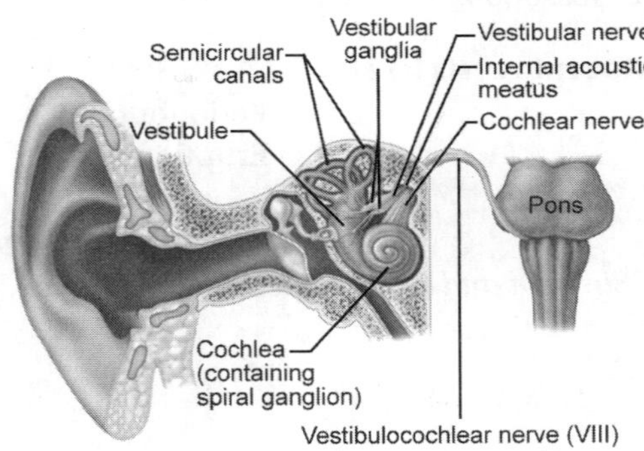

Fig. 7: Vestibulocochlear nerve.

- ❑ The vestibulocochlear nerve is the eighth cranial nerve.
- ❑ It comprises of two parts—vestibular fibers and cochlear fibers. Both have a purely sensory function.
- ❑ The vestibular fibers arise from the vestibular nuclei complex in the pons and medulla.
  - ▪ Concerned with equilibrium and represent the central processes of nerve cells of ***vestibular ganglion***.
  - ▪ This is located in outer part of internal acoustic meatus.
- ❑ The cochlear fibers are concerned with hearing.
  - ▪ Arise from the ventral and dorsal cochlear nuclei, situated in the inferior cerebellar peduncle.
  - ▪ Represent the central processes of nerve cells of ***spiral ganglion of cochlea.***
- ❑ Both sets of fibers combine in the pons to form the vestibulocochlear nerve. The nerve emerges from the brain at the cerebellopontine angle and exits the cranium via the internal acoustic meatus of the temporal bone.

10. Which of the following is true about epiglottis?

a. Oval in shape
b. Made up of elastic cartilage
c. Contains mucus glands
d. Contains serous glands
e. Bilateral lymphatic drainage

Ans. b, c, e *Ref: Snell's Anatomy, 9th/ed*

Option a	False	Leaf shaped
Option b	True	Yes
Option c	True	Yes
Option d	False	Contains mucus glands
Option e	True	Midline structure, so bilateral drainage

The **epiglottis** is a leaf-shaped elastic cartilage situated behind the root of the tongue. It is connected in front to the body of the hyoid bone, and by its stalk to the back of the thyroid cartilage. The sides of the epiglottis are connected to the arytenoid cartilages by the aryepiglottic folds. The upper edge of the epiglottis is free, and the covering of mucous membrane is reflected forward onto the posterior surface of the tongue. Here, there are a **median glossoepiglottic fold** and **lateral pharyngoepiglottic folds.** The **valleculae** are depressions of mucous membrane present on either side of the glossoepiglottic fold.

11. Inflammatory odontogenic cysts is/are:

a. Periapical cyst
b. Periodontal cyst
c. Residual cyst
d. Eruption cyst
e. Primordial cyst

Ans. a, c *Ref: Inflammatory odontogenic cysts Journal of Surgical and Clinical Dentistry Vol. 2, n.1, pp.20-28 (Jul – Sep 2014)*

Option a	True	
Option b	False	Cyst of development
Option c	True	
Option d	False	Occurs on the soft tissue over an erupting tooth
Option e	False	Cyst of development

Odontogenic cyst are a group of jaw cysts that are formed from tissues involved in odontogenesis (tooth development).

The ***inflammatory cysts*** are lesions that originate from the infection of root canals from caries or occurrence of a trauma that generated pulp changes.

- The appearance of these cysts occurs from the pre-existence of a periapical granuloma or by induction of epithelial rests of Malassez.
- The inflammatory cysts can be classified as:
  - Inflammatory periapical cyst (apical radicular cyst and lateral periodontal cyst or apical),
  - Residual cyst
  - Cyst paradental
  - These cysts require a source of infection for the remaining epithelial root sheath of Hertwig (or epithelial remnants of Malassez).

- Some of these cysts, such as periapical cysts, inflammatory and lateral root cyst, depend on endodontic infection, while paradental require periodontal cyst or pericoronal infection.
- The odontogenic inflammatory cysts constitute about 70.1 to 85% of maxillary cysts.

12. True statement for embryonic development of cochlea:

a. Development starts by 20 weeks of gestation
b. Michel aplasia may occur
c. Develops from endoderm
d. Adult cochlea has snail shape appearance
e. None

Ans. b, d

Option a	False	Cochlear duct starts developing during week 6 of embryonic development
Option b	True	Congenital abnormality of the inner ear
Option c	False	Develops from ectoderm
Option d	True	
Option e	False	

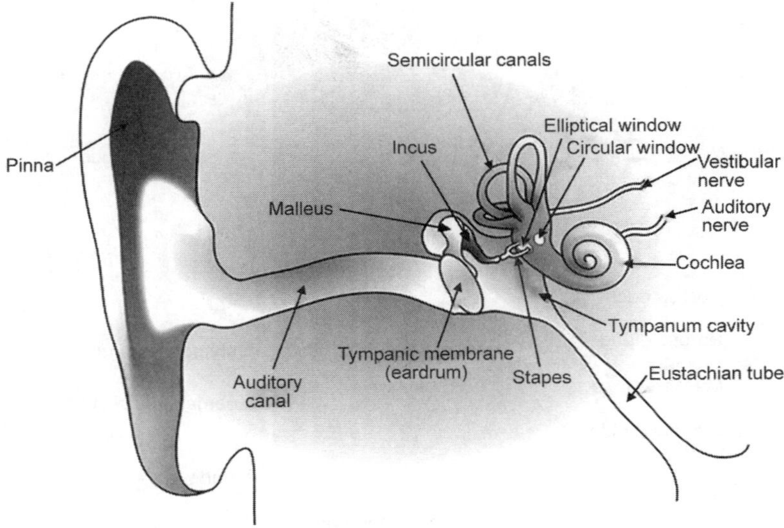

Fig. 8: Human ear.

- The human inner ear develops during week 4 of embryonic development from the auditory placode, a thickening of the ectoderm which gives rise to the bipolar neurons of the cochlear and vestibular ganglions.
- The adult human cochlea has a "snail-shell" appearance and is typically described as having 2.5 turns.
- ***Michel aplasia***, also known as complete labyrinthine aplasia (CLA), is a congenital abnormality of the inner ear and is characterized by bilateral absence of differentiated inner ear structures with resultant anacusis.
- ***Michel dysplasia***, in which arrest of embryologic development occurs later.

- Structural stage corresponding to the onset of cochlear function starts at 18–20 weeks of gestation.

13. True regarding parotid gland:
   a. Separated by facial nerve
   b. 2nd largest salivary gland
   c. Stensen's duct open in front of the 3rd upper molar
   d. Lymph nodes are situated in deep parotid lobe
   e. Retromandibular vein lies within the gland

Ans. a, d, e *Ref: Snell's, 9th/ed*

Option a	True	In fully formed gland, the facial nerve can be said to divide the parotid gland into superficial and deep parts
Option b	False	Largest of the salivary glands
Option c	False	Duct opens opposite the upper second molar tooth
Option d	True	
Option e	True	

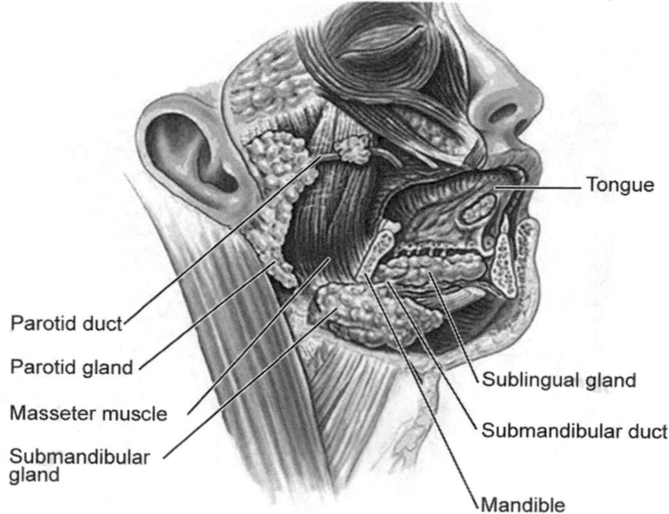

Fig. 9: Salivary glands.

Parotid gland:

- Largest of the salivary glands and composed entirely of serous acini.
- Situated below the external auditory meatus and lies in deep hollow behind ramus of mandible and in front of sternocleidomastoid, bilateral and paired.
- There it is encapsulated by the masseteric fascia deriving from the deep cervical fascia.
- During development, parotid gland covers the lateral surface of facial nerve. As the development proceeds, deep part of the gland extends medially between branches of facial nerve (parotid plexus).
- "In the fully formed gland, the facial nerve can be said to divide the parotid gland into superficial and deep parts." *Ref: Snell's, 9th/ed*

- ❑ The parotid duct (also known as Stensen's duct) drains the saliva into the oral cavity opposite the ***upper second molar tooth*** via the parotid papilla. In its course it crosses the masseter and pierces through the buccinator.
- ❑ Gland tissues along the parotid duct and lying on the masseter muscle are referred to as accessory parotid glands.

Blood supply:

- ❑ The maxillary arteries and superficial temporal arteries—two terminal branches of the external carotid artery—provide the major blood supply.
- ❑ The venous blood drains to the retromandibular (or posterior facial) vein which runs lateral to the carotid artery.
- ❑ Retromandibular vein is formed within the parotid gland by union of superficial temporal and maxillary veins.

Lymphatic drainage:

- ❑ Parotid lymph nodes are situated on or with in the parotid gland.
- ❑ They receive lymph from scalp above parotid gland, lateral surface of auricle, anterior wall of external auditory meatus, and lateral parts of eyelids.
- ❑ Nodes deeply placed into parotid gland receive lymph from the middle ear.
- ❑ Efferent lymph vessels drain into deep cervical lymph nodes.

14. Abduction of arms:

a. Supraspinatus is the main abductor
b. Serratus anterior and trapezius act together
c. Acromial fibers of deltoid help in pulling of arm
d. Axillary nerve injury does not affect abduction
e. Rotator cuff stabilizes the humerus head

Ans. b, c, e *Ref: Snell's 9th/ed; MedCharts Anatomy—Thomas R. Gest and Jaye Schlesinger*

Option a	False	Deltoid muscle is the principle abductor of arm
Option b	True	
Option c	True	
Option d	False	Axillary nerve damage/palsy causes loss of abduction at shoulder
Option e	True	

Abduction is any motion of the limbs or other body parts that pulls away from the midline of the body.

This motion actually can be divided into *two motions*:

a. True abduction of the arm at the shoulder, and
b. Upward rotation of the scapula.

Muscles:

a. Supraspinatus (initiates abduction - first 15 degrees),
b. Deltoid (up to 90 degrees),
c. Trapezius and serratus anterior (scapular rotation, for abduction beyond 90 degrees).

Muscle	Origin	Insertion	Innervation	Action	Imp Points
Deltoid	Lateral one-third of the clavicle, acromion, the lower lip of the crest of the spine of the scapula	Deltoid tuberosity of the humerus	Axillary nerve (C5,6) from the posterior cord of the brachial plexus	Abducts arm; anterior fibers flex and medially rotate the arm; posterior fibers extend and laterally rotate the arm	The deltoid muscle is the principle abductor of the arm but due to poor mechanical advantage it cannot initiate this action; it is assisted by the supraspinatus muscle
Supraspinatus	Supraspinatus fossa	Greater tubercle of the humerus (highest facet)	Suprascapular nerve (C5, 6) from the superior trunk of the brachial plexus	Abducts the arm (initiates abduction)	Supraspinatus initiates abduction of the arm, then the deltoid muscle completes the action; a member of the rotator cuff group
Trapezius	Medial third of the superior nuchal line, external occipital protuberance, ligamentum nuchae, spinous processes of vertebrae C7-T12	Lateral third of the clavicle, medial side of the acromion and the upper crest of the scapular spine, tubercle of the scapular spine	Motor: spinal accessory (XI), proprioception: C3-C4	Elevates and depresses the scapula (depending on which part of the muscle contracts); rotates the scapula superiorly; retracts scapula	Named for its shape; trapezius is an example of a muscle that migrates during development from its level of origin (cervical) to its final position, pulling its nerve and artery along behind
Serratus anterior	Ribs 1–8 or 9	Medial border of the scapula on its costal (deep) surface	Long thoracic nerve (from ventral rami C5-C7)	It draws the scapula forward; the inferior fibers rotate the scapula superiorly	Lesion of long thoracic nerve will cause winging of the scapula (i.e., the medial border of the scapula falls away from the posterior chest wall and looks like an angel's wing)

15. True about thyroid anatomy is:

a. Capsule is tightly adherent
b. Recurrent laryngeal nerve has a variable course on both the sides
c. Deep cervical fascia is connected to the Berry's ligament
d. Thyroid is present between deep and superficial cervical fascia
e. Lymphatic drainage is unidirectional

Ans. a, b, d *Ref: Snell's 9th/ed; Last's Anatomy 12th/ed*

Option a	True	
Option b	True	
Option c	False	Ligament of berry connects the lobe to cricoid cartilage

Option d	True	
Option e	False	Lymphatic drainage is multidirectional

Thyroid gland:

- Highly vascular, located in anterior neck extending from the level of C5 vertebra down to T1.
- H or U shaped, divided into two lobes (right and left) which are connected by an isthmus.
- The gland is in visceral compartment of the neck, along with the trachea, esophagus and pharynx. The compartment is bound by pretracheal fascia.
- The gland is covered by:
  - An adherent fibrous capsule, and
  - A sheath ("false capsule") derived from the deep cervical fascia.
- Each lobe has an apex, which ascends between the sternothyroid muscle and the inferior constrictor of the pharynx; a base directed inferiorly; and three surfaces.
  - The lateral surface is covered by infrahyoid muscles
  - The medial surface is related to the larynx, pharynx, trachea, and esophagus
  - The posterior surface is related to the carotid sheath and its contents and to the prevertebral muscles.
  - The isthmus connects the right and left lobes and lies anterior to rings 2 to 4 of the trachea.
  - The inconstant pyramidal lobule (or "lobe") ascends from the isthmus and may be anchored to the hyoid bone by fibrous or muscular tissue (levator glandulae thyroideae).

Blood supply:

- Supplied mainly by:
  - The superior thyroid artery (from the external carotid), and
  - The inferior thyroid artery (from the thyrocervical trunk of the subclavian).
  - The thyroid gland is drained by superior and middle thyroid veins into the internal jugular vein and by inferior thyroid veins into the brachiocephalic vein.

Lymphatic drainage:

- The lymph vessels drain:
  - Upward to the deep cervical nodes, and
  - Downward to the paratracheal nodes.
  - The isthmus drains into the prelaryngeal and pretracheal nodes.
- **Development:** The thyroid gland develops largely as a median diverticulum from the tongue (foramen cecum). Parts of the embryonic thyroglossal duct may remain as cysts, the pyramidal lobule, and accessory thyroid tissue.

Clinical relevance: Recurrent laryngeal nerve

- There are two recurrent laryngeal nerves; one left and one right.
- They arise from their respective vagus nerves, and descend into the chest.
- In the chest, they hook around the subclavian artery (right RL nerve), or the arch of aorta (left RL nerve).
- The nerves then ascend back up the neck, running between the trachea and esophagus.
- They pass underneath the thyroid gland to innervate the larynx.

During surgery on the thyroid gland, care must be taken not to ligate or damage the recurrent laryngeal nerves.

16. True about anterior interosseous nerve:

a. Supplies flexor pollicis longus
b. Supplies flexor carpi ulnaris
c. Supplies extensor digitorum
d. Supplies pronator teres
e. Supplies flexor digitorum profundus

Ans. a, e *Ref: Snell's 9th/ed; Last's Anatomy 12th/ed*

Option a	True	
Option b	False	
Option c	False	
Option d	False	Supplies pronator quadratus
Option e	True	

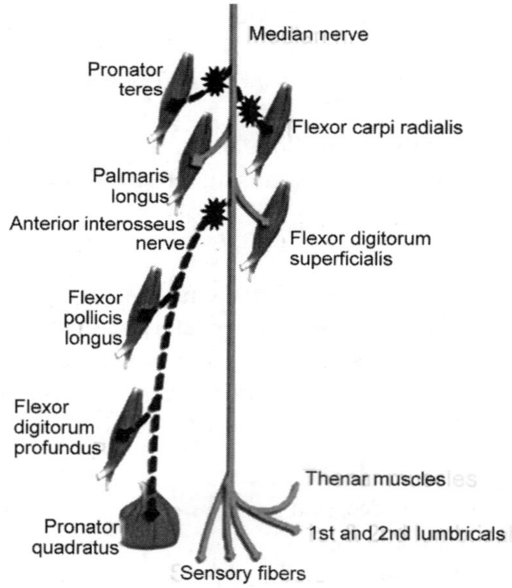

Fig. 10: Anterior interosseous nerve (AIN).

Anterior interosseous nerve:

- Motor nerve
- Arises from median nerve, 5 cm above medial epicondyle.
- Runs on volar surface of flexor digitorum profundus and along interosseous membrane between ulna and radius.
- Supplies flexor pollicis longus, lateral half of flexor digitorum profundus and pronator quadratus.
- Sensory fibers to volar wrist joint capsule.

17. True about meiosis in Prophase I is:
   a. Separation of homologous chromosomes
   b. Duplication of sister chromatids
   c. Exchange of material within chromatids
   d. Reduction in number of chromosomes
   e. Separation of sister chromatids

Ans. c *Ref: Langman's Medical Embryology, 13th/ed*

Option a	False	Pairing of homologous chromosomes and crossing over takes place
Option b	False	Chromosomes have already duplicated
Option c	True	Gives rise to genetic variability
Option d	False	Occurs in telophase
Option e	False	Occurs in anaphase I

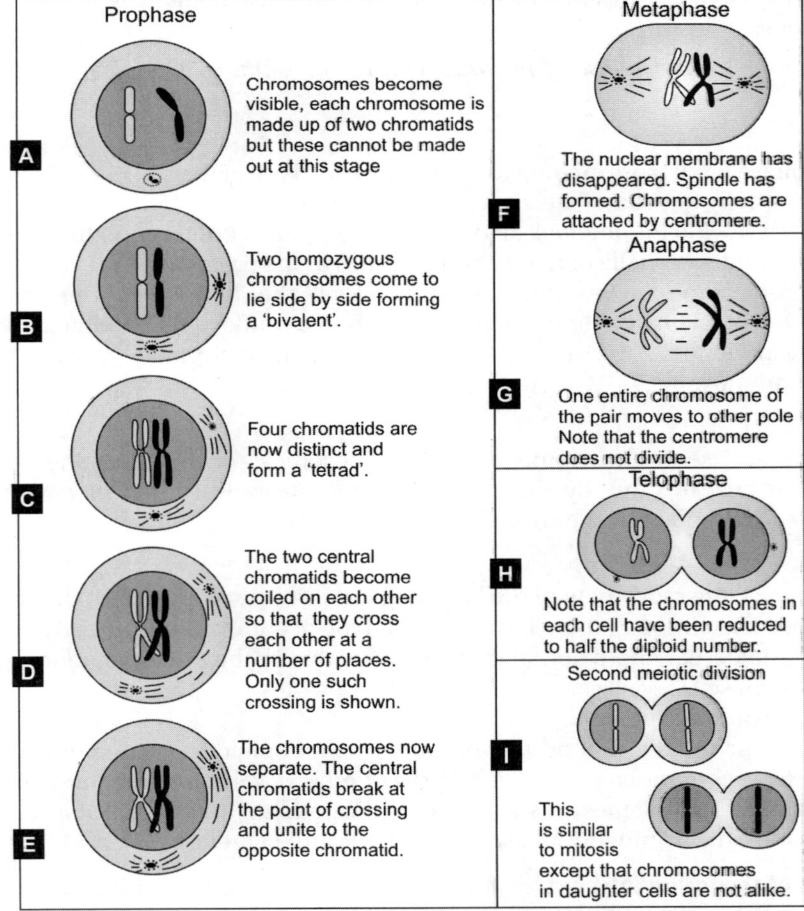

Fig. 11: Scheme to show the main steps of meiosis. Only the telophase of the second division is shown.

Meiosis I: Prophase I

Chromosomes become visible, crossing-over occurs, the nucleolus disappears, the meiotic spindle forms, and the nuclear envelope disappears.

- At the start of prophase I, the chromosomes have already duplicated.
- During prophase I, they coil and become shorter and thicker and visible under the light microscope.
- The duplicated homologous chromosomes pair, and *crossing-over* (the physical exchange of chromosome parts) occurs.
- Crossing-over is the process that can give rise to genetic recombination.
- At this point, each homologous chromosome pair is visible as a *bivalent (tetrad)*, a tight grouping of two chromosomes, each consisting of two sister chromatids.
- The sites of crossing-over are seen as crisscrossed non-sister chromatids and are called chiasmata (singular: chiasma).
- The nucleolus disappears during prophase I.
- In the cytoplasm, the meiotic spindle, consisting of microtubules and other proteins, forms between the two pairs of centrioles as they migrate to opposite poles of the cell.
- The nuclear envelope disappears at the end of prophase I, allowing the spindle to enter the nucleus.

Prophase I is the longest phase of meiosis, typically consuming 90% of the time for the two divisions.

Metaphase I

- In metaphase I, the pairs migrate to the equatorial plane of the cell.
- The spindle fully forms and attaches to the centromeres.
- The pattern in which homologs align during metaphase I determine the combination of maternally and paternally derived chromosomes in the progeny cells.
- Each chromosome moves independently of all the others—a phenomenon called *independent assortment*. For example, the copy of chromosome 1 that a gamete receives in no way influences if the same gamete will receive the maternally-derived or paternally-derived chromosome 4.

Anaphase I

- During anaphase I, the homologous chromosomes—each consisting of two sister chromatids held together by a centromere—*separate* and begin to *move to the opposite poles of the cell,* pulled by the shrinking spindle fibers.

Telophase I

- In telophase I, the movement of the homologous chromosomes to the poles is completed. Remember that although there is one of each type of chromosome at each pole, there is a mixture of maternal and paternal chromosomes due to the recombination that occurred during prophase I.
- The spindle now disappears.
- Cytokinesis, or cell division occurs, producing two haploid (n) daughter cells, each with *only one set of chromosomes* (1n) i.e. *half the number of chromosomes* per nucleus.
- However, the chromosomes are still in their replicated state and consist of sister chromatids.
- The cells move back into interphase, marking the end of meiosis I.

18. Which of the following are true for medial longitudinal fasciculus (MLF)?

a. It connects 6th and 3rd nerve nucleus on ipsilateral side
b. It causes ipsilateral adduction palsy
c. Helps in the conjugate eye movement
d. Saccadic movements
e. Cause contralateral adduction

Ans. b, c, d *Ref: Snell's, 9th/ed; Last's Anatomy, 12th/ed*

Option a	False	Connects the interneurons of the abducens nucleus with the motoneurons of the contralateral oculomotor nucleus
Option b	True	
Option c	True	
Option d	True	
Option e	False	Ipsilateral adduction

- The medial longitudinal fasciculus is a white matter tract that rides the midline dorsally, while the spinothalamic tract maintains its anterolateral position in the brainstem, immediately dorsal to the olive in the medulla.
- It links the three main nerves which control eye movements, i.e. the *oculomotor, trochlear* and the *abducent nerves,* as well as the *vestibulocochlear nerve.*
- The purpose of the medial longitudinal fasciculus is to integrate movement of the eyes and head movements.
- It connects the interneurons of the abducens nucleus with the motoneurons of the contralateral oculomotor nucleus and yokes the two eyes together.
- It also carries fibers from the vestibular nuclei directed toward the oculomotor and trochlear nuclei as well as the interstitial nucleus of Cajal.
- Unilateral lesions in the medial longitudinal fasciculus disconnect the two nuclei, so that when the patient attempts lateral gaze, the adducting eye *ipsilateral* to the abnormal medial longitudinal fasciculus is unable to move medially, but the *abducting eye is able to move laterally.*

19. Inferior ophthalmic vein:

a. Begins in anterior border of eye
b. Connected to pterygoid plexus
c. More connections than superior ophthalmic vein (SOV)
d. Joins SOV in cavernous sinus
e. Drains floor and lateral wall of orbit

Ans. a, b, d *Ref: Snell's, 9th/ed; Last's Anatomy, 12th/ed*

Option a	True	
Option b	True	
Option c	False	Smaller than the SOV
Option d	True	
Option e	False	Vein of inferior orbit. Drains blood from the lower and lateral muscles, the inferior conjunctiva, the lacrimal sac, and the inferior vortex veins

- The inferior ophthalmic vein (IOV) is a vein of the *inferior orbit* and is *smaller* than the more well known superior ophthalmic vein.
- It drains blood from the lower and lateral muscles, the inferior conjunctiva, the lacrimal sac, and the inferior vortex veins.
- Superior ophthalmic vein (SOV) communicates in front with the facial vein.
- The inferior ophthalmic vein communicates through inferior orbital fissure with pterygoid venous plexus.
- Both IOV and SOV pass backward through the superior orbital fissure and drain into the cavernous sinus.

Physiology

1. Renin-angiotensin system

a. Renin secreted by epithelial cells of efferent arterioles
b. Renin helps in angiotensin I secretion
c. ACE in lungs converts angiotensin I to angiotensin II
d. Angiotensin II acts on body for 2-3 hours and functions for long-term control of blood pressure
e. Angiotensin increases the tubular reabsorption of sodium and water.

Ans. a,c,e *Ref: JP Montani. General Physiology and Pathophysiology of the Renin–Angiotensin System. p8-10; Guyton, 11th/ed p224*

Option a	False	No, it is secreted by the juxtaglomerular cells
Option b	True	Yes, correct
Option c	True	Yes, correct
Option d	False	No, angiotensin II is active for few minutes (<2-3 minutes)
Option e	True	Yes, correct

Renin-angiotensin-aldosterone system

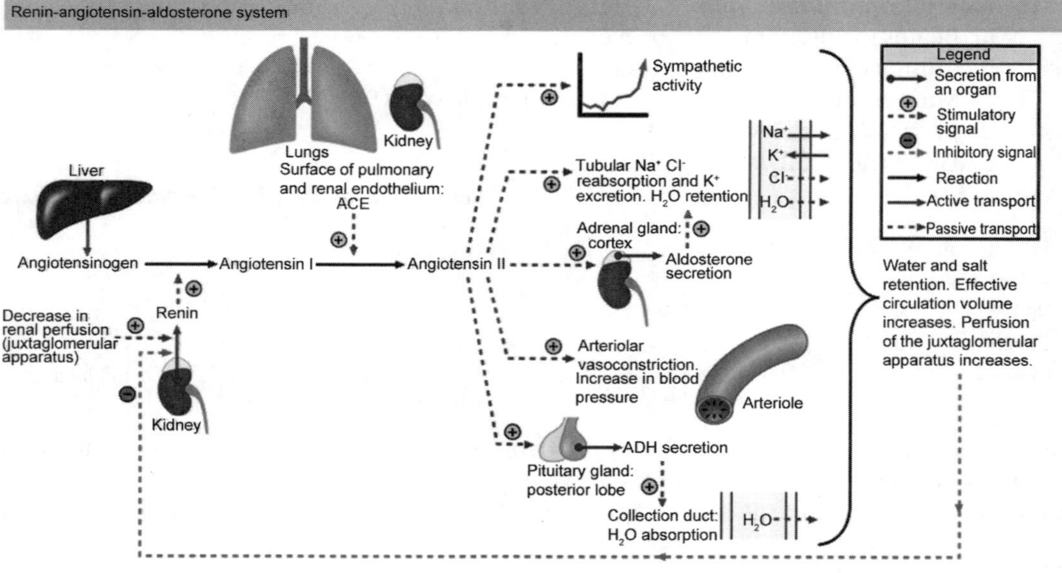

RAS in Nut-shell

- If the perfusion of the juxtaglomerular apparatus in the kidney's macula densa decreases, then the juxtaglomerular cells (granular cells, modified pericytes in the *walls of the afferent arterioles immediately proximal to the glomeruli*) release the enzyme renin.
- Renin is synthesized and stored in an inactive form called *prorenin.*
- Renin itself is an enzyme, not a vasoactive substance. Renin acts enzymatically on another plasma protein, a globulin called *renin substrate* (or *angiotensinogen*), to release a 10-amino acid peptide, *angiotensin I.*
- Angiotensin I has mild vasoconstrictor properties but not enough to cause significant changes in circulatory function.
- The renin persists in the blood for 30 minutes to 1 hour and continues to cause formation of still more angiotensin I during this entire time.
- Angiotensisn further splits to form the angiotensin II (8 amino acid peptide) in the lungs.
- Angiotensin II is an extremely powerful vasoconstrictor, and it also affects circulatory function in other ways as well. However, it persists in the blood only for 1 or 2 minutes because it is rapidly inactivated by multiple blood and tissue enzymes collectively called *angiotensinases*

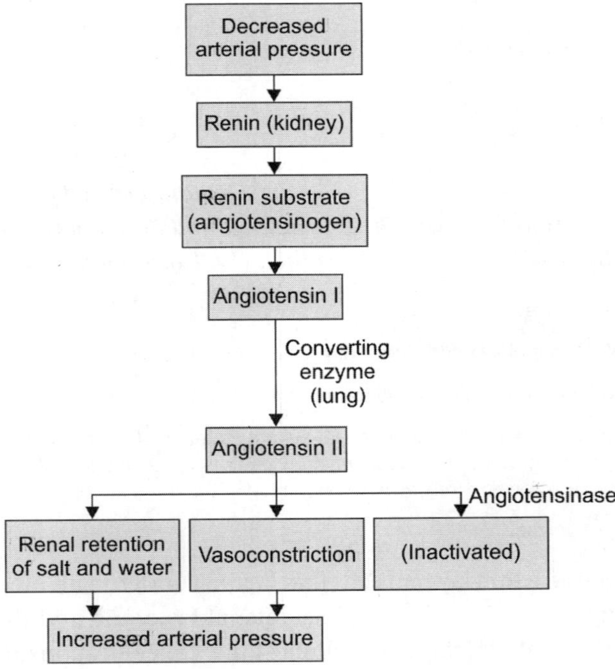

Effect of angiotensin (on kidney):

1. Constrict renal arterioles to decrease the blood flow.
2. Less fluid filters to the glomeruli and the tubules.
3. Direct effect on renal tubules for increased tubular reabsorption of sodium and water.

Decreased salt intake with negative feedback mechanism:

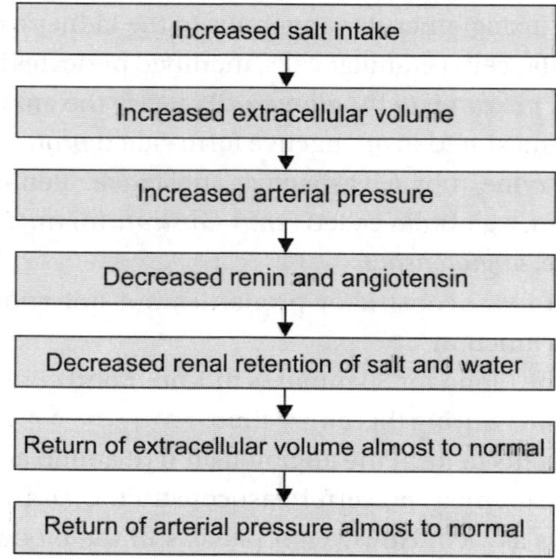

2. ACTH helps in metabolic conversion of:

a. DHEA
b. 11-Deoxycorticosterone
c. Aldosterone
d. Angiotensinogen
e. Melanin

Ans. a,e *Ref: Guyton, 11th/ed p956-959; Ahsan Husain, Robert M Graham. Drugs, Enzymes and Receptors of the Renin-Angiotensin System. CRC press, p72; Anthony W. Hormones; academic press 2014, p329*

Option a	True	Yes, correct
Option b	False	No, it is mainly under effect of potassium and sodium
Option c	False	No, it is under effect of potassium and sodium
Option d	False	No, Plasma angiotensinogen levels are increased by plasma corticosteroid, estrogen, thyroid hormone, and angiotensin II levels and not under ACTH control. It is precursor for angiotensin I formation under action of renin
Option e	True	Yes, correct

- The *zona glomerulosa,* a thin layer of cells that lies just underneath the capsule, constitutes about 15 percent of the adrenal cortex. Secrete: aldosterone and the secretion of these cells is controlled mainly by the extracellular fluid concentrations of *angiotensin II* and *potassium,* both of which stimulate aldosterone secretion
- The *zona fasciculata,* the middle and widest layer, constitutes about 75 percent of the adrenal cortex and secretes the glucocorticoids *cortisol* and corticosterone. The secretion of these cells is controlled in large part by the hypothalamic-pituitary axis via *adrenocorticotropic hormone (ACTH).*

- The *zona reticularis,* the deep layer of the cortex, secretes the adrenal androgens *dehydroepiandrosterone (DHEA)* and *androstenedione,* as well as small amounts of estrogens and some glucocorticoids. ACTH also regulates secretion of these cells, although other factors such as *cortical androgen-stimulating hormone,* released from the pituitary, may also be involved.

ACTH, because it contains an MSH sequence, has about 1/30 as much melanocyte-stimulating effect as MSH. Furthermore, because the quantities of pure MSH secreted in the human being are extremely small, whereas those of ACTH are large, it is likely that ACTH normally is more important than MSH in determining the amount of melanin in the skin.

3. Skeletal muscle contraction features:

a. Extracellular calcium used
b. T-tubule is used
c. DHPR receptor
d. Ryanodine receptor
e. Actin pulls myosin

Ans. a,b,c,d *Ref: Guyton, 11th/ed, pg74; Rodney A. Rhoades Medical physiology: Principals for clinical medicine. p141*

Option a	True	Yes, correct
Option b	True	Yes correct. T tubule: Extension of the sarcolemma that extends into the muscle fiber and conveys impulses that causes Calcium to be released from the sarcoplasmic reticulum
Option c	True	Yes, these are the voltage-gated L-type calcium channels
Option d	True	Yes, Ryanodine receptors mediate the release of calcium ions from the sarcoplasmic reticulum and endoplasmic reticulum, an essential step in muscle contraction
Option e	False	No, it's the myosin protein which binds to actin and pulls it thus shortening the sarcomere.

Neuromuscular contraction:

1. Action Potential (AP) in motor nerve axon terminal
2. Opening of voltage gated Ca2+ channels and entry of Calcium in axon terminal
3. Calcium activates calmodulin which activates protein kinase
4. Protein kinase phosphorylates synapsins (which regulate neurotransmitter release at the synapse) which aid in the fusion of synaptic vesicles
5. Diffusion of ACh from vesicles into synaptic cleft
6. Attachment of ACh with receptors (with 5 subunits) in the sarcolemma
7. Opening of voltage gated Na+ channel and Na+ entry in the sarcolemma
8. End plate potential
9. AP in sarcolemma
10. Hydrolysis of Ach by cholinesterase

- In skeletal muscle, excitation–contraction coupling relies on a direct coupling between key proteins, the sarcoplasmic reticulum (SR) calcium release channel (ryanodine receptor, RyR) and voltage-gated L-type calcium channels (dihydropyridine receptors, DHPRs).

- DHPRs are located on the sarcolemma (which includes the surface sarcolemma and the transverse tubules), while the RyRs reside across the SR membrane.

The sliding of actin over the myosin filaments is caused by forces generated by interaction of the cross-bridges from the myosin filaments with the actin filaments. Under resting conditions, these forces are inactive, but when an action potential travels along the muscle fiber, this causes the sarcoplasmic reticulum to release large quantities of calcium ions that rapidly surround the myofibrils. The calcium ions in turn activate the forces between the myosin and actin filaments, and contraction begins. But energy is needed for the contractile process to proceed. This energy comes from high-energy bonds in the ATP molecule, which is degraded to adenosine diphosphate (ADP) to liberate the energy.

Physiology

1. True statement(s) about Olfactory system:

a. Olfactory mucosa cover upper 1/3rd of nasal cavity
b. Olfactory pathway passes via thalamus to orbitofrontal cortex
c. Adaptation to odor develop only after 1–2 minutes
d. Olfactory receptors act via cAMP
e. Rate of Olfactory nerve impulses change approximately in proportion to the logarithm of stimulus strength

Ans. a, b, d, e *Ref: Guyton and Hall Medical Physiology, 12th/ed; Ganong's review of Medical Physiology, 24th/ed*

Option a	True	It covers an area of 10 cm^2 in the roof of nasal cavity near the septum
Option b	True	
Option c	False	The olfactory receptors adapt about 50% in the first second or so after stimulation
Option d	True	
Option e	True	

The sense of smell:

- Olfactory sensory neutrons are located in a specialised portion of nasal mucosa, the yellowish pigmented olfactory epithelium. It covers an area of 10 cm^2 in the roof of nasal cavity near the septum. This covers the upper one third of lateral wall, corresponding area on the septum and roof of nasal cavity.
- The olfactory epithelium is said to be the place in the body where the nervous system is closest to the external world.
- The olfactory epithelium contains about 50 million bipolar olfactory sensory neutrons interspersed with glia like supporting (sustentacular) cells and basal stem cells. Supporting cells and bowman's glands lying beneath the epithelium secrete mucus which covers the olfactory epithelium.
- Each olfactory sensory neutron has a short, thick dendrite that projects into the nasal cavity where it terminates in a knob containing 6–12 cilia. The cilia are 5–10 micron long and 0.1–2 micron in diameter and protrude into the mucus overlying the epithelium. Odorants molecules dissolve in the mucus and bind the odorant receptors on these cilia.
- The axons of olfactory sensory neurons (the first cranial nerve) pass through the cribriform plate of ethmoid bone to enter the olfactory bulbs.
- In the olfactory bulbs—The axons of olfactory sensory neurons contact the dendrites of mitral cells and tufted cells to form 'olfactory glomeruli'. Olfactory bulbs also contain inhibitory neurons called periglomerular cells and GABA releasing inhibitory cells called granule cells.
- The axons of mitral and tufted cells pass posteriorly through lateral olfactory stria to terminate on apical dendrites of pyramidal cells in five regions of the olfactory cortex: anterior olfactory nucleus, olfactory tubercle, piriform cortex, amygdaloid and entorhinal cortex.

- From these regions information travels directly to frontal cortex or via thalamus to orbitofrontal cortex.

The olfactory receptors:

- There are approximately 500 functional olfactory genes in humans accounting for about 2% of the human genome.
- All olfactory receptors are G protein coupled receptors. When an odorant molecule binds to its receptor, the G protein subunits (alpha, beta, gamma) dissociate. The alpha subunit activates adenylate cyclase to catalyze the second messenger cAMP. cAMP opens cation channels increasing permeability to Na, K and Ca. The net effect is inward directed Ca current which produces graded receptor potential.

Membrane potential and action potential:

- The membrane potential inside unstimulated olfactory cells as measured by microelectrodes averages about -55 millivolts. At this potential, most of the cells generate continuous action potentials at a very slow rate, varying from once every 20 seconds to up to 2 to 3 per second.
- Most odorants cause depolarisation of the olfactory cell membrane, decreasing the negative potential in cell to –30 millivolts or less. Along with this, the number of action potential increases to 20–30 per second, which is a high rate for the tiny olfactory nerve fibers.
- Over a wide range the rate of olfactory nerve impulses changes approximately in proportion to the logarithm of the stimulus strength, which demonstrates that the olfactory receptors obey principles of transduction similar to those of other sensory receptors.

Adaptation

The olfactory receptors adapt about 50% in the first second or so after stimulation. Additional adaptation takes place in the central nervous system. After the onset of olfactory stimulus the CNS quickly develops strong feedback inhibition to suppress relay of smell signals through olfactory bulbs. Hence smell sensations adapt almost to extinction within a minute or so after entering a strongly odorous atmosphere.

2. Vomiting centers involved in postoperative vomiting is/are:

a. Area postrema
b. Chemoreceptor trigger zone (CTZ)
c. Basal ganglia
d. Reticular formation located in medulla
e. Nucleus tractus solitaries

Ans. a, b, d, e *Ref: Pharmacology and Physiology in anesthetic practice, 5th/ed; Guyton and Hall Medical Physiology, 12th/ed; Ganong's review of Medical Physiology, 24th/ed*

Option a	True	
Option b	True	
Option c	False	Mainly involved in motor function
Option d	True	
Option e	True	

Vomiting centre is located in the reticular formation of medulla.

Stimuli like Irritation of mucosa of gastrointestinal tract (GI), overdistension of GI, delayed gastric emptying, nauseous odor are carried through nucleus tractus solitarius to the reticular formation in medulla.

Signals arising in areas of the brain like vestibular labyrinth of the inner ear are transmitted by vestibular nuclei into the cerebellum, then to the 'chemoreceptor trigger zone (CTZ)' located bilaterally on the floor of fourth ventricle in the area called area postrema. This structure is not protected by blood brain barrier. Administration of drugs like apomorphine, morphine, some digitalis derivatives, emetogenics in CSF can directly stimulate the CTZ.

Postoperative nausea and vomiting (PONV)

A patient who experiences nausea or has emesis within 24 hrs of a surgical procedure that required anesthesia meets the criteria for diagnosis of PONV.

Operative procedure and anesthesia can trigger vomiting by either or both of the above mentioned pathways, decreased gastric motility may send impulses via tractus solitarius, while anaesthetic drugs like morphine or spinal anaesthesia may trigger the CTZ.

3. Rapidly adapting receptors are:

a. Pain
b. Paccinian
c. Golgi tendon organ
d. Muscle spindle
e. Meissner corpuscles

Ans. b, e *Ref: Guyton and Hall Medical Physiology, 12th/ed*

Option a	False	
Option b	True	
Option c	False	
Option d	False	
Option e	True	

Adaptation of sensory receptors

A characteristic of all sensory receptors is that they adapt either partially or completely to any constant stimulus after a period of time. That is when a continuous sensory stimulus is applied, the receptors first respond at a high impulse rate and then at a progressively slower rate until finally the rate of action potentials decreases to very few or often none at all.

Slowly adapting receptors or Tonic receptors

These receptors continue to transmit impulses to the brain as long as the stimulus is present (or at least for many minutes or hours). They keep the brain apprised of the status of the body and its relations to its surroundings, e.g.

- Muscle spindle receptors
- Golgi tendon apparatuses
- Baroreceptors of the arterial tree

- Pain receptors
- Chemoreceptors of the carotid and aortic bodies
- Ruffini's endings

Rapidly adapting receptors/Rate receptors/Phasic receptors/Movement receptors

These receptors are stimulated only when the stimulus strength changes that cannot be used to transmit a continuous signal, e.g.

- Pacinian receptors
- Meissner's corpuscle

4. Which of the following is true about lung mechanics?

a. Surfactant prevent collapse of small alveoli into larger one
b. Larger alveoli collapse more than smaller ones in the absence of surfactant
c. Decrease in surfactant decreases chance of collapse
d. Surfactant increases surface tension
e. With surfactant, large alveoli tend to become smaller and smaller ones tend to become larger

Ans. a, e *Ref: Guyton and Hall Medical Physiology, 12th/ed; Johnson Essential Medical Physiology, 3rd/ed*

Option a	True	
Option b	False	The pressure generated in alveoli is directly proportional to the surface tension of the lining fluid and inversely proportional to its radius
Option c	False	Decrease in surfactant will increase the chances of alveolar collapse
Option d	False	Surfactant decreases surface tension
Option e	True	

Surfactant and surface tension

Surface tension: When water forms a surface with the air, it is attempting to contract. This is called surface tension. Inner surfaces of alveoli are lined by water. Here also the water surface is attempting to contract. This results in an attempt to force the air out of alveoli through the bronchi, and in doing so causes the alveoli to try to collapse. The net effect is to cause an elastic contractile force of the entire lungs which is called the surface tension elastic force.

Surfactant: Surfactant is a surface active agent in water. It reduces the surface tension of water. It is secreted by type II alveolar epithelial cells which constitute 10% surface area of the alveoli.

By decreasing the surface tension of the fluid lining the alveoli, surfactant prevents collapse of alveoli into smaller ones.

Decrease in surfactant will increase the chances of alveolar collapse. Decreased surfactant production in the lungs of premature babies results in respiratory distress due to tendency of alveoli to collapse and their inability to remain open, thus decreasing oxygen exchange through alveoli.

Fluid	Surface tension
Water	72 dynes/cm
Fluid lining alveoli without surfactant	50 dynes/cm
Fluid lining alveoli with normal amount of surfactant	5-30 dynes/cm

Positive Pressure in an alveolus caused by surface tension is calculated by the following formula.

Pressure = 2 × Surface tension/Radius of alveolus. (LaPlace formula)

Thus the pressure generated in alveoli is directly proportional to the surface tension of the lining fluid and inversely proportional to its radius. This implies, smaller the alveolus, greater the alveolar pressure. Which in turn implies smaller alveoli collapse more than the larger ones in the absence of surfactant.

Surfactant promotes alveolar stability. Look at the picture below. According to the formula previously stated the positive pressure is higher in smaller alveoli. So the smaller alveolus here will collapse and empty into the larger alveolus, owing to its greater positive pressure. Thus in the absence of surfactant all small alveoli in the lung will collapse and empty into adjacent larger alveoli, creating alveolar instability (large alveoli become larger and smaller ones become smaller).

Surfactant negates this effect. It reduces the surface tension and hence the positive pressure in smaller alveoli, thus small alveoli tend to remain open and become larger while the larger ones tend to become smaller creating alveolar stability.

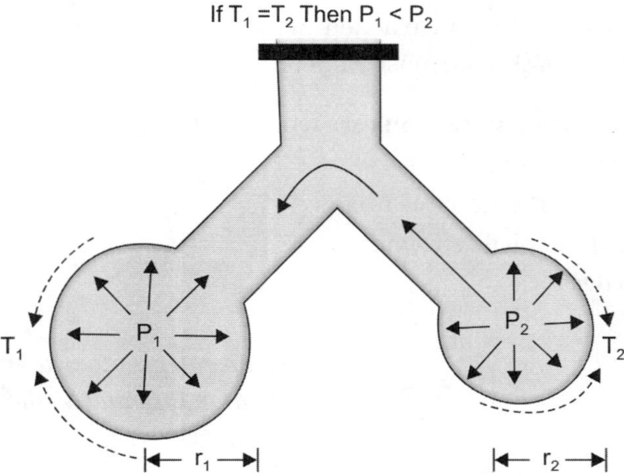

5. True about action potential in skeletal muscle fibers and nerve fibers:

a. Skeletal muscle fibers conduction velocity is $\frac{1}{4}$ of thick myelinated nerve fiber

b. Action potential of both is qualitatively similar to each other

c. Resting membrane potential is almost same

d. Duration of action potential remains same in both
e. Action potential of both differ quantitatively from each other

Ans. b, c *Ref: Guyton and Hall, Medical Physiology, 12th/ed; Ganong review of Medical Physiology, 24th/ed*

Option a	False	
Option b	True	
Option c	True	
Option d	False	
Option e	False	

"The electrical events in the skeletal muscle and the ionic fluxes that underlie them share distinct similarities to those in nerve, with quantitative differences in timing and magnitude". ..."*Ganong*".

"Almost everything regarding initiation and conduction of action potentials in the nerve fibers applies equally to skeletal muscle fibers except for quantitate differences". ..."*Guyton*"

	Nerve action potential	Muscle action potential
Resting membrane potential	– 70 mV	– 80 to – 90 mV
Duration of action potential	0.2 – 0.3 m/sec	1 – 5 m/sec
Velocity of conduction	70 – 120 m/sec	3 – 5 m/sec

Conduction velocity in thick myelinated nerve fiber is 100 m/sec which is more than 30 times higher than that of skeletal muscle fibers.

6. Which of the following statements are true about ovulation?

a. Prostaglandins increase
b. Gonadotropin hormone surge occurs
c. Activation of proteolytic enzymes occurs
d. GnRH level decreases
e. hCG surge

Ans. a, b, c *Ref: Speroff gynecologic endocrinology, 8th/ed; Johnson Essential Medical Physiology, 3rd/ed*

Option a	True	
Option b	True	
Option c	True	
Option d	False	GnRH does not decrease, but increases during ovulation
Option e	False	hCG is a pregnancy hormone and not normally present in a menstruating female

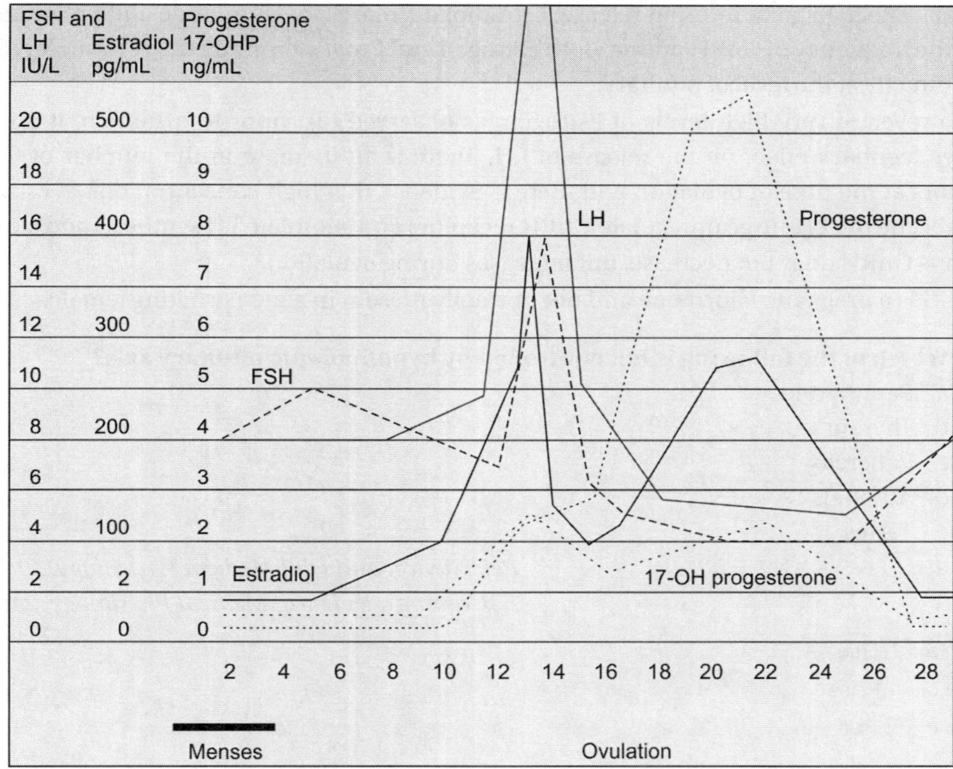

Ovulation

LH Surge is responsible for ovulation

The peak levels of FSH, LH and Estrogen occur around the time of ovulation.

Rapidly rising Estrogen gives positive feedback to the pituitary to increase secretion of LH -> LH acts on a mature follicle primed by FSH in the follicular phase.

Action of LH:

- Resumption of meiosis in oocyte.
- Stimulates release of progesterone by granulosa cells.
- FSH, LH, and progesterone stimulate the activity of proteolytic enzymes, resulting in digestion of collagen in the follicular wall and increasing its distensibility.
- Prostaglandins, and other eicosanoids increase markedly in the preovulatory follicular fluid in response to the LH surge, reaching a peak concentration at ovulation.
- Prostaglandins and eicosanoids act to free proteolytic enzymes within the follicular wall, and may promote angiogenesis and hyperemia.

GnRH in menstrual cycle

During normal menstrual cycle, GnRH pulses are more frequent in the follicular phase than in the luteal phase. At the average blood levels both Estrogen and Progesterone exert a negative feedback effect on gonadotropin release. Estradiol decreases the amplitude and progesterone slows the frequency of GnRH pulses. Both Estrogen and Progesterone also exert their feedback effect directly at the level of pituitary.

However, at very high levels of Estrogen, as observed just prior to ovulation, it exerts a positive feedback effect on the release of LH. There is an increase in the number of GnRH receptors at the time of ovulation and there is evidence that high concentrations of estradiol that precede the LH surge upregulate GnRH receptors and stimulate LH synthesis and storage.

Thus GnRH does not decrease, but increases during ovulation.

hCG is a pregnancy hormone and not normally present in a menstruating female.

7. Which of the following is not controlled by hypothalamic pituitary axis?

a. Parathyroid
b. Thyroid
c. Pancreas
d. Adrenals
e. Testes

Ans. a, c *Ref: Guyton and Hall Medical Physiology, 12th/ed; Ganong's review of Medical Physiology, 24th/ed*

Option a	True	
Option b	False	
Option c	True	
Option d	False	
Option e	False	

Hypothalamic hormones	Effect on anterior pituitary hormones	Actions	
Thyrotropin-releasing hormone	Stimulates TSH secretion by thyrotropes	Stimulates Thyroid to secrete T3 andT4	
Gonadotropin releasing hormone	Stimulates FSH, LH secretion by gonadotropes	Male (testes) FSH – spermatogenesis LH –Testosterone secretion	Female (ovaries) FSH – Estrogen secretion LH – Androgen and progesterone secretion
Corticotropin-releasing hormone	Stimulates ACTH secretion by corticotrophs	Stimulates adrenal cortex to secrete corticosteroids	
Growth hormone releasing hormone	Stimulates GH secretion by somatotrophs	Several metabolic effects over cells of the body resulting in overall growth	
Prolactin inhibiting hormone/dopamine	Inhibits synthesis and secretion of prolactin by lactotropes		

The bodies of cells that secrete Posterior pituitary hormones are located in the hypothalamus. These hormones are transported in the axoplasm of the neurons passing from hypothalamus to posterior pituitary.

Antidiuretic hormone - increases permeability of collecting ducts and tubules of renal cortex to water, thus allowing most water to be reabsorbed as tubular fluid passes through these ducts, thereby resulting in antidiuresis.

Oxytocin -contraction of pregnant uterus and milk ejection by breasts.

8. Erythropoietin is produced by:

a. Juxtaglomerular apparatus
b. Proximal tubular cells
c. Para recta
d. Interstitium
e. Peritubular capillaries

Ans. e *Ref: Ganong's review of Medical Physiology, 24th/ed*

Option a	False	
Option b	False	
Option c	False	
Option d	False	
Option e	True	Produced by interstitial cells in the peritubular capillary bed of the kidneys

In adults, about 85% erythropoietin comes from the kidneys and 15% from the liver.

Erythropoietin is produced by:

- Interstitial cells in the peritubular capillary bed of the kidneys.
- Perivenous hepatocytes in liver.

It is also produced in (insignificant sources)

- Brain—where it exerts protective effect against excitotoxic damage triggered by hypoxia.
- Uterus and oviducts—where it is induced by Estrogen and appears to mediate Estrogen dependent angiogenesis.

9. Increase in 2, 3 DPG causes:

a. Right shift of HODC
b. Left shift
c. Higher affinity for oxygen
d. Lower affinity for oxygen
e. Higher offloading of oxygen at the tissues

Ans. a, d, e *Ref: Guyton and Hall Medical Physiology, 12th/ed; Ganong's review of Medical Physiology, 24th/ed*

Option a	True	
Option b	False	Right shift
Option c	False	Causes lower affinity for oxygen
Option d	True	
Option e	True	

Factors affecting the affinity of hemoglobin for oxygen

Decrease O_2 affinity of hemoglobin

- Low pH (Bohr effect)
- 2, 3-Diphosphoglycerate

Factors that shift hemoglobin-oxygen dissociation curve (HODC) to right:

- Increase in hydrogen ions, fall in pH
- Increased CO_2
- Rise in temperature
- Increased 2, 3-Diphosphoglycerate

Shift of HODC to right indicates decreased O_2 affinity of hemoglobin. This allows release of oxygen from blood to the tissues.

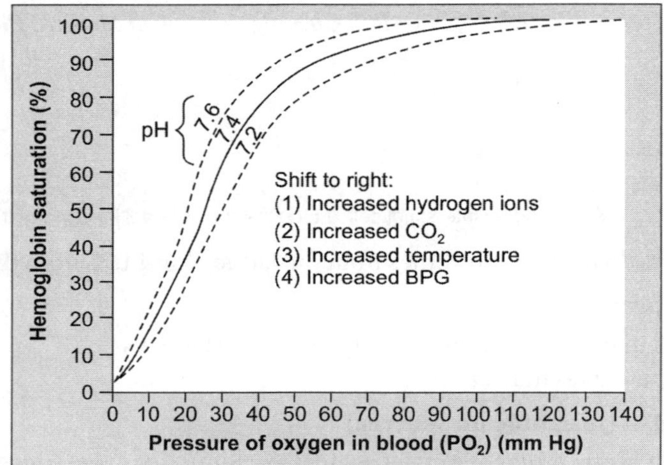

10. Taste sensation is carried by:

a. Facial nerve
b. Hypoglossal nerve
c. Trigeminal nerve
d. Vagus nerve
e. Glossopharyngeal nerve

Ans. a, d, e *Ref: Guyton and Hall Medical Physiology, 12th/ed*

Option a	True
Option b	False
Option c	False
Option d	True
Option e	True

Transmission of taste signals to the CNS

- Taste impulses from the anterior two thirds of the tongue pass first into the lingual nerve then through the chords tympani into the **facial nerve** and finally into tractus solitarius in the brain stem.

- Taste sensations from the circumvallate papillae on the back of tongue and from other posterior regions of mouth an throats are transmitted through the **glossopharyngeal nerve** also into the tractus solitarius, but more posteriorly.
- Taste sensations from base of tongue and other parts of pharyngeal regions travel via the **vagus nerve.**

11. Myocardial oxygen demand is dependent on:

a. Heart rate
b. Contractility
c. BMR
d. Shortening of muscle
e. Ventricular wall tension

Ans. All *Ref: Guyton and Hall Medical Physiology, 12th/ed; Ganong's review of Medical Physiology, 24th/ed*

Option a	True
Option b	True
Option c	True
Option d	True
Option e	True

Myocardial oxygen consumption by the myocardium is about 2 mL/100 g/min. Oxygen consumption by the beating heart is 9 mL/100 g/min.

- Myocardial oxygen consumption is increased by increasing:
  - Tension-time index = Intramyocardial tension during contraction multiplied by duration of time that the contraction persists (shortening of muscle implies contraction).
  - Intramyocardial tension~pressure multiplied by diameter of ventricle (stretching of myocardial fibers).
  - Heart rate.
  - Contractile state of the myocardium.
  - Ventricular work per beat: Work is the product of **stroke volume** and **mean arterial pressure** in the pulmonary artery or aorta, for the right and left ventricle respectively. However, pressure work (i.e. after load) produces a greater increase in oxygen consumption than volume work (i.e. preload).
  - During exercise.

BMR

The minimum level of energy required to exist is called the basal metabolic rate and accounts for about 50–70% of daily energy expenditure in most sedentary individuals.

The method of determining BMR is to measure the oxygen utilization over a given period of time after a night of restful sleep, no food for at least previous 12 hours, no activity for at least 1 hour before the test, comfortable temperature.

Skeletal muscle even under resting conditions, accounts for 20–30% of BMR. The BMR averages 65–70 Calories per hour in an average 70 kg man.

A rise in BMR will increase cardiac output and hence myocardial oxygen consumption.

12. True about carotid sinus:

a. At the starting of internal carotid artery
b. Stimulated by chemoreceptors
c. High elastin and receptors
d. Most sensitive in changes in arterial pressure at 100 mm Hg
e. Stimulated by baroreceptors

Ans. a, c, d, e *Ref: Medical physiology by Boron and Boulpaep, 2nd/ed; C.C. Chatterjee's Human Physiology, 11th/ed; Guyton and Hall Medical Physiology, 12th/ed; Ganong's review of Medical Physiology, 24th/ed*

Option a	True	
Option b	False	They are stimulated when stretched
Option c	True	
Option d	True	
Option e	True	

Baroreceptors are spray type nerve endings that lie in the walls of arteries. They are stimulated when stretched. A few baroreceptors are located in the wall of almost every large artery of the thoracic and the neck regions.

Baroreceptors are extremely abundant in:

1. The wall of each internal carotid artery slightly above the carotid bifurcation, an area known as the **carotid sinus,** and
2. The wall of aortic arch.

Signals from the carotid sinus baroreceptors are transmitted through small Hernig's nerves to the glossopharyngeal nerves in the high neck, and then to tractus solitarius in the medullary area of the brain stem. Signals from the aortic baroreceptors in the arch of aorta are transmitted through the vagus nerve also to the tractus solitarius of the medulla.

After the baroreceptor signals have entered the tractus solitarius of medulla, secondary signals inhibit the vasoconstrictor center of the medulla and excite the Vagal parasympathetic center. The net effects are:

1. Vasodilation of veins and arterioles throughout the peripheral vascular system.
2. Decreased heart rate and strength of heart contraction.

Conversely low pressure has opposite effects, reflexly causing the pressure to rise backwards towards normal. In the normal operating range of arterial pressure, around 100 mm Hg, even a slight change in pressure causes a strong change in baroreceptor signal to readjust arterial pressure back to normal.

Closely related with the baroreceptor pressure control system is the chemoreceptor reflex that operates in the much same way. The chemoreceptors are chemosensitive cells sensitive to oxygen lack, carbon dioxide excess and hydrogen ion excess. They are located in several small chemoreceptor organs about 2 mm in size.

1. Two **carotid bodie**s, one of which lies in the bifurcation of each common carotid artery.
2. One to three aortic bodies adjacent to the aorta. The chemoreceptors excite nerve fibers that, along with baroreceptor fibers, pass through hering's nerves and vagal nerves to the

Vasomotor centre of brain stem. Each carotid or aortic body is supplied with an abundant blood flow through a small nutrient artery, so that the chemoreceptors are always in close contact with arterial blood. Whenever the arterial pressure falls below a critical level, the chemoreceptors become stimulated because diminished blood flow causes decreased oxygen, build up of carbon dioxide and hydrogen ions. The signals transmitted via chemoreceptors excite the Vasomotor centre and this elevates arterial pressure back to normal. Chemoreceptors are not very powerful arterial pressure controller unless arterial pressure falls below 80 mm Hg.

	Carotid sinus	Carotid body
Receptors	Baroreceptor	Chemoreceptor
Location	Wall of each internal carotid artery slightly above the carotid bifurcation	Bifurcation of each common carotid artery
Sensitivity	Very sensitive around 100 mm Hg. Even a slight change in pressure causes a strong change in baroreceptor signal to readjust arterial pressure back to normal.	Not very powerful arterial pressure controller unless arterial pressure falls below 80 mm Hg

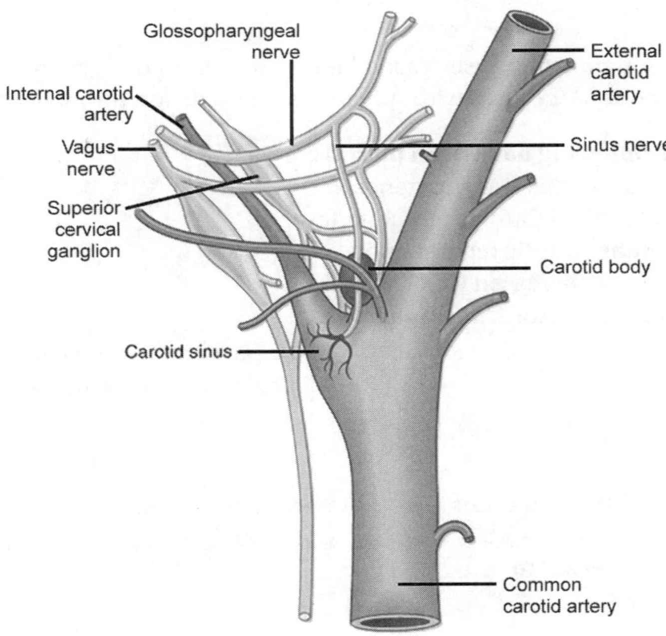

13. Local vasoconstriction occurs in presence of:

a. Calcium
b. Sodium
c. Potassium
d. Hydrogen
e. Magnesium

Ans. a *Ref: Guyton and Hall, Textbook of Medical Physiology, 12th/ed*

Option a	True	
Option b	False	
Option c	False	Causes vasodilation
Option d	False	Causes vasodilation
Option e	False	Causes powerful vasodilation

Many different ions and other chemical factors can either dilate or constrict local blood vessels. Most of them have little function in overall regulation of circulation, but some specific effects are:

Increase in	Action	Mechanism
Calcium ion	Vasoconstriction	Stimulation of smooth muscle contraction
Potassium ion	Vasodilation	Inhibition of smooth muscle contraction
Magnesium ion	Powerful vasodilation	Inhibition of smooth muscle contraction
Hydrogen ion (decreased pH)	Vasodilation	
Increased pH (decreased hydrogen ion)	Vasoconstriction	
Acetate	Mild vasodilation	
Citrate	Mild vasodilation	
Carbon dioxide	Moderate vasodilation in most tissues but marked vasodilation in brain	

Note that local carbon dioxide causes vasodilation. But through chemoreceptor mechanism (carotid and aortic bodies) it causes widespread vasoconstriction throughout the body.

14. Which of the following have been paired correctly?

a. Pulsus parvus/tardus—Aortic stenosis
b. Paradoxical pulse—Cardiac tamponade
c. Pulsus alterans—Aortic regurgitation
d. Dicrotic pulse—Increased PVR
e. Pulsus bisferiens—Aortic regurgitation

Ans. a, b, e *Ref: Harrison's Manual of Medicine, 19th/ed; Clinical examination by Harmanjit Singh Hira*

Option a	True	
Option b	True	
Option c	False	Pulsus alternans is seen in severe LV dysfunction
Option d	False	Dicrotic pulse is seen in Conditions associated with low peripheral vascular resistance
Option e	True	

Character of arterial pulse

Type of carotid artery pulse	Character	Seen in
Pulsus parvus	Weak upstroke due to decreased stroke volume	Hypovolemia, LV failure, aortic and mitral stenosis
Pulsus tardus	Delayed upstroke	Aortic stenosis

Contd...

Contd...

Type of carotid artery pulse	Character	Seen in
Pulsus parvus et tardus	Delayed weak upstroke (small amplitude delayed peak)	Severe aortic stenosis
Hyperkinetic pulse	Bounding	Hyperkinetic circulation, aortic regurgitation, patent ductus arteriosus, marked vasodilation
Pulsus bisferiens	Double systolic pulsation	Aortic regurgitation, hypertrophic cardiomyopathy
Pulsus alternans	Regular alteration in pulse pressure amplitude	Severe LV dysfunction
Pulsus paradoxus	Exaggerated inspiration fall (> 10 mm Hg) in systolic BP	Pericardial tamponade, severe obstructive lung disease
Dicrotic pulse	One peak in systole and one in diastole. (A percussion wave in systole and a prominent dicrotic wave in diastole)	Conditions associated with low peripheral vascular resistance (PVR) like fever, sepsis, reduced stroke volume

15. True about JVP waves is/are:

a. A wave is due to late diastolic filling
b. Cannon a waves are due to AV dissociation
c. V wave is due to isovolumetric contraction after systole
d. Constrictive pericarditis show 30% steep x and y descent
e. C wave is seen in the later part of diastole

Ans. b, d *Ref: Harrison's Principles of Internal Medicine, 19th/ed*

Option a	False	a wave is due to atrial systole
Option b	True	
Option c	False	v wave is due to atrial diastole
Option d	True	
Option e	False	c wave corresponds to tricuspid valve closure and bulging

Jugular venous pulse: Fluctuations in right atrial pressure during cardiac cycle generate a pulse that is transmitted backwards into the jugular veins.

Waveform of jugular venous pulses

In sinus rhythm, the jugular venous pulse has a double waveform attributable to the 'a' and 'v' waves separated by 'x' and 'y' descents. JVP normally falls with inspiration. Normally the venous pressure should fall by 3 mm Hg with inspiration.

Wave	Caused by	Relation with cardiac cycle
a	Right atrial presystolic contraction or atrial systole	Occurs before S1 and just after the P wave of ECG.
c	Tricuspid valve closure and bulging/isovolumetric contraction plus impact of adjoining carotid artery	
x	Descent of tricuspid valve ring	
v	Rise in atrial pressure due to passive filling during ventricular systole, atrial diastole	Ventricular systole, coincides with S2
y	As tricuspid valve opens to allow ventricular filling	Ventricular diastole

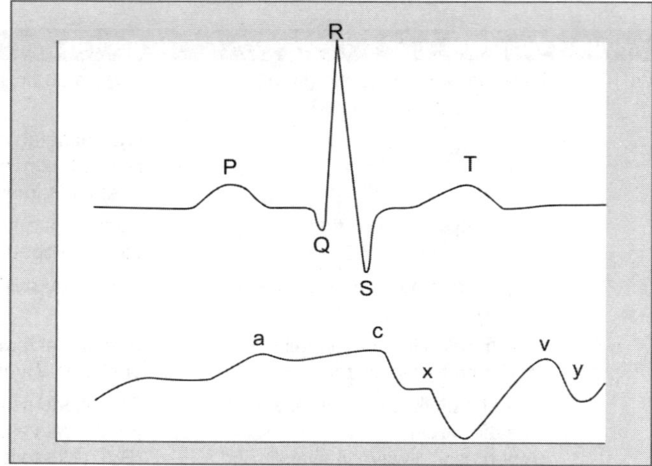

Abnormal JVP	Cause
Rise in JVP with inspiration (Kussmaul sign)	Constrictive pericarditis
Absent 'a' wave	Atrial fibrillation
Giant 'a' wave	Forceful atrial contraction against a stenosed tricuspid valve or a non compliant hypertrophied right ventricle
Cannon 'a' wave	Atrial systole against a closed tricuspid valve seen in atrioventricular dissociation when there is coincident atrial and ventricular systole (e.g. Complete heart block, ventricular tachycardia)
Giant 'v' wave	Tricuspid regurgitations, atrial septal defect.
Steep 'y' descent	Constrictive pericarditis
Steep 'x' and 'y' descents	Constrictive pericarditis
Exaggerated 'x' descent	Cardiac tamponade
Slow 'y' descent	Tricuspid stenosis

16. Which of the following ions move intracellularly?

a. K^+
b. Mg^+
c. Na_2^+
d. Bicarbonate
e. Chloride

Ans. a, b *Ref: Guyton and Hall, Medical Physiology, 12th/ed; Ganong's review of Medical Physiology, 24th/ed*

Option a	True
Option b	True
Option c	False
Option d	False
Option e	False

The intercellular fluid (ICF) is separated from the extracellular fluid (ECF) by a cell membrane that is highly permeable to water but not to most of the electrolytes in body. In contrast to the

ECF, ICF contains only small amounts of sodium, chloride, bicarbonate ions and almost no calcium ions.

Instead it contains large amounts of potassium, phosphate, proteins, and moderate amounts of magnesium and sulfate ions. All of these are in low concentrations in the ECF.

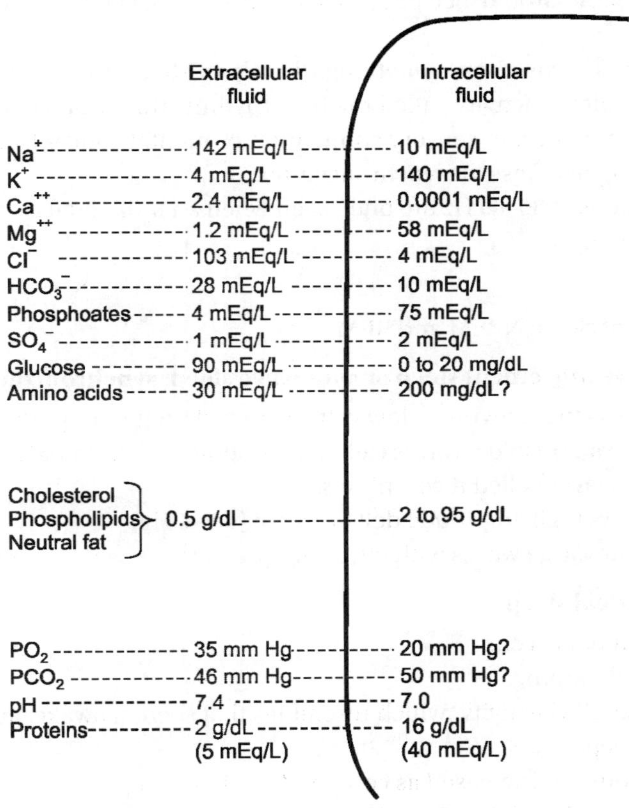

17. Which of the following is true for sleep?

a. Disappearance of alpha waves
b. K-complex
c. Pontogeniculo-occipital (PGO) spikes
d. Gamma oscillations
e. High amplitude low frequency pattern of EEG during most of sleep

Ans. a, b, c, e *Ref: Ganong's review of Medical Physiology, 24th/ed*

Option a	True	
Option b	True	
Option c	True	
Option d	False	Gamma oscillations at 30–80 Hz are often seen when an individual is aroused and focuses attention on something
Option e	True	

Sleep wake cycle and the EEG waves.

EEG in the awake

- In adult humans who are awake but at rest with the mind wandering and eyes closed, the most prominent component of the EEG is a fairly regular pattern of waves at a frequency of 8–13 Hz and amplitude of 50–109 micro V. This pattern is the alpha rhythm. It is most marked in the parietal and occipital lobes and is associated with decreased levels of attention.
- When attention is focused on something, the alpha rhythm is replaced by an irregular (13–39 Hz) low voltage activity called the beta rhythm. This is called alpha block and can be produced by any form of sensory stimulation or mental concentration. Other names : arousal or alerting response, desynchronization.
- Gamma oscillations at 30–80 Hz are often seen when an individual is aroused and focuses attention on something.

Sleep stages

There are two kinds of sleep: NREM and REM.

NREM, non rapid eye movement sleep or slow wave sleep, synchronization in EEG.

- Stage 1: EEG shows theta rhythm – low voltage, mixed frequency pattern (4–7 Hz).
- Stage 2: EEG shows sinusoidal waves called sleep spindles (12–14 Hz), and occasional high voltage biphasic waves called K complexes.
- Stage 3: EEG shows high amplitude delta rhythm (0.5–4 Hz)
- Stage 4: EEG shows large waves with lowest frequency.

REM sleep, paradoxical sleep

- Rapid eye movements occur.
- Associated with dreaming.
- Rapid low voltage EEG activity, which resembles that seen in awake, aroused state and in stage 1 NREM sleep.
- Threshold for arousal is increased as compared to REM sleep.
- **Ponto-geniculo-occipital (PGO) spikes:** Occurrence of large phasic potentials in the cholinergic neurons in the pons, which pass rapidly to the lateral geniculate body and from there to occipital cortex.
- Tone of skeletal muscles in the neck is markedly reduced.
- PET scans show increased activity in pons, amygdala, and anterior cingulate gyrus, visual association areas but decreased activity in prefrontal and parietal cortex, primary visual cortex.

18. At physiological conditions, which of the following features are not shown by plasma membrane?

a. Lateral diffusion of ions
b. Transmembrane diffusion of uncharged molecules
c. Rotation of transmembrane proteins along their own axis
d. Movements of cholesterol particles throughout the membrane
e. Movement of water molecules throughout the membrane

Ans. b, c, d *Ref: Molecular cell biology by Lodish, 6th/ed; Medical cell biology by Goodman, 2nd/ed; Guyton and Hall Medical Physiology, 12th/ed*

Option a	False	
Option b	True	
Option c	True	
Option d	True	
Option e	False	

Biomembranes:

- The basic structural unit of all biomembranes is the phospholipid bilayer, which is a two dimensional lipid sheet with hydrophilic faces and hydrophobic core, which is impermeable to water soluble molecules and ions.
- The primary lipid components of biomembranes are phosphoglycerides, sphingolipids, and sterols such as cholesterol.
- Membrane phospholipids are capable of several types of motion within the biological membrane. The phospholipids can rotate very rapidly around a central long axis.
- In pure membrane bilayer, phospholipids and sphingolipids rotate and move laterally but they do not spontaneously migrate or flip flop from one leaflet to the other.
- Flip flop movement of phospholipids from one leaflet to other is very rare but does occur. Special membrane proteins are required for this flip flop motion.
- Most lipids and many proteins are laterally mobile in biomembranes (lateral diffusion).
- Membranes can undergo phase transition from fluid to gel like states depending on temperature and composition of the membrane.
- In general, membrane fluidity is decreased by sphingolipids and increased by phosphoglycerides.
- Membrane proteins can be classified into three categories: (1) integral or transmembrane, (2) lipid anchored, (3) peripheral.
- Integral membrane proteins can also rotate along their axis within the membrane but cannot flip flop from one leaflet to the other.
- Small uncharged molecules can pass through lipid bilayer by simple diffusion, e.g. Oxygen, carbon dioxide, nitrogen and small uncharged polar molecules such as ethanol, glycerol and urea.
- Water is highly insoluble in the membrane lipids but it readily passes through channels in transmembrane proteins. Similarly small lipid insoluble and water soluble substance like ions can cross the membrane through these channels.

19. Comprehension is preserved in:

a. Conduction aphasia
b. Global aphasia
c. Anomic aphasia
d. Wernicke's aphasia
e. Broca's aphasia

Ans. a, c, e *Ref: Harrison's principles of Internal Medicine, 19th/ed*

Option a	True	
Option b	False	Comprehension impaired
Option c	True	

Option d	False	Comprehension impaired
Option e	True	

Aphasia

Abnormalities of language functions that are not because of defects in vision, hearing or to motor paralysis.

Clinical features of aphasia and related conditions commonly seen in cerebrovascular hemorrhages

	Comprehension	*Repetition of spoken language*	*Naming*	*Fluency*
Wernicke's	Impaired	Impaired	Impaired	Preserved or increased
Broca's	Preserved (except grammar)	Impaired	Impaired	Decreased
Global	Impaired	Impaired	Impaired	Decreased
Conduction	Preserved	Impaired	Impaired	Preserved
Nonfluent (anterior) transcortical	Preserved	Preserved	Impaired	Impaired
Fluent (posterior) transcortical	Impaired	Preserved	Impaired	Preserved
Isolation	Impaired	Echolalia	Impaired	No purposeful speech
Anomic	Preserved	Preserved	Impaired	Preserved except for word-finding pauses
Pure word deafness	Impaired only for spoken language	Impaired	Preserved	Preserved
Pure alexia	Impaired only for reading	Preserved	Preserved	Preserved

20. True statement(s) is/are:

a. ADH increases only water reabsorption, not solute reabsorption
b. Aldosterone mainly leads to sodium reabsorption and not water
c. Glomerular filtrate of PCT has similar osmolarity as of plasma
d. Hypertonic fluid is passed from early DCT
e. Generally urine osmolarity equals to plasma osmolarity

Ans. a, c *Ref: Guyton and Hall, Medical Physiology, 12th/ed*

Option a	True	
Option b	False	Causes increased NaCl and water reabsorption
Option c	True	
Option d	False	Hypertonic fluid passes from thin descending limb of loop of Henle
Option e	False	

The most important renal action of ADH is to increase water permeability of the distal tubule, collecting tubule, and the collecting duct epithelia. Increase in ADH permits large amount of water to be resorted in distal and collecting tubules and duct, but does not markedly alter the rate of renal excretion of the solute.

Hormones that regulate tubular reabsorption in the renal cortex

Hormone	Site of action	Effects
Aldosterone	Collecting tubule and duct	Increased NaCl and water reabsorption, Increased potassium secretion
Angiotensin II	Proximal tubule, thick ascending loop of Henle/distal tubule, collecting tubule	Increased NaCl and water reabsorption, Increased H^+ secretion
Antidiuretic hormone (ADH)	Distal tubule, collecting tubule and duct	Increase water reabsorption
Atrial natriuretic peptide	Distal tubule, collecting tubule and duct	Decreased NaCl reabsorption
Parathyroid hormone	Proximal tubule, thick ascending loop of Henle/distal tubule	Decreased phosphate reabsorption, increased calcium reabsorption

21. True about normal blood levels is:

a. TSH level: 0.1–3.1 mIU/L
b. Sodium: 135–145 mmol/L
c. Potassium: 3.5–5.1 mmol/L
d. Creatinine: 0.6–2.6 mg/dL
e. Total Calcium: 8.5–10.5 mg/dL

Ans. b, c, e *Ref: Harrison's principles of Internal Medicine, 19th/ed*

Option a	False	0.34–4.25 mIU/L
Option b	True	
Option c	True	
Option d	False	0.5–0.9 mg/dL in females and 0.6–1.2 mg/dL in males
Option e	True	

Testosterone, free Female, adult Male, adult	S	 10.4–65.9 pmol/L 312–1040 pmol/L	 3–19 pg/mL 90–300 pg/mL
Testosterone, total, Female Male	S	 0.21–2.98 nmol/L 9.36–37.10 nmol/L	 6–6 ng/dL 270–1070 ng/dL
Thyroglobulin	S	13–318 μg/L	1.3–31.8 ng/dL
Thyroid-binding globulin	S	13–30 mg/L	1.3–3.0 mg/dL
Thyroid-stimulating hormone (thyrotropin)	S	0.34–4.25 mIU/L	0.34–4.25 μIU/mL
Thyrotropin receptor antibody	S	≤ 1.75 IU/L	≤ 1.75 mIU/mL
Thyroxine, free (fT_4)	S	9.0–16 pmol/L	0.7–1.24 ng/dL
Thyroxine, total (T_4)	S	70–151 nmol/L	5.4–11.7 μg/dL
Thyroxine index (free)	S	6.7–10.9	6.7–10.9
Sex hormone-binding globulin (adult) Male Female	S	 11–80 nmol/L 30–135 nmol/L	 11–80 nmol/L 30–135 nmol/L

Contd...

Contd...

Sodium	S	136–146 mmol/L	136–146 mEq/L
Creatinine Female Male	S	44–80 µmol/L 53–106 µmol/L	0.5–0.9 mg/dL 0.6–1.2 mg/dL
Bilirubin Total Direct Indirect	S	5.1–22 µmol/L 1.7–6.8 µmol/L 3.4–15.2 µmol/L	0.3–1.3 mg/dL 0.1–0.4 mg/dL 0.2–0.9 mg/dL
Calcium	S	2.2–2.6 mmol/L	8.7–10.2 mg/dL
Calcium, ionized	WB	1.12–1.32 mmol/L	4.5–5.3 mg/dL
Potassium	S	3.5–5.0 mmol/L	3.5–5.0 mEq/L

S – Serum
WB – Whole blood

Biochemistry

1. ω-6 fatty acids are all except:

a. γ-linolenic acid
b. Linoleic acid
c. Arachidonic acid
d. α-Linolenic acid
e. Elaidic Acid

Ans. d,e *Ref: Harper 30/e p214 & 29/e p142; Lippincotts 5/e p362*

Option a	True	Yes, it a ω-6 fatty acids
Option b	True	Yes, it a ω-6 fatty acids
Option c	True	Yes, it a ω-6 fatty acids
Option d	False	No, it is a ω-3 fatty acids
Option e	False	No, it is a ω-9 (MUFA) fatty acids

Triacylglycerols containing primarily fatty acids with more than one double bond are referred to as polyunsaturated fats.

Unsaturated fats are classified as:

ω-3 fatty acids	ω-6 fatty acids	ω-9 fatty acids
α-Linolenic acid	Linoleic acid	Oleic acid
Clupandonic acid	γ-linolenic acid	Nervonic acid
Cervonic acid	Arachidonic acid	Elaidic acid

ω-6 fatty acids

These are long-chain, PUFAs, with the first double bond beginning at the sixth bond position when starting from the methyl end of the fatty acid molecule.

Source: vegetable oils

Effect: lower LDL and HDL

ω-3 Fatty acids: These are long-chain, PUFAs, with the first double bond beginning at the third bond position from the methyl end.

Effect: Dietary ω-3 polyunsaturated fats suppress cardiac arrhythmias, reduce serum triacylglycerols, decrease the tendency for thrombosis, lower blood pressure, and substantially reduce risk of cardiovascular mortality.

Acceptable intake range: 0.6-1.2% of total calorie intake

Source: vegetable oils – flaxseed

Note: Fish oils contain long chain, ω-3 docosahexaenoic acid (DHA) and eicosapentaenoic acid (EPA)

Trans fatty acids: Trans fatty acids are chemically classified as unsaturated fatty acids, but behave more like saturated fatty acids in the body, that is, they elevate serum LDL (but not HDL), and they increase the risk of CHD. Trans fatty acids do not occur naturally in plants, but occur in small amounts in animals.

Trans fatty acids are formed during the hydrogenation of liquid vegetable oils, for example, in the manufacture of margarine and partially hydrogenated vegetable oil.

Metabolic effects of fatty acids

Type of Fat	Metabolic Effects	Effects on Disease Prevention
Trans fatty acid	↑ LDL ↓ HDL	↑ Incidence of coronary heart disease
Saturated fatty acid	↑ LDL Little effect on HDL	↑ Incidence of coronary heart disease: may increase risk of prostate, colon cancer
Monounsaturated fatty acid	↓ LDL ↓ HDL	↓ Incidence of coronary heart disease
Polyunsaturated fatty acid ω-6	↓ LDL ↓ HDL Provide arachidonic acid which is an important precursor of prostaglandinas and leukotrienes	↓ Incidence of coronary heart disease
Polyunsaturated fatty acids ω-3	Little effect on LDL; Little effect on HDL Suppress cardiac arrhythmias, reduce serum triacylglycerols, decrease the tendency for thrombosis, lower blood pressure	↓ Incidence of coronary heart disease ↓ Risk of sudden cardiac death

2. Apolipoproteins present in HDL:

a. Apo-AI
b. Apo-AII
c. Apo B-100
d. Apo B-48
e. Apo C

Ans. a,b,e *Ref: Harper 30th/ed p255 & 29th/ed p238; Lippincots 5th/ed p228*

Option a	True	Yes, correct
Option b	True	Yes, correct
Option c	False	No, it is in LDL, VLDL and IDL
Option d	False	No, it is in chylomicron remnants
Option e	True	Yes, correct

- The major apolipoprotein of HDL is Apo-A, whereas major apolipoprotein of VLDL, LDL and chylomicron is apo-B, apo – B100 in VLDL and LDL and apo B-48 in chylomicrons.

Lipoprotein	Apolipoprotein	
Chylomicrons	A-I, A-II, A-IV, B-48, C-I, C-II, C-III, E	Transport dietary triglyceride and cholesterol from intestine to tissues
Chylomicron remnants	B-48, E	
VLDL	B-100, C-I, C-II, C-III	Transports triglyceride from liver to tissues
IDL	B-100, E	Picks up cholesterol from HDL to become LDL Picked up by liver

Contd...

Contd…

Lipoprotein	Apolipoprotein	
LDL	B-100	Delivers cholesterol into cells
HDL	A-I, A-II, A-IV, C-I, C-II, C-III, D, E	Picks up cholesterol accumulating in blood vessels Delivers cholesterol to liver and steroidogenic tissues via scavenger receptor (SR-B1) Shuttles apo C-II and apo E in blood

Function of important apoproteins:

Apoproteins	Functions
apo B-48 apo C-II apo E	Secreted by intestine Activates lipoprotein lipase Uptake of remnants by the liver
apo B-100 apo C-II apo E	Secreted by liver Activate lipoprotein lipase Uptake of remnants (IDL) by liver
apo E apo B-100	Uptake by liver
apoB-100	Uptake by liver and other tissues via LDL receptor (apoB-100 receptor)
apo A-1	Activates lectition cholesterol acyltransferase (LCAT) to produce cholesterol esters

Overview of lipoprotein metabolism

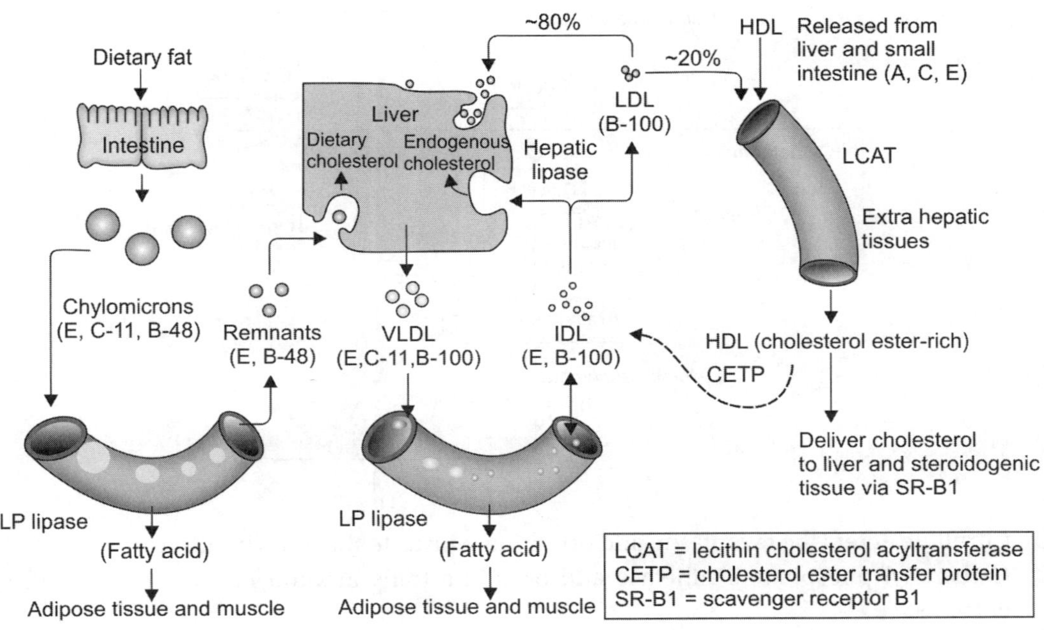

3. Urea cycle enzyme present in cytosol:

a. CPS I
b. CPS II
c. Arginase
d. Arginosuccinase
e. Ornithine transcarbomylase

Ans. c,d *Ref: Harper 30th/ed p293-294 & 29th/ed p276-278; Li pincotts 5th/ed p253*

Option a	False	No, CPS I is present in mitochondria
Option b	False	No, CPS II is cytosolic but not involved in urea cycle. It is involved in pyrimidine synthesis
Option c	True	Yes correct
Option d	True	Yes correct
Option e	False	No, it is in mitochondrial matrix

Salient points to remember in urea cycle:

- Overall summary:

$$\text{Aspartate} + NH_3 + CO_2 + 3\,ATP + H_2O \rightarrow$$
$$\text{urea} + \text{fumarate} + 2\,ADP + AMP + 2\,P_i + PP_i$$

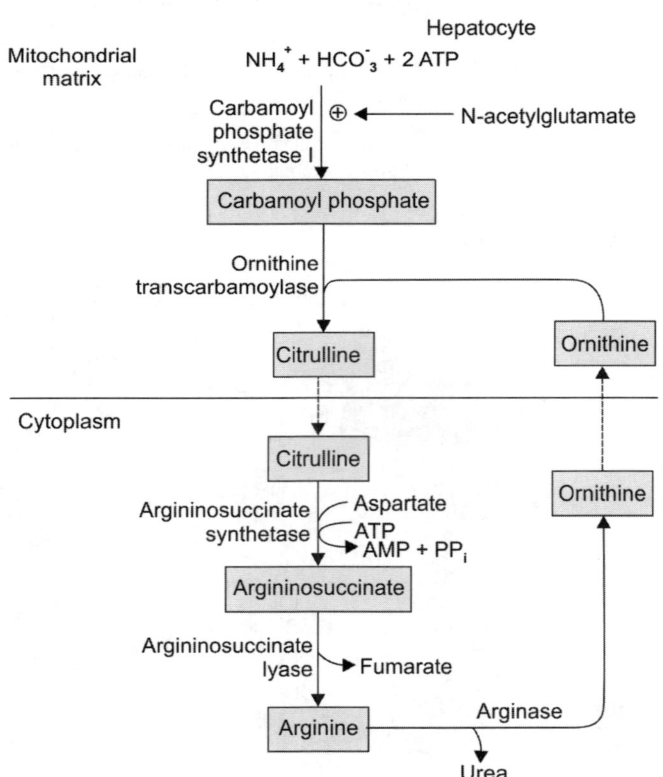

- Citrulline enters the cytoplasm, and ornithine returns to the mitochondria.
- Carbamoyl phosphate synthetase and ornithine transcarbamoylase are mitochondrial enzymes.

- Aspartate enters the cycle in the cytoplasm and leaves the cycle (minus its amino group) as fumarate. If gluconeogenesis is active, fumarate can be converted to glucose.
- The product urea is formed in the cytoplasm and enters the blood for delivery to the kidney.
- One nitrogen of the urea molecule is supplied by free ammonia, and the other nitrogen by aspartate. [Note: Glutamate is the immediate precursor of both ammonia (through oxidative deamination by glutamate dehydrogenase) and aspartate nitrogen (through transamination of oxaloacetate by AST)]. The carbon and oxygen of urea are derived from CO_2. Urea is produced by the liver, and then is transported in the blood to the kidneys for excretion in the urine.
- The urea diffuses from the liver, and is transported in the blood to the kidneys, where it is filtered and excreted in the urine. A portion of the urea diffuses from the blood into the intestine, and is cleaved to CO_2 and NH_3 by bacterial urease. This ammonia is partly lost in the feces, and is partly reabsorbed into the blood.

Good to Remember:

Genetic deficiency in urea synthesis:

Carbamoyl Phosphate Synthetase	Ornithine Transcarbamoylase
↑ $[NH_4^+]$; hyperammonemia	↑ $[NH_4^+]$; hyperammonemia
Blood glutamine is increased	Blood glutamine is icnreased
BUN is decreased	BUN is decreased
No orotic aciduria Autosomal recessive	Orotic aciduria X-linked recessive
Cerebral edema	Cerebral edema
Lethargy, convulsions, coma, death	Lethargy, convuilsions, coma, death

4. Vit B12 deficiency results in:

a. Peripheral neuropathy
b. Microcytic hypochromic anemia
c. Demyelination
d. Decreased Methylmalonyl CoA
e. Isolated paresthesia

Ans. a,c,e *Ref: Harper 30th/ed p559 & 29th/ed p537; Michael Jeffrey aminoff, Neurology and General Medicine, Elsevier Health Sciences, 2008; 228 g; Sid Gilman, Neurobiology of Disease, Elsevier, 2011, p650*

Option a	True	Yes, correct
Option b	False	No, it leads to megaloblastic anemia
Option c	True	Yes, correct
Option d	False	No, Methylmalonyl CoA is increased in vitamin B12 deficiency
Option e	True	Yes, correct

- Vitamin B 12 deficiency causes peripheral neuropathy, demyelination of nerve fibres, subacute combined degeneration, megaloblastic anemia.
- Methylmalonyl CoA is increased in vitamin B12 deficiency.

$$\underset{\text{(R)-Methylmalonyl-CoA}}{{}^{-}OOC-\overset{H}{\underset{\underset{O}{\overset{|}{CoAS-\overset{\|}{C}}}}{C}}-\overset{H}{\underset{H}{C}}-H} \xrightleftharpoons[\text{(5'-deoxyadenosylcobalamin as cofactor\_}]{\text{methylmalonyl-CoA mutase}} \underset{\text{Succinyl-CoA}}{{}^{-}OOC-\overset{H}{\underset{H}{C}}-\overset{H}{\underset{\underset{O}{\overset{\|}{C}}-SAoC}{C}}-H}$$

Note: *As significant amount of vitamin B12 is stored in the body hence the most cause for deficiency of this vitamin is not insufficient dietary intake, but failure of the body to absorb vitamin B12 from the intestine.*

Vitamin B_{12} deficiency: Pernicious anemia

- Most commonly due to autoimmune destruction of gastric parietal cells, which secrete intrinsic factor.
- Patients with cobalamin deficiency are usually anaemic, but later in the development of the disease they show neuropsychiatric symptoms. However, central nervous system (CNS) symptoms may occur in the absence of Anemia.

Neurologic manifestations in vitamin B12 deficiency:

- Paresthesias (most common) - due to demy lination of nerve fibers,
- Gait abnormalities
- Psychiatric or cognitive symptoms, subacute combined degeneration
- Symptoms include subacute progressive decrease in visual acuity, usually caused by bilateral optic neuropathy and rarely pseudotumor cerebri or optic neuritis.
- Autonomic features include orthostasis, sexual dysfunction, and bowel and bladder incontinence (rare)
- Other symptoms include light headedness and impaired taste and smell.
- Non-neurologic symptoms, some of which may also reflect autonomic nervous system involvement: (common presentations)
  - Constitutional symptoms — anorexia and weight loss
  - Cardiovascular symptoms include syncope, dyspnea, orthopnea, palpitations, and angina.
  - Gastrointestinal symptoms include heartburn, flatulence, constipation, diarrhea, sore tongue, and early satiety.

Vitamin	Other Names	Active Form	Function
Folic acid	–	Tetrahydrofolic acid	Transfer one-carbon units: Synthesis of methlionine, purines, and thymidine monophosphate
Vitamin B_{12}	Cobalamin	Methylcobalamin Deoxyadenosyl cobal main	Coenzyme for reactions: Homocysteine → methionine Methylmalonyl CoA → succinyl CoA
Vitamin C	Ascorbic acid	Ascorbic acid	Antioxidant Coenzyme for hydroxylation reactions, for example; in procollagen; Proline → hydroxyproline Lysine → Hydroxylysine
Vitamin B6	Pyridoxine Pyridoxamine Pyridoxal	Pytridoxal phosphate	Coenzyme for enzymes, particularly in amino acid metabolism

Contd...

Contd...

Vitamin	Other Names	Active Form	Function
Vitamin B1	Thiamine	Thiamine Pyrophosphate	Coenzyme of enzymes catalyzing: Pyruvate → acetyl CoA α–Ketoglutarate → Succinyl CoA Ribose 5–P + xylulose 5–P → Sedoheptulose 7–P + Glyceraldehyde
Niacin	Nicotinic acid Nicotinamide	NAD+, NADP⁺,	Electron transfer
Vitamin B2	Riboflavin	FMN, FAD	Electron transfer
Biotin	–	Enzyme-Bound biotin	Carboxylation reactions
Pantothenic acid	–	Coenzyme A	Acyl Carrier Water-Soluble
Vitamin A	Retinol Retinal Retinoic acid β-Carotene	Retinol Retinal Retinoic acid	Maintenance of reproduction Vision Promotion of growth Differentiation and maintenance of epithelial tissue Gene expression
Vitamin D	Cholecalciferol Ergocalciferol	1, 25-Dihydroxycholecalciferol	Calcium uptake
Vitamin K	Menadione Menaquinosne Phylioquinone	Menadione Manaquinosne Phylioquinon	γ-Carboxylation of glutamate residue in clotting and other proteins
Vitamin E	α-Tocopherol	Any of several tocopherol derivatives	Antioxidant

Deficiency	Signs and Symptoms	Toxicity	Notes
Megaloblastic anemia Nueral tube defects	Anemia Birth defects	None	Administration of high leveles of folate can mask vitamin B12, deficiency
Pernicious anemia Dementia Spinal degeneration	Megaloblastic anemia Neuropsychilatric symptoms	None	Pernicious anemia is treated with IM or high-dose oral vitamin B12
Scurvy	Sore, spongy gums Loose teeth Poor wound healing	None	Benefits of supplementation not established in controlled trials
Rare	Glossitis Neuropathy	Yes	Deficiency can be induced by isoniazid Sensory neuropathy occurs at high doses
Beriberi	Tachycardia, vomiting, convulsions Apathy, loss of memory, eye movements	None	–
Pellagra	Dermatitis Diarrhea Dementia	None	High doses of niacin used to treat hyperlipidemia
Rare	Dermatitis Angular stomatitis	None	–
Rare	–	None	Consumption of large amounts of raw egg whites (which contains a protein, avidin, that binds biotin) can induce a biotin deficiency

Contd...

Contd...

Deficiency	Signs and Symptoms	Toxicity	Notes
Rare	–	None	– Water-soluble`
Infertility Night blindness Retardation of growth Xerophthalmia	Increased visual threshold Dryness of cornea	Yes	β-Carotene not acutely toxic, but supplementation is not recommended Excess vitamin A can increase incidence of fractures
Rickets (in children) Osteomalacia (in adults)	Soft, pliable bones	Yes	Vitamin D is not a true vitamin because it can be synthesized in skin. Application of sunscreen locations or presence of dark skin color decrease this synthesis,
Newborn Rare in adults	Bleeding	Rare	Vitamin K produced by intestinal bacteria, Virtamin K deficiency common in newborn intramuscular treatment with vitamin K is recommended at birth
Rare	Red blood cell fragility leads to hemolytic anemia	None	Benefits of supplementation not established in controlled trials

5. Vitamin K dependent coagulation factor include:

a. VII
b. IX
c. X
d. XI
e. XIII

Ans. a,b,c *Ref: Harper 30th/ed p554 & 29th/ed p533*

Option a	True	Yes, correct
Option b	True	Yes, correct
Option c	True	Yes, correct
Option d	False	No, not correct
Option e	False	No, not correct

Important Vitamin K dependent proteins are:

- **Coagulation proteins:** Factor II (prothrombin), factor VII (proconvertin), factor IX (Christmas factor), and factor X (Stuart- Rower factor)
- **Anticoagulation proteins:** Protein C, S and Z
- Gas 6

Formation of gamma-carboxyglutamate (Gla): Vitamin K is required in the hepatic synthesis of prothrombin and blood clotting factors II, VII, IX, and X.

These proteins need to be post translationally modified by carboxylation of glutamic acid residues forming gamma-carboxyglutamic acid in order to become biologically active. The so formed gama carboxyglutamate acts as binding site for calcium ions. After binding to Gla residues on activated clotting factors, calcium binds with negatively charged phospholipids present on platelet cell membrane. In this way these occurs a bridging of the phospholipids with the Gla residues of prothrombin via calcium ion.

Gas6 is a gamma-carboxyglutamic acid (Gla) domain—containing protein which is actively involved in cell survival, chemotaxis, mitogenesis, and cell growth of neurons and glial cells.

The presence of Gla needs a vitamin K-dependent enzymatic reaction that carboxylates the gamma carbon of certain glutamic residues of the protein during its production in the endoplasmic reticulum.

- The main role of vitamin K is post translational modification of various blood clotting factors, where it functions in carboxylation of certain glutamic acid residues present in these proteins
- **Interaction of prothrombin with platelets:** The Gla residues of prothrombin are good chelators of positively charged calcium ions, because of the two adjacent, negatively charged carboxylate groups. The prothrombin–calcium complex is then able to bind to phospholipids essential for blood clotting on the surface of platelets.

Source: cabbage, kale, spinach, egg yolk, and liver

Requirement – 120 and 90 mcg/day for males and females respectively

Deficiency of Vit K results in bleeding tendency. Newborns with Vit K deficiency may suffer from hemorrhagic disease of newborn. (HDN).

6. Which of the following is/are reglatory enzymes in glycolysis:

A. PFK-1
b. Pyruvate kinase
c. PDH
d. Hexokinase
e. Glucose1,6-bisphosphatase

Ans. a,b,d *Ref: Lippincots 5th/ed p97*

Option a	True	Yes, it is Glycolysis controlling enzyme
Option b	True	Yes, it is Glycolysis controlling enzyme
Option c	False	No, pyruvate dehydrogenase contributes to linking the glycolysis metabolic pathway to the citric acid cycle and releasing energy via NADH.
Option d	True	Yes, it is Glycolysis controlling enzyme
Option e	False	No, it is not regulatory enzyme

Hexokinase/Glucokinase:

- Glucose entering the cell is trapped by phosphorylation using ATP.
- Hexokinase is widely distributed in many tissues, whereas glucokinase is found only in hepatocytes and pancreatic β-islet cells

Hexokinase	Glucokinase
Most tissues	Hepatocytes and pancreatic β-islet cells (along with GLUT-2, acts as the glucose sensor)
Low K_m (0.05 mM in erythrocytes)	High K_m (10 mM)
Inhibited by glucose 6-Phosphate	Induced by insulin in hepatocytes

Phosphofructokinases (PFK-1 and PFK-2): PFK-1 is

- It is the main rate-limiting enzyme
- It is the main control point in glycolysis.
- **Action:** fructose 6-phosphate is phosphorylated to fructose 1,6-bisphosphate using ATP.
  - PFK-1 is inhibited by ATP and citrate, and activated by AMP.
  - Insulin stimulates and glucagon inhibits PFK-1 in hepatocytes by an indirect mechanism involving PFK-2 and fructose 2,6-bisphosphate

Glyceraldehyde 3-phosphate dehydrogenase:

- Catalyzes an oxidation and addition of inorganic phosphate (P_i) to its substrate.
- **Action:** Production of a high-energy intermediate 1,3-bisphosphoglycerate and the reduction of NAD to NADH

3-Phosphoglycerate kinase:

- Transfers the high-energy phosphate from 1,3-bisphosphoglycerate to ADP, forming ATP and 3-phosphoglycerate.

Pyruvate kinase:

- Last enzyme in aerobic glycolysis,
- **Action:** Catalyzes a substrate-level phosphorylation of ADP using the high-energy substrate phosphoenolpyruvate (PEP)

Lactate dehydrogenase:

- Used only in anaerobic glycolysis.
- **Action:** Reoxidizes NADH to NAD, replenishing the oxidized coenzyme for glyceraldehyde 3-phosphate dehydrogenase

Glycolysis is Irreversible

Three enzymes in the pathway catalyze reactions that are irreversible. When the liver produces glucose, different reactions and therefore different enzymes must be used at these three points:

- Glucokinase/hexokinase
- PFK-1
- Pyruvate kinase

7. UDP glucose is used for:

A. Glycogen synthesis
b. Galactose metabolism
c. HMP pathway
d. Bilirubin metabolism
e. Gangliosides synthesis

Ans. a,b,d,e

Option a	True	Yes, correct
Option b	True	Yes, correct
Option c	False	No, not correct
Option d	True	Yes, correct
Option e	True	Yes, correct

Role of UDP galactose in biosynthetic reactions:

UDP-galactose can serve as the donor of galactose units in a number of synthetic pathways, including synthesis of lactose, glycoproteins, glycolipids and glycosaminoglycans.

1. Role of UDP-glucose in galactose metabolism

Epimerization of galactose-1-phosphate to glucose-1-phosphate (G1P) requires the transfer of UDP from UDP-glucose catalyzed by galactose-1-phosphate uridylyl transferase (GALT) (gene locate on 9p13.3)

Galactosemia:

- Galactosemia type 1: Classical galactosemia - deficiency of the enzyme galactose-1-phosphate uridyltransferase (GALT)

- ❑ Galactosemia type 2: Deficiency of galactokinase (GALK1)
- ❑ Galactosemia type 3: Deficiency of UDP-galactose-4-epimerase (GALE)

2. Role of UDP-glucose in Glycogenesis:

Glycogenin serves as acceptor of glucose residues from UDP glucose

α-D-Glucose attached to uridine diphosphate (UDP) is the source of all the glucosyl residues that are added to the growing glycogen molecule.

3. Role of UDP-glucose in bilirubin metabolism:

Unconjugated bilirubinin is lipophilic. Its conjugation with glucuronic acid renders it hydrophilic, thus, it can be eliminated in the bile. Many other agents are eliminated by conjugation with glucuronic acid: steroids, thyroid hormone, catecholamines, estradiol, testosterone, bile acids, phenols, morphine, which can be conjugated by other cells besides hepatocytes.

GLUCOSE + UDP-Glucose-dehydrogenase = UDP-GLUCURONIC ACID (UDPGA)

UDPGA + BILIRUBIN + Glucuronyl transferase = BILIRUBIN MONO & DI- GLUCURONIDES.

4. Role of UDP-glucose in ganglioside metabolism:

The first step in the biosynthesis of most gangliosides is the transfer of a glucose residue from UDP glucose to ceramide catalysed by UDP-glucose:ceramide glucosyltransferase

8. In PCR, proof reading is done by:

a. Pfu Polymerase
b. Taq Polymerase
c. Telomerase
d. DNA topoisomerase
e. Polymerases γ and θ (gamma and theta)

Ans. a,b *Ref: Lippincots 5th/ed p479-483; Michael A Innis. PCR Applications: Protocols for Functional Genomics. Academic Press, 1999, p13; Joe O'Connell. RT-PCR Protocols. Springer Science & Business Media, 2002, p176*

Option a	True	Yes, correct (however, it is better than Taq polymerase)
Option b	True	Yes, correct
Option c	False	No, Telomerase is an RNA-dependent DNA polymerase that synthesizes telomeric DNA sequences (for replication and not for proof reading)
Option d	False	No, Topoisomerases are enzymes that participate in the overwinding or underwinding of DNA and not for error repair
Option e	False	No, it is a proof reading enzyme for many bacteria and/or viruses but not used in PCR

Pfu DNA polymerase has superior thermostability and proofreading properties compared to *Taq* DNA polymerase. Unlike *Taq* DNA polymerase, *Pfu* DNA polymerase possesses 3' to 5' exonuclease proofreading activity, meaning that as the DNA is assembled from the 5' end to 3' end, the exonuclease activity immediately removes nucleotides misincorporated at the 3' end of the growing DNA strand. Consequently, *Pfu* DNA polymerase-generated PCR fragments will have fewer errors than *Taq*-generated PCR inserts.

***Thermus thermophiles*: rTth DNA polymerase** is a recombinant thermostable DNA polymerase derived from *Thermus thermophilus*, with optimal activity at 70–80 °C, used in some PCR applications. The enzyme possesses efficient reverse transcriptase activity in the presence of manganese. It is not known to have proof reading capacities.

Types of DNA polymerase

Polymerases β, λ, σ and μ (beta, lambda, sigma, and mu): Used for a DNA repair pathway that is essential for repairing alkylated or oxidized bases as well as a basic sites.

1. Polymerases α, δ and ε (alpha, delta, and epsilon): main polymerases involved with nuclear DNA replication
2. Polymerases η, ι and κ (eta, iota, and kappa): involved in the DNA repair by translesion synthesis. Associated with xeroderma pigmentosum
3. Polymerases Rev1 and ζ (zeta): increases the catalytic function of the polymerase
4. Telomerase: replicate ends of linear chromosomes for elongation and proliferation
5. Polymerases γ and θ (gamma and theta): DNA polymerase III holoenzyme is the primary enzyme involved in DNA replication in *E. coli* and belongs to family C polymerases. The core consists of three subunits: α, the polymerase activity hub, ε, exonucleolytic proofreader, and θ, which may act as a stabilizer for.

9. Components/genes involved in RISC complex:

a. miRNA
b. rRNA
c. RNase Dicer
d. Drosha
e. Pasha

Ans. a,c,d,e *Ref: Lippincotts 5th/ed p459; Stanley T Crooke. Antisense Drug Technology 2nd/ ed, p78; John J RossiMicroRNA Methods. Academic Press, 2007 p92-96*

Option a	True	Yes correct
Option b	False	No, it is not part of RNA silencing complex
Option c	True	Yes correct
Option d	True	Yes correct
Option e	True	Yes correct

RNA interference—slicing of genes

RNA interference (RNAi) is a genetic regulatory system that functions to silence the activity of specific genes.

RNAi occurs naturally, through the production of nuclear-encoded pre-microRNA (pre-miRNA), and can be induced experimentally, using short segments of synthetic double-stranded RNA (dsRNA).

In both the natural and the experimental pathways, an enzyme known as DICER is necessary for the formation of miRNA from pre-miRNA or of siRNA from shRNA. The miRNA or siRNA then binds to an enzyme-containing molecule known as RNA-induced silencing complex (RISC). The miRNA-RISC or siRNA-RISC complex binds to target, or complementary, messengerRNA (mRNA) sequences, resulting in the enzymatic cleavage of the target mRNA. The cleaved mRNA is rendered nonfunctional and hence is "silenced."

The RNA-induced silencing complex, or RISC, is a multiprotein (ribonucleoprotein) complex. It incorporates one strand of:

- Single-stranded RNA (ssRNA) fragment, such as microRNA (miRNA) or
- Double-stranded small interfering RNA (siRNA)

Good to remember:

1. RNA Inference (RNAi): is cleaving the mRNA by a protein called as "Argonauate", a component of RISC
2. RNAse III dicer (protein of RISC) – helps in cleaving the dsRNA as an important function of RNAi.
3. mRNA degradation: is localised in cytoplasmic bodies called *P-bodies*

4. Translational repression: RISC can modulate the loading of ribosome and accessory factors in translation to repress expression of the bound mRNA transcript.
5. Heterochromatin formation
6. Both Drosha and Dicer can function as master regulators of miRNA processing and have been observed to be down-regulated in some types of breast cancer.
7. Drosha is a type III RNase, which plays a critical role in miRNA biogenesis.
8. Drosha and its double-stranded RNA-binding partner protein Pasha/DGCR8 likely recognize and cleave miRNA precursor RNAs or pri-miRNA hairpins cotranscriptionally.

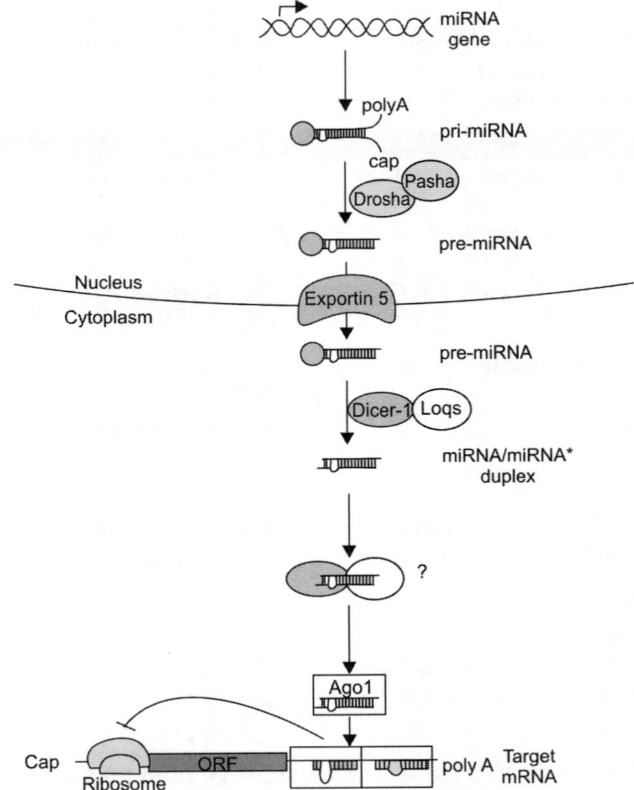

10. Which of the following are non-reducing sugar ?

A. Glucose
b. Maltose
c. Isomaltose
d. Sucrose
e. Trehalose

Ans. d,e

Option a	False	No, it is reducing sugar
Option b	False	No, it is reducing sugar
Option c	False	No, it is reducing sugar
Option d	True	Yes, It is non-reducing sugar
Option e	True	Yes, It is non-reducing sugar

Any carbohydrate which is capable of being oxidized and causes the reduction of other substances without having to be hydrolysed first is known as reducing sugar, but those which are unable to be oxidised and do not reduce other substances are known as non-reducing sugars. Generally, all the free monosaccharides having free aldehyde or hydroxyl ketonic group are capable of being oxidised. After being oxidised they cause the reduction of the other substances and so known as reducing sugars.

- Hence, A reducing sugar is any sugar that is capable of acting as a reducing agent because it has a free aldehyde group or a free ketone group.
- This includes common monosaccharides like galactose, glucose, glyceraldehyde, fructose, ribose, and xylose.
- Nonreducing disaccharides like sucrose and trehalose have glycosidic bonds between their anomeric carbons and thus cannot convert to an open-chain form with an aldehyde group; they are stuck in the cyclic form

No	Reducing Sugars	Non-reducing Sugars
1.	Such sugar bear a free aldehyde (–CHO) or ketonic (–CO) group.	These sugars do not have such groups
2.	Reducing sugars have the capacity to reduce cupric ions of Benedict's or Fehling solution to cuprous ions	Non reducing sugar fail to reduce the cupric ions of Benedict's solution to cuprous ions
3.	Examples: Maltose, Lactose, Melibiose, Cellobiose, Gentiobiose	Examples: Sucrose, Trehalose

11. 30S pre-initiation complex used:

a. GTP
b. ATP
c. Elongation factor
d. Initiation factor
e. mRNA

Ans. a, d and e

Ref: George M Malacinski. Essentials of Molecular Biology, Jones & Bartlett Learning, 2005, p182; Hans Trachsel. Translation in eukaryotes, CRC press 1991, p358

Option a	True	Yes, correct
Option b	False	No, not correct
Option c	False	No, not correct
Option d	True	Yes, correct
Option e	True	Yes, correct

Translation of prokaryotes involve - getting together of components of translation system:

1. Two ribosomal subunits (50S and 30S)
2. Mature mRNA to be translated
3. tRNA charged with N-formylmethionine
4. GTP as source of energy
5. Prokaryotic initiation factors (IF1,2,3)

The ribosome has three active sites:

A site - point of entry of amino acyl tRNA
P site - formation of peptidyl tRNA in the ribosome
E site - exit of the tRNA and formation of the peptide chain

Elongation of the polypeptide chain involves addition of amino acids to the carboxyl end of the growing chain. The growing protein exits the ribosome through the polypeptide exit tunnel in the large subunit.

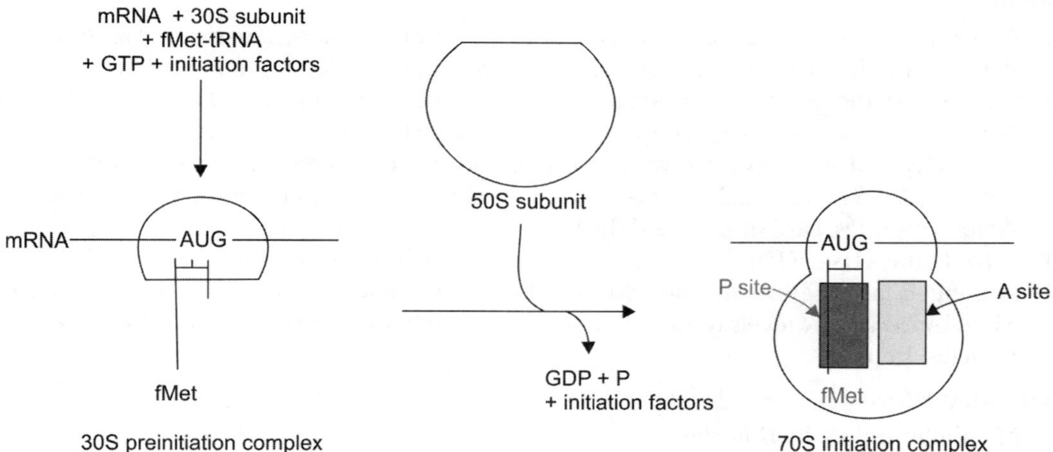

12. Starvation leads to

a. Low hepatic glucose and oxidation in 24 hrs
b. Ketogenesis max at 7 days
c. Death occurs when 50-60% skeletal muscle is lost
d. Protein is the major contributor of energy during starvation
e. 30 gms of protein breaks down to yield approx. 10 gms of glucose

Ans. a, b, c and e

Option a	True	Yes, correct
Option b	True	Yes, correct
Option c	True	Yes, correct
Option d	False	No, glycogen reserve, fatty acids, ketone bodies, and then protein is used in prolonged starvation
Option e	True	Yes, correct

Changes during prolonged fasting

1. Levels of glucagon and epinephrine are markedly elevated during starvation.
2. Lipolysis is rapid, resulting in excess acetyl-CoA that is used for ketone synthesis. Levels of both lipids and ketones are therefore increased in the blood.
3. Muscle uses fatty acids as the major fuel, and the brain adapts to using ketones for some of its energy.
4. After several weeks of fasting, the brain derives approximately two thirds of its energy from ketones and one third from glucose.
5. The shift from glucose to ketones as the major fuel diminishes the amount of protein that must be degraded to support gluconeogenesis. There is no "energy-storage form" for protein because each protein has a specific function in the cell. Therefore, the shift from using glucose to ketones during starvation spares protein, which is essential for these other functions.
6. Red blood cells (and renal medullary cells) that have few, if any, mitochondria continue to be dependent on glucose for their energy.

Features:

- As the human brain can use ketone, the body does not force down to use glucose from the skeletal muscles at a very high rate, at least in the initial part of starvation phase.
- **0-2/3 days:** The normal body glycogen stores are however consumed within the first 24 hours. In normal body the glycogen stores from muscles is the next to be utilized.
- **> 2/3 days till 6/7 days:** However the main source of energy during starvation is the triglycerides. The fatty acids undergo beta oxidation in the mitochondria mostly of the skeletal muscles, cardiac cells and the liver cells.
- **7-10/12 days** Use of fats, ketone and starting of use of protein muscles
- Prolonged fasting leads to more degradation of the skeletal muscles. Late in starvation, when blood ketone levels reach 5-7 mM, ketone use in the brain rises, while ketone use in muscles drops.

Starvation effects:

1. Metabolic and endocrine effects
   - Slow growth rate
   - Delayed puberty
2. Hypotension
3. Low GFR
4. Immune suppression
5. Hypothermia
6. Amenorrhoea

Good to Remember:

Organ	Well-Fed	Fasting
Liver	Glucose and amino acids	Fatty acids
Resting skeletal muscle	Glucose	Fatty acids, ketones
Cardiac muscle	Fatty acids	Fatty acids, ketones
Adipose tissue	Glucose	Fatty acids
Brain	Glucose	Glucose (ketones in prolonged fast)
Red blood cells	Glucose	Glucose

13. Which of the following helps in maintaining the tertiary structure of proteins?

a. Disulphide bonds
b. Hydrogen bonds
c. Organic solvents
d. SSB Proteins
e. Chaperons

Ref: Lippincotts, 5th/ed p16

Ans. a, b and e

Option a	True	Yes, correct
Option b	True	Yes, correct
Option c	False	No, it causes denaturation of proteins
Option d	False	No, Binds to single-stranded DNA and prevents annealing of single-stranded DNA into double-stranded DNA
Option e	True	Yes, correct

Protein stability

Various forces and bonds helps stabilise a protein molecule.

Various forces could be:

1. A **disulphide bond** contributes to the stability of the three-dimensional shape of the protein molecule, and prevents it from becoming denatured in the extracellular environment
2. **Hydrophobic interactions** helps to stabilise the protein structure
3. Formation of **hydrogen bonds** between polar groups on the surface of proteins and the aqueous solvent enhances the solubility of the protein
4. Electrostatic interactions
5. **Chaperons:** Special group of proteins required for the proper folding of protein molecule

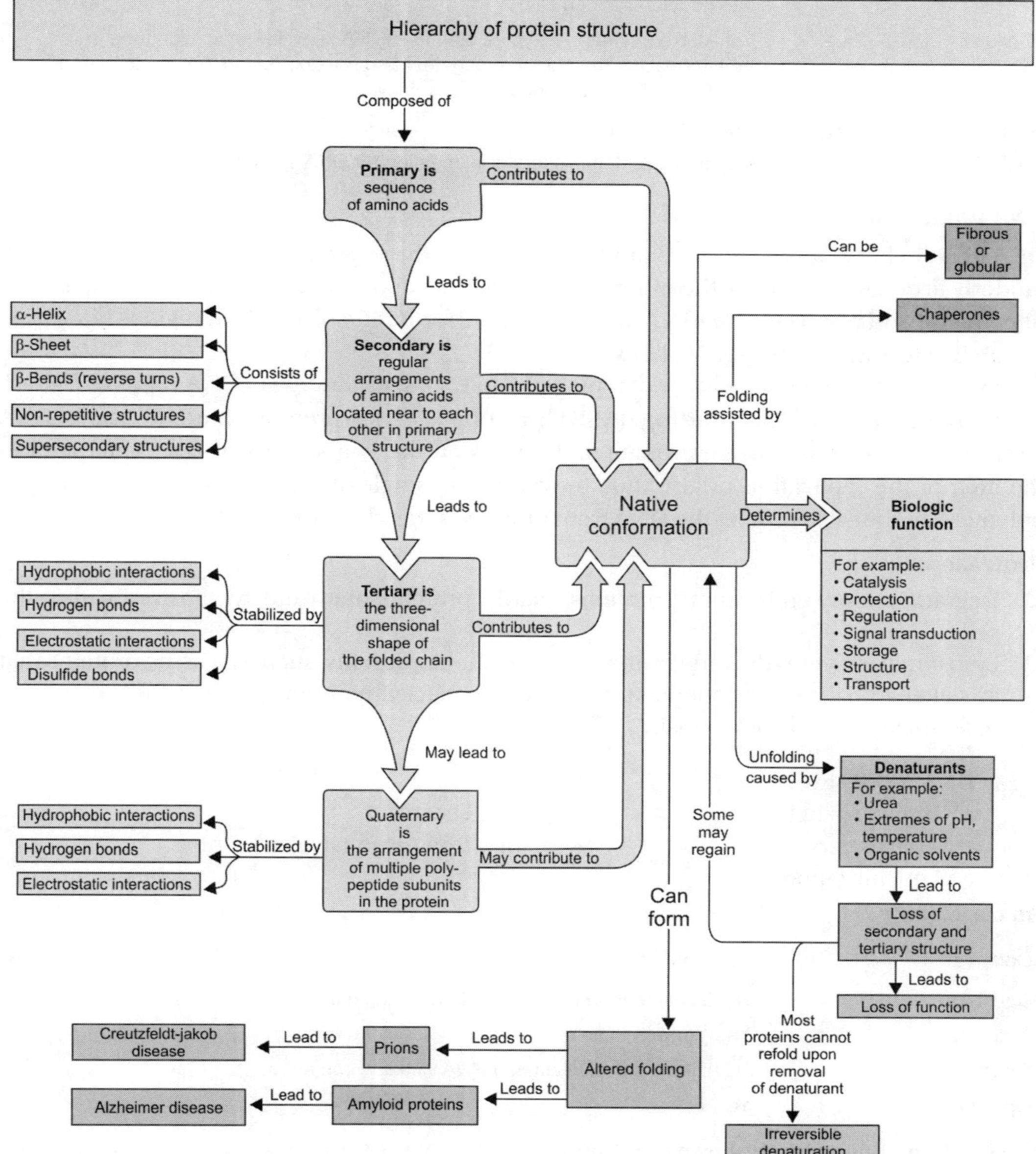

Fig: Hierarchy of protein structure

14. Unwinding of double helix of DNA is by:

a. DNA protein
b. ssB protein
c. Helicase
d. Proteasomes
e. Primase

Ans. a, b and c

Option a	True	Yes, correct
Option b	True	Binds to single-stranded DNA and prevents annealing of single-stranded DNA into double-stranded DNA
Option c	True	Yes, correct. These enzymes bind to ssDNA near the replication fork, and then move into the neighbouring double- stranded region, forcing the strands apart—in effect, unwinding the double helix
Option d	False	No, these are used for protein degradation
Option e	False	No, not correct. It is used for elongation for DNA synthesis

DNA separation:

DNA protein binds to specific nucleotide sequences at the origin of replication, causing short, tanderly arranged (one after the other) AT-rich regions in the origin to melt. Melting is ATP-dependent, and results in strand separation with the formation of localized regions of ssDNA

Helicase: unwind the double helix.

- DNA B is the principal helicase of replication in E. coli. Its binding to DNA requires DNA C.

Single-stranded DNA-binding (SSB) proteins: These proteins bind to the ssDNA generated by helicases. These proteins not only keep the two strands of DNA separated in the area of the replication origin, thus providing the single-stranded template required by polymerases, but also protect the DNA from nucleases that degrade ssDNA.

Proteasomes

- Degrade mainly endogenous proteins, that is, proteins that were synthesized within the cell.
- Lysosomal enzymes degrade primarily extracellular proteins, such as plasma proteins that are taken into the cell by endocytosis, and cell-surface membrane proteins that are used in receptor-mediated endocytosis.

15. DNA motifs are:

a. Helix turn helix
b. Dicers
c. Zinc finger
d. Iron responsive element
e. Leucine zippers

Ans. a, c and e

Option a		Yes, correct
Option b		No, it is an endonuclease for cleaving the miRNA
Option c		Yes, correct
Option d		No, it is for stabilization of mRNA with low iron stores
Option e		Yes, correct

The binding of proteins and transcription factors to DNA is through structural motifs such as the zinc finger leucine zipper, or helix-turn-helix in the protein.

16. Seen in prophase of meiosis II:

a. Sister chromatids separate
b. Number is reduced to half
c. Chromosome duplicate
d. Centriole duplicate
e. Centromere separate

Ans. d

Option a	False	No, this is in anaphase
Option b	False	No, not correct. The chromosome become half in no in m1
Option c	False	No, no new chromosome duplication occurs in meiosis II. It takes place in meiosis I
Option d	True	Yes, correct
Option e	False	No, this is in anaphase

Meiosis:

1. Meiosis I segregates homologous chromosomes, which are joined as tetrads (2n, 4c), producing two haploid cells (n chromosomes, 23 in humans) which each contain chromatid pairs (1n, 2c). Because the ploidy is reduced from diploid to haploid, meiosis I is referred to as a *reductional division.*
2. Meiosis II is the second meiotic division, and usually involves equational segregation, or separation of sister chromatids. Mechanically, the process is similar to mitosis, though its genetic results are fundamentally different. The end result is production of four haploid cells (n chromosomes, 23 in humans) from the two haploid cells (with in chromosomes, each consisting of two sister chromatids) produced in meiosis I.

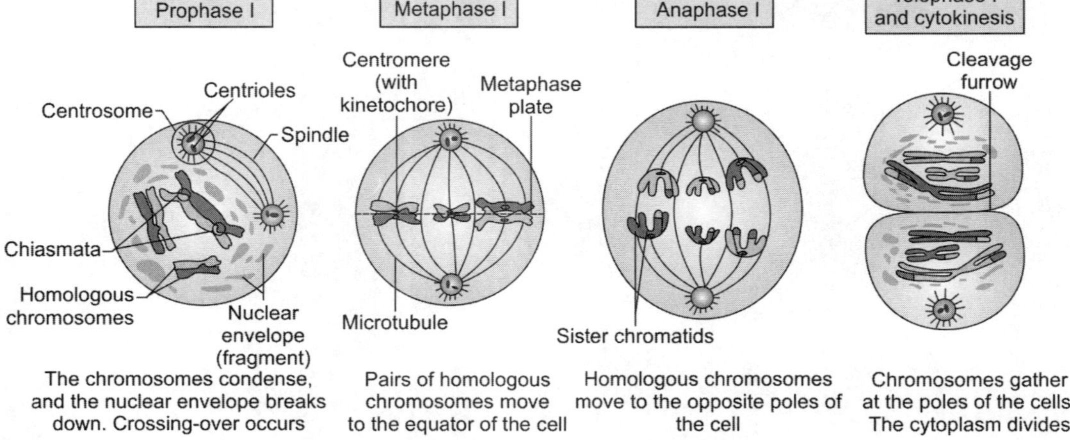

Source: https://en.wikipedia.org/wiki/Meiosis#/media/File:Meiosis_Stages.svg

Meiosis II

Prophase II

While chromosome duplication took place prior to meiosis I, no new chromosome replication occurs before meiosis II.

The centrioles duplicate. This occurs by separation of the two members of the pair, and then the formation of a daughter centriole perpendicular to each original centriole. The two pairs of centrioles separate into two centrosomes.

The nuclear envelope breaks down, and the spindle apparatus forms.

Metaphase II

Each of the daughter cells completes the formation of a spindle apparatus.

Single chromosomes align on the metaphase plate, much as chromosomes do in mitosis. This is in contrast to metaphase I, in which homologous pairs of chromosomes align on the metaphase plate.

For each chromosome, the kinetochores of the sister chromatids face the opposite poles, and each is attached to a kinetochore microtubule coming from that pole.

Anaphase II

The centromeres separate, and the two chromatids of each chromosome move to opposite poles on the spindle. The separated chromatids are now called chromosomes in their own right.

Telophase II

A nuclear envelope forms around each set of chromosomes.

Cytokinesis takes place, producing four daughter cells (gametes, in animals), each with a haploid set of chromosomes.

Because of crossing-over, some chromosomes are seen to have recombined segments of the original parental chromosomes.

Biochemistry

1. Amino acid with hydroxyl group is:

a. Serine
b. Threonine
c. Valine
d. Lysine
e. Tyrosine

Ans. a, b, e *Ref: Lippincott Biochemistry, 6th/ed*

Option a	True	
Option b	True	
Option c	False	Nonpolar alkyl group
Option d	False	Amino group
Option e	True	

Nonpolar alkyl groups—contain alkyl side chains.

1. Glycine (side chain consists of a single hydrogen atom)
2. Alanine (methyl side chain)
3. Valine (isopropyl side chain)
4. Leucine and isoleucine (alkyl side chains).

Hydroxyl groups:

1. Serine
2. Threonine
3. Tyrosine

Sulfur groups:

1. Cysteine, and
2. Methionine

Carboxylic acid groups:

1. Aspartic acid, and
2. Glutamic acid

Amide groups: The amide formed from glutamic acid is called **glutamine** and the amide formed from aspartic acid is called **asparagine**.

Amino groups: Amino acids that contain one or more amino groups in the side chain:

1. Lysine,
2. Arginine, and
3. Histidine

Aromatic groups: Side chains contain aromatic ring structures:

1. Phenylalanine (nonpolar)
2. Tyrosine (polar)
3. Tryptophan (nonpolar)

Looped group: Proline

2. Hyperuricemia is/are associated with:
   a. HGPRT deficiency
   b. Glucose 6-phosphatase deficiency
   c. Glucose phosphate dehydrogenase deficiency
   d. HGPRT over activity
   e. PRPP synthetase deficiency

Ans. a, b *Ref: Lippincott Biochemistry, 6th/ed*

Option a	True	Inborn error of purine metabolism
Option b	True	
Option c	False	Glucose 6-phosphatase deficiency
Option d	False	HGPRT deficiency
Option e	False	Elevated activity of PRPP synthetase

There are at least three different inherited defects that lead to early development of severe hyperuricemia and gout:
1. Glucose-6-phosphatase (G6PT) deficiency
2. Severe and partial HGPRT deficiency
3. Elevated 5'-phosphoribosyl-1'-pyrophosphate synthetase (PRPP synthetase) activity.

- ❑ **Deficiency of hypoxanthine-guanine phosphoribosyltransferase (HGPRT)** activity is an inborn error of purine metabolism associated with uric acid overproduction and a continuum spectrum of neurological manifestations depending on the degree of the enzymatic deficiency.
- ❑ A complete or virtually complete loss of HGPRT activity results in the severe disorder, *Lesch-Nyhan syndrome.*
- ❑ **Deficiencies in glucose-6-phosphatase** result in *type I glycogen storage disease* (von Gierke disease). However, associated with this defect is increased uric acid production and symptoms of gout.
- ❑ **Increased levels of PRPP**, drive enhanced de novo synthesis of purine nucleotides in excess of the needs of the body. Thus, the excess purine nucleotides are catabolized resulting in elevated production of uric acid and consequent hyperuricemia and gout.

3. Hyperphenylalaninemia occurs due to:
   a. Dihydrobiopterin reductase deficiency
   b. Tyrosine hydroxylase deficiency
   c. Phenylalanine hydroxylase deficiency
   d. Phenylalanine hydroxylase overactivity
   e. Defect in dihydrobiopterin biosynthesis

Ans. a, c, e *Ref: Harper's Biochemistry, 30th/ed*

Option a	True	
Option b	False	
Option c	True	
Option d	False	Phenylalanine hydroxylase deficiency
Option e	True	

Hyperphenylalaninemia

- Metabolic disorders associated with impaired ability to convert phenylalanine to tyrosine are classified into three broad groups:
  - Due to defects in Phenylalanine hydroxylase (*Hyperphenylalaninemia* type I or classic phenylketonuria)
  - Defects in Dihydrobiopterin reductase (*Hyperphenylalaninemia type II and III*)
  - Defects in Dihydrobiopterin biosynthesis (*Hyperphenylalaninemia type IV and V*).

Hyperphenylalaninemias[1]

Type	*Condition*	*Defect*	*Treatment*
I	Phenylketonuria	Phe hydroxylase absent	Low Phe diet
II	Persistent hyperphenylalaninemia	Decreased Phe hydroxylase	None, or temporary dietary therapy
III	Transient mild hyperphenylalaninemia	Maturational delay of hydroxylase	Same as type II
IV	Dihydrobiopterin reductase deficiency	Deficient or absent dihydropteridine reductase	Dopa, 5-hydroxytryptophan, carbidopa
V	Abnormal dihydrobiopterin function	Dihydrobiopterin synthesis defect	Dopa, 5-hydroxytryptophan, carbidopa
VI	Persistent hyperphenylalaninemia and tyrosinemia	Catabolism of tyrosine	Reduced Phe intake
VII	Transient neonatal tyrosinemia	*p*-Hydroxyphenylpyruvic oxidase inhibition	Vitamin C
VIII	Hereditary tyrosinemia	Deficiency: 1. *p*-Hydroxyphenylpyruvate oxidase 2. Cytoplasmic tyrosine aminotransferase 3. Fumarylacetoacetate hydrolase	Low Tyr diet plus glutathione injections

[1]Modified and reproduced, with permission, from Tourian A, Sidbury JB: Phenylketonuria and hyperphenylalaninemia. In: Scriver CR et al. (editors): The Metabolic Basis of Inherited Disease, 6/e McGraw-Hill, 1989.

4. Component of 50S ribosomal subunit:

a. 5S RNA
b. 18S RNA
c. 16S RNA
d. 23S RNA
e. 5.8 RNA

Ans. a, d *Ref: Harper's Biochemistry, 30th/ed*

Option a	True	
Option b	False	
Option c	False	
Option d	True	
Option e	False	

- A 70S ribosome can be dissociated into a large subunit (50S) and a small subunit (30S).
- These subunits can be further split into their constituent proteins and RNAs.
- The 30S subunit contains 21 different proteins (referred to as S1 through S21) and a 16S RNA molecule.
- The 50S subunit contains 34 different proteins (L1 through L34) and two RNA molecules, a 23S and a 5S species.

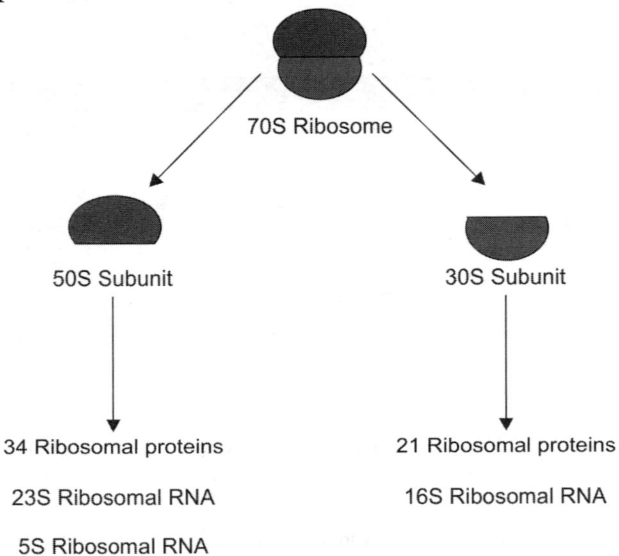

5. DNA-transcription factor interaction can be detected by:

a. Chromatin immunoprecipitation b. Northern blot
c. South-western blot d. Western blot
e. DNA footprinting

Ans. a, c, e *Ref: Harper's Biochemistry, 30th/ed*

Option a	True	Monitor transcriptional regulation
Option b	False	
Option c	True	Detects specific DNA-binding proteins
Option d	False	
Option e	True	Identify the specific site of binding of a protein to DNA

Transcription factors are proteins involved in the process of converting, or transcribing, DNA into RNA. Transcription factors include a wide number of proteins, excluding RNA polymerase, that initiate and regulate the transcription of genes.

The coordinated expression of genes drives a majority of cellular processes. This coordination is in part regulated by interactions between proteins, called transcription factors (TFs) and sequence-specific DNA elements, called TF-binding sites (TFBS).

Methods to detect DNA-transcription factor interactions:

1. **Chromatin immunoprecipitation (ChIP) assays:** used to monitor transcriptional regulation through histone modification or transcription factor-DNA binding interactions.

2. **DNA Electrophoretic mobility shift assay (EMSA):** The EMSA is used to study proteins binding to known DNA oligonucleotide probes and can be used to assess the degree of affinity or specificity of the interaction.
3. **DNA pull-down assay:** Pull-down assays are used to selectively extract a protein-DNA complex from a sample.
4. **DNase footprinting assay:** can be used to identify the specific site of binding of a protein to DNA.
5. **Southwestern blotting:** detects specific DNA-binding proteins by incubating radiolabeled DNA with a gel blot, washing, and visualizing through autoradiography.
6. Structure determination using **X-ray crystallography** has been used to give a highly detailed atomic view of protein–DNA interactions.

6. Inhibitors of oxidative phosphorylation are:

a. 2, 4-dinitrophenol (DNP)
b. Fluoride
c. Ouabain
d. Oligomycin
e. Carboxin

Ans. d, e *Ref: Harper's Biochemistry, 30th/ed*

Option a	False	
Option b	False	
Option c	False	
Option d	True	ATP synthase inhibitor
Option e	True	Block electron transport in Complex II

Oxidative phosphorylation:

- Process by which ADP is phosphorylated to Pi to ATP in respiratory chain.
- The process is limited to mitochondria.
- There are several well-known drugs and toxins that inhibit oxidative phosphorylation.

Inhibitors:

Site specific inhibitors:

Complex I:

Rotenone: Interferes with the electron transport chain in mitochondria. It inhibits the transfer of electrons from iron-sulfur centers in complex I to ubiquinone. This interferes with NADH during the creation of usable cellular energy (ATP).

Amytal: Barbiturate that inhibits the electron transport of complex I.

Demerol: It is painkiller that also inhibits complex I.

Complex II:

2-Thenoyltrifluoroacetone (TTFA) and *carboxin*: Specifically block electron transport in complex II.

Malonate: Competitive inhibitor of complex II.

Complex III:

Antimycin A: Inhibits electron transfer in complex III by blocking the transfer of electrons between Cyt bH and coenzyme Q bound at the QN site.

Complex IV:

Cyanide, Azide, Carbon Monoxide: Inhibit electron transport in Complex IV. They all inhibit electron transfer by binding tightly with the iron coordinated in Cyt a3.

ATP synthase:

Oligomycin: Oligomycin binds directly to ATP synthase F0 subunit and blocks the flow of protons through the channel.

ATP-ADP translocase: Atractyloside (plant glycoside).

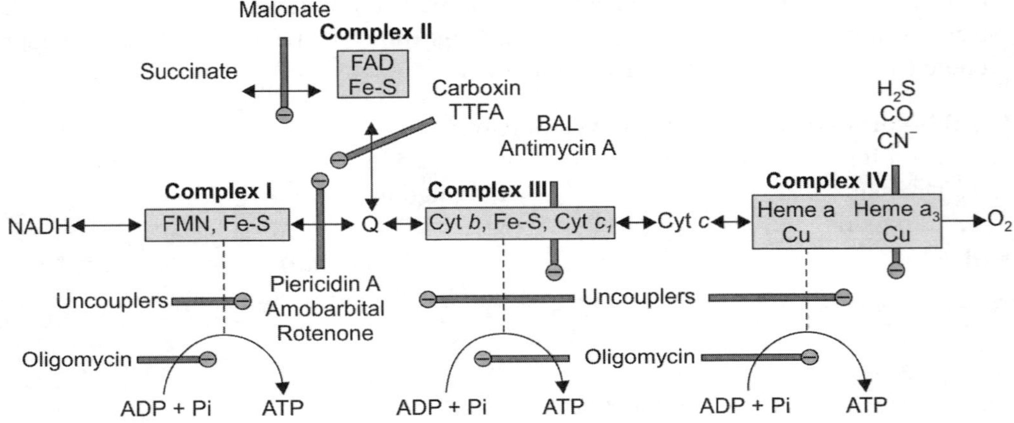

Fig. 1: Site specific inhibition of oxidative phosphorylation.

7. **All of the following are true about Apolipoproteins *except*:**
   a. Apo A-I is the major protein component of HDL
   b. Constitute peripheral region of plasma lipoproteins
   c. Role in enzyme activation
   d. Apo a, b and c are divided further
   e. Divided into a, b, c only

Ans. e *Ref: Harper's Biochemistry, 30th/ed*

Option a	True	True, major protein component of HDL
Option b	True	True, consist of a core of triglyceride and cholesterol esters and a peripheral region of phospholipid, sphingolipid and protein
Option c	True	True, Role in enzyme activation
Option d	True	True, Apo A, B, C are further subdivided
Option e	False	-

- Apolipoproteins are proteins that bind to and help solubilize hydrophobic lipids in the blood.
- Together with phospholipids, apolipoproteins form lipoprotein particles into which different lipids can be packed.
- Lipoprotein—Apolipoproteins have pivotal functions as structural components in lipoprotein particles, as ligands for receptors, and as co-factors for enzymes.

- Lipoprotein particles are necessary for transportation of lipids used for energy and for synthesis of hormones, vitamins, and bile acids.
- The apolipoproteins apoB and apoE are important in the transport of dietary and endogenous lipids to the peripheral tissues where these lipids are used as an energy source, whereas apoA1 is crucial for returning excess cholesterol from peripheral tissues to the liver.
- Apolipoproteins also have an essential role in neurological processes; for example, apoE and apoJ are involved in the transportation of lipids in the brain.
- Apolipoproteins consist of a core of triglyceride and cholesterol esters and a peripheral region of phospholipid, sphingolipid and protein.
- They are designated as:
  - Apo A-I, apo A-II, apo A-IV
  - Apo B-48, apo B-100
  - Apo C-I, apo C-II, apo C-III
  - Apo D
  - Apo E-I, apo E-II, apo E-III, apo E-IV
  - Apo F
  - Apo G, and
  - Apo H.
- **Apo A-I** is the major protein component of *high density lipoprotein (HDL)* and a minor component of chylomicrons and very low density lipoprotein (VLDL).
- **Apo A-II** is the second most abundant protein in HDL, thus, high levels of apo A-I or A-II, or both, are predictive of a decreased risk of coronary artery disease (CAD).
- **Apo A-IV** synthesis and secretion are significantly increased during fat absorption.
- **Apo B** is the largest of the carrier proteins and is a major protein constituent of low density lipoprotein (LDL), VLDL, and chylomicrons.
- **Apo C-II** is the specific activator of lipoprotein lipase which hydrolyzes the triglyceride component of chylomicrons and VLDL.
- Virtually nothing is known of apo D.
- Apo E, or 'arginine-rich apo,' has been found in all major classes of plasma lipoproteins

8. Cytochrome P450 is involved in:

a. Hydroxylation of xenobiotics
b. Methylation of xenobiotics
c. Drug interaction
d. Involved in hydroxylation of steroids
e. Deamination reaction

Ans. a, c, d, e *Ref: Harper's Biochemistry, 30th/ed*

Option a	True	
Option b	False	Involved in hydroxylation of xenobiotics
Option c	True	
Option d	True	
Option e	True	

- Cytochrome P450 enzymes are the most important enzymes in Phase I metabolism in mammals, and are primarily responsible for the metabolism of drugs.

- Six different P450 isozymes—CYP1A2, CYP2C19, CYP2C9, CYP2D6, CYP2E1, and CYP3A4—that play important roles in drug metabolism have been identified.
- **In phase 1 reactions**, xenobiotics are converted to more polar, hydroxylated derivatives. In phase 2 reactions, these derivatives are conjugated with molecules such as glucuronic acid, sulfate or glutathione. They involve either adding or unmasking a hydroxyl group, or some other hydrophilic group such as an amine or sulfhydryl group, and usually involve hydrolysis, oxidation or reduction mechanisms. This renders them even more water soluble and they are ultimately excreted in urine or bile.
- Cytochrome P450 enzymes are responsible for most phase I reactions.

Some properties of Cytochrome P450s

- Involved in the metabolism of many xenobiotics and also endogenous compounds such as steroids.
- All are hemoproteins.
- Often exhibit broad substrate specificity.
- Catalyze reactions involving introduction of one atom of oxygen into the substrate and one into water.
- Their hydroxylated products are more water-soluble than their generally lipophilic substrates.
- Liver contains highest amounts, but found in most tissues.
- Located in the smooth endoplasmic reticulum or in mitochondria (steroidogenic enzymes).
- In some cases, their products are mutagenic or carcinogenic.
- Most have molecular mass of about 55 kDa.
- Many are inducible.
- Some exhibit polymorphisms, which can result in atypical drug metabolism.

9. Which RNA contains highest amount of abnormal purine and pyrimidine bases?

a. 16S rRNA
b. mRNA
c. RNA
d. 5S rRNA
e. 23S rRNA

Ans. c *Ref: Molecular Cell Biology by Lodish and Baltimore*

Option a	False	
Option b	False	
Option c	True	
Option d	False	
Option e	False	

- **Transfer RNA (tRNA)** is unique among nucleic acids in its content of "unusual" bases.
- An unusual base is any purine or pyrimidine ring except the usual A, G, C, and U from which all RNAs are synthesized. All other bases are produced by modification of one of the four bases after it has been incorporated into the polyribonucleotide chain.
- All classes of RNA display some degree of modification, but in all cases except tRNA this is confined to rather simple events, such as the addition of methyl groups.
- In tRNA, there is a vast range of modifications, ranging from simple methylation to wholesale restructuring of the purine ring.
- Modifications occur in all parts of the tRNA molecule. There are >50 different types of modified bases in tRNA.
- Modifications of pyrimidines (C and U) are less complex than those of purines (A and G).

10. True about Chromatin remodeling:

a. Chromatin remodeling is a dynamic process
b. Histone modifications occur by specific enzyme
c. Aberrations in chromatin remodeling proteins may be associated with cancer
d. Do not involve enzymes
e. Energy is required to displace the histone octamers from DNA or translocate them onto neighboring DNA segments

Ans. a, b, c, e *Ref: Molecular Cell Biology by Lodish and Baltimore*

Option a	True	
Option b	True	A histone modification is a covalent post-translational modification (PTM) to histone proteins which includes methylation, phosphorylation, acetylation, ubiquitylation, and sumoylation
Option c	True	Alternations in chromatin remodeling could lead to changes in gene expression, and hence causing cancer
Option d	False	It does involve enzymatic action
Option e	True	Yes, the process is energy dependent

- Chromatin remodeling is a dynamic process involving rearrangement of chromatin from a condensed state to a transcriptionally accessible state, allowing transcription factors or other DNA binding proteins to access DNA and control gene expression.
- Chromatin is the complex of DNA and proteins that are packed within the nucleus of mammalian cells.
- To form chromatin, DNA is tightly condensed by being wrapped around nuclear proteins called histones. This repeating DNA-histone complex, which consists of 146 base pairs of double-stranded DNA wrapped around eight histone proteins, is called a nucleosome. The repeating nucleosomal units are commonly referred to appear as "beads on a string" when seen under a microscope.
- Chromatin structure is regulated by enzymes that affect histone structure and function by chemically modifying the histone proteins (through acetylation, methylation, and phosphorylation)
- Alternations in chromatin remodeling could lead to changes in gene expression, in some cases causing cancer.

11. Which of the following is true about role of phospholipids?

a. Cell to cell recognition
b. Regulate membrane permeability
c. Precursor of second messengers
d. Mediators of inflammation
e. Help in cell signaling

Ans. b, c, d, e *Ref: Harper's Biochemistry, 30th/ed*

Option a	False	
Option b	True	Main lipid constituent of membranes
Option c	True	Phosphatidylinositol is a precursor of second messenger or internal cell signal
Option d	True	Oxidized phospholipids act as modulators of inflammation
Option e	True	Phosphatidylinositol is a precursor of second messenger or internal cell signal

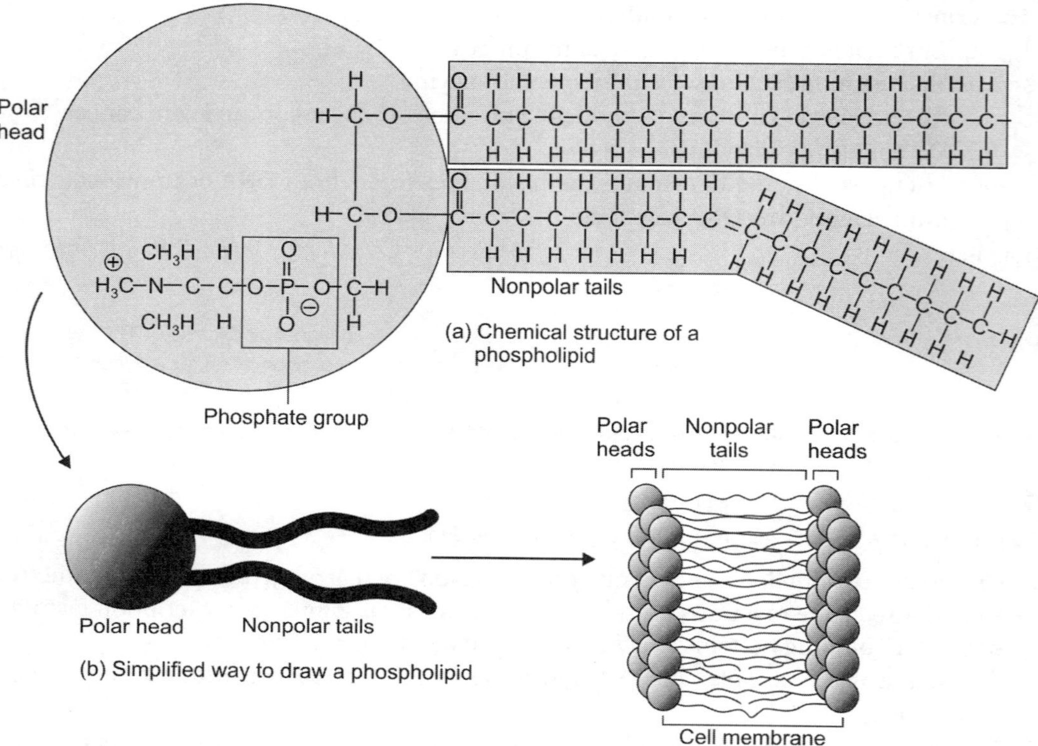

Fig. 2: Phospholipid structure.

Phospholipids

- Lipids containing in addition to fatty acid and alcohol, a phosphoric acid residue.
- Phospholipids include:
  - Phosphatidic acid (important intermediate in the synthesis of triacylglycerol and phosphoglycerols) and phosphatidylglycerol.
  - Phosphatidylcholine—most abundant phospholipids of cell membrane. Choline is important in nervous transmission.
  - Phosphatidylethanolamine
  - Phosphatidylinositol—is a precursor of second messengers.
  - Phosphatidylserine—found in most of the tissues.
  - Lysophospholipid—intermediates in metabolism of phosphoglycerols.
  - Plasmalogen—occur in brain and muscle.
  - Sphingomyelin—found in nervous system.
- Cardiolipin is major lipid of mitochondrial membrane.
- Lipid oxidation products accumulate in inflamed and oxidatively damaged tissue, where they are derived from oxidative modification of lipoproteins, but also from membranes of cells undergoing apoptosis. Thus, increased oxidative stress as well as decreased clearance of apoptotic cells lead to accumulation of oxidized phospholipids in chronically inflamed tissues.

12. During DNA replication which of the following bond breaks?

a. Phosphodiester bonds
b. Phosphate bond
c. N-base to N-base
d. Hydrogen bond
e. Glycosidic

Ans. d *Ref: Harper's Biochemistry, 30th/ed*

Option a	False
Option b	False
Option c	False
Option d	True
Option e	False

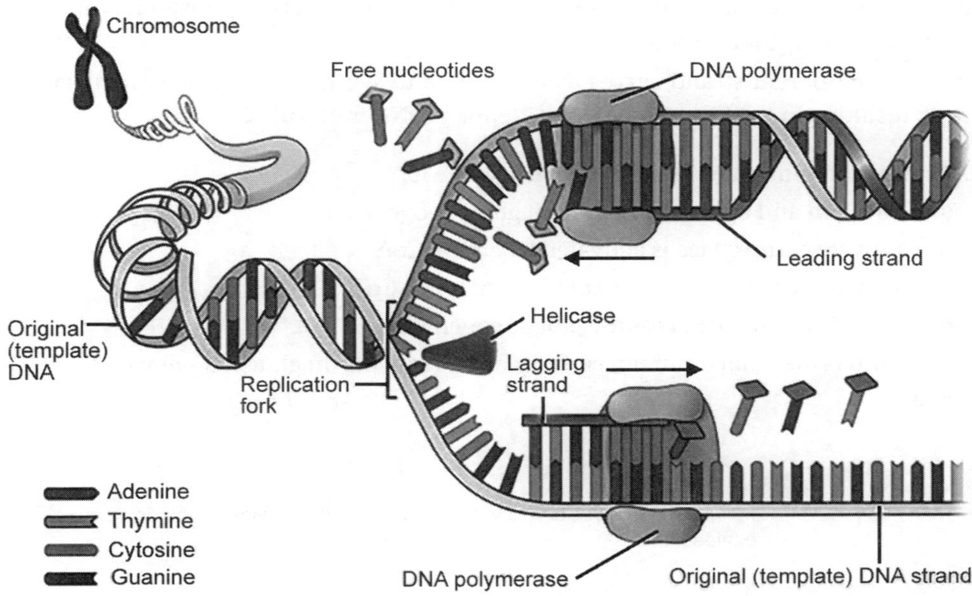

Fig. 3: DNA replication process.

DNA replication:

- DNA is replicated by uncoiling of the helix, strand separation by breaking of the ***hydrogen bonds*** between the complementary strands, and synthesis of two new strands by complementary base pairing.
- Replication begins at a specific site in the DNA called the origin of replication.
- DNA replication is bidirectional from the origin of replication.
- To begin DNA replication, unwinding enzymes called *DNA helicases* cause the two parent DNA strands to unwind and separate from one another at the origin of replication to form two "Y-shaped" replication forks.

- These replication forks are the actual site of DNA copying.
- Helix destabilizing proteins bind to the single-stranded regions so the two strands do not rejoin.
- Enzymes called *topoisomerases* produce breaks in the DNA and then rejoin them in order to relieve the stress in the helical molecule during replication.
- As the strands continue to unwind and separate in both directions around the entire DNA molecule, the hydrogen bonding of free DNA nucleotides with those on each parent strand produce new complementary strands.
- As the new nucleotides line up opposite each parent strand by hydrogen bonding, enzymes called *DNA polymerases* join the nucleotides by way *of phosphodiester bonds*.
- As the phosphodiester bond forms between the 5' phosphate group of the new nucleotide and the 3' OH of the last nucleotide in the DNA strand, two of the phosphates are removed providing energy for bonding.
- Finally each parent strand serves as a template to synthesize a complementary copy of itself, resulting in the formation of two identical DNA molecules.

13. True about gluconeogenesis in fasting state is:

a. Glucagon and epinephrine inhibit gluconeogenesis
b. Pyruvate carboxylase is activated by acetyl-CoA
c. Pyruvate carboxylase is activated by malonyl-CoA
d. Non-esterified fatty acids are gluconeogenic
e. Biotin is the cofactor in the carboxylation reactions in gluconeogenesis

Ans. b, e *Ref: Harper's Biochemistry, 30th/ed*

Option a	False	
Option b	True	Increase in acetyl CoA activates pyruvate carboxylase to synthesize more oxaloacetate
Option c	False	
Option d	False	
Option e	True	Biotin carboxylation is catalyzed at one active site of pyruvate carboxylase

- During short-term fasting periods, the liver produces and releases glucose mainly through glycogenolysis.
- During prolonged fasting (periods of fasting, starvation, low-carbohydrate diets, or intense exercise), glycogen is depleted, and hepatocytes synthesize glucose through gluconeogenesis using lactate, pyruvate, glycerol, and amino acids.
- When gluconeogenesis is active in liver, oxaloacetate is diverted to form glucose (via PEP). Oxaloacetate depletion hinders **acetyl CoA** entry into Krebs Cycle. The resulting increase in **acetyl CoA activates pyruvate carboxylase** to synthesize more oxaloacetate.
- Biotin acts as a cofactor in the carboxylation reactions.

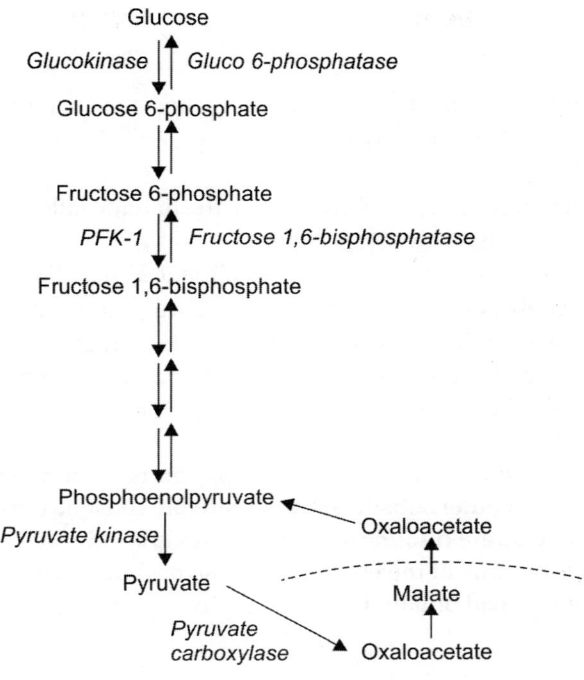

Fig. 4: Gluconeogenesis.

Gluconeogenesis vs Glycogenolysis	
Gluconeogenesis	***Glycogenolysis***
Substrates are non carbohydrate substance like lactate and amino acids.	Substrate is glycogen which is a complex carbohydrate.
Occur in liver and kidney and a small extent in muscle.	Occur in liver and muscles.
There are 4 key enzymes—Pyruvate carboxylase, Phosphoenolpyruvate carboxykinase, Fructose 1, 6-bisphosphatase and Glucose 6-phosphatase.	Key enzyme is glycogen phosphorylase
Pyruvate is the first step.	Glucose 6-phosphate is the first step

14. True about long chain fatty acids is:

a. Linoleic acid is an essential fatty acid
b. Hydrogenation converts unsaturated fatty acids to saturated fatty acids
c. Neutralization of oils is done with fuller's earth
d. Elongation of fatty acids take place in endoplasmic reticulum
e. Arachidonic acid can be produced from linoleic acid

Ans. a, b, d, e *Ref: Harper's Biochemistry, 30th/ed*

Option a	True	
Option b	True	
Option c	False	Crude oil is neutralized using a mild alkaline solution

Option d	True	
Option e	True	

Fatty acid chains differ by length, often categorized as short to very long.

Short-chain fatty acids (SCFA) are fatty acids with aliphatic tails of five or fewer carbons (e.g. butyric acid).

Medium-chain fatty acids (MCFA) are fatty acids with aliphatic tails of 6 to 12 carbons, which can form medium-chain triglycerides.

Long-chain fatty acids (LCFA) are fatty acids with aliphatic tails of 13 to 21 carbons.

Very long chain fatty acids (VLCFA) are fatty acids with aliphatic tails of 22 or more carbons.

Elongation of fatty acid chains occurs in **endoplasmic reticulum.**

- Unsaturated fatty acids have one or more double bonds between carbon atoms. Hydrogenation converts double bonds of unsaturated fatty acid to single bonds, making it an unsaturated fatty acid.
- Essential fatty acids are the ones required by the human body but cannot be made in sufficient quantity from other substrates, and therefore must be obtained from food.
- Two essential fatty acids are **linoleic acid (LA)** and **alpha-Linolenic acid (ALA).**
- Arachidonic acid is not one of the essential fatty acids, but it becomes essential if there is a deficiency in linoleic acid or if there is an inability to convert *linoleic acid to arachidonic acid.*

15. Secondary hypertriglyceridemia is associated with:

a. Nephritic syndrome
b. Diabetes mellitus
c. Alcoholism
d. Cholestasis
e. Congestive heart disease

Ans. b, c *Ref: Harper's Biochemistry, 30th/ed*

Option a	False	Associated with nephrotic syndrome
Option b	True	
Option c	True	
Option d	False	
Option e	False	

- Hypertriglyceridemia can be divided into primary and secondary types.
- People who develop secondary hypertriglyceridemia generally have inherited metabolic defect that confers susceptibility.
- Major factors associated with secondary hypertriglyceridemia include:
  - Obesity
  - Poorly controlled type 2 diabetes, and
  - Excessive alcohol consumption
- Hypertriglyceridemia, both in the *metabolic syndrome* and in *type 2 diabetes,* results from increased plasma concentrations of VLDL, with or without chylomicronemia; deficient lipoprotein lipase activity; increased cholesterylester transfer protein activity; and increased flux of free fatty acids to the liver.
- Hypertriglyceridemia due to *excessive alcohol consumption* results from increased plasma VLDL, with or without chylomicronemia.

- ❑ *Nephrotic syndrome* is also characterized by increases in apo B-containing lipoproteins, including VLDL.
- ❑ *Nonalcoholic fatty-liver disorder*—reflects the increasing prevalence of obesity, insulin resistance and metabolic syndrome.
- ❑ Other less common causes of secondary hypertriglyceridemia include:
  - Hypothyroidism
  - Drugs—corticosteroids, estrogen, tamoxifen, non-cardioselective beta blockers etc.

16. True about stress-induced hyperglycemia:

a. Increased insulin resistance
b. Increased glycogenolysis
c. Increased cortisol
d. Decreased corticotropin-releasing hormone
e. Increased norepinephrine levels

Ans. a, c, e *Ref: Harper's Biochemistry, 30th/ed*

Option a	True	
Option b	False	There is increased gluconeogenesis
Option c	True	
Option d	False	Increased CRH
Option e	True	

- ❑ Stress-induced hyperglycemia also known as hyperglycemia without diabetes is a common problem in patients admitted to the ICU due to any reason, even when glucose homeostasis has previously been normal.
- ❑ The stress response is mediated largely by the hypothalamic-pituitary-adrenal (HPA) axis and the sympathoadrenal system. The HPA axis, sympathoadrenal system and proinflammatory cytokines (TNF-α, IL-1 and IL-6) act collectively and synergistically to induce stress hyperglycemia.
- ❑ **Adrenal cortisol** output **increases** up to ten-fold with severe stress (approximately 300 mg hydrocortisone per day).
- ❑ In patients with shock, plasma concentrations of **epinephrine increase** 50-fold and **norepinephrine levels increase** 10-fold.
- ❑ The adrenal medulla is the major source of these released catecholamines.
- ❑ The neuroendocrine response to stress is characterized by **excessive gluconeogenesis, glycogenolysis** and **insulin resistance.**

17. Photolyase identifies thymine dimers by:

a. Palindromic sequence
b. Triple hydrogen bond in bases
c. Cyclobutane dimer
d. Configurational change in the DNA
e. Restriction sequence

Ans. c, d

Option a	False	
Option b	False	
Option c	True	

Option d	True	
Option e	False	

18. True about gene or function of gene:

a. Not capable of independent expression
b. Cistron is the smallest functional unit of gene expression
c. Attachment to larger ribosome
d. Attachment to tRNA
e. RNA polymerase attachment

Ans. b, e *Ref: Harper's Biochemistry, 30th/ed*

Option a	False	Capable of independent expression
Option b	True	
Option c	False	Ribosomes attach to mRNA strand
Option d	False	Building the mRNA strand
Option e	True	

- Genes are the working subunits of DNA.
- Each gene contains a particular set of instructions, usually coding for a particular protein or for a particular function.
- In order to be expressed, genes require a promoter sequence. The promoter is recognized and bound by transcription factors and RNA polymerase to initiate transcription.
- RNA polymerase is responsible for reading the gene, and building the mRNA strand. It reads only the 3′ to 5′ strand.
- Many prokaryotic genes are organized into operons, with multiple protein-coding sequences that are transcribed as a unit.
- The genes in an operon are transcribed as a continuous messenger RNA, referred to as a polycistronic mRNA.
- The term cistron in this context is equivalent to gene and is the smallest functional unit of gene expression.

19. Which of the following are post-translational modification of polypeptides?

a. Addition of base pairs at the end
b. Deletion of base pairs at the end
c. Phosphorylation of serine
d. Excision of a peptide
e. Ubiquitination of lysine

Ans. c, d, e *Ref: Harper's Biochemistry 30th/ed; Lippincott's Biochemistry, 6th/ed*

Option a	False	
Option b	False	
Option c	True	
Option d	True	
Option e	True	

- Most of the proteins that are translated from mRNA undergo chemical modifications before becoming functional in different body cells, known as post-translational modifications.

- Post-translational modifications play an important part in modifying the end product of expression and contribute towards biological processes and diseased conditions.
- The amino terminal sequences are removed by proteolytic cleavage when the proteins cross the membranes.
- Protein post-translational modifications may happen in several ways. Some of them are:
  - Glycosylation: Results in addition of a glycosyl group to either asparagine, hydroxylysine, serine, or threonine.
  - Acetylation: The addition of an acetyl group, usually at the N-terminus of the protein.
  - Alkylation: The addition of an alkyl group (e.g. methyl, ethyl).
  - Methylation: The addition of a methyl group, usually at lysine or arginine residues (this is a type of alkylation).
  - Biotinylation: Acylation of conserved lysine residues with a biotin appendage.
  - Glutamylation: Covalent linkage of glutamic acid residues to tubulin and some other proteins.
  - Glycylation: Covalent linkage of one to more than 40 glycine residues to the tubulin C-terminal tail of the amino acid sequence.
  - Isoprenylation: The addition of an isoprenoid group.
  - Lipoylation: The attachment of a lipoate functionality.
  - Phosphorylation: The addition of a phosphate group, usually to serine, tyrosine, threonine or histidine.
  - Sulfation: The addition of a sulfate group to a tyrosine.
  - Selenation
  - C-terminal amidation
  - Ubiquitination: Covalently attaching one or more ubiquitin monomers via an isopeptide bond.

20. True about proteoglycans:

a. Always positively charged
b. Glycosaminoglycans covalently attached to core proteins
c. Always found on cell surface
d. Part of extracellular matrix and connective tissue
e. Holds lot of water

Ans. b, d, e *Ref: Lippincott Biochemistry, 6th/ed*

Option a	False	
Option b	True	
Option c	False	
Option d	True	
Option e	True	

- Proteoglycans are proteins that contain covalently linked glycosaminoglycans.
- Proteoglycans are a major component of the extracellular matrix
- The amount of carbohydrate in a proteoglycan is much higher than is found in a glycoprotein and may comprise up to 95% of its weight.
- The point of attachment is a serine (Ser) residue to which the glycosaminoglycan is joined through a tetrasaccharide bridge.

- The combination of proteoglycans and collagen form cartilage, that is usually heavily hydrated (mostly due to the negatively charged sulfates in the glycosaminoglycan chains of the proteoglycans).
- The major biological function of proteoglycans derives from the physicochemical characteristics of the glycosaminoglycan component of the molecule, which provides hydration and swelling pressure to the tissue enabling it to withstand compressional forces. This function is best illustrated by the most abundant proteoglycan in cartilage tissues, aggrecan.
- They are also involved in binding cations (such as sodium, potassium and calcium) and water, and also regulating the movement of molecules through the matrix.
- The various proteoglycans have been divided into several major classes which are defined by their function, tissue distribution, and protein homologies. The major classes are: *interstitial proteoglycans*, the *basement membrane proteoglycans*, the *secretory granule proteoglycans*, and the *membrane-bound proteoglycans*.

Characteristics of glycosaminoglycans (GAG)		
GAG	***Localization***	***Comments***
Hyaluronate	• Synovial fluid • Articular cartilage • Skin • Vitreous humor • ECM of loose connective tissue	• High shock absorbing character • Synthesized in plasma membrane by three hyaluronan synthases: HAS1, HAS2, and HAS3
Chondroitin sulfate	• Cartilage • Bone • Heart valves	• Most abundant GAG • Principally associated with protein to form proteoglycans • Loss of chondroitin sulfate from cartilage is a major cause of osteoarthritis
Heparan sulfate	• Basement membranes • Components of cell surfaces	• Contains higher acetylated glucosamine than heparin • Found associated with protein forming heparan sulfate proteoglycans (HSPG)
Heparin	• Component of intracellular granules of mast cells • Lining the arteries of the lungs • Liver and skin	• More sulfated than heparan sulfates • Clinically useful as an injectable anticoagulant
Dermatan sulfate	• Skin • Blood vessels • Heart valves • Tendons • Lung	• May function in coagulation, wound repair, fibrosis, and infection • Excess accumulation in the mitral valve can result in mitral valve prolapse
Keratan sulfate	• Cornea • Bone • Cartilage aggregated with chondroitin sulfates	• Usually associated with protein forming proteoglycans • Keratan sulfate proteoglycans include lumican, keratocan, fibromodulin, aggrecan, and prolargin

21. True about HMP shunt:

a. Takes place in cytosol
b. Does not produce ATP
c. NADH is produced in oxidative phase
d. Found in liver, adipose tissue, gonads
e. Pyruvate is produced in the non-oxidative phase

Ans. a, b, d *Ref: Lippincott Biochemistry, 6th/ed*

Option a	True	
Option b	True	
Option c	False	Oxidative phase, end products are D-ribose 5-phosphate and NADPH
Option d	True	
Option e	False	Non-oxidative phase leads to inter-conversion of 3, 4, 5 and 7- carbon sugars

The hexose monophosphate pathway is used for production of NADPH from NADP.

The NADPH is required for biosynthetic reactions such as fatty acid synthesis, cholesterol synthesis, drug reduction, and as a cofactor for some non-synthetic enzymatic reactions.

Hexose monophosphate shunt is the alternative glucose oxidative pathway.

The hexose monophosphate shunt also allows the entry of carbohydrates into the glycolytic pathway.

The HMP shunt occurs in the cytoplasm. Steroidogenic tissues, red blood cells, and the liver are the prominent sector of hexose monophosphate pathway.

It is a source of NADPH and ribose-5-phosphate for nucleic acid biosynthesis.

It has an oxidative phase (NADPH generation) and a non-oxidative (non-oxidative sugar interconversion).

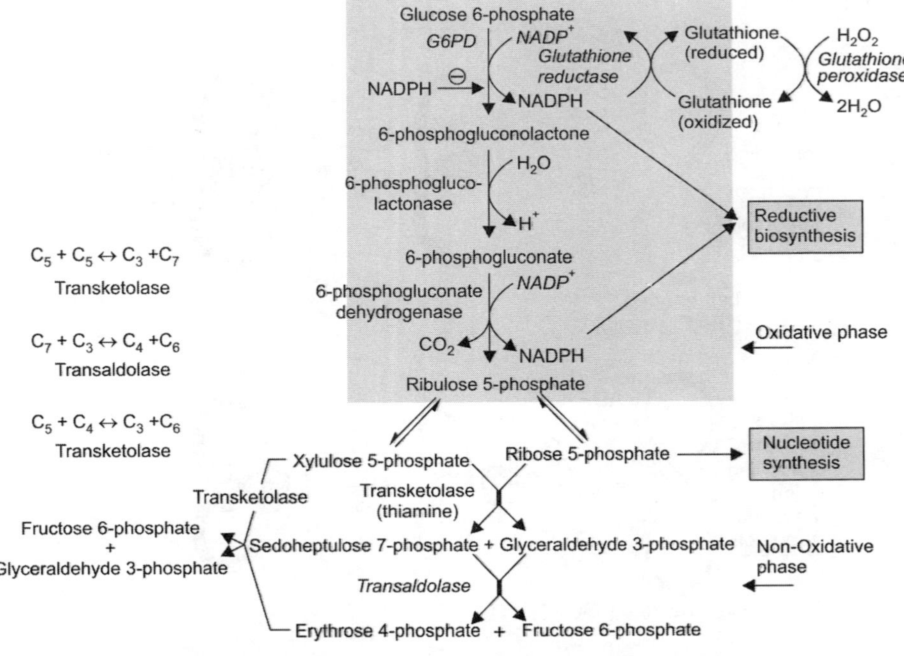

Fig. 5: Pentose phosphate pathway (Hexose monophosphate shunt).

Oxidative phase:

The oxidative portion of HMP shunt composes of 3 chemical reactions that lead to the production of ribulose-5-phosphate, carbon dioxide and 2 additional molecules of NADPH, for each molecule of glucose-6-phosphate would get oxidized.

Non-oxidative phase:

The non-oxidative reactions accelerate the inter-conversion of 3, 4, 5 and 7-carbon sugars. The non-oxidative source of the pentose phosphate pathway beguns when the cell demands extra NADPH than ribose-5-phosphate.

22. True about DNA gyrase:

a. Prokaryotic topoisomerase-I
b. Prokaryotic topoisomerase-II
c. Reverse transcriptase
d. Restriction endonuclease
e. RNA polymerase

Ans. b *Ref: Harper's Biochemistry 30/e; Lippincott's Biochemistry, 6th/ed*

Option a	False	
Option b	True	
Option c	False	
Option d	False	
Option e	False	

- DNA gyrase is a bacterial type II DNA topoisomerase with a tetrameric structure made up of 2 gyrA (97 kDa) subunits and 2 gyrB (90 kDa) subunits.
- Gyrase is apparently needed in replication systems for initiation, chain elongation, and termination.

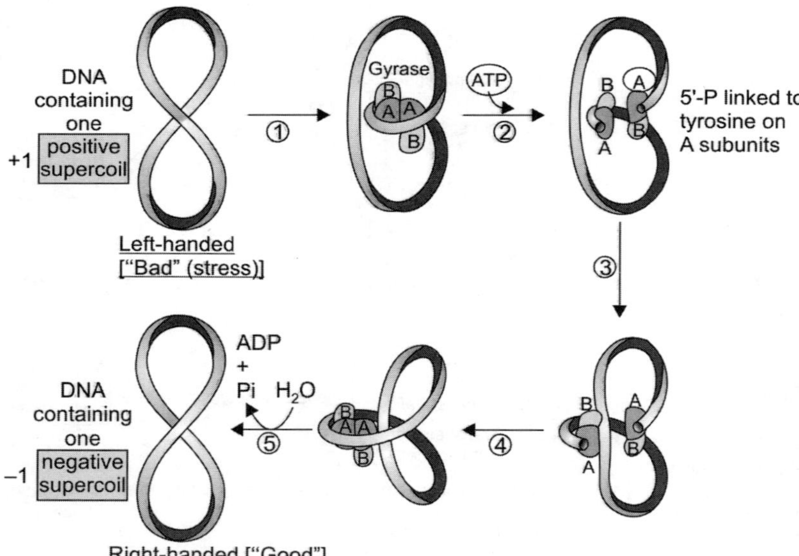

Fig. 6: Mechanism of DNA Gyrase (a Topoisomerase II).

- DNA gyrase catalyzes the ATP-dependent negative super-coiling of double-stranded closed-circular DNA.
- Blocking gyrase activity in whole cells, with inhibitors or temperature-sensitive mutations, thus arrests DNA replication.

23. Pyrimidine is a part of:

a. Adenosine
b. Cytosine
c. Uridine
d. Cysteine
e. Guanosine

Ans. b, c *Ref: Harper's Biochemistry 30th/ed; Lippincott's Biochemistry, 6th/ed*

Option a	False	
Option b	True	Pyrimidine derivative
Option c	True	Glycosylated pyrimidine-analog
Option d	False	
Option e	False	

- ❑ One of the important specialized pathways of a number of amino acids is the synthesis of purine and pyrimidine nucleotides.
- ❑ Purines consist of a six-membered and a five-membered nitrogen-containing ring, fused together.
- ❑ Pyrimidines have only a six-membered nitrogen-containing ring.
- ❑ There are 4 purines and 4 pyrimidines that are of concern to us.

Purines:

Adenine = 6-aminopurine
Guanine = 2-amino-6-oxy purine
Hypoxanthine = 6-oxy purine
Xanthine = 2,6-dioxy purine

Pyrimidines:

Uracil = 2,4-dioxy pyrimidine (found only in RNA)
Thymine = 2,4-dioxy-5-methyl pyrimidine (found in DNA)
Cytosine = 2-oxy-4-amino pyrimidine (found in both DNA and RNA)
Orotic acid = 2,4-dioxy-6-carboxy pyrimidine
Sometimes tRNA will contain some thymine as well as uracil.

24. Enzyme activity is regulated by:

a. Covalent modification
b. Allosteric inhibition
c. Allosteric activation
d. Zymogen activation
e. Regulated by increased synthesis

Ans. a, b, c, d, e *Ref: Harper's Biochemistry 30th/ed; Lippincott's Biochemistry, 6th/ed*

Option a	True	
Option b	True	
Option c	True	
Option d	True	
Option e	True	

- ❑ Enzymatic activity is controlled at the enzyme content level through the synthesis and degradation of enzymes as well as at the level of individual enzymatic molecules by low molecular substances (effectors) such as metabolites, ATP and ADP.

- When effectors are attached to sites other than the active centers of enzymes, these sites are known as *allosteric sites*, and the enzymes regulated by them are called allosteric enzymes (allo means "other" and steric means "space").
- Allosteric activators/positive effectors result in increasing the reaction velocity and in increasing the affinity of an allosteric enzyme to its substrate.
- Phosphofructokinase (PFK)—a major enzyme in glycolysis is a typical allosteric enzyme and is inhibited by ATP and citric acid and activated by adenosine monophosphate (AMP), Adrenomedullin (ADM) and fructose 6-phosphate.
- Allosteric inhibitors/negative effectors result in decreasing the reaction velocity and in decreasing the affinity of an allosteric enzyme to its substrate.
- Enzymatic activity is also regulated through enzyme-molecule-level modification by covalent bonds. The phosphorylation involved in signal transduction is a typical example of this.
- One of the basic regulation mechanisms of metabolism is *feedback regulation,* in which a metabolic pathway is stopped when the amount of final product becomes *excessive.* With such regulation, not all enzymes involved in the pathway need to be inhibited, and it is common for the most important enzyme in the pathway to be inhibited instead.

25. Telomerase is:

a. Reverse transcriptase
b. Ribonucleoprotein
c. Ribozyme
d. Active in cancer cells and germ cells
e. Carry its own RNA template

Ans. a, b, d, e *Ref: Harper's Biochemistry 30th/ed; Lippincott's Biochemistry, 6th/ed*

Option a	True	
Option b	True	
Option c	False	
Option d	True	
Option e	True	

- Telomerase is an enzyme containing its own RNA template. So, it is a ribonucleoprotein.
- It extends the 3' G-rich telomeric DNA using its own RNA as a template. So, it is a reverse transcriptase.
- Telomerase is expressed predominantly in germ cells and cancer cells making these cells immortal.
- Ribozymes are catalytic RNAs. Catalysis of telomerase is due to protein part, not due to RNA. RNA is just a template here.

Pathology

1. BRCA 1 affects which phase of cell cycle:

a. G1-G2
b. G2M
c. S PHASE
d. G2S PHASE
e. Centrosome duplication

Ans. b,c,e *Ref: Deng C-X. BRCA1: cell cycle checkpoint, genetic instability, DNA damage response and cancer evolution. Nucleic Acids Research. 2006;34(5):1416-1426. doi:10.1093/nar/gkl010.*
Timothy K. BRCA1 Effects on the Cell Cycle and the DNA Damage Response Are Linked to Altered Gene Expression. J. Biol. Chem. 2000, 275:2777-2785.
Robbins/7th,307

Option a	False	No, not correct
Option b	True	Yes, correct
Option c	True	Yes, correct
Option d	False	No, not correct
Option e	True	Yes, correct

Germline mutations of the breast cancer associated gene 1 (*BRCA1*) predispose women to breast and ovarian cancers

BRCA1 deficiency, consequently causes abnormalities in the S-phase checkpoint, the G2/M checkpoint, the spindle checkpoint and centrosome duplication. The genetic instability caused by BRCA1 deficiency, however, also triggers cellular responses to DNA damage that blocks cell proliferation and induces apoptosis. During late G_1 and early S phases, BRCA1 protein increases and becomes phosphorylated . Upon exit from mitosis, the protein becomes progressively dephosphorylated and decreases in expression.

2. True about splenosis is:

a. Histologically resembles normal spleen
b. Also known as accessory spleen
c. Gold standard for splenosis depends on pathological diagnosis which can be obtained by needle aspiration prior to operation
d. Preoperative diagnosis of splenosis could be acquired by using of nuclear imaging studies
e. Can occur after trauma

Ans. a,c,d,e

Option a	True	Yes, correct
Option b	False	No, accessory spleen is splenunculi
Option c	True	Yes, correct
Option d	True	Yes, correct
Option e	True	Yes, correct

Splenosis is a condition in which ectopic spleen tissue may be found in the peritoneal cavity or in other unusual locations due to heterotopic auto-transplantation and implantation of splenic tissue after spleen trauma or splenectomy. It is a benign condition that is often misdiagnosed as a tumor. Therefore, knowledge of this condition is important when evaluating patients with a previous history of splenic trauma or splenectomy and newly appearing peritoneal lesions.

Sites:
- Peritoneal cavity - m/c
- Thorax
- Abdomen
- Subcutaneous tissues

Diagnosis:
- CT / MRI for initial test
- Tc 99m sulphar colloid scan - confirmatory
- Needle aspiration biopsy - Gold standard

Differential diagnosis:
- Splenenculi - or accessory spleen
- Spleen pathology - metastases
- Endometriosis
- Lymphadenopathy

3. Not a extranodal lymphoma:

a. Waldenstroms macroglobulinemia
b. Burkit lymphoma
c. Maltoma
d. Mycosis fungoides
e. Mantle cell lymphoma

Ans. a, e

Option a	False	No, it has lymph node involvement as primary component
Option b	True	Yes, correct (Jaw, GIT, CNS)
Option c	True	Yes, correct (GIT)
Option d	True	Yes, correct (skin)
Option e	False	No, it has lymph node involvement as primary component

At least one quarter of non-Hodgkin's lymphomas (NHL) arise from tissue other than lymph nodes and even from sites which normally contain no lymphoid tissue. These forms are referred to as primary extranodal lymphomas.

Extra nodal presentation is commonly seen in:
- Burkit (jaw and git)
- Maltoma (git)
- Mycosis(skin)
- Primary GI lymphomas

*uncommon in WM (Waldenstroms macroglobulinemia) and MCL (mantle cell lymphoma)

Waldenstroms macroglobulinemia:

- Is a subset type of Lymphoplasmacytic lymphoma (LPL)
- It is a chronic, lymphoproliferative neoplasm characterized by small B lymphocytes, plasmacytoid lymphocytes, and plasma cells typically involving the bone marrow, lymph nodes, and spleen.
- Most common presentation – anemia, chronic fatigue

Differential diagnosis

- Chronic Lymphocytic Leukemia (CLL)
- Monoclonal Gammopathies of Undetermined Significance
- Multiple Myeloma

Non-Hodgkin Lymphoma. The 2008 World Health Organization criteria for classification of hematologic diseases characterizes Waldenstrom macroglobulinemia (WM) as a subset of LPL that has ¨a detectable level of monoclonal immunoglobulin (Ig) M gammopathy, with bone marrow involvement by LPL. In rare instances, diffuse lymphoplasmacytic infiltration of the lung, stomach, or bowel may occur.

Mantle cell Lymphoma

- B-cell NHL, age > 60 years
- Associated with increased level of cyclin D1 (most sensitive investigation for diagnosis of MCL)
- BM biopsy is diagnostic and confirmatory

4. True statement about Muccopolysaccharidosis is:

a. All are AR except type 4
b. Enzyme replacement therapy is approved by FDA for MPS IV
c. All are AR except type 2
d. Type 2 is x linked
e. Type III has little somatic involvement

Ans. b, c, d

Option a	False	All are AR except type 2 which is X linked recessive
Option b	True	
Option c	True	
Option d	True	
Option e	True	

Disease	Alternative name	Enzyme	Neurological involvement
Mucopolysaccharidosis type I	Hurler's syndrome, Scheie's syndrome	α-L-iduronidase	Mental retardation
Mucopolysaccharidosis type II	Hunter's syndrome	iduronate-2-sulfatase	Hydrocephalus, mental retardation, seizures

Contd...

Contd…

Disease	Alternative name	Enzyme	Neurological involvement
Mucopolysaccharidosis type IIIA	Sanfilippo's syndrome	Heparan-N-sulfatase	Hyperactivity, mental retardation, seizures, sleep disturbances
Mucopolysaccharidosis type IIIB	Sanfilippo's syndrome	Alpha-N-acetylglucosaminidase	
Mucopolysaccharidosis type IIIC	Sanfilippo's syndrome	AcetylCOA:N-acetyltransferase	
Mucopolysaccharidosis type IIID	Sanfilippo's syndrome	N-acetylglucosamine 6-sulfatase	
Mucopolysaccharidosis type IVA	Morquio syndrome	Galactose 6-sulfatase	Cervical myelopathy
Mucopolysaccharidosis type IVB	Morquio syndrome	Beta-galactosidase	
Mucopolysaccharidosis type VI	Maroteaux-Lamy Morquio syndrome	N-acetylgalactosamine 4-sulfatase	Cervical myelopathy, hydrocephalus
Mucopolysaccharidosis type VII	Sly syndrome	Beta-glucuronidase	Mental retardation, hydrocephalus, neurodegeneration

Type	Gene/locus	Enzyme deficient	GAG accumulation
MPS 1 (Hurler, Hurler-Scheie, Scheie syndromes	IDUA (4p16)	α-L-iduronidase	Dermatan sulphate Heparan sulphate
MPS II (Hunter syndrome)	IDS (Xq28)	Iduronate 2-sulphatase	Dermatan sulphate Heparan sulphate
MPS III (Sanfilippo) Type A Type B Type C Type D	 SGSH (17q25) NAGLU (17q21) HGSNAT (8p11) GNS (12q14)	 Heparan sulphatase N acetylglucosaminidase Acetyl coA: Glucosaminide acetyltransferase Acetylglucosamine-6- sulphatase	Heparan sulphate
MPS IV (Morquio) Type A Type B		 Galactose-6-sulphatase β Galactosidase	 Keratan sulphate Chondroitin sulphate
MPS VI (Maroteaux-Lamy)	ARSB (5q14)	Arylsulphatase B	Dermatan & Chondriotin sulphate
MPS VII (Sly)	GUSB (7q11)	β Glucoronidase	Dermatan/Heparan/ Chondriotin sulphate
MPS IX	HYAL1 (3p21)	Hyaluronidase	Hyaluronan
http://www.genetics4medics.com/mucopolysaccharidoses.html			

MPS I

- Includes **severe MPS (Hurler syndrome) & Attenuated MPS (Hurler-Scheie & Scheie syndromes)**. Symptoms and signs are less severe in the attenuated form.
- **Craniofacial:** Appear normal at birth but coarsen with age. This is caused by accumulation go GAGs in the soft issue and bone dysostosis. Characterised by full lips, thickening of alar nasi, ear lobes and skull bones.

- **Dysostosis multiplex:** Progressive skeletal dysplasia.
- Thickened ribs, clavicles and calvarium.
- Vertebral abnormalities including gibbous deformity (due to excessive thoraco-lumbar kyphosis).
- Short stature, genu valgum/varum.
- Joint stiffness, restricted mobility.
- Phalangeal dysostosis which present as claw hand deformity.
- **Eyes:** Corneal clouding which can cause significant visual impairment. Other features include glaucoma and retinal degeneration.
- **ENT:** Hearing loss, obstructive sleep apnoea.
- **CNS:** Hydrocephalus, developmental delay.
- **CVS:** Valves are thickened and stiff, which lead to regurgitation (mitral/aortic). Cardiomyopathy, arrhythmias.
- Abdomen: Hepatosplenomegaly, umbilical & inguinal hernia.

MPS II (Hunter syndrome)

Includes severe and attenuated forms.

- Severe form has many features similar to that seen in Hurler syndrome including the coarse facial features, airway/ENT problems, CVS, CNS, abdomen findings and skeletal features.
- **Specific features** include:
  - Corneal opacity not a usual feature. Some flecks may be seen on slit lamp examination.
  - Chronic diarrhoea is a common problem.
  - Distinctive skin lesion (pebbling).

MPS III (Sanfilippo Syndrome)

- Usually presents around 2-6 years of age with developmental delay and behavioural problems. Progressive neurocognitive decline in severe cases.
- Little or no somatic involvement.

MPS IV (Morquio Syndrome)

- Severe cases become apparent by 1-3 years of age.
- **Skeletal dysplasia:**
  - Kyphoscoliosis, genu valgum, chest wall deformities. Short stature.
  - Ligamentous laxity/joint hypermobility.
  - Odontoid hypoplasia leading to atlantoaxial instability.
  - Spinal cord compression leading to cervical myelopathy.
- Normal intellect (unless complicated by spinal cord compression). Very little or no facial dysmorphism.
- Other systemic features occur as seen in MPS1, but less severe.

MPS VI (Maroteaux-Lamy Syndrome)

- Somatic features quite similar to MPS I.
- Present with a spectrum of clinical severity.
- Normal intellect (unless complicated by spinal cord compression).

Treatment

Enzyme replacement therapy:
1. Idursulfase – tried for MPS II (Hunter's)
2. Laronidase – tried for MPS I (Hurler's)
3. Elosulfase alfa – FDA approved for MPS IVA

BMT – esp MPS I (hurler)

5. True about Chest wall tumours is/are:
- a. Fibrous dysplasia is the most common skeletal soft tissue sarcoma
- b. Lipoma is the most common...
- c. Desmoid is usually not malignant
- d. Completely cured if resected with margin and no mets
- e. Neurogenic tumour are the commonest

Ans. a, b, c, d

Ref: 1. Fraser RG, Paré JAP, Paré PD, Fraser RS, Genereux GP. Diseases of the diaphragm and chest wall. In: Fraser RG, Paré JAP, Paré PD, Fraser RS, Genereux GP, eds. Diagnosis of diseases of the chest. 3rd ed. Philadelphia, Pa: Saunders, 1991; 2921-2973.
2. Mi-Young Jeung, Afshin gangi. Imaging of chest wall disorders. RSNA 1999, 19:3.

Option a	True	Yes, correct
Option b	True	Yes, correct
Option c	True	Yes, correct. Desmoid tumors are non-malignant growths that occur in the connective tissue.
Option d	True	Yes, correct
Option e	False	No, not correct, hemangiomas and lymphomas are most common

- ❑ Almost 50% of chest wall tumors are benign
- ❑ The most common benign chest wall tumors are – skeletal in origin
  - Lipoma (m/c soft tissue tumor of chest wall)
  - Fibrous dysplasia (m/c skeletal tumor - non malignant - of chest wall / ribs)
  - Fibrosarcomas (m/c primary malignant tumor from the soft tissue of chest wall)
  - Osteochondroma (m/c benign tumor of the cartilage and bone in chest wall)
  - Chondrosarcomas (m/c primary malignant chest wall sarcoma – especially sternum)

Soft Tissue Tumors

Lipoma: Lipomas of the chest wall are benign and do not require treatment until they become large. Some of these lesions are dumbbell-shaped, having both intrathoracic and extrathoracic components.

Neurogenic tumors may originate from the intercostal nerves of the thoracic cage or from the paraspinal ganglion of the sympathetic chain.

1. Tumors that arise from nerve roots include neurilemmoma (benign schwannoma, neurinoma), neurofibroma, neurofibrosarcoma, and neuroma.

2. Tumors that affect the sympathetic ganglion include neuroblastoma, ganglioneuroma, and ganglioneuroblastoma
3. Neurofibromas develop as multiple tumors located throughout the body and associated with the pigmented "café-au-lait" skin lesions of von Recklinghausen disease (neurofibromatosis).

Hemangiomas are occasionally found in the soft tissues of the chest wall. They are usually cavernous and may contain a significant amount of fat. Hemangiomas may be visible at radiography if they contain phleboliths.

Desmoid tumors are distinctly uncommon lesions and may involve the chest wall. Although they can be locally aggressive and tend to recur after resection, these firm, fibroblastic tumors are considered benign and do not metastasize. However, desmoid tumours most often occur in the abdomen, arms and legs.

Hemangiopericytomas: Slow growing vascular tumor arising from pericytes of Zimmerman which surround the capillary walls.

Lymphomas: Hodgkins or NHL may involve chest wall with or without mediastinal or lung parenchymal disease.

- ❑ Best modality to diagnose chest wall tumors is MRI > CT, biopsy is confirmatory
- ❑ Treatment
  - Surgical resection and reconstruction
  - Small cell malignant tumors such as ewings sarcoma would require multi-modality approach – chemotherapy + radiotherapy + surgery

6. Lipoma true is:

a. Most common benign tumor of soft tissue
b. Subcutaneous lipoma more distinct then intradermal as it commonly affect women
c. Hibernomas arise from brown fat tissue
d. Jejunum is most common site for GI lipoma
e. Complete excision of lipoma with capsule is done

Ans. a, b, c, e

Option a	True	Yes, correct
Option b	True	Yes, correct
Option c	True	Yes, correct.
Option d	False	No, They are more common in the ileum than in the duodenum or jejunum
Option e	True	Yes, correct, complete excision is advised to prevent recurrence

- ❑ Most common soft tissue tumor - 16% of all mesenchymal neoplasms
- ❑ Adults, age 40+
- ❑ No gender or ethnic preference
- ❑ Rare in children
- ❑ Associated with obesity
- ❑ Multiple lipomas: 5%, more common in women, often familial, associated with neurofibromatosis, multiple endocrine neoplasia syndromes, Bannayan syndrome (macrocephaly, hemangiomas and lipomas

- ❑ Usually trunk, back, shoulder, neck, proximal extremities
- ❑ Rare on hands, feet, face, lower leg, retroperitoneum
- ❑ Usually subcutaneous (liposarcomas are usually deep seated)
- ❑ Unusual sites include oral cavity, pancreas, breast, intestines.

Treatment: Treatment is indicated only if causing symptoms or pain or for cosmetic reasons. Surgical excision with capsule removal is adequate.

7. NK cells marker is/are:

a. CD 4 b. CD 1
c. CD 16 d. CD 56
e. CD 20

Ans. c and d

Option a	False	Marker for T-helper cells
Option b	False	Marker for various APCs
Option c	True	Yes, correct.
Option d	True	Yes, correct
Option e	False	No, it is general marker all leucocytes

NK cells differ from natural killer T cells (NKTs) phenotypically, by origin and by respective effector functions; often, NKT cell activity promotes NK cell activity by secreting interferon gamma. In contrast to NKT cells, NK cells do not express T-cell antigen receptors (TCR) or pan T marker CD3 or surface immunoglobulins (Ig) B cell receptors, but they usually express the surface markers CD16 (FcγRIII) and CD56 in humans, NK1.1 or NK1.2 in C57BL/6 mice.

Remember:

Type of cell	CD markers
Stem cells	CD34+, CD31-, CD117
All leukocyte groups	CD45+
Granulocyte	CD45+,CD11B,CD15+, CD24+, CD114+, CD182+[16]
Monocyte	CD4, CD45+, CD14+, CD114+, CD11a, CD11b, CD91+,[16] CD16+ [17]
T lymphocyte	CD45+, CD3+
T helper cell	CD45+, CD3+, CD4+
T regulatory cell	CD4, CD25, FOXP3 (a transcription factor)
Cytotoxic T cell	CD45+, CD3+, CD8+
B lymphocyte	CD45+, CD19+, CD20+, CD24+, CD38, CD22
Thrombocyte	CD45+, CD61+
Natural killer cell	CD16+, CD56+,CD3-,CD31,CD30,CD38

8. Premalignant condition is/are:

a. Erythroplakia b. Oral lichen planus
c. Leucoplakia d. Oral submucous fibrosis
e. COPD

Ans. a,b,c,d

Option a	True	Yes, correct
Option b	True	Yes, correct, it is common condition leading to oral cancers
Option c	True	Yes, correct
Option d	True	Yes, correct, it is common condition leading to oral cancer
Option e	False	No, COPD is not a pre-malignant condition

Many oral SCCs develop from premalignant conditions of the oral cavity. A wide array of conditions have been implicated in the development of oral cancer, including leukoplakia, erythroplakia, palatal lesion of reverse cigar smoking, oral lichen planus, oral submucous fibrosis, discoid lupus erythematosus, and hereditary disorders such as dyskeratosis congenital and epidermolysis bullosa.

Points to remember for Oral submucus fibrosis:

Oral Submucous Fibrosis

- Induced by chewing areca nut
- Particularly common in Asian communities
- Probably a genetic predisposition for OSF
- Have an increased risk of developing oral carcinoma
- There does not seem to be any satisfactory treatment for OSF although intralesional steroids have been used.
- Primary prevention by reducing the use of areca nut products would appear to be the best way forward to reduce the incidence of OSF

9. Reticulocyte count is low in:

a. Aplastic anemia
b. Megaloblastic
c. Iron deficiency
d. Hereditary spherocytosis
e. Acute blood loss

Ans. a, b, c

Option a	True	Yes, correct
Option b	True	Yes, correct
Option c	True	Yes, correct
Option d	False	Not correct, reticulocyte count is higher
Option e	False	Not correct, reticulocyte count is higher

The **reticulocyte** count is decreased in megaloblastic anaemia due to destruction of fragile and abnormal megaloblastic erythroid precursor.

When there is an increased production of red blood cells to overcome chronic or severe loss of mature red blood cells, such as in a **haemolytic anaemia**, there is often a markedly high number and percentage of reticulocytes.

Abnormally low numbers of reticulocytes can be attributed to **chemotherapy, aplastic anaemia, pernicious anaemia**, bone marrow malignancies, problems of **erythropoietin** production, various vitamin or mineral deficiencies (**iron, vitamin B_{12}, folic acid**), disease states (**anaemia of chronic disease**) and other causes of anaemia due to poor RBC production.

Retic count differentials:

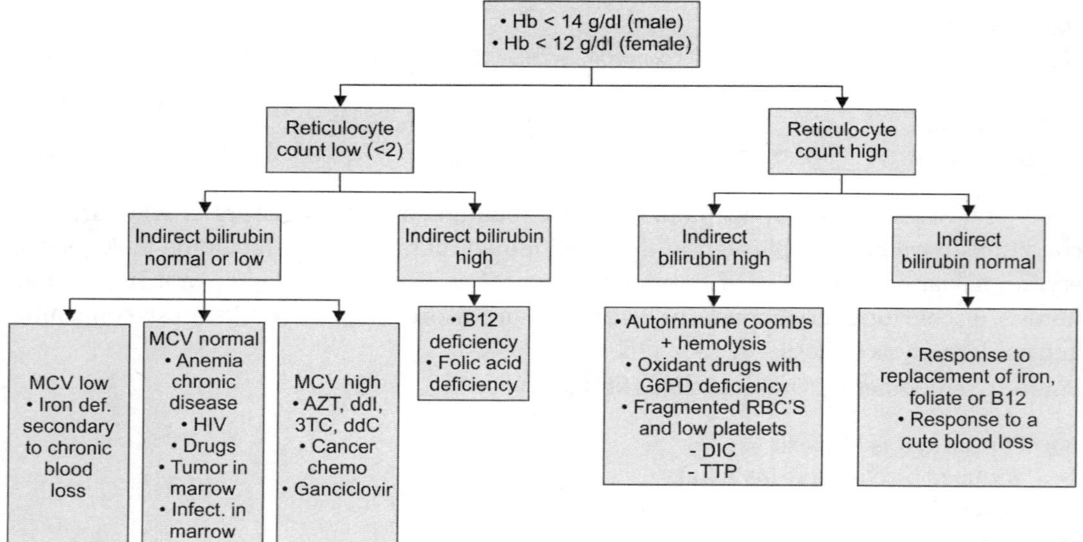

Must remember: (FAQ)

Comparing disorders of iron

Iron panel	Iron panel tests					
	Serum Iron	Serum Ferritin	Transferrin Iron saturation percentage	Total Iron Binding capacity (TIBC)	Transferrin	Hemoglobin
Hemochromatosis	↑	↑	↑	↓	↓	Normal
Iron Deficiency Anemia	↓	↓	↓	↑	↑	↓
Sideroblastic Anemia	↑	↑	↑	↓	↓	↓
Thalassemia	↑	↑	↑	↓	↓	↓
Porphyria Cutanea Tarda (PCT)	↑	↑	↑	↓	↓	Normal
Anemia of Chronic Disease (ACD)	↓	↑	↓	↓	↓	↓
African Siderosis (AS)	↑	↑ Or Normal	↑	↓	↓	Normal
Vitamin B12 Deficiency (pernicious anemia)	↑ Or Normal	↑ Or Normal	↑ Or Normal	↓ Or Normal	↓ Or Normal	↓

Iron study test name	Explanation	Iron as an analogy to money
Serum iron	Unbound serum iron	Loose change in your pocket
Total iron binding capacity	Ability to bind even more iron	Greedinesss for more money
Transferrin saturation	• Iron absorbed from duodenum bound to a transport protein • One molecule of transferrin binds two atoms of iron	Money kept in your wallet
Serum ferritin	• Iron within a storage protein • One molecule of ferritin binds 4500 atoms of iron	The savings you have in your bank

10. Which is true regarding pathological features of rheumatic heart disease?

a. Aschoff body
b. Mc cullams lesion
c. Usually pericarditis is commonly seen
d. Endocarditis involves mainly the valves, which show a finely nodular "verrucous" appearance at the line of closure
e. Aortic valve is most common valve involvement in acute RHD

Ans. a, b, d

Option a	True	Yes, correct. They are diagnostic - fibrinoid necrosis surrounded by anitschkow cells (caterpillar cells)
Option b	True	Yes, correct, common in posterior wall of left atria
Option c	False	No, myocarditis or valve dysfunction is most severe sequel of RHD
Option d	True	Yes, correct
Option e	False	No, in acute RHD – myocarditis is most common. Although the chances of mitral valve involvement is higher than aortic valve in RHD.

Acute Rheumatic Carditis

- Acute rheumatic heart disease is a pancarditis, involving all three layers of the heart.
- The myocarditis is most typically involved in the acute stage of the disease.
- A diffuse non-specific myocarditis is present in some cases, together with a unique type of interstitial inflammation, the Aschoff body.
- The main cause of death in the acute stage of rheumatic heart disease is heart failure from the myocarditis.
- Also seen during the acute stage of the disease is a prominent pericarditis, characterized by tenacious deposits of fibrin that resemble the shaggy irregular surfaces of two slices of buttered bread that have been pulled apart- the so called bread-and-butter appearance.
- The pericarditis may be recognized clinically by a friction rub, but the involvement has little functional effect and only rarely leads to constrictive pericarditis.
- During the acute stage, an endocarditis involves mainly the valves, which show a finely nodular "verrucous" appearance at the line of closure.

Chronic Rheumatic Heart Disease

- A patient who has an attack of rheumatic fever is more susceptible to recurrent episodes following infections by beta-hemolytic streptococci.
- Such recurrent attack result in repeated progressively increasing damage to the heart valves.
- Thus in chronic recurrent rheumatic heart disease the valve involvement, which was of little clinical significance during the acute attack, becomes the major problem. For example the mitral valve which is most frequently and severely involved valve, shows conspicuous, irregular thickening and calcification of its leaflets, often with fusion of its commissures and thickening and fusion of the chordae tendineae.
- As a result the valve is often severely stenotic and when viewed from the atrial aspect has a narrowed orifice described as having a "fish mouth" appearance.
- The aortic valve, the second most commonly involved valve, shows typical fusion of the commissures and later pronounced thickening and calcification of the cusps, with resulting stenosis or insufficiency.
- The subendocardial collections of Aschoff nodules, usually in the left atrium, induce thickenings called MacCallum plaques (patch).

Also MUST REMEMBER: various histological bodies frequently asked in exams:

Important histological bodies seen

Psammoma bodies	Papillary carcinoma thyroid Papillary serous tumors of ovary Meningioma
Russel body	Multiple myeloma
Dutcher body	Waldenstrom's macroglobulinemia Multiple myeloma
Councilman body	Viral hepatitis
Mallory body	Alcoholic hyaline Indian childhood cirrhosis Wilson's disease Primary biliary cirrhosis Focal nodular hyperplasia Hepatocellular carcinoma Chronic cholestatic syndrome
Cowdry a body	Herpes infection
Aschoff body	Rheumatic fever
Ferruginous body	Asbestos
Negri body	Rabies
Lewy body	Parkinsonism
Heinz bodies	G6PD deficiency
Orphan Annie nuclei	Papillary carcinoma of thyroid

11. Prothrombin time is not increased in:

a. Hemophilia A
b. DIC
c. Liver disease
d. Factor 7 deficiency
e. Vitamin A supplementation

Ans. a, e

Option a	True	Yes, PT is not increased in haemophilia. There is normal PT, BT with increase in aPTT
Option b	False	No, PT is increased
Option c	False	No, PT is increased
Option d	False	No, PT is increased
Option e	True	Yes, PT is decreased in case of Vit A supplementation

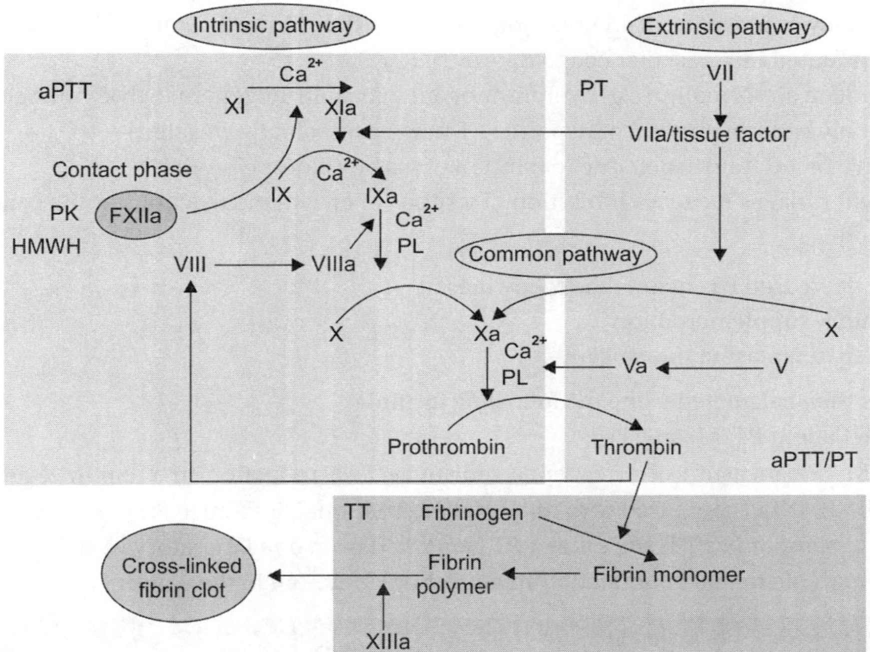

The prothrombin time is the time it takes plasma to clot after addition of tissue factor (obtained from animals such as rabbits, or recombinant tissue factor, or from brains of autopsy patients).

This measures the quality of the extrinsic pathway (as well as the common pathway) of coagulation. The speed of the extrinsic pathway is greatly affected by levels of functional factor VII in the body. Factor VII has a short half-life and the carboxylation of its glutamate residues requires vitamin K. The prothrombin time can be prolonged as a result of deficiencies in vitamin K, warfarin therapy, malabsorption, or lack of intestinal colonization by bacteria (such as in newborns). In addition, poor factor VII synthesis (due to liver disease) or increased consumption (in disseminated intravascular coagulation) may prolong the PT. In general, the prothrombin time is more sensitive to factor VII deficiency than factor deficiencies within the final common pathway.

- The reference range for prothrombin time is 9.5–13.5 seconds.
- The reference range for international normalized ratio (INR) is less than 1.3

- However, the normal range is highly variable and dependent on the laboratory performing the test.

Various conditions may prolong or shorten prothrombin time.

Causes of prolonged PT include the following:

- Warfarin use
- Vitamin K deficiency from malnutrition, biliary obstruction, malabsorption syndromes, or use of antibiotics
- Liver disease, due to diminished synthesis of clotting factors
- Deficiency or presence of an inhibitor to factors VII, X, II/prothrombin, V, or fibrinogen
- Disseminated intravascular coagulopathy (DIC)
- Fibrinogen abnormality (e.g. hypofibrinogenemia, afibrinogenemia, dysfibrinogenemia)
- After bolus administration of heparin (PT may be transiently elevated)
- Massive blood transfusion due to dilution of plasma clotting proteins
- Hypothermia, as it causes inhibition of a series of enzymatic reactions of the coagulation cascade

Causes of decreased PT include the following:

- Vitamin K supplementation
- Fresh frozen plasma transfusion

The INR is then calculated using the following formula:

- INR = $[\text{Patient PT}/\text{Mean PT}]^{ISI}$

The ISI is a measure of a reagent's sensitivity to a reduction in Vitamin K-dependent factors (II, VII, IX, X) compared with the WHO International Reference Preparation. The INR is intended to standardize PT, such that a PT generated from one laboratory would yield an INR value comparable to that generated from any other laboratory in the world.

Test	Possible conditions
Prolonged PT	Factor VII deficiency, early oral anticoagulation therapy
APTT	Deficiency of factors, VIII, IX, XI, XII, and prekallikrien, Von Willebrand disease, Lupus anticoagulant
Prolonged PT and APTT	Deficiency of factors V, X, II, oral anticoagulants, vitamin K deficiency, liver disease
Prolonged PT, APTT and TT	Fibrinogen deficiency/disorder, liver disease, heparin
Prolonged bleeding time or abnormal PFA result	Platelet function defect, Von Willebrand disease

12. Diagnostic criteria for Aplastic Anaemia include

a. Absolute neutrophil count < 500 / micro L
b. Platelet < 20,000 / micro L
c. Hb< 8 gm/dL
d. Bone marrow hypocellular, with no abnormal cells and no fibrosis
e. Absolute retic count <60 × 10^9/L

Ans. d

Option a	False	No, this is criteria for severe aplastic anemia
Option b	False	No, this is criteria for severe aplastic anemia
Option c	False	No, this is criteria for severe aplastic anemia
Option d	True	Yes correct, this is essential criteria for diagnosis of aplastic anemia
Option e	False	No, this is criteria for severe aplastic anemia

Diagnosis Criteria

- CBC, reticulocyte count
- Bone marrow examination
  - Bone marrow hypocellular, with no abnormal cells and no fibrosis.
  - At least 2 among the following:
    - Hb <10 g/dL
    - Platelet count <50 × 10^9/L
    - Absolute neutrophil count <1.5 × 10^9/L.

Severity Criteria

Severe AA

- Bone marrow cellularity <25% or cellularity <50% with <30% residual hematopoietic cells
- At least 2 among the following:
  - Absolute reticulocyte count <20 × 10^9/L (<60 × 10^9/L using an automated analysis)
  - Platelet count <20 × 10^9/L
  - Absolute neutrophil count <0.5 × 10^9/L (or 500 / microL)

Very Severe AA

- Absolute neutrophil count <0.2 × 10^9/L (or < 200/microL)
- AND fulfills rest of the criteria for severe AA

Non-severe AA

Patients not fulfilling the criteria for severe or very severe AA.

Treatment

- Hematopoietic stem cell transplantation is first-line therapy. It is curative and treatment of choice.
- If transplantation is not an option, immunosuppression with equine antithymocyte globulin and cyclosporine is given.

13. Adenomyosis features

a. Uterus is irregular and large
b. It is estrogen dependent
c. It is presence of ectopic endometrial gland outside the uterus
d. It is presence of endometrial gland within the muscle layer of uterus
e. Adenomyosis is premalignant condition

Ans. a,b,d

Option a	True	Yes, correct
Option b	True	Yes, correct
Option c	False	No, it is present inside the myometrium
Option d	True	Yes, correct
Option e	False	No, it is not pre-malignant

Adenomyosis is characterised by island of endometrial tissue within the myometrium resulting in tender boggy uterus.

- The diagnosis is formed by exclusion of other causes of dysmenorrhea.
- Histologic examination is confirmatory.

Endometriosis: endometrial tissue present outside the uterus.

14. True about Rett's syndrome is/are:

a. Perinatal microcephaly
b. Postnatal microcephaly
c. Normal brain development at birth
d. Regression starts at 5th to 30 months
e. Sensory features remains intact

Ans. b, c, d, e *(Ref: Judith P. Hudson, A Practical Guide to Congenital Developmental Disorders and Learning Difficulties: Routledge, 2014, pg 100)*

Option a	False	No, the new-born is usually normal at birth
Option b	True	Yes, correct, the child develops deceleration of head growth, most prominent in stage 2
Option c	True	Yes correct
Option d	True	Yes, correct
Option e	True	Yes, correct

Classic Rett syndrome is seen in girls who are normal at birth and achieve expected developmental milestones until reaching 6–18 months of age. These affected females then develop deceleration of head growth, leading to microcephaly, with a loss of acquired language, cognitive, social, and motor skills.

It involves a gene defect MeCP2 on the 'x' chromosome

Rett syndrome is most often misdiagnosed as autism, cerebral palsy, or nonspecific developmental delay

Stage 1 (6-18 months age)

- Early onset
- Delay in gross motor skills as crawling or walking
- Less eye contact

Stage 2 (1-4 years age)

- Rapid deterioration
- Loss of hand coordination, less speech
- Breath holding, hyperventilation spells

Stage 3 (2-10 years age)
- Slow/plateau phase
- Apraxia, seizures

Stage 4 (after 10 years of age)
- Late deterioration of gross motor skills
- Spine disorders as scoliosis +/- muscle rigidity
- Gait abnormalities to complete inability to walk

DSM V Criteria for Diagnosis

A. All of the following:
- Apparently normal prenatal and perinatal development
- Apparently normal psychomotor development through the first 5 months after birth
- Normal head circumference at birth

B. Onset of all of the following after the period of normal development:
- Deceleration of head growth between ages 5 and 48 months
- Loss of previously acquired purposeful hand skills between ages 5 and 30 months with the subsequent development of stereotyped hand movements (e.g., hand-wringing or hand washing)
- Loss of social engagement early in the course (although often social interaction develops later)
- Appearance of poorly coordinated gait or trunk movements
- Severely impaired expressive and receptive language development with severe psychomotor retardation.

15. Middle mediastinal mass could be due to:

a. Oesophageal cyst
b. Bronchogenic cyst
c. Thymomas
d. Pericardial cysts
e. Descending aorta aneurysm

Ans. a, b, d

Option a	True	Yes correct
Option b	True	Yes correct
Option c	False	No, it is an anterior mediastinum mass
Option d	True	Yes correct
Option e	False	No, it is posterior mediastinal mass

Masses in children
- Lymphadenopathy
- Fore gut duplication cysts
- Bronchogenic cysts
- Oesophageal duplication cysts
- Neurenteric cysts
- Cystic hygroma
- Hiatus hernia
- Achalasia

Masses in adults

- Lymph nodes
- Carcinoma of bronchus
- Bronchogenic cyst
- Aneurysm

DD for Mediastinal Masses

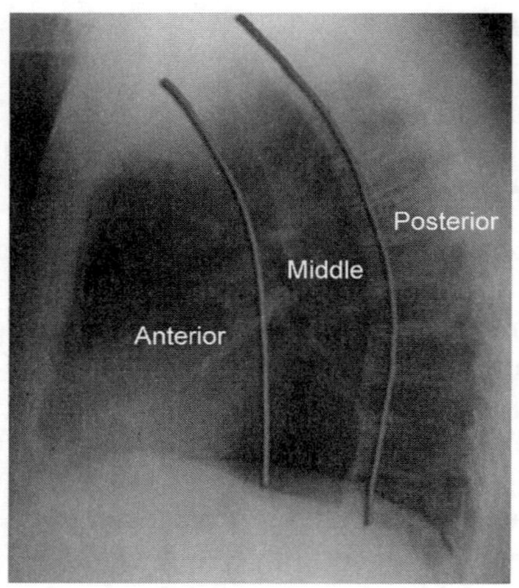

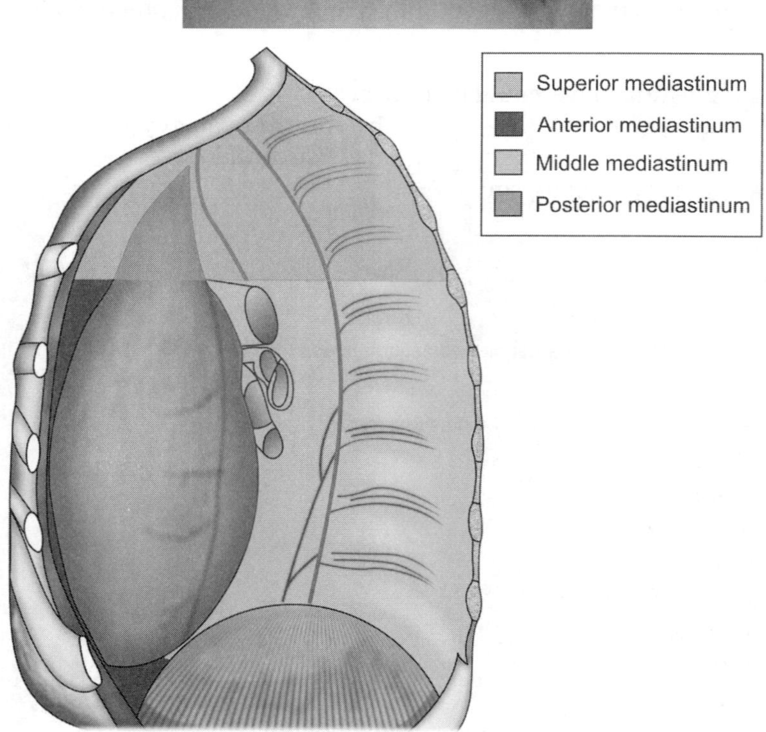

	Lesions	Fluid	Fat	Vascular
Anterior	Thymic Lymphoma Germ cell Goiter	Thymic C Thymoma Pericardial C Germ cell Lymphoma	Germ cell-b Thymolipoma Fat pad	Thyroid Cardiac Coronary
Middle	Lymph nodes Duplication C Arch anomaly	Duplication C Necrotic nodes Pericard recess Retroperitoneal	Lipoma Esophageal FV polyp	Arch anomaly Azygous vein Vascular nodes
Posterior	Neurogenic Bone and marrow	Neuroenteric C Schwannoma Meningocoele	Extramedullary Hematopoiesis	Desc aorta
>1 comp	Infection Hemorrhage Lung cancer	Lymphangioma Mediastinitis	Liposarcoma	Hemangioma

Statistically, it is important to remember the following:

- Most masses (> 60%) are:
  - Thymomas
  - Neurogenic tumors
  - Benign cysts
  - Lymphadenopathy (LAD)
- In children the most common (> 80%) are:
  - Neurogenic tumors
  - Germ cell tumors
  - Foregut cysts
- In adults the most common are:
  - Lymphomas
  - LAD
  - Thymomas
  - Thyroid masses

Remember

Anterior mediastinum: 5T's

T: Thymus

T: Thyroid

T: Thoracic aorta

T: Terrible lymphoma

T: Teratoma

16. Monogenetic disorder is/are:

a. Sickle cell disease
b. Marfans syndrome
c. Cystic fibrosis
d. Turner syndrome
e. Familial adenomatous polyposis

Ans. a, b, c, e

Option a	True	Yes, correct, its 11p defect
Option b	True	Yes, correct, its chromosome 15 defect (fibrillin protein gene defect)
Option c	True	Yes, correct, it is 7q defect
Option d	False	It is chromosomal defect (45, XO)
Option e	True	Yes, correct, it is defect in APC gene on chr 5q22.2

Some common gene defects asked in exams:

Disease	Gene mutated
Ataxia-telangiectasia syndrome	ATM
Bloom syndrome	RecQ2
Chédiak-Higashi syndrome	LSYT
Cowden syndrome	PTEN
Fanconi anemia	FANCA, FANCC, FANCG
Gardner syndrome	APC
Hereditary leiomyomatosis/renal cell cancer syndrome	Fumarate hydratase
Howel-Evans	TOC
Melanoma/pancreatic cancer syndrome	CDKN2A
Multiple mucosal neuroma syndrome (multiple endocrine neoplasia 2B, and 3 Howel-Evans)	RET protooncogene
Neurofibromatosis	NF1/NF2
Peutz-Jeghers syndrome	STK11/LKB1
Seckel syndrome	SCKL1, ATR, SCKL2, SCKL3, Pericentrin
Tuberous sclerosis	TSC1/TSC2
Werner syndrome	RecQ3

Disorder	Chromosome or gene	Type
Achondroplasia	4p16.3	S
Acute intermittent porphyria	HMBS	
Alkaptonuria	HGD	
Angelman syndrome	UBE3A	
Ataxia telangiectasia	ATM	
CADASIL syndrome	NOTCH3	P
CARASIL syndrome	HTRA1	
Cystic fibrosis	CFTR (7q31.2)	D or S
Charcot–Marie–Tooth disease	PMP22, MFN2	
Chédiak–Higashi syndrome	LYST	recessive
Cri du chat	5p	D

Contd...

Contd...

Disorder	Chromosome or gene	Type
Crohn's disease	16q12	P
Darier's disease	ATP2A2	
Denys–Drash syndrome	WT1	
Di George's syndrome	22q11.2	D
Fabry disease	GLA (Xq22.1)	P
Familial adenomatous polyposis	APC	
Friedreich's ataxia	FXN	
Galactosemia	GALT, GALK1, GALE	
Gaucher disease	GBA (1)	
Gillespie syndrome	PAX6	
Hailey-Hailey disease	ATP2C1 (3)	
Harlequin type ichthyosis	ABCA12	
Hemophilia		
Hepatoerythropoietic porphyria	UROD	
Hereditary coproporphyria	3q12	P
Huntington's disease	HD	T
Hunter syndrome	IDS	
Hurler syndrome	IDUA	
Hypochondroplasia	FGFR3 (4p16.3)	
Krabbe disease	GALC	
LCAT deficiency	LCAT	
Lesch-Nyhan syndrome	HPRT (X)	
Li-Fraumeni syndrome	TP53	
Marfan syndrome	15	dominant
Maroteaux–Lamy syndrome	ARSB	recessive
McCune–Albright syndrome	20 q13.2-13.3	
Microcephaly	ASPM (1q31)	P
Morquio syndrome	GALNS, GLB1	
Patau Syndrome (Trisomy 13)	(13)	trisomy
Porphyria cutanea tarda (PCT)	UROD	dominant
Pendred syndrome	PDS (7)	recessive
Peutz-Jeghers syndrome	STK11	dominant

Contd...

Contd...

Disorder	Chromosome or gene	Type
phenylketonuria	PAH	recessive
Prader-Willi syndrome	15	paternal imprinting
Rett syndrome	MECP2	dominant, often de novo
sickle cell anemia	11p15	P
Tay-Sachs disease	HEXA (15)	recessive
Turner syndrome	X	monosomy
von Hippel-Lindau disease	VHL	dominant
Williams syndrome	chromosome 7	dominant
Wilson disease	ATP7B	recessive
Xeroderma pigmentosum	15 ERCC4	
X-linked severe combined immunodeficiency(X-SCID)	X	

A few, mutation types:

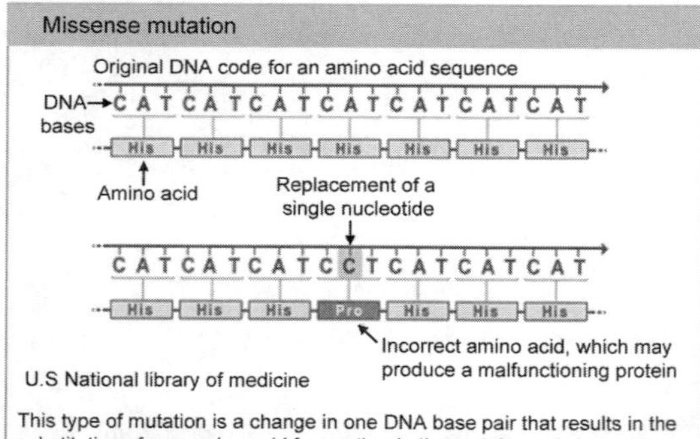

U.S National library of medicine

This type of mutation is a change in one DNA base pair that results in the substitution of one amino acid for another in the protein made by a gene

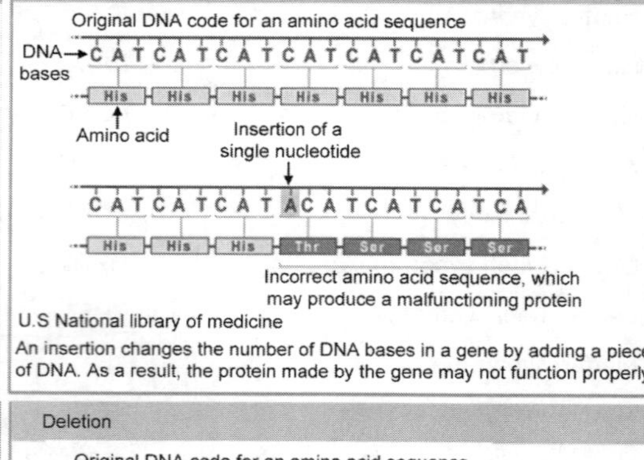

U.S National library of medicine

An insertion changes the number of DNA bases in a gene by adding a piece of DNA. As a result, the protein made by the gene may not function properly

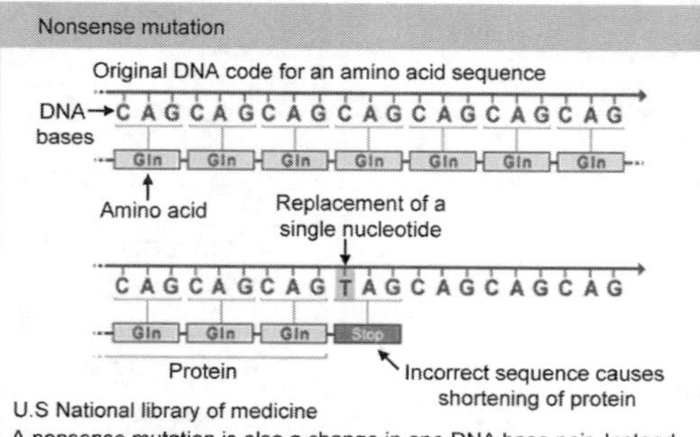

U.S National library of medicine

A nonsense mutation is also a change in one DNA base pair. Instead of sub sttuting one amino acid for another, howver, the altered DNA sequence prematurely signals the cell to stop building a protien. This type of mutation results in a shortened protein that may function improperly or not at all

Deletion

Original DNA code for an amino acid sequence

DNA bases

C A T C A T C A T C A T C A T C A T C A T

His His His His His His His

Amino acid

Deletion of a single nucleotide (A)

C A T C A T C A T C T C A T C A T C A T C

His His His Leu Ile Ile Ile

Incorrect amino acid sequence, which may produce a malfunctioning protein

U.S National library of medicine

A deletion changes the number of DNA bases by removing a piece of DNA. Small deletions may remove one or a few base pairs within a gene, shile larger deletions can remove an entire gene or several neighboring genes. The deleted DNA may alter the function of the resulting protein(s)

Repeat expansion

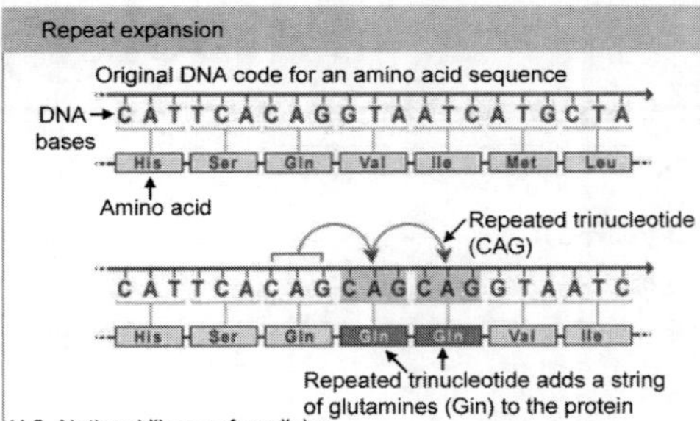

U.S. National library of medicine

Nucleotide repeats are short DNA sequences that are repeated a number of times in a row. For example, a trinucleotide repeat is made up of 3-base-pair sequences, and a tetranucleotide repaeat is made up of 4-base-pair sequences. A repeat expansion is a mutation that increases the number of time sthat the shor DNA sequence is repeated.This type of mutation can cause the resulting protein to function improperly

Frameshift mutation

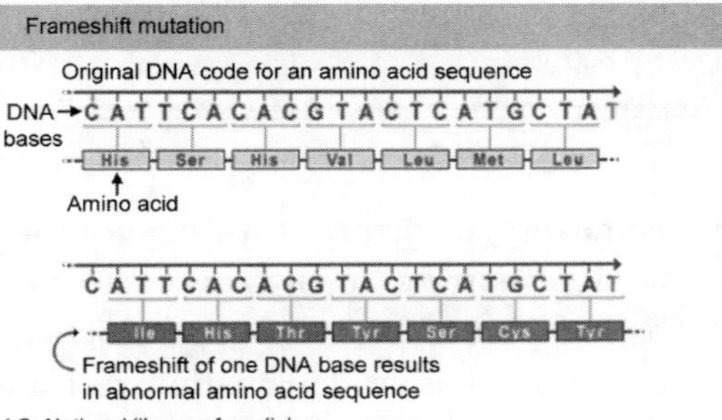

U.S. National library of medicine

This type of mutation occurs when the addition or loss of DNA bases changes a gene's reading frame. A reading frame consists of groups of 3 base that each code for one amino acid. A frameshift mutation shifts the grouping of these bases and changes the code for amino acids. The resulting protein is usually nonfunctional. Insertions, deletions, and duplications can all be frameshift mutations

Pathology

1. **Feature(s) of chronic myelogenous leukemia (CML):**
   a. Bone narrow biopsy is necessary for diagnosis
   b. Presence of BCR-ABL gene which directs the synthesis of BCR-ABL tyrosine kinase
   c. Dasatinib is used in imatinib resistant cases
   d. Generalized painful lymphadenopathy is presenting feature in most cases
   e. Myeloblasts usually constitute more than 10% of all white cells in most cases

Ans. b, c *Ref: Concepts in Pathology, Devesh Mishra, 3rd/ed, p 335*

Option a	False	Histopathological findings of peripheral blood smear are required
Option b	True	
Option c	True	
Option d	False	No peripheral lymph node enlargement
Option e	False	Myeloblasts are less than 10% of the total circulating cells

Chronic myelogenous/Myeloid leukemia (CML):

- Neoplasm of pluripotent hematopoietic stem cells leading to preferential proliferation of granulocytic progenitors.
- Presence of active BCR-ABL tyrosine kinase.
- ***Philadelphia chromosome*** is formed due to translocation of ABL gene from chromosome 9 q to BCR gene on chromosome 22 q. The resultant BCR-ABL gene forms 210-kD fusion protein with tyrosine kinase activity.

Clinical features:

- Affects mostly adults from 50–60 years of age.
- Splenomegaly.
- No peripheral lymph node enlargement.
- Sudden, painful enlargement of lymph node in a known case of CML suggests blast crisis.

Diagnosis: Based on the histopathologic findings in the peripheral blood and the Philadelphia (Ph1) chromosome in bone marrow cells.

- *Peripheral smear* shows leukocytosis (> 100,000 cells).
- Blast cells are usually less than 10% of the total circulating cells.
- Leukocyte alkaline phosphatase stains score very low to absent in most cells (except for accelerated phase and blast crisis), due to decreased apoptosis of mature neutrophils or granulocytes. Hence, the cells are long-lived with low or absent enzymes.
- *Bone marrow* is hypercellular, with presence of sea-blue histiocytes (pseudo-Gaucher cells).
- Hyperuricemia.
- Elevated serum vitamin B-12–binding protein (TC-I).

Treatment:

Imatinib mesylate 400 mg per day orally, inhibits proliferation and induces apoptosis in cells positive for BCR/ABL.

Newer BCR/ABL inhibitors, *dasatinib, nilotinib,* and *bosutinib* are more potent inhibitors of BCR/ABL than imatinib. Moreover, they exhibit significant activity against all resistant mutations except the BCR/ABL/T315I mutation.

2. True about caspases:

a. Caspases initiate apoptosis by extrinsic and intrinsic pathway
b. Caspases are protease enzyme
c. Caspases are receptor molecules
d. Caspases inhibit apoptosis and inflammation
e. Causes non enzymatic degradation of critical cellular components

Ans. a, b *Ref: Concepts in Pathology, Devesh Mishra, 3rd/ed; Robbins, 9th/ed*

Option	Answer	Explanation
Option a	True	
Option b	True	
Option c	False	Family of aspartate-specific, cysteine proteases, primary mediators of apoptosis
Option d	False	Primary mediators of apoptosis and inflammation
Option e	False	Activate endonuclease for nuclear DNA breakdown into internucleosomal fragments

- Caspases are a family of aspartate-specific, cysteine proteases that serve as the primary mediators of apoptosis.
- Caspases involved in apoptosis have been subclassified by their mechanism of action and are either initiator caspases (caspase-8 and -9) or executioner caspases (caspase-3, -6, and -7).

Initiation caspase:

- Most apoptotic programs fall into either the extrinsic or intrinsic category.

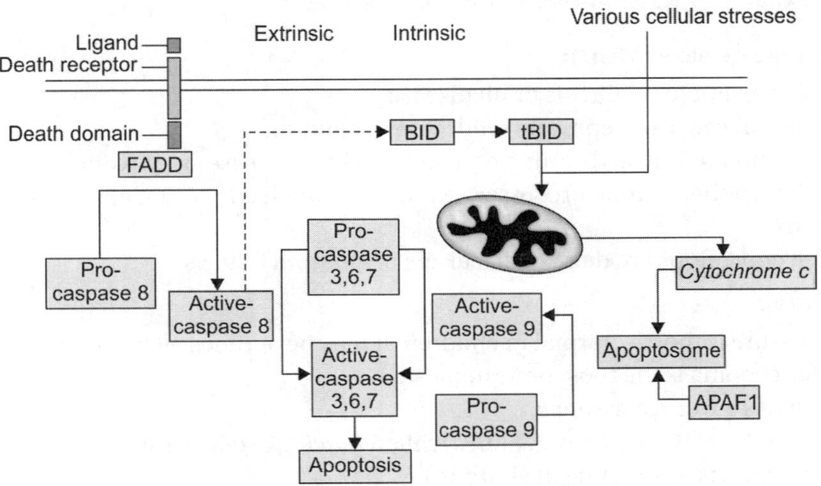

Fig. 1: Extrinsic and intrinsic pathways of apoptosis.

- The extrinsic apoptosis pathway (also known as Death Receptor pathway) is activated through the binding of a ligand to a death receptor, which in turn leads, with the help of the adapter proteins (FADD/TRADD), to recruitment, dimerization, and activation of caspase-8.
- Active caspase-8 then either initiates apoptosis directly by cleaving and thereby activating executioner caspase (–3, –6, –7), or activates the intrinsic apoptotic pathway through cleavage of BID to induce efficient cell death.
- The intrinsic or mitochondrial apoptosis pathway can be activated through various cellular stresses that lead to cytochrome c release from the mitochondria and the formation of the apoptosome, comprised of APAF1, cytochrome c, ATP, and caspase-9, resulting in the activation of caspase-9. Active caspase-9 then initiates apoptosis by cleaving and thereby activating executioner caspases.

Execution caspase:

- Initiator caspase (C-9 and C-8) activate executioner caspases (C3, 6, 7).
- Caspases activate endonuclease and induce double stranded breaks in DNA.

3. True about minimal change disease:

a. Most common cause of nephritic syndrome in adults
b. Hypertension is commonly present in children
c. Highly responsive to steroids
d. Reversible loss of podocyte function
e. Commonly progress to chronic renal failure

Ans. c, d *Ref: Concepts in Pathology, Devesh Mishra, 3rd/ed; Robbins 9th/ed*

Option a	False	Most common cause of nephrotic syndrome in children
Option b	False	Absent/rare
Option c	True	Dramatic response
Option d	True	Reversible loss
Option e	False	No chronic sequel. Excellent prognosis

Minimal change disease (MCD):

- Also known as lipoid nephrosis or nil disease.
- Most common cause of nephrotic syndrome in children.
- MCD is postulated as a disorder of T cells, which release a cytokine that injures the glomerular epithelial foot processes, which in turn leads to a decreased synthesis of polyanions.
- When the polyanions are damaged, leakage of albumin follows.

Clinical features:

- Blood pressure is mostly normal in children, it may be at times elevated in adults.
- Dependent edema is the most prominent sign.
- The retina has a wet appearance.
- Subungual edema with horizontal lines (called *Muehrcke lines*) also may occur.
- Heavy proteinuria (consisting of albumin).
- Dramatic response to corticosteroid therapy.

Diagnosis:

- In children, the critical level for diagnosis is proteinuria of more than 40 mg/h/m^2.
- A 24-hour urine measurement should be obtained for protein and creatinine clearance.
- Immunofluorescence shows no immune deposits.
- Light microscopy shows normal glomeruli.
- Electron microscopy shows retraction of the epithelial foot processes.

4. Feature(s) of Adult polycystic kidney disease is/are:

a. Renal enlargement
b. Small kidney
c. Spider leg deformity on intravenous urography
d. Ultrasound shows multiple cysts
e. Berry aneurysms

Ans. a, c, d, e *Ref: Concepts in Pathology, Devesh Mishra, 3rd/ed; Robbins 9th/ed*

Option a	True	
Option b	False	Large multicystic kidneys
Option c	True	
Option d	True	
Option e	True	

Adult polycystic kidney disease:

- Inherited as Autosomal dominant disease.
- Adult AD-PKD is universally bilateral in occurrence.
- Main feature is a bilateral progressive increase in the number of cysts, which may lead to End Stage Renal Disease.

Pathogenesis:

- Caused by 2 mutations:
  1. PKD1 mutations (chromosome 16 p 13.3)
  - This account for about **85%** of cases.
  - PKD1 encodes **polycystin-1 protein** that localizes to tubular epithelial cells and usually involved in cell-cell and cell-matrix interactions.

  2. PKD2 mutations (chromosome 4q21)
  - They are responsible for 15% of cases.
  - PKD2 encodes **polycystin-2** protein (a cation channel).
  - Its mutation can derange the regulation of intracellular calcium.

Investigations:

- Ultrasonography is the procedure of choice and shows multiple cysts.
- CT, MRI, Magnetic resonance angiography can be done in selected cases.
- MRI is the best imaging tool for monitoring kidney size after treatment to assess progress.
- Intravenous urography shows spider leg deformity, diagnostic only in advanced-stage ADPKD when distortion of calyces has developed.

Cystic diseases of kidney				
Disease	***Inheritance***	***Pathology***	***Clinical features***	***Outcome***
1. **Adult polycystic**[Q] **kidney disease**[Q] **(APKD)**	Autosomal dominant Berry's aneurysms	Large multicystic kidneys, **liver cysts**[Q]	Hematuria UTI, renal stones, hypertension	Chronic renal failure begins at **40–60 yrs**[Q]
2. Childhood polycystic kidney disease	Autosomal recessive	Enlarged cystic kidney at birth	**Hepatic fibrosis**[Q]	Variable outcome death in infancy or childhood
3. **Medullary sponge**[Q] **kidney**[Q]	None	**Medullary cysts**[Q]	• Hematuria • Urinary tract infection • **Recurrent renal stones**[Q]	Benign
4. **Familial juvenile**[Q] **nephronophthisis**[Q]	Autosomal recessive	Corticomedullary cysts, Shrunken kidneys	• **Salt wasting polyuria**[Q] • Growth retardation	Progressive renal failure beginning in childhood and anemia
5. **Adult onset medullary cystic disease**[Q]	Autosomal dominant	• **Corticomedullary cysts**[Q]	• **Salt wasting**[Q] • Polyuria • Shrunken kidneys	Chronic renal failure beginning in adulthood
6. Multicystic renal dysplasia	None	• Irregular kidneys with variable sized cysts	Associated with other renal anomalies	• Unilateral is curable • Bilateral will have renal failure

Ref: Concepts in Pathology, Devesh Mishra, 3/e

5. True about proliferative phase of wound healing:

a. Neutrophils increases gradually
b. Macrophage increases gradually
c. Collagen type I present predominantly
d. Collagen type III present predominantly
e. Angiogenesis occurs

Ans. b, d, e *Ref: Concepts in Pathology, Devesh Mishra, 3rd/ed; Robbins 9th/ed*

Option a	False	Neutrophil count decreases
Option b	True	Macrophages replace neutrophils
Option c	False	Collagen Type I predominates in Maturation Phase
Option d	True	Collagen Type III predominates in Proliferation Phase
Option e	True	Neovascularization occurs

Wound healing is divided into 3 or 4 phases:

1. Hemostasis:

a. Starts within the very first moments of the injury.
b. Platelets play a role by aggregating, as well as by releasing cytokines, chemokines, and hormones.

c. Vasoconstriction.
d. Clot formation.
e. Chemokines released by platelet activation attract inflammatory cells to the area.

2. **Inflammatory phase:**
   a. Migration of inflammatory cells to the site of injury by increasing vascular permeability.
   b. More persistent period of vasodilation mediated by histamine, prostaglandins, kinins, and leukotrienes.
   c. Neutrophils are the predominant cell type for the first 48 hours after injury.
   d. T lymphocytes migrate into the wound during the inflammatory phase, approximately 72 hours following injury.
3. **Proliferative phase:**
   a. Formation of granulation tissue is a central event during the proliferative phase. Its formation occurs 3–5 days following injury and overlaps with the preceding inflammatory phase.
   b. Granulation tissue includes *inflammatory cells, proliferative fibroblasts*, and *neovasculature* in a matrix of fibronectin, collagen, glycosaminoglycans, and proteoglycans.
   c. The synthesis and deposition of collagen is a critical event in the proliferative phase.
   d. Collagen is secreted to the extracellular space in the form of procollagen. This form is then cleaved of its terminal segments and called tropocollagen. Tropocollagen can aggregate with other tropocollagen molecules to form collagen filaments.
   e. Type III collagen is the primary component of early granulation tissue.
   f. Angiogenesis results in greater blood flow to the wound and, consequently, increased perfusion of healing factors.
4. **Maturation phase:**
   a. Myofibroblasts allow wound contraction. Simultaneously, collagen deposits around to form the scar tissue.
   b. Collagen becomes increasingly organized.
   c. Type III collagen is replaced by type I collagen.
   d. Intramolecular and intermolecular collagen cross-links result in increased wound bursting strength.

6. Correct match of stain with tissue is/are:

a. Perls' Prussian blue-iron in tissue
b. von Kossa-collagen
c. Masson's trichrome-connective tissue
d. PAS-glycogen
e. PAS-Acidic and neutral mucin

Ans. a, c, d *Ref: Concepts in Pathology, Devesh Mishra, 3rd/ed; Robbins 9th/ed*

Option a	True	
Option b	False	von Kossa is for Calcification
Option c	True	
Option d	True	
Option e	False	PAS is for glycogen

Perls' Prussian blue iron (Liver): This stain is used to detect and identify ferric (Fe^{3+}) iron in tissue preparations, blood smears, or bone marrow smears.

Minute amounts of ferric iron (hemosiderin) are commonly found in bone marrow and in the spleen. Abnormal amounts of iron can indicate hemochromatosis and hemosiderosis.

von Kossa stain (Calcium): A silver reduction method that demonstrates phosphates and carbonates, but these are usually present along with calcium. This stain is most useful when large amounts are present, as in bone.

Masson's trichrome (skin): This stain is intended for use in histological observation of collagenous connective tissue fibers in tissue specimens.

It is used to assist in differentiating collagen and smooth muscle in tumors and assists in the detection of diseases or changes in connective/muscle tissue.

Periodic Acid Schiff (PAS) (Kidney): PAS staining is mainly used for staining structures containing a high proportion of carbohydrates such as glycogen, glycoproteins, proteoglycans typically found in connective tissues, mucus and basement membranes.

Often used to stain kidney biopsies, liver biopsies, certain glycogen storage diseases in striated muscles and suspected fungal infections.

7. **True about Fat necrosis in the breast is/are:**
    a. Mostly due to trauma
    b. Decreased incidence in lactating
    c. FNAC differentiates from carcinoma
    d. It can present as a painless mass
    e. Nipple retraction

Ans. a, d, e *Ref: Concepts in Pathology, Devesh Mishra, 3rd/ed; Robbins 9th/ed*

Option a	True	
Option b	False	Unrelated to lactation
Option c	False	Needle core biopsy is required to rule out malignancy
Option d	True	
Option e	True	

- Fat necrosis in breast may result from *surgical trauma, radiation*, or *incidental trauma.*
- Characterized histologically by *foamy histiocytes, lipid-laden macrophages*, inflammatory cells with *peripheral fibrosis* and *necrosis.*
- Clinically, it may produce a *superficial painless mass* with skin retraction that may be difficult to distinguish from recurrent carcinoma in patients who have undergone surgery and radiation therapy.
- It may be associated with ecchymosis, erythema, inflammation, pain, skin retraction or thickening, *nipple retraction* and lymphadenopathy simulating carcinoma
- Sections show disruption of fat, lipid-laden macrophages, chronic inflammation and *foreign body giant cell reaction.*
- Hemosiderin deposition may also be seen.
- In late stages, fibrosis, calcifications, and *squamous metaplasia* may ensue.
- A *biopsy* is usually required to distinguish fat necrosis from carcinoma.

Diagnosis:

- *Fine needle aspiration cytology (FNAC)*- high sensitivity and specificity—87% and 99%, respectively.

- ❑ *Needle core biopsy* is required to rule out malignancy.
- ❑ Imaging techniques such as Mammography, Ultrasonography, MRI, etc. can show findings pertaining to fat necrosis.

8. Features of hemolytic anemia include:

a. Raised indirect bilirubin
b. Raised direct bilirubin
c. Hemoglobinuria seen in intravascular hemolysis
d. Increased bilirubin in the urine
e. Raised urobilinogen

Ans. a, c, e *Ref: Concepts in Pathology, Devesh Mishra, 3rd/ed; Robbins 9th/ed*

Option a	True	
Option b	False	Raised indirect bilirubin
Option c	True	
Option d	False	Hemoglobinuria may be seen
Option e	True	

Hemolytic anemia:

- ❑ Premature destruction of RBCs.
- ❑ Elevated erythropoietin levels with increased erythropoiesis.
- ❑ Increased hemoglobin catabolites.
- ❑ Hemolysis in hemolytic anemia could be extravascular or intravascular.
  - ■ Extravascular hemolysis
    - It occurs in macrophages of spleen.
    - **Clinical features:**
      - ♦ Anemia, splenomegaly and jaundice.
      - ♦ Mild decrease in haptoglobin (a serum protein that binds hemoglobin).
  - ■ **Intravascular hemolysis**
    - **It will show:**
      - ♦ Anemia, hemoglobinemia, hemoglobinuria, hemosiderinuria, and jaundice.
      - ♦ Severe decrease in serum haptoglobin.
      - ♦ Free hemoglobin can be oxidized to methemoglobin.

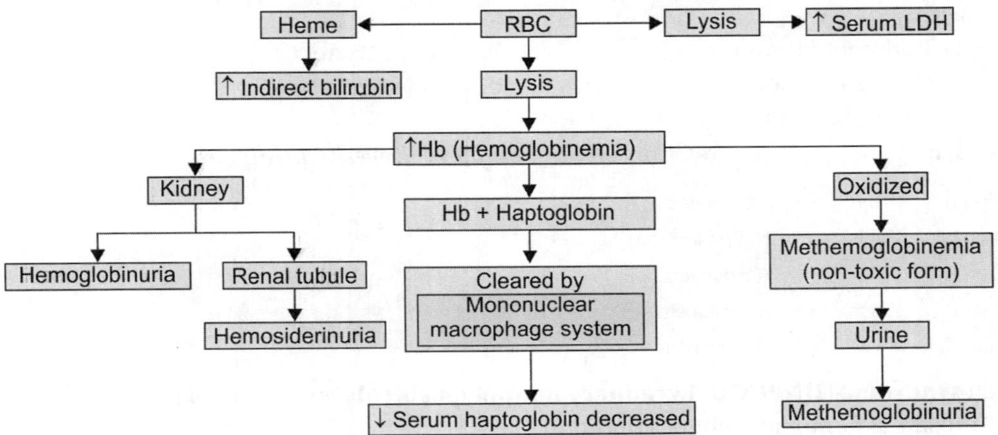

9. True about Creutzfeldt-Jakob disease:

a. Gliosis in thalamus
b. Spongiform swelling in cerebral cortex
c. Brain atrophy in late stage
d. Slow and irregular background rhythm on EEG
e. Inflammation invariably present

Ans. a, b, c *Ref: Concepts in Pathology, Devesh Mishra, 3rd/ed; Robbins 9th/ed*

Option a	True	
Option b	True	
Option c	True	
Option d	False	In early stages, EEG is normal. At later stages, Periodic sharp waves on EEG
Option e	False	Inflammation is absent

Creutzfeldt-Jakob disease (CJD):

- Rapidly progressive, fatal neurodegenerative disorder believed to be caused by an abnormal isoform of a cellular glycoprotein known as the prion protein.
- A distinctive finding in a subacute, progressive dementia.
- EEG may be normal early in the course of CJD.
- At the point of evolution of clinically overt myoclonus, periodic sharps appear, at times subtle or confined to a focal region (especially posteriorly); but with full-blown dementia and myoclonus, periodic sharp waves of 1- to 2-Hz frequency appear in a generalized distribution.
- Spongiform change seen in the frontal cortex.
- Gliosis and neuronal loss throughout the frontal cortex, basal ganglia, thalamus, peri-aqueductal gray matter and tectum of the mid brain, pontine nuclei and dorsal medulla but no evidence of inflammation.
- Extensive atrophy and gliosis of the cerebellar cortex with widespread loss of neurons from the internal granular layer but relative sparing of Purkinje cells.

10. Hereditary non-polyposis colorectal cancer (HNPCC) is/are commonly associated with:

a. Endometrial cancer
b. Cervical cancer
c. Ovarian cancer
d. Breast cancer
e. Thyroid cancer

Ans. a, c *Ref: Concepts in Pathology, Devesh Mishra, 3rd/ed; Robbins 9th/ed*

Option a	True	Associated
Option b	False	Not associated
Option c	True	Associated
Option d	False	Not associated
Option e	False	Not associated

Lynch syndrome (**HNPCC** or **hereditary nonpolyposis colorectal cancer**)

- Autosomal dominant genetic condition that has a high risk of colon cancer.

- ❑ Increased risk of other cancers including endometrial cancer (second most common), ovary, stomach, small intestine, hepatobiliary tract, upper urinary tract, brain, and skin.
- ❑ The increased risk for these cancers is due to inherited mutations that impair DNA mismatch repair.
- ❑ It is a type of cancer syndrome.

11. Feature of non-bacterial thrombotic endocarditis (NBTE):

a. Common is SLE
b. Present on undersurface of valve
c. Vegetative growth is large and loosely attached to valve
d. May occur after post-cardiac catheterization
e. Source of systemic emboli

Ans. a, b, d, e *Ref: Concepts in Pathology, Devesh Mishra, 3rd/ed; Robbins, 9th/ed*

Option a	True	
Option b	True	
Option c	False	Vegetative growth is tiny to large mass
Option d	True	
Option e	True	

Non-bacterial thrombotic endocarditis:

- ❑ Also known as *Libman-Sacks endocarditis.*
- ❑ Characterized by endocardial vegetations made up of accumulations of sterile blood platelets and fibrin which do not usually involve inflammatory responses.
- ❑ Are typically small, friable, white or tan masses.
- ❑ < 1 cm in diameter.
- ❑ Broad based and irregular.
- ❑ Most commonly involves the mitral and aortic valves, usually along lines of valve closure on leaflets, which may be normal or previously damaged.
- ❑ Valvular abnormalities occur as masses (classic Libman-Sacks vegetations), diffuse leaflet thickening, valvular regurgitation, and, infrequently, stenosis.
- ❑ Vary from tiny lesions to large and exuberant masses.
- ❑ More frequent in patients with connective tissue and autoimmune diseases and rheumatic heart disease. Most common association is with systemic lupus erythematosus *(SLE).*
- ❑ In SLE, usually involves *undersurface* of valve.
- ❑ High incidence of accompanying embolic events.
- ❑ Prognosis dependent on the underlying disease activity of SLE and associated renal and myocardial dysfunction.

12. True about Alzheimer's disease:

a. Most common cause of dementia in elderly
b. Unusual before 45 years of age
c. Plaques consists of tau protein
d. May have family history
e. Short term memory is affected less than long-term memory

Ans. a, b, d *Ref: Concepts in Pathology, Devesh Mishra, 3rd/ed; Robbins 9th/ed*

Option a	True	
Option b	True	
Option c	False	Neurofibrillary tangles are hyperphosphorylated tau protein
Option d	True	
Option e	False	Short term memory is the first one to get affected

Alzheimer's disease:

- Most common cause of dementia among ***elderly.***
- Cortical atrophy with narrowed gyri and widened sulci in frontal, temporal and parietal lobes.
- Earliest sites involved are ***medial temporal lobe structures*** (hippocampus, entorhinal cortex and amygdala).
- Neuritic plaques are a non-specific finding and contain ***beta amyloid protein.***
- Increased number of neuritic plaques correlate with advanced age and severity of dementia.
- Neurofibrillary tangles are ***hyperphosphorylated tau protein***, seen in other dementias as well.
- Number of increased NFT correlates severity of dementia.
- Cerebral Amyloid Angiopathy—accompanies alzheimer's disease, showing *granulovacuolar degeneration.* ***Hirano bodies***, composed of actin are seen.
- Alzheimer's does not affect all memory capacities equally:
  - ***Short-term memory*** (the ability to hold information in mind in an active, readily-available state for a short period of time) is the first to go;
  - Next comes ***episodic memory*** (memory of autobiographical events);
  - Then ***semantic memory*** (memory of the meanings of words and facts about the world); and
  - Finally ***procedural memory*** (how to perform tasks and skills).
  - As the disease advances, parts of memory which were previously intact also become impaired, and eventually all reasoning, attention, and language abilities are disrupted.

13. Negri bodies in animal can be best seen in:

a. Hippocampus
b. Basal ganglia
c. Cerebral cortex
d. Cerebellum
e. Thalamus

Ans. a *Ref: Concepts in Pathology, Devesh Mishra, 3rd/ed; Robbins 9th/ed*

Option a	True	
Option b	False	
Option c	False	
Option d	False	
Option e	False	

Rabies:

- Rabies is a severe encephalitis transmitted by the bite of a rabid animal.
- After **1 to 3 months**[Q] the virus ascends from the wound site to the CNS along the peripheral nerves. It causes extraordinary CNS excitability, **hydrophobia** and **flaccid paralysis**.
- Death occurs due to **respiratory center failure**[Q].
- Widespread neuronal necrosis and inflammation are present.
- Most severe affected areas are **basal ganglia, midbrain**[Q]**, and medulla**[Q].
- Pathognomonic **Negri bodies**[Q] **(intracytoplasmic eosinophilic inclusions)** are found in **hippocampal pyramidal cells and Purkinje cells** without associated inflammation.

Negri bodies are eosinophilic, sharply outlined, pathognomonic inclusion bodies (2–10 μm in diameter) found in the cytoplasm of certain nerve cells containing the virus of rabies, especially in pyramidal cells within Ammon's horn of the hippocampus.

They are also often found in the purkinje cells of the cerebellar cortex from postmortem brain samples of rabies victims.

They consist of ribonuclear proteins produced by the virus.

They are named for Adelchi Negri.

14. True about p53:

a. Has tyrosine kinase activity
b. Has pro-apoptotic activity
c. Tumor suppressor gene
d. Has anti-apoptotic activity
e. p53 gene is located on chromosome 21

Ans. b, c *Ref: Robbins 9th/ed; http://www.bioinformatics.org/p53/introduction/html*

Option a	False	Important role in cell cycle control and apoptosis
Option b	True	
Option c	True	
Option d	False	Important role in cell cycle control and apoptosis
Option e	False	Located on the seventeenth chromosome (17p13.1)

- ***p53, also known as TP53 or tumor protein (EC: 2.7.1.37)*** is a gene that codes for a protein that regulates the cell cycle and hence functions as a *tumor suppression.*
- P53 has been described as "the guardian of the genome", referring to its role in conserving stability by preventing genome mutation.
- The name is due to its molecular mass: it is in the 53 kilodalton fraction of cell proteins.
- The human p53 gene is located on the seventeenth chromosome (17p13.1).
- It consists of four units (or domains):
  - A domain that activates transcription factors.
  - A domain that recognizes specific DNA sequences (core domain).
  - A domain that is responsible for the tetramerization of the protein.
  - A domain that recognized damaged DNA, such as misaligned base pairs or single-stranded DNA.
- It plays an important role in cell cycle control and *apoptosis.*

15. Cause(s) of non-megaloblastic macrocytic anemia:

a. Folate deficiency
b. Lead toxicity
c. Hypothyroidism
d. Liver disease
e. Vit B12 deficiency

Ans. c, d *Ref: Concepts in Pathology, Devesh Mishra, 3rd/ed; Robbins 9th/ed*

Option a	False	Megaloblastic anemia
Option b	False	Hypochromic/hemolytic anemia
Option c	True	
Option d	True	
Option e	False	Megaloblastic anemia

Causes of non-megaloblastic macrocytic anemia are not related to defective DNA synthesis. Non-megaloblastic macrocytic anemia is less common and is characterized by the absence of megaloblasts, and instead, the presence of mature but large red blood cells.

Non-megaloblastic cause of macrocytic anemia are:

- Hypothyroidism
- Liver disease
- Alcoholism
- Aplastic anemia.

16. Which of the following is not classified as Primitive neuroectodermal tumor (PNET)?

a. Neuroblastoma
b. Medulloblastoma
c. Rhabdomyosarcoma
d. Ewing sarcoma
e. Carcinoid tumor

Ans. a, b, c, e *Ref: Concepts in Pathology, Devesh Mishra, 3rd/ed; Robbins 9th/ed*

Option a	True	Tumors derived from the autonomic nervous system (PNET)
Option b	True	
Option c	True	
Option d	False	Ewing's sarcoma is PNET
Option e	True	

Primitive neuroectodermal tumors (PNETs):

- Are a group of highly malignant tumors composed of small round cells of neuroectodermal origin that affect soft tissue and bone.
- CNS primitive neuroectodermal tumors (PNETs)—Tumors derived from the central nervous system.
- Neuroblastoma—Tumors derived from the autonomic nervous system.
- Peripheral primitive neuroectodermal tumors (pPNETs)—Tumors derived from tissues outside the central and autonomic nervous system.
- The following tumors are classified as peripheral primitive neuroectodermal tumors (pPNETs):
  - Ewing sarcoma (osseous and extraosseous).
  - Malignant peripheral primitive neuroectodermal tumors (pPNETs) or peripheral neuroepithelioma of bone and soft tissues.

- Askin tumor (peripheral neuroepithelioma of the thoracopulmonary region).
- Other less common tumors (e.g. neuroectodermal tumor, ectomesenchymoma, peripheral medulloepithelioma).

17. Glucose level in CSF is/are reduced in:

a. Bacterial meningitis
b. Fungal meningitis
c. Viral meningitis
d. Tubercular meningitis
e. Multiple sclerosis

Ans. a, b, d *Ref: Concepts in Pathology, Devesh Mishra, 3rd/ed; Robbins 9th/ed* [Lumbar Puncture (LP) Interpretation of Cerebrospinal Fluid; Gil Z Shlamovitz].

Option a	True	Low CSF Glucose levels
Option b	True	Low CSF Glucose levels
Option c	False	Normal CSF Glucose levels
Option d	True	Low CSF Glucose levels
Option e	False	Normal CSF Glucose levels

Cerebrospinal fluid analysis:

1. **Normal results in adults**
   Appearance: Clear
   Opening pressure: 10–20 cm H_2O
   WBC count: 0–5 cells/μL [< 2 polymorphonucleocytes (PMN); normal cell counts do not rule out meningitis or any other pathology]
   Glucose level: > 60% of serum glucose
   Protein level: < 45 mg/dL.
2. **Bacterial meningitis**
   Appearance: Clear, cloudy, or purulent
   Opening pressure: Elevated (> 25 cm H_2O)
   WBC count: > 100 cells/μL (> 90% PMN); partially treated cases may have as low as 1 WBC/μL
   Glucose level: Low (< 40% of serum glucose)
   Protein level: Elevated (> 50 mg/dL).
3. **Aseptic (viral) meningitis**
   Appearance: Clear
   Opening pressure: Normal or elevated
   WBC count: 10–1000 cells/μL (lymph but PMN early)
   Glucose level: > 60% serum glucose (may be low in HSV infection)
   Protein level: Elevated (> 50 mg/dL).
4. **Fungal meningitis**
   Appearance: Clear or cloudy
   Opening pressure: Elevated
   WBC count: 10–500 cells/μL
   Glucose level: Low
   Protein level: Elevated.

5. **Tuberculosis**
   Appearance: Clear or opaque
   Opening pressure: Elevated
   WBC count: 50–500 cells/μL (early PMN then lymph)
   Glucose level: Low
   Protein level: Elevated.
6. **Multiple sclerosis**
   Appearance: Clear
   Opening pressure: Normal
   WBC count: 0–20 cells/μL (lymph)
   Glucose level: Normal
   Protein level: Mildly elevated (45–75 mg/dL).
7. **Guillain-Barré syndrome**
   Appearance: Clear or xanthochromia
   Opening pressure: Normal or elevated
   WBC count: Normal or elevated
   Glucose level: Normal
   Protein level: Elevated.

18. Which of the following acute phase reactants decrease in inflammation?

a. Fibrinogen
b. C-reactive protein
c. Transferrin
d. Albumin
e. Antithrombin.

Ans. c, d, e *Ref: Concepts in Pathology, Devesh Mishra, 3rd/ed; Robbins 9th/ed*

Option a	False	Increase
Option b	False	Increase
Option c	True	Decrease
Option d	True	Decrease
Option e	True	Decrease

Positive acute phase proteins: Proteins which increase by 25% of normal level in response to inflammation.

Negative acute phase proteins: Proteins which decrease by 25% of normal level in response to inflammation.

Positive acute phase proteins	Negative acute phase proteins
C-reactive protein	Albumin
Highly sensitive CRP	Prealbumin
Fibrinogen	Transferrin
Plasminogen activator inhibitor	Insulin-like growth factor I
Serum amyloid A	Antithrombin
Ferritin	
Ceruloplasmin	

Negative acute phase proteins decrease in inflammation.

19. Factors causing increase in both PT and aPTT:

a. Factor V
b. VIII
c. VII
d. X
e. XII

Ans. a, d *Ref: Robbins, 9th/ed; Kitchens CS. Approach to the bleeding patient. Hematol Oncol Clin North Am 1992; 6:983–989.*

Option a	True	
Option b	False	Deficiency increases only aPTT
Option c	False	Deficiency increases only PT
Option d	True	
Option e	False	Deficiency increases only aPTT

- The ***aPTT*** represents the time for clot formation after adding calcium, phospholipids, and kaolin to a sample of citrated blood.
- It is prolonged by heparin, direct thrombin inhibitors, a deficiency of or inhibitor of factors in the intrinsic and common pathways (e.g., factors II, V, VIII, IX, X, XI, and XII) as well as lupus anticoagulant, vitamin K deficiency, or severe liver disease.
- Lupus anticoagulants interfere with the activity of the phospholipids used to trigger the clotting in the laboratory, and results may vary for different commercial preparations.
- The ***PT*** represents the time for clot formation after the addition of thromboplastin (tissue factor) and calcium to citrated blood.
- It is prolonged with deficiencies of factors II, V, VII, and X or fibrinogen, liver disease, vitamin K deficiency, and warfarin use.
- Currently, this time is accompanied by the International Normalized Ratio, which compares it to the laboratory's baseline normal.

Causes of prolonged prothrombin time (PT) and activated partial thromboplastin time (aPTT)		
Prolonged PT	***Prolonged aPTT***	***Prolonged PT and aPTT***
Inherited		
Factor VII deficiency	vWF, factor VIII, IX, XI, or XII deficiency	Prothrombin, fibrinogen, factor V, X or combined factor deficiency
Acquired		
Vitamin K deficiency	Heparin use	Liver disease
Liver disease	Inhibitor of vWF, factors VIII, IX, XI or XII	DIC
Warfarin use	Antiphospholipid antibodies	Supratherapeutic heparin or warfarin
Factor VII inhibitor		• Combined heparin or warfarin use • Inhibitor of prothrombin, fibrinogen factor V or X • Direct thrombin inhibitor

20. True about bleeding:

a. In DIC, PT and aPTT are prolonged
b. In ITP, i/v immunoglobulin is used

c. In hemophilia B, factor VIII is given as treatment
d. Diffuse alveolar hemorrhage is seen in Wegener granulomatosis
e. None of the above

Ans. a, b, d *Ref: Robbins 9th/ed*

Option a	True	
Option b	True	
Option c	False	Factor VIII is given in Hemophilia A. In Hemophilia B, factor IX is given
Option d	True	
Option e	False	

1. **Disseminated intravascular coagulation (DIC):**
   a. Suspected in patients with unexplained bleeding or venous thromboembolism, especially if a predisposing condition exists.
   b. Rapidly evolving DIC results in more severe thrombocytopenia, more prolonged PT and PTT, a rapidly declining plasma fibrinogen level, and a high plasma d-dimer level.
   c. Factor VIII is reduced in DIC because of the thrombin-induced generation of activated protein C, which proteolyses the activated form of factor VIII.
2. **Idiopathic thrombocytopenic purpura (ITP):**
   a. In the patient with known ITP, high-dose parenteral glucocorticoids and IV immunoglobulin (IVIG), with or without platelet transfusions, are appropriate. Platelet transfusion is indicated for controlling severe hemorrhage.
   b. PT and aPTT are normal.
3. **Hemophilia B, or Christmas disease**:
   a. An inherited, X-linked, recessive disorder that results in deficiency of functional plasma coagulation factor IX.
   b. The hallmark of hemophilia is hemorrhage into the joints.
   c. This bleeding is painful and leads to long-term inflammation and deterioration of the joint (typically the ankles in children, and the ankles, knees, and elbows in adolescents and adults), resulting in permanent deformities, misalignment, loss of mobility, and extremities of unequal lengths.
   d. The main treatment for hemophilia is called replacement therapy. Concentrates of clotting factor VIII (for hemophilia A) or clotting factor IX (for hemophilia B) are slowly injected into the vein.
4. **Granulomatosis with polyangiitis (GPA),** formerly known as **Wegener granulomatosis**:
   a. Rare multisystem autoimmune disease of unknown etiology.
   b. Its hallmark features include necrotizing granulomatous inflammation and pauci-immune vasculitis in small- and medium-sized blood vessels.
   c. Diffuse alveolar hemorrhage due to alveolar capillaritis is seen.

21. AML translocation

a. t15:17
b. t9:22
c. t14:18
d. t11:18
e. t8:21

Ans. a, e *Ref: Robbins 9th/ed*

Option a	True	
Option b	False	
Option c	False	
Option d	False	
Option e	True	

WHO Classification—AML with recurrent genetic abnormalities:

- AML with translocations between chromosome 8 and 21 - [t(8;21)(q22;q22);]RUNX1/RUNX1T1; (ICD-O 9896/3);
- AML with inversions in chromosome 16 - [inv(16)(p13.1q22)] or internal translocations in it - [t(16;16)(p13.1;q22);] CBFB/MYH11; (ICD-O 9871/3);
- Acute promyelocytic leukemia with translocations between chromosome 15 and 17 - [t(15;17)(q22;q12);] RARA/PML; (ICD-O 9866/3);
- AML with translocations between chromosome 9 and 11 - [t(9;11)(p22;q23);]MLLT3/MLL;
- AML with translocations between chromosome 6 and 9 - [t(6;9)(p23;q34);]DEK/NUP214;
- AML with inversions in chromosome 3 - [inv(3)(q21q26.2)] or internal translocations in it - [t(3;3)(q21;q26.2);] RPN1/EVI1;
- Megakaryoblastic AML with translocations between chromosome 1 and 22 - [t(1;22)(p13;q13);] RBM15/MKL1;
- AML with mutated NPM1
- AML with mutated CEBPA.

22. In synovial sarcoma, following features are true:

a. Most common in third decade
b. t(11:22)
c. Fusion gene SS18
d. t(x;18)
e. Painful mass

Ans. a, c, d *Ref: Concepts in Pathology, Devesh Mishra, 3rd/ed; Robbins 9th/ed*

Option a	True	
Option b	False	tX;18
Option c	True	SS18-SSX1-SSX2 or SSX4 fusion genes
Option d	True	
Option e	False	Slow growing painless mass

- Common age of presentation is 20–50 years.
- Most common site of occurrence is deep soft tissue of lower extremities (knee and thigh) as slow growing painless mass.
- Characteristic chromosomal translocation t(x:18) producing SS18-SSX1-SSX2 or SSX4 fusion genes. The resulting fusion protein brings together the transcriptional activating domain of SS18 and the transcriptional repressor domains of SSX.
- SS18-SSX is thought to underlie synovial sarcoma pathogenesis through dysregulation of gene expression.
- It also incorporates into the SWI/SNF chromatin remodeling complex, a well known tumor suppressor.

- Most common site of metastasis is lungs.
- The diagnosis is typically made based on histology and is confirmed by the presence of t(X;18).

23. Antigen presenting cells are:

a. Macrophage
b. Kupffer cells
c. Langerhans cells of epidermis
d. Thymic epithelial cells
e. Dendritic cells

Ans. a, b, c, d, e *Ref: Concepts in Pathology, Devesh Mishra, 3rd/ed; Robbins 9th/ed*

Option a	True	Professional APC
Option b	True	Professional APC; macrophages present in liver sinusoids
Option c	True	Professional APC
Option d	True	Non-professional APC
Option e	True	Professional APC

- ***Antigen-presenting cells (APCs)*** are a heterogeneous group of immune cells that mediate the cellular immune response by processing and presenting antigens for recognition by certain lymphocytes such as T-cells.
- The T-cell receptor is restricted to recognizing antigenic peptides only when bound to appropriate molecules of the major histocompatibility complex (MHC), also known in humans as human leukocyte antigen (HLA).
- Helper T-cells receive antigens from MHC II on an APC, while cytotoxic T-cells receive antigens from MHC I. Helper T-cells present their antigen to B cells as well. Dendritic cells, B cells, and macrophages play a major role in the innate response, and are the primary antigen-presenting cells (APC).
- There are two categories of APC—Professional and non-professional.

Antigen presenting cells (APC)	
Professional APCs	***Non-professional APCs***
• They express **MHC class II molecules** along with **co-stimulatory molecules and pattern recognition receptors.** - **Dendritic cells (DCs)**[Q]	• **Non-professional APCs** express **MHC class I molecules.** • Stimulation of non-professional APC by cytokines like **IFN-γ**.
- Immature dendritic cells (immature dendritic cells) - **Macrophages**[Q] - **B-cells**[Q]	• It includes: - **Fibroblasts**[Q] (skin) - Thymic epithelial cells - Thyroid epithelial cells - **Glial cells**[Q] (brain) - Pancreatic beta cells - **Endothelial cells**[Q]

- **Most potent**[Q] **and effective** antigen presenting cells in the body is **dendritic cells**[Q].
  a. Professional antigen presentation.

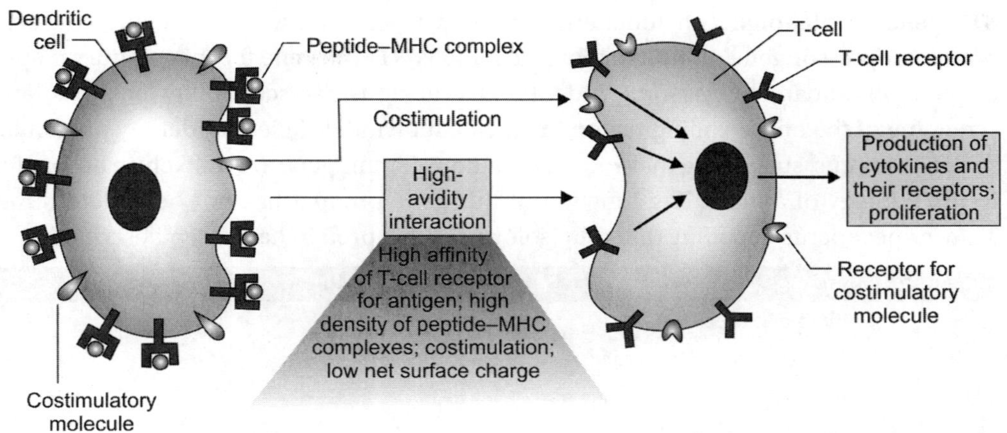

b. Amateur antigen presentation

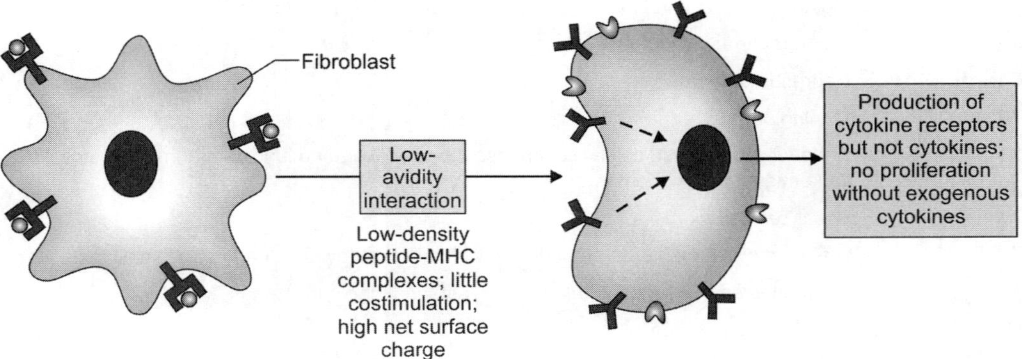

24. Which of the following is not a tumor suppressor gene?

a. pRB
b. p53
c. CD95
d. RAS
e. ST7

Ans. c, d *Ref: Robbins, 9th/ed*

Option a	False	Is a tumor suppressor gene for Retinoblastoma. First tumor suppressor gene to be ever identified
Option b	False	Is a tumor suppressor gene
Option c	True	Not a tumor suppressor gene
Option d	True	Not a tumor suppressor gene
Option e	False	Is a tumor suppressor gene

- **The RB gene**—is an archetypal tumor suppressor gene that was first identified in a malignant tumor of the retina known as retinoblastoma.
- **P53**—The second tumor suppressor gene to identified is p53, which is frequently inactivated in a wide variety of human cancers, including leukemias, lymphomas, sarcomas, brain tumors, and carcinomas of many tissues, including breast, colon, and lung.

- **ST7 gene**—Mutational and functional analyses reveal that ST7 is a highly conserved tumor-suppressor gene on human chromosome ***7q31***. The gene for this product maps to a region on human chromosome 7 identified as an autism-susceptibility locus. Mutation screening of the entire coding region in autistic individuals failed to identify phenotype-specific variants, suggesting that coding mutations for this gene are unlikely to be involved in the etiology of autism. The function of this gene product has not been determined. Transcript variants encoding different isoforms of this protein have been described.

Tumor suppressor genes	
Gene	***Type of cancer***
APC	Colon/rectum *carcinoma*
BRCA1	Breast and ovarian carcinomas
BRCA2	Breast *carcinoma*
DPC4	Pancreatic *carcinoma*
INK4	Melanoma, lung *carcinoma*, brain tumors, leukemias, lymphomas
MADR2	Colon rectum *carcinoma*
NF1	Neurofibrosarcoma
NF2	Meningioma
p53	Brain tumors; breast, colon/rectum, esophageal, liver, and lung carcinomas; sarcomas; leukemias and lymphomas
PTC	Basal cell *carcinoma*
PTEN	Brain tumors; melanoma; prostate, endometrial, kidney, and lung carcinomas
RB	Retinoblastoma; sarcomas; bladder, breast, and lung carcinomas
VHL	Renal cell *carcinoma*
WT1	Wilms' *tumor*

25. True about primary myelofibrosis is/are:

a. Dry tap
b. Allogeneic bone marrow transplantation is the definitive treatment
c. Increase myeloblasts in peripheral blood
d. Splenectomy is never indicated
e. Extramedullary hematopoiesis

Ans. a, b, e *Ref: Concepts in Pathology, Devesh Mishra, 3rd/ed; Robbins 9th/ed*

Option a	True	Due to bone marrow fibrosis
Option b	True	
Option c	False	Leukoerythroblastosis and tear drop-shaped red blood cells (RBCs) in peripheral blood
Option d	False	Splenomegaly may be an indication for splenectomy
Option e	True	

- ***Primary myelofibrosis (PMF)*** is a myeloproliferative neoplasm characterized by stem cell-derived clonal myeloproliferation, abnormal cytokine expression, bone marrow fibrosis, anemia, splenomegaly, extramedullary hematopoiesis (EMH), constitutional symptoms, cachexia, leukemic progression, and shortened survival.

- Primary myelofibrosis is categorized as a chronic myeloproliferative disorder, along with chronic myelogenous leukemia (CML), polycythemia vera, and essential thrombocytosis.
- Characterized by:
    - Anemia
    - Bone marrow fibrosis (myelofibrosis)
    - Extramedullary hematopoiesis
    - Leukoerythroblastosis and teardrop-shaped red blood cells (RBCs) in peripheral blood
    - Hepatosplenomegaly
- Mild cases may require only supportive therapy. Higher-risk disease may respond to ***ruxolitinib***. Splenomegaly may be an indication for splenectomy. Finally, ***allogeneic stem cell transplantation*** is a potentially curative.

26. True about sideroblastic anemia is/are:

a. Dimorphic cells are found
b. Cause basophilic stippling in lead poisoning
c. Increased MCHC
d. Congenital condition
e. Sideroblasts stained by H and E stain

Ans. a, b, d *Ref: Concepts in Pathology, Devesh Mishra, 3rd/ed; Robbins 9th/ed*

Option a	True	
Option b	True	
Option c	False	MCV is generally low
Option d	True	
Option e	False	Stained with Prussian blue

Sideroblastic anemia:

- Bone marrow produces ringed sideroblasts.
- Under normal circumstances, iron is used to make heme. Inside mitochondria, iron fails to combine with protoporphyrin for heme synthesis and remains in mitochondria as ringed sideroblast.
- On a marrow stained with Prussian blue, a sideroblast is an erythroblast that has stainable deposits of iron in cytoplasm.
- This ineffective erythropoiesis results in iron overload.
- Sideroblastic anemia could be hereditary or acquired.

Hereditary	Acquired
X-linked recessive (more common)	Hematological conditions- leukemia, myeloma, polycythemia vera, myelodysplastic syndrome
Autosomal recessive	Drugs—isoniazid, lead, alcohol, chloramphenicol
	Autoimmune disorders—SLE, RA
	Iron overload, porphyria, etc.

- ❑ Major causes of death in cases of sideroblastic anemia are secondary hemochromatosis from transfusions and leukemia.
- ❑ On a peripheral smear, the mean corpuscular volume (MCV) is usually low, with a microcytic picture.
- ❑ Siderocytes with ***Pappenheimer bodies*** (hypochromic erythrocytes with basophilic iron deposits) are seen.
- ❑ The peripheral smear may also exhibit ***basophilic stippling*** in cases of lead poisoning.
- ❑ Increased iron level with decreased TIBC.
- ❑ A urine porphyrin profile may reveal erythropoietic porphyria.

27. True about adenocarcinoma of lungs is/are:

a. Cytokeratin 5 positive
b. Cytokeratin 7 positive
c. Cytokeratin 20 negative
d. Transthyretin positive
e. Cytokeratin 5 negative

Ans. b, c, e *Ref: Robbins, 9th/ed*

Option a	False	Cytokeratin 5 negative
Option b	True	
Option c	True	
Option d	False	Transthyretin is associated with amyloidosis
Option e	True	

- ❑ Non-small cell lung carcinoma represents 85% of lung carcinomas, with the two major subtypes being adenocarcinoma and squamous cell carcinoma.
- ❑ CK7 positive and 5 and 20 negativity is seen in lung adenocarcinoma.
- ❑ The CK7+/CK20– profile is typical of carcinomas of the lung, breast, and gynecologic tract.
- ❑ The CK7–/CK20+ profile is typical of carcinoma of colorectal origin.

Transthyretin (TTR):

- ❑ Is a protein that functions as a transporter of thyroxine and retinol and is produced chiefly by the liver (> 95%).
- ❑ Also produced within the choroid plexus of the brain and the retinal pigment epithelium.
- ❑ However, it is also associated with the formation of amyloid fibrils, leading to TTR-related amyloidosis (ATTR).

Pharmacology

1. Which of the following antidiabetic drugs correctly match with their mechanism of action?

a. Acarbose – Alpha glucosidase inhibitor
b. Sitagliptin – GLP analogue
c. Dapagliflozin – DPP-4 inhibitor
d. Metformin – PPAR gamma stimulator
e. Pioglitazone – AMPK stimulator

Ans. a. *Ref: Goodman Gilman, 12th/ed p1258–65)*

Option a	True	Yes, correct
Option b	False	No, sitagliptin is DPP-4 inhibitor
Option c	False	No, it is SGLT-2 inhibitor
Option d	False	No, it is a biguanide
Option e	False	No, it is PPAR gamma activator

Antidiabetic drugs	Mechanism of action
Acarbose Voglibose Miglitol	Alpha glucosidase inhibitors
Exenatide Liraglutide Albiglutide Dulaglutide	GLP-1 Agonists
Sitagliptin Saxagliptin Alogliptin Linagliptin Vildagliptin	DPP-4 Inhibitors
Sulfonylurea Meglitinide	Inhibit ATP sensitive potassium channels
Biguanide	Stimulate AMPK
Thiazolidenidiones	Stimulate PPAR gamma
Canagliflozin Dapagliflozin Empagliflozin	Inhibit SGLT-2

2. Drugs used in XDR-TB:

a. Amikacin
b. Fluroquinolone
c. Pyrazinamide
d. Streptomycin
e. Ethionamide

Ans. a and b *(Ref: Park's PSM 24th/ed p199)*

Option a	True	Yes, correct
Option b	True	Yes, correct
Option c	False	No, not used in XDR
Option d	False	No, not used in XDR
Option e	False	No, not used in XDR

Drugs used in MDR and XDR-TB are given in the box

MDR-TB	XDR-TB
Kanamycin Levofloxacin Ethambutol Pyrazinamide Ethionamide Cycloserine	Capreomycin Moxifloxacin Linezolid PAS Clofazimine High dose INH Amoxicillin + Clavulinic acid

3. True about bedaquilline is:

a. New antibacterial class
b. MOA is ATP synthase inhibitor
c. Given for 12 month schedule
d. Highly efficient as solo-drug regime
e. Used for XDR-TB

Ans. a, b and e *Ref: Park's PSM, 24th/ed p197, 200*

Option a	True	Yes, correct
Option b	True	Yes, correct
Option c	False	No, it is given for 6 months as a daily dose and 22 weeks as weekly dose, not to be given for more than 1 year
Option d	False	No, NOT recommended as single drug regime
Option e	True	Yes, correct

- Bedaquiline is a new antimycobacterial drug that acts by inhibiting ATP synthase.
- It is indicated currently in the following cases:
  - MDR TB or rifampicin resistant TB with resistance to all fluoroquinolones or all second line injectables
  - XDR TB with resistance to all fluoroquinolones and second line injectables
  - XDR TB with resistance to all fluoroquinolones and any second line injectables
  - XDR TB with resistance to all second line injectables and any fluoroquinolone
  - Treatment failure of MDR TB with fluoroquinolone or second line injectables resistance
  - Treatment failure of XDR TB
- Beqdaquiline is combined with other drugs depending on the resistance pattern. It is given for 6 months with the dose being 400 mg OD for the first two weeks, followed by 600 mg per week (200 mg three times with 48 hours gap between two doses) for 22 weeks.
- Bedaquiline is contraindicated in:

- Age < 18 years
- Pregnant
- Cardiac arrhythmia – As it can cause QT prolongation.

4. Drugs which do not suppress bone marrow:

a. 5FU
b. Cisplatin
c. Chlorambucil
d. Vincristine
e. Vinblastine

Ans. b and d *Ref: CMDT 2018, Pages 1677–84*

Option a	False	Yes, it suppresses the BM
Option b	True	No, it is BM sparing
Option c	False	Yes, it suppresses the BM
Option d	True	No, it is BM sparing
Option e	False	Yes, it suppresses the BM

- Most anticancer drugs which act on cell cycle cause bone marrow suppression and it is the most common dose limiting toxicity of anticancer drugs.
- However, some anticancer drugs which are bone marrow sparing are:
  - Cisplatin
  - Vincristine
  - Bleomycin

5. Norepinephrine reuptake inhibitor:

a. Fluoxetine
b. Duloxetine
c. Paroxetine
d. Atomoxetine
e. Milnacipran

Ans. d *Ref: Goodman Gilman, 12th/ed p405*

Option a	False	No, it is SSRI
Option b	False	No, it is selective NE reuptake inhibitors
Option c	False	No, it is SSRI
Option d	True	Yes, correct
Option e	False	No, it is selective NE reuptake inhibitors

- Atomoxetine is the only selective NE inhibitor available and is used for the treatment of ADHD.
- Fluoxetine and paroxetine are selective serotonin reuptake inhibitors.
- Duloxetine and milnacipran are serotonin norepinephrine reuptake inhibitors.

6. Drugs given in mania:

a. Mood stabilizers
b. Antipsychotics
c. Antidepressants
d. Antiepileptics
e. Sedative hypnotics

Ans. a, b, d, e *Ref: Goodman Gilman 12th/ed p448*

Option a	True	Yes, lithium is the DOC
Option b	True	Yes, they are used for acute mania
Option c	False	No, they are contraindicated

Option d	True	Yes, correct, they are used in mania
Option e	True	Yes, correct, they are used in mania

Drugs used in mania:

- **Mood stabilizers:** Lithium is the best drug available for mania and is the drug of choice for the prevention of mania and bipolar disorder.
- **Antipsychotics:** These are the fastest acting antimania drugs and are the drug of choice for the treatment of an acute attack of mania.
- **Antiepileptics:** Valproate, carbamazepine, topiramate and gabapentin are the antiepileptics that are used in mania and bipolar disorder.
- **Sedative hypnotics:** Benzodiazepines are used in an acute attack of mania.

Note: Antidepressants increase brain derived neurotropic factors (BDNF) and hence can precipitate mania. Thus antidepressants are contraindicated in mania.

7. Diarrhea is caused by:

a. PPI
b. Ca2+ channel blockers
c. Antacids containing magnesium
d. Antacids containing Aluminum
e. Antibiotics

Ans. a,c,e *Ref: Harrison 19th/ed p268*

Option a	True	Yes, correct
Option b	False	No, may lead to constipation
Option c	True	Yes, correct
Option d	False	No, may lead to constipation
Option e	True	Yes, correct

Drugs causing diarrhea

- Antibiotics
- Anticancer drugs
- PPI and H2 blockers
- Laxatives
- Antiarrhythmics like quinidine and digoxin
- Antihypertensives like propranolol, guanethidine and methyl Dopa
- Indomethacin
- Theophylline
- Antacids containing magnesium

Note: Calcium channel blockers and antacids containing aluminum cause constipation.

8. True about 1st order kinetics:

a. Variable t1/2
b. Fraction eliminated is constant
c. Amount eliminated is constant
d. Variable clearance
e. Elimination process is saturatable

Ans. b, e *Ref: Goodman Gilman, 12th/ed p28*

Option a	False	No, it is constant fraction (or proportion) of drug is eliminated per unit time
Option b	True	Yes, correct
Option c	False	No, it is constant fraction (or proportion) of drug is eliminated per unit time
Option d	False	No, it is constant fraction (or proportion) of drug is eliminated per unit time
Option e	True	Yes, correct

Zero order kinetics	First order kinetics
As dose increases t1/2 increases and clearance decreases	Both t1/2 and clearance are constant
A constant amount is eliminated per unit time	A constant fraction is eliminated per unit time
Elimination process is saturated	Elimination process is non-saturable
Ethanol, Phenytoin, Salicylates, Cisplatin, Fluoxetin, Omeprazol	Most drugs
Non-linear kinetics	Linear kinetics

9. Competitive antagonist true is:

a. Shift of the drug response curve parallel to right
b. Low efficacy
c. Low potency, dose is higher
d. Shift of drug response curve to left non-parallel
e. Action at the same drug site

Ans. a, c, e *Ref: Goodman Gilman 12th/ed p44*

Option a	True	Yes, correct
Option b	False	No, the efficacy does not change
Option c	True	Yes, correct
Option d	False	No, it is shift to the right
Option e	True	Yes, correct

Competitive antagonism	Noncompetitive antagonism
At same site	At different sites
DRC shifts to right side	Slope of DRC decreases
Efficacy and V_{max} does not change	Efficacy and V_{max} decreases
Dose and K_m increases as **potency decreases**	Dose, potency and K_m does not change

10. B1 agonist features are:

a. No cardiac involvement
b. No vasoconstriction
c. Increased lipolysis
d. Bronchodilation
e. Tachycardia

Ans. b,c,e. *Ref: Lippincott's Illustrated Review: Pharmacology, 6th/ed p80*

Option a	False	No, Beta 1 is located in the heart and has cardiac stimulation effect
Option b	True	Yes, correct
Option c	True	Yes, correct
Option d	False	No, bronchodilation is the feature of beta 2 receptor
Option e	True	Yes, correct

- For α receptors, the rank order of potency and affinity is *epinephrine ≥ norepinephrine >> isoproterenol.*
- The rank order for Beta receptor is: *isoproterenol > epinephrine >norepinephrine.*

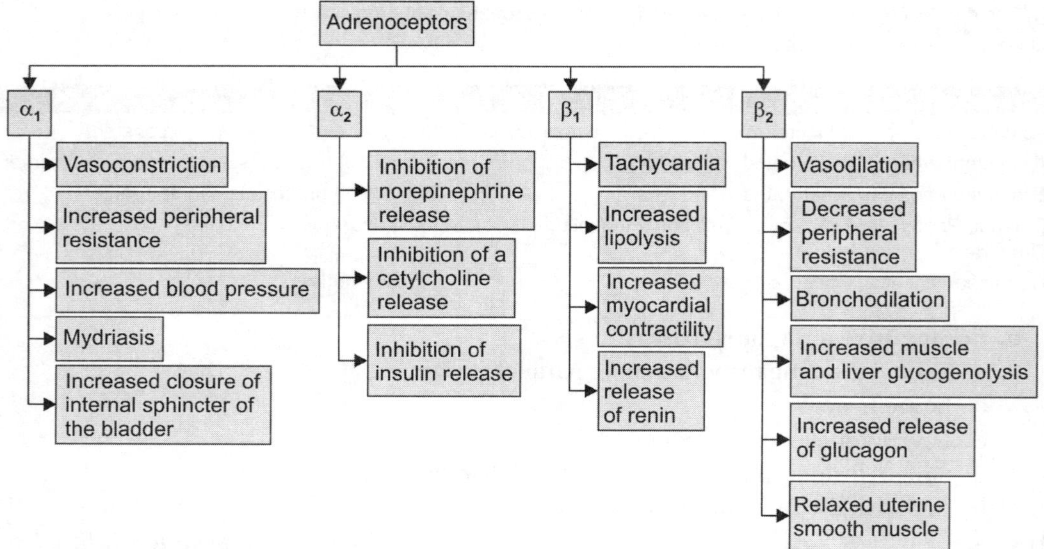

	Beta 1	Beta 2	Beta 3
Feature	Approximately equal affinities for *epinephrine* and *norepinephrine*	Higher affinity for *epinephrine* than for *norepinephrine*	Involved in lipolysis and also have effects on the detrusor muscle of the bladder
2nd messenger	cAMP	cAMP	cAMP
Predominant organ	Heart	Skeletal muscle vasculature	Bladder, uterus
Response by adrenoreceptor stimulation	Cardiac stimulation – tachycardia and contractility	Vasodilation and smooth muscle relaxation	

11. Side effects of clonazepam:

a. Hypothermia
b. Sedation
c. Not given along with valproate
d. Develops tolerance
e. Hepatotoxicity

Ans. b, c, d *Ref: KDT 7th/ed p418*

Option a	False	No, not correct
Option b	True	Yes, correct
Option c	True	Yes, correct
Option d	True	Yes, correct
Option e	False	No, liver enzymes are frequently raised with valproate, not clonazepam

The most important side effect are of clonazepam sedation and dullness. This can be minimized by starting at low dose; some tolerance develops with chronic therapy.

Other side effects:

- ❑ Lack of concentration
- ❑ Irritability
- ❑ Temper and other behavioral abnormalities may occur in children
- ❑ Motor disturbances and ataxia are dose-related adverse effects
- ❑ Salivation and increased respiratory secretions
- ❑ Tolerance to drug after use for 5–7 months.

Good to remember

Uses:

- ❑ Used as second line in absence seizures. It is also useful as an adjuvant in myoclonic and akinetic epilepsy and may afford some benefit in infantile spasms.
- ❑ It has also been used to suppress acute mania.

Table 1: Choice of antiseizure drugs

S. No.	Type of seizure	First choice drugs	Second choice drugs	Alternative/Add-on drugs
1	Generalized tonic-cionic/simple partial with without generalization	Carbamazepine, phenytoin	Valproate, phenobarbitone	Lamotrigine, gabapentin, topiramate, primidone, levetiracetam
2	Complex partial with without generalization	Carbamazepine, valproate, phenytoin	Gabapentin, lamotrigine, levetiracetam	Clobazam, zonisamide, topiramate
3	Absence	Valproate	Ethosuximide, lamotrigine	Clobazam, clonazepam
4	Myocionic	Valproate	Lamotrigine, topiramate	Levetiracetam, clonazepam
5	Atonic	Valproate	Clonazepam, clobazam	Lamotrigine
6	Febrile seizures	Diazepam (rectal)	--	--
7	Status epilepticus	Lorazepam (iv), diazepam (iv)	Fosphenytoin (iv), phenobarbitone (iv, im)	General anaesthetics

12. Isotretinoin adverse side effects include:

a. Hyperglycemia
b. Hydrocephalus
c. Hyperlipidemia
d. Cheilitis
e. Photosensitivity

Ans. b,c,d *(Ref: KDT, 7th/ed p894)*

Option a	False	No, not correct
Option b	True	Yes, correct, Isotretinoin may cause hydrocephalus as a teratogenic adverse effect
Option c	True	Yes, correct
Option d	True	Yes, correct
Option e	False	No, not correct

Side effects include:

- Cheilitis, dryness of skin, eyes, nose and mouth - frequent
- Epistaxis
- Pruritus, paronychia
- Conjunctivitis
- Hyperlipidemia
- Raised ICT

Teratogenicity:

- Highly teratogenic; up to 25% exposed fetuses had birth defects—craniofacial, heart and CNS abnormalities
- It is contraindicated in women likely to become pregnant during therapy and one month after.

Indications:

- Unresponsive cases of severe acne.
- Prevention and treatment of skin cancers. Oral leukoplakia, actinic keratosis and other premalignant lesions can be treated, but benefit-risk ratio is not clear.

13. Homocystinuria, correct statement is/are:

a. Pyridoxine associated treatment
b. No mental retardation
c. Predisposed to stroke
d. Ectopia lentis
e. Defective methylcobalamine synthesis

Ans. a, c, d, e *(Ref: Julia A, Oski's Pediatrics: Principles & Practice, lippincotts; Page 2158)*

Option a	True	Yes, correct, pyridoxine is the DOC
Option b	False	No, MR is present
Option c	True	Yes, correct
Option d	True	Yes, correct
Option e	True	Yes, correct

Homocystinuria

Pathology

- The accumulation of homocysteine and its metabolites is caused by disruption of any of the 3 interrelated pathways of methionine metabolism—deficiency in the cystathionine B-synthase (CBS) enzyme, defective methylcobalamin synthesis, or abnormality in methylenetetrahydrofolate reductase (MTHFR)
- Higher chances of carotid stenosis and stroke.

Clinical presentation

- Ectopia lentis - downward dislocation of lens - characteristic
- Marfanoid habitus
- Pectus excavatum, pectus carinatum, and genu valgum
- Mental retardation
- Signs and symptoms of strokes in any vascular distribution.

*The DOC is pyridoxine @ 100-500 mg/d with low methionine diet.

Pharmacology

1. All are true about bisphosphonates except:

a. Prevent reabsorption of bone by osteoclast
b. Structurally similar to pyrophosphate
c. Absorption increases with food
d. Use is contraindicated in liver disease
e. Contraindicated in cases of kidney disease

Ans. c, d *Ref: Goodman and Gilman's, 12th/ed*

Option a	True	True, they reduce osteoclast activity
Option b	True	True, they are analogues of pyrophosphate
Option c	False	False, food decreases their absorption
Option d	False	False, can be safely given in liver disease
Option e	True	True, If given, the risk of renal failure increases by many folds

- Bisphosphonates are analogues of pyrophosphate that slow down or prevent bone loss, strengthening bones.
- Bisphosphonates also reduce osteoclast activity by decreasing osteoclast progenitor development and recruitment and by promoting osteoclast apoptosis and hence prevent bone resorption.
- Bone formation is often reduced by bisphosphonates, which is probably an indirect effect of inhibition of bone resorption. In normal bone remodeling, bone resorption and formation are coupled together. However, bisphosphonates allow osteoblasts to work more effectively, thereby improving the bone mass.

Uses:

1. Osteoporosis
2. Paget's disease
3. Tumor osteolytic syndrome
4. Breast and prostate cancer
5. Hypercalcemia

Factors decreasing their absorption in intestine:

1. Calcium supplements
2. Antacids
3. Food
4. Drugs containing divalent cations
5. Iron

In cases of liver disease, these drugs can be given safely, however in the presence of kidney disease with creatinine clearance less than 30 mL/min, the use of bisphosphonates is contraindicated. If given, the risk of renal failure increases by many folds.

2. All are true about oral iron therapy in anemia except:
   a. May worsen inflammatory bowel disease
   b. It takes minimum 2 weeks for reticulocyte count to increase
   c. Generally 3–6 month therapy is required to replenish iron stores
   d. Gastrointestinal side-effects limit its dose
   e. Hb level is generally attained in 1-3 months

Ans. a, b, d *Ref: Goodman and Gilman's, 12th/ed*

Option a	False	May improve the inflammatory bowel disease
Option b	False	Reticulocyte count takes atleast 4-7 days to increase
Option c	True	Yes, this is correct
Option d	False	GI side effects donot limit its use
Option e	True	Yes, this is correct

- ❑ Clinically, the effectiveness of iron therapy is best evaluated by tracking the reticulocyte response and the rise in hemoglobin and hematocrit.
- ❑ Red cell mass is usually reconstituted within 1–2 months.
- ❑ Iron stores are replenished in more than 3–4 months.
- ❑ Reticulocyte count takes at least 4–7 days to increase.
- ❑ Since iron deficiency leads to repeated inflammatory attacks in the intestine, the therapy with oral iron supplements may improve the inflammatory bowel disease.
- ❑ Main side effect of oral iron therapy is the GI side effects, but these do not limit its use as these side effects can be avoided by:
  - Dividing the dose in three parts
  - Initiating therapy at a smaller dose and then gradually increasing the dose as desired.

3. True about Low-molecular-weight heparin (LMWH):
   a. Anti-factor Xa assay monitoring is required
   b. It increases aPTT more than unfractionated heparin
   c. Can be safely given in renal failure
   d. Toxicity is totally reversed by protamine sulphate
   e. Inactivate factor Xa selectivity

Ans. a, e *Ref: Goodman Gilman's, 12th/ed*

Option a	True	Yes, true
Option b	False	LMWHs barely increase aPTT as compared to UFH
Option c	False	Relatively contraindicated in patients with renal failure
Option d	False	No, this is false
Option e	True	Yes, true

- ❑ LMWHs are derived from Unfractionated Heparin (UFH) by chemical or enzymatic depolymerization to yield fragments that are approximately one third the size of heparin.
- ❑ Compared with UFH, LMWHs have:
  - Reduced ability to catalyze inactivation of thrombin because the smaller fragments cannot bind to thrombin but retain their ability to inactivate factor Xa.
  - Reduced nonspecific binding to plasma proteins, with a corresponding improvement in the predictability of their dose-response relationship.

- Reduced binding to macrophages and endothelial cells, with an associated increase in their plasma half-life.
- Lower incidence of Heparin induced thrombocytopenia due to reduced binding to platelets and PF4.
- Possibly reduced binding to osteoblasts, which results in less activation of osteoclasts and an associated reduction in bone loss.

- Like UFH, LMWHs produce their major anticoagulant effect by activating antithrombin (AT).
- The anti–factor Xa assay is designed to measure plasma heparin [unfractionated heparin (UFH) and low molecular weight heparin (LMWH)] levels and to monitor anticoagulant therapy.
- The LMWHs barely increase aPTT as compared to UFH.
- Unlike UFH, the low-molecular-weight heparin is excreted mainly by the kidneys and is relatively contraindicated in patients with renal failure because of concerns of increased bleeding risks.

LMWH Toxicity

- Accidental overdose following administration of LMWH may lead to hemorrhagic complications. In such cases, it should be immediately discontinued, in cases of significant excess dosage.
- The anticoagulant effect of LMWH is inhibited by protamine. This effect may be largely neutralized by slow intravenous injection of ***protamine sulfate***. However, even with higher doses of protamine, the aPTT may remain prolonged to a greater extent than usually seen with unfractionated heparin. Anti-factor Xa activity is *never completely neutralized* (maximum about 60%).

4. Adverse effects of mirtazapine is/are:

a. Insomnia
b. Sedation
c. Sexual dysfunction
d. Anorexia
e. Weight gain

Ans. a, b, c, e *Ref: Goodman Gilman's, 12th/ed; KDT, 7th/ed*

Option a	True	
Option b	True	
Option c	True	
Option d	False	
Option e	True	

- Mirtazapine is a tetracyclic antidepressant acting as an antagonist at presynaptic a2-autoreceptors on noradrenergic and serotoninergic neurons, thereby increasing norepinephrine and serotoninergic activity.
- It also has significant sedative properties, probably mediated by its antihistaminergic action.
- Additionally, it is a 5-HT2- and 5-HT3-receptor antagonist.
- Commonly reported side effects of mirtazapine include:
  - Severe sedation

- Constipation
- Drowsiness
- Increased serum cholesterol
- Weight gain
- Fatigue
- Insomnia
- Increased appetite
- Xerostomia, and
- Decreased appetite.

❑ Other side effects include: dizziness, increased serum triglycerides, tremor, dyspepsia, hot flash, palpitations, vertigo, abnormal dreams, bitter taste, decreased libido, and diaphoresis.

5. Drug which can be given by inhalation route:

a. Zileuton
b. Steroid
c. Salbutamol
d. Tobramycin
e. Oseltamivir

Ans. b, c, d *Ref: Goodman Gilman's, 12th/ed; KDT, 7th/ed*

Option a	False	Given as an oral drug
Option b	True	
Option c	True	
Option d	True	
Option e	False	Given as an oral drug

Zileuton: It is a 5-COX inhibitor which is given as an ***oral drug***. It is a hepatotoxic drug.
Steroids: Inhaled steroids are used in the treatment of Asthma and COPD. Side effects include oropharyngeal candidiasis and Dysphonia.
Salbutamol: It is a β_2 agonist which is given as by inhalational route. It is the shortest and fastest acting out of all its class drugs.
Tobramycin: Apart from other routes, tobramycin is given in inhalational form as well. It is used to treat the chronic pseudomonas aeruginosa lung infections in cases of cystic fibrosis.
Oseltamivir: It is given as an oral tablet. Zanamivir is available in the powder form and is used as an inhalational drug.

6. Liver function test (LFT) monitoring is/are required in use of which of the following?

a. Methotrexate
b. Hydroxychloroquine
c. Sulfasalazine
d. Leflunomide
e. Gold

Ans. a, d, e *Ref: Goodman Gilman's, 12th/ed; KDT, 7th/ed*

Option a	True	Causes hepatic fibrosis
Option b	False	Cause retinal and corneal toxicity
Option c	False	Hepatitis occurs very rarely
Option d	True	Causes profound liver toxicity when combined with methotrexate
Option e	True	It is hepatotoxic

Methotrexate: For the treatment of Rheumatoid arthritis, Methotrexate is the first DMARD (Disease-modifying anti-rheumatic drug) of choice. It has a rapid onset of action, efficacy to effect sustained improvement and higher level of patient retention.

Adverse effects:

- GI upset
- Oral ulceration
- Abnormal liver functions (may need liver biopsy)
- Hepatic fibrosis
- Drug induced pneumonitis

Hydroxychloroquine: It is known to cause retinal and corneal toxicity.

- Retinal damage
- Corneal opacity
- Graying of hair
- Irritable bowel syndrome
- Myopathy and neuropathy

Sulfasalazine: Hepatitis can occur, but very rare.

Leflunomide: It is a synthetic isoxazole derivative with immunosuppressive and anti-inflammatory properties. It is a potential hepatotoxic drug. If used alone LFT enzymes raise by 5% and when used in combination with methotrexate, the liver enzymes may increase by >50%. It has properties, so contraindicated in pregnancy.

Gold: It is the oldest drug known for the treatment of rheumatoid arthritis and is seen to be hepatotoxic.

7. **Drugs which can be used in gestational hypertension:**
   a. Metoprolol
   b. Labetalol
   c. Methyldopa
   d. Sustained release nifedipine
   e. Losartan

Ans. a, b, c, d *Ref: Goodman Gilman's, 12th/ed; KDT, 7th/ed*

Option a	True	
Option b	True	
Option c	True	
Option d	True	
Option e	False	Contraindicated in pregnancy

- Anti-hypertensive drugs that can be used safely in pregnancy are:
  - Cardioselective beta blockers: When used for short periods (<6 weeks) during the third trimester, β-blockers are effective and well tolerated.
  - Central sympatholytics (alpha-2 agonists)
  - Calcium channel blockers (Dihydropyridines): Among the calcium blockers, nifedipine has been best studied in pregnancy and the drug has been used extensively in later pregnancy.
  - Hydralazine: Oral hydralazine, a direct vasodilator, is effective as monotherapy or as add-on therapy to methyldopa in the long term management of chronic hypertension in pregnancy.
  - Alpha blockers.

- Drugs not to be given in pregnancy are:
  - ACE Inhibitors: Administration of ACE inhibitors during the second and third trimesters can result in a number of fetal adverse effects, including growth retardation, renal failure, persistent patent ductus arteriosus, respiratory distress syndrome, fetal hypotensive syndrome, and prepartum death.
  - Angiotensin receptor blockers
  - Diuretics: reduce maternal plasma volume and can cause electrolyte disturbances.
  - Sodium nitroprusside.
- Drug of Choice for PIH:
  - Labetalol followed by Methyldopa.

8. Newer drugs for TB include:

a. Bedaquiline
b. Clofazimine
c. Ceftaroline
d. Rifapentine
e. Etanercept

Ans. a, d *Ref: Goodman Gilman's, 12th/ed; KDT, 7th/ed*

Option a	True
Option b	False
Option c	False
Option d	True
Option e	False

Bedaquiline: Diarylquinoline derivative which is indicated as a part of combination treatment in adults in cases of MDR- Tuberculosis.

Mode of action: Inhibits ATP synthase enzyme in mycobacteria. This enzyme is used by the bacteria to generate energy. Without the ability to generate energy, the TB bacteria die and the patient's condition can start to improve.

It should only be used when an effective treatment cannot otherwise be provided. It is also sometimes used when other drugs cannot be used because of their side effects.

Bedaquiline should not be used for the treatment of:

- Latent infections due to Mycobacterium tuberculosis
- Drug sensitive tuberculosis
- Extrapulmonary tuberculosis
- Infections caused by non tuberculosis mycobacteria.

The recommended dose is 400 mg a day for two weeks and then 200 mg taken three times a week (with at least 48 hours between doses) for the next 22 weeks.

Clofazimine: Antileprotic drug.

Ceftaroline: Is a 5th generation cephalosporin.

Rifapentine: Rifapentine is a rifamycin antimycobacterial indicated for the treatment of pulmonary tuberculosis caused by Mycobacterium tuberculosis in combination with one or more antituberculosis drugs.

Dosage: 600 mg twice weekly for two months by direct observation of therapy, with an interval of no less than 3 consecutive days (72 hours) between doses, in combination with other antituberculosis drugs. 600 mg once weekly for 4 months by direct observation therapy with isoniazid or another appropriate antituberculous agent.

Etanercept: Is a TNF inhibitor and is used in the treatment of autoimmune diseases.

9. True about mafenide acetate is/are:

a. Used in burns
b. Does not cause burning sensation when applied to raw surface
c. Can be used orally
d. May cause metabolic acidosis
e. Broad spectrum

Ans. a, d *Ref: Goodman Gilman's, 12th/ed; KDT, 7th/ed*

Option a	True	
Option b	False	Common side effect
Option c	False	Used as a topical antibiotic
Option d	True	
Option e	False	This is not true

- Mafenide acetate is a sulfonamide derivative which is used as a topical antibiotic to prevent infection in severe burn wounds and is absorbed rapidly from the raw surface.
- It is active in the presence of pus.
- It is highly effective for Pseudomonas infection.

Common side effects of sulfamylon include:

- Skin rash,
- Redness, or
- Itching, or
- Pain,
- Burning, or
- Redness of the treated skin areas.

It inhibits carbonic anhydrase due to which metabolic acidosis can be caused.

10. Carbonic anhydrase inhibitor(s) is/are:

a. Acetazolamide
b. Amiloride
c. Nitrofurantoin
d. Topiramate
e. Nifedipine

Ans. a, d *Ref: Goodman Gilman's, 12th/ed; KDT, 7th/ed*

Option a	True	
Option b	False	It is a potassium-sparing diuretic
Option c	False	Belongs to nitrofuran group of antibiotics
Option d	True	
Option e	False	It is a calcium-channel blocker

Acetazolamide:

- Causes sodium bicarbonate diuresis and a reduction in total body bicarbonate stores.

- Its effectiveness is limited by the development of hyperchloremic metabolic acidosis.
- The bicarbonaturia induces phosphaturia, whereas the metabolic acidosis increases calcium excretion. Both factors are responsible for renal stone formation and nephrocalcinosis during prolonged use of acetazolamide.
- It can cause severe K^+ wasting, especially during the acute bicarbonaturic phase.
- Uses:
  - Chronic treatment of glaucoma,
  - In alkalinization of the urine,
  - In the treatment of acute mountain sickness,
  - To stimulate ventilation in central sleep apnea,
  - To reduce endolymph formation in Meniere's disease, and
  - In the treatment of refractory hydrocephalus.

Topiramate:

- Potent anti-epileptic drug with a broad spectrum of activity.
- Carbonic anhydrase inhibiting properties have been demonstrated by topiramate.

Uses of carbonic anhydrase inhibitors:

Disease condition	Drug(s)
Glaucoma	Acetazolamide
	Dorzolamide
	Brinzolamide
	Methazolamide
Diuretic	Acetazolamide
Epilepsy	Acetazolamide (Catamenial Epilepsy)
	Topiramate
	Zonisamide
Altitude Sickness	Acetazolamide

11. Which of the following is/are true about tacrolimus:

a. Renal elimination
b. Structure similar to cyclosporine
c. Derived from a fungus
d. T-cell inhibitor
e. Hirsutism less evident than cyclosporine

Ans. d, e *Ref: Goodman Gilman's, 12th/ed; KDT, 7th/ed*

Option a	False	Eliminated by feces
Option b	False	Not a fungus like cyclosporine
Option c	False	
Option d	True	
Option e	True	

Tacrolimus is an immunosuppressive agent which is used for the prevention of rejection of transplanted kidneys, liver, or heart. It is:

- Produced from Streptomyces
- Not a fungus like cyclosporine
- Chemically different from cyclosporine.

Mode of action: It binds to FK506 Binding protein and causes inhibition of T-cells via calcineurin.

- The drug is eliminated via feces
- Toxicity profile of tacrolimus is similar to cyclosporine except for;
  - Lesser occurrence of following side effects than cyclosporine:
    - Hypertension
    - Hirsutism
    - Hyperplasia of gums
    - Hyperuricemia
  - Greater occurrence of following side effects than cyclosporine:
    - Diabetes mellitus
    - Neurotoxicity
    - Alopecia
    - Diarrhea

12. Which of the following is/are true about pharmacodynamics of drugs?

a. Affinity means how strongly drug binds to receptor
b. Efficacy means maximal effect by a drug
c. Irreversible antagonist mainly forms ionic bonds with receptor
d. Agonist potency depends on two parameters: affinity and efficacy
e. For antagonists, efficacy is zero

Ans. a, b, d, e *Ref: Goodman Gilman's, 12th/ed; KDT, 7th/ed*

Option a	True	
Option b	True	
Option c	False	Irreversible antagonists form covalent bond with receptors
Option d	True	
Option e	True	

Action through receptors:

- Affinity means the binding capacity of a drug to its receptor.
- Intrinsic activity denotes the action of the drug. Intrinsic activity is a relative term that describes drug's efficacy.
- Efficacy is the maximum response achieved from the drug.
- Irreversible antagonists form covalent bond with receptors.
- For antagonists, the intrinsic activity is zero, i.e. efficacy is zero.
- Potency: amount of drug needed to produce certain response. It depends on both affinity and efficacy.

13. All are true about plasma binding except:

a. Acidic drugs generally bind to plasma albumin and basic drugs to α_1 acid glycoprotein
b. Plasma binding determines volume of distribution
c. More plasma protein binding means storage in liver
d. More plasma protein binding less penetration in vascular membrane
e. High degree of protein binding generally makes the drug long acting

Ans. c *Ref: Goodman Gilman's, 12th/ed; KDT, 7th/ed*

Option a	True	Yes, this is true
Option b	True	Yes, this is true
Option c	False	More the plasma protein binding, lesser is the distribution of a drug
Option d	True	Yes, this is true
Option e	True	Yes, this is true

Plasma protein binding:

- ❑ Acidic drugs bind to albumin and basic drugs bind to alpha-1-acidic glycoprotein
- ❑ Bound form of the drug:
  - ▪ Can not be distributed
  - ▪ Remains in plasma/blood
  - ▪ Can not be removed by dialysis
  - ▪ Can not be filtered in the kidneys
- ❑ Plasma protein binding is an important factor in volume of distribution of a drug
- ❑ More the plasma protein binding, lesser is the distribution of a drug
- ❑ More plasma protein binding makes the drug longer acting because of its slow excretion by the kidneys.

14. First pass metabolism is a significant problem when the drug is given through:

a. Sublingual route b. Rectal route
c. Intramuscular route d. Subcutaneous route
e. Directly into the intestine

Ans. e *Ref: Essentials of Medical Pharmacology, KD Tripathi 7th/ed*

Option a	False	
Option b	False	
Option c	False	
Option d	False	
Option e	True	Across the gut wall, drug goes into the portal circulation and hence faces extensive first pass metabolism

First pass (Presystemic) metabolism

This refers to metabolism of a drug during its passage from the site of absorption into the systemic circulation.

- ❑ All orally administered drugs are exposed to drug metabolizing enzymes in the intestinal wall and liver. They first reach liver through the portal vein before entering the systemic circulation.
- ❑ The extent of first pass metabolism differs for different drugs and is an important determinant of oral bioavailability.

Transport sequence:

1. Across the gut wall into the portal circulation
2. Portal blood transports of the drug to the liver
3. The drug may then reach the systemic circulation.

Bioavailability may be affected by steps 1 – 3:

- ❑ Drug metabolism may occur in the intestinal wall or in the blood
- ❑ Drug metabolism (potentially extensive) may occur in liver
- ❑ Liver may excrete drug into the bile.

Overall process that contributes to bioavailability reduction is the first-pass metabolism or elimination.

Attributes of drugs with high first pass metabolism:

1. Oral dose is considerably higher than the sublingual or parenteral dose.
2. There is a great individual variation in the oral dose due to differences in the extent of first pass metabolism.
3. Oral bioavailability is apparently increased in patients with severe liver disease.
4. Oral bioavailability of a drug is increased if another drug competing with it in first pass metabolism is given concurrently, e.g. Chlorpromazine and propranolol.

15. True about osmotic diuretics:

a. Osmotic diuretics have their major effect in the distal convoluted tubule
b. Contraindicated in congestive heart failure
c. Causes Hyperkalemia
d. Increases renal blood flow
e. Maintain GFR

Ans. b, d, e *Ref: Goodman Gilman's, 12th/ed; KDT, 7th/ed*

Option a	False	Inhibit transport process in the thick ascending Loop of Henle
Option b	True	
Option c	False	Increased excretion of potassium
Option d	True	
Option e	True	

Osmotic diuretics: are freely filtered at the glomerulus, undergo minimal reabsorption by the renal tubules, and are relatively pharmacologically and metabolically inert. Examples are intravenous mannitol and urea.

Mannitol:

- ❑ Non-electrolyte of low molecular weight, pharmacologically inert.
- ❑ Given in large quantities.
- ❑ Not metabolized in the body, freely filtered at glomerulus and undergoes limited reabsorption.

Mode of action:

1. **Expands extracellular fluid volume** by increasing GFR and inhibiting rennin release.
2. **Increases** renal blood flow
3. Retains water isoosmotically in the **proximal tubule**
4. Inhibits transport process in the **thick ascending loop of Henle.**
5. Along with increased urine volume, excretion of all cations and anions is also enhanced (excretion of sodium, potassium, calcium, magnesium, bicarbonate and chloride is increased).

Uses:

1. To maintain GFR and urine flow in impending acute renal failure, e.g. Shock, severe trauma, cardiovascular surgery, haemolytic reactions, etc.
2. Forced diuresis in hypnotic or other poisonings. Promote excretion of nephrotoxic substances such as cisplatin.
3. Increased intracranial or intraocular tension (acute congestive glaucoma, head injury, or stroke). Also used before or after the ocular and brain surgery to prevent acute rise in intraocular or intracranial pressure.
4. To counteract low osmolality of plasma/ECF due to rapid hemodialysis or peritoneal dialysis.

Contraindications:

1. Acute tubular necrosis
2. Anuria
3. Acute left ventricular failure
4. Cerebral hemorrhage
5. Because it increases circulatory volume, mannitol is contraindicated in congestive cardiac failure and pulmonary oedema.

16. Drug that can potentiate Torsades de pointes:

a. Amiodarone
b. Sotalol
c. Chlorpromazine
d. Cisapride
e. Aspirin

Ans. a, b, d *Ref: Goodman Gilman's, 12th/ed; KDT, 7th/ed*

Option a	True	
Option b	True	
Option c	False	
Option d	True	
Option e	False	

- **Amiodarone:** is used for treating ventricular and supraventricular arrhythmias.
  - Fall in BP and myocardial depression can occur on iv injection.
  - The potential to precipitate *torsades de pointes* is very *low (rare)* despite prolongation of action potential duration.
- **Sotalol:** is a beta blocker having prominent class III action of prolonging repolarization by blocking cardiac K^+ channels.
  - Delays AV Conduction
  - Effective in Ventricular Tachycardia and atrial fibrillation/flutter.
  - Due to prolongation of action potential duration and Q-T, the risk of developing *torsades de pointes* is high.
- **Cisapride:** prokinetic drug without antidopaminergic side effects.
  - It restores and facilitates the motility throughout the GIT including colon.
  - Primary indication is gastroesophageal reflux, Also been used in constipation.
  - At high blood levels, and in the presence of hypokalemia, it causes Q-T prolongation leading to *Torsades de pointes.*

Microbiology

1. **Which of the following is/are correct for dengue fever:**
    a. Classified on basis of WHO guidelines as mild, moderate and severe dengue infection
    b. Dengue virus belongs to flaviviridae family of Arbovirus
    c. Antibody dependent enhancement seen.
    d. Breteau index should be less than 1
    e. MAC-ELISA testing is positive in first 2 days.

Ans. a,b,c *Ref: Lange, Review of Medical Microbiology, 13th/ed p777; http://www.who.int/mediacentre/factsheets/fs117/en/ accessed on 25 Jan 2018; Scott B. Halstead. Dengue: Tropical Medicine: Science and Practice. Volume 5 of Tropical Medicine. Imperial College Press (2008). Pg 239-241; Whitehead, S S, et al. Prospects for a Dengue Virus Vaccine. Nature Reviews Microbiology 2007;5:518-28.*

Option a	True	Yes correct
Option b	True	Yes correct
Option c	True	Yes correct
Option d	False	No, it should be less than 5, indicating low level transmission
Option e	False	No, MAC ELISA is to be done after 5 days of fever history. NS1 Antigen is done with first 5 days on onset of infection.

Dengue:

- Dengue is a mosquito-borne viral infection.
- Immunity to a single dengue virus is lifelong, but infection with 2nd, 3rd and 4th serotypes can occur.
- When a person has had classical dengue (by one serotype), a second infection later increases the likelihood of DHF.
- The infection causes flu-like illness, and occasionally develops into a potentially lethal complication called severe dengue.
- There is no specific treatment for dengue/severe dengue, but early detection and access to proper medical care lowers fatality rates below 1%.
- Dengue prevention and control depends on effective vector control measures.
- A dengue vaccine has been licensed by several National Regulatory Authorities for use in people 9-45 years of age living in endemic settings.
- Severity of dengue is less in patients with Protein Calorie Malnutrition (yet to be evaluated using better statistical methods and evidence-based medicine).

Antibody dependent enhancement with dengue infection:

In case of a previous dengue infection, the pre-existing antibodies present in the body bind to an infecting DENV particle during a subsequent infection with a different dengue serotype.

The antibodies from the primary infection cannot neutralize the virus, but the Ab-virus complex attaches to receptors called Fcγ receptors (FcγR) on circulating monocytes. The antibodies help the virus infect monocytes more efficiently.

This instead leads to an increase in the overall replication of the virus and a higher risk of severe dengue.

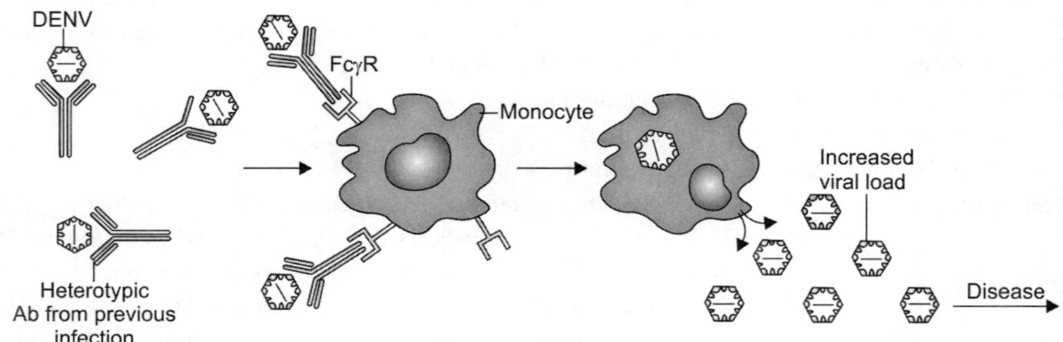

Aedes mosquito

- Vector—*Aedes aegypti* mosquito (female)
- Breeding water: artificial, man-made stored water collections
- Endophilic (indoors predominently)
- Small flight range (~ 100-200 mt)
- Peak biting time: 2 hrs after sunrise, 2 hours before sunset
- Mc site of bite: lower leg, ankle, socks area.

Transmission

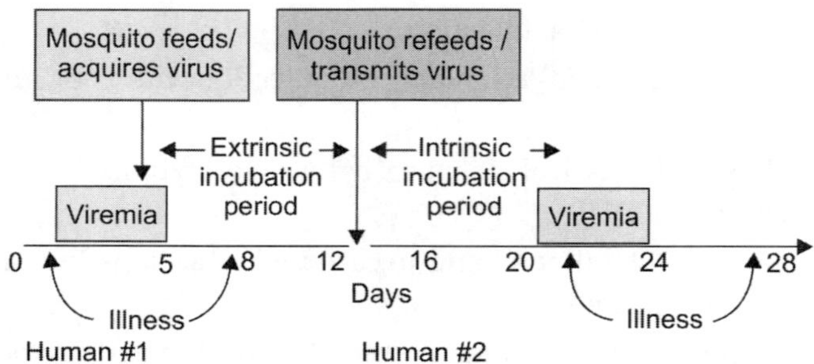

Clinical features

1. Dengue (classical) fever:
   - It's a viral disease, characterized by high grade fever, intense myalgia, arthralgia and typical retro-orbital pain
   - Other symptoms may include intense headache, rash, nausea, vomiting.
2. Dengue hemorrhagic fever: Hemorrhagic tendencies-one or more of following:
   - Positive tourniquet test
   - Petechiae, ecchymosis or purpura

- Bleeding from buccal mucosa, GIT, injection site, nasal bleeding
- Hematemesis or malena
- Thrombocytopenia (<1 lakh /mm^3) and plasma leakage manifested by one or more of following:
  - $\geq$ 20% rise in average hematocrit for age and sex
  - Signs of plasma leakage (pleural effusion, ascitis, hypoproteinemias).

3. Dengue shock syndrome: DHF with circulatory failure manifested by:
   - Rapid and weak pulse
   - Narrow pulse pressure
   - Cold and clammy skin
   - Restlessness and lethargy
   - Altered sensorium.

Severe dengue is a potentially deadly complication due to plasma leaking, fluid accumulation, respiratory distress, severe bleeding, or organ impairment.

Treatment is supportive. Maintenance of the patient's body fluid volume is critical to severe dengue care.

Dengue larval survey indicators:

House Index: Number of houses +ve for aedes larvae/number of houses checked

Container Index: Number of containers +ve for aedes larvae/number of containers checked

Breteau Index: Number of containers +ve for aedes larvae/number of houses checked.

Indices	High risk of transmission	Low risk of transmission
Breteau Index	> 50	<5
House Index	>10%	<1%

However, a single water container found positive for aedes breeding warrants for immediate action for source reduction.

2. True about Ebola virus:

a. Flavivirus
b. Post Ebola infection, semen testing should be done every year till negative
c. Fruit bat is the natural Ebola host
d. Biosafety level 4 is used for diagnosis
e. Air borne transmission is main mode of transmission of Ebola

Ans. a,c,d *Ref: http://www.who.int/mediacentre/factsheets/fs103/en/ accessed on 25 Jan 2018; https://www.cdc.gov/vhf/ebola/about.html*

Option a	True	Yes, correct
Option b	False	No, in previous EBOLA infected persons, it is recommended for three monthly (and not annual) semen analysis or till declared negative. The risk of sexual mode of transmission is particularly high
Option c	True	Yes, correct
Option d	True	Yes, correct
Option e	False	No, it has predominant mode of transmission via body fluids or direct human to human transmission

- Ebola virus disease (EVD), formerly known as Ebola hemorrhagic fever, is a severe, often fatal illness in humans.
- The virus is transmitted to people from wild animals and spreads in the human population through human-to-human transmission.
- The average EVD case fatality rate is around 50%. Case fatality rates have varied from 25% to 90% in past outbreaks.
- The first EVD outbreaks occurred in remote villages in Central Africa, near tropical rainforests. The 2014–2016 outbreak in West Africa involved major urban areas as well as rural ones.

Ebola virus:

- Belong to flaviviridae
- Family Filoviridae includes three genera: Cuevavirus, Marburg virus, and Ebolavirus.
- Genus Ebolavirus, five species have been identified:
  - Bundibugyo ebolavirus
  - Reston ebolavirus
  - Sudan ebolavirus
  - Taï Forest ebolavirus
  - Zaire ebolavirus (largest outbreak in Africa)

A biosafety level is a set of biocontainment precautions required to isolate dangerous biological agents in an enclosed laboratory facility. The levels of containment range from the lowest biosafety level 1 (BSL-1) to the highest at level 4 (BSL-4)

At the lowest level of biosafety, precautions may consist of regular hand-washing and minimal protective equipment. At higher biosafety levels, precautions may include airflow systems, multiple containment rooms, sealed containers, positive pressure personnel suits, established protocols for all procedures, extensive personnel training, and high levels of security to control access to the facility.

Biosafety level 1

- For all pathogenic, no pathogenic organisms with low damage level.

Biosafety level 2

- Suitable for work involving agents of moderate potential hazard to personnel and the environment
- Cause milder disease or are difficult to be transmitted by air or aerosols.

Examples include Hepatitis A, B, and C viruses, human immunodeficiency virus (HIV), pathogenic Escherichia coli, Staphylococcus aureus, Salmonella, Plasmodium falciparum, and Toxoplasma gondii.

Biosafety 3

For research and diagnostic work involving microorganisms which may cause serious disease and spread by aerosol or inhalation.

Francisella tularensis, Mycobacterium tuberculosis, Chlamydia psittaci, Venezuelan equine encephalitis virus, Eastern equine encephalitis virus, SARS coronavirus, Coxiella burnetii, Rift Valley fever virus, Rickettsia rickettsii, several species of Brucella, chikungunya, yellow fever virus, and West Nile virus.

Biosafety level 4 laboratories are used for diagnostic work and research on easily transmitted pathogens which can cause fatal disease.

Marburg virus	Ebola virus,	Crimean-Congo hemorrhagic fever	Lassa virus,	Hendra virus,	Nipah virus

3. *Staph aureus* and *E.coli* are put on a single culture plate The *E.coli* grows on Macconkey agar because:

a. *E.coli* secretes colicin
b. Differential media
c. Selective media
d. Indicator media
e. Enriched media

Ans. b,c *Ref: Author Subhash Chandra Parija. Textbook of Microbiology and Immunology. 2nd/ed. Elsevier Health Sciences (2014). Pg 36; Patrick R. Murray, Ken S. Rosenthal Review of Medical Microbiology. Elsevier Health Sciences (2005). Pg 55-57.*

Option a	False	No, Colicin is definitely produced by *E. coli*, but is not responsible for selective growth of *E. coli* on the MacConkey agar
Option b	True	Yes, correct
Option c	True	Yes, correct
Option d	False	No, not correct. It is differential and selective media
Option e	False	No, not correct. It is differential and selective media

Different media used in microbiology:

1. **Nutritive media** are defined as media types that support the growth of a wide range of microorganisms. These types are typically considered nonselective due to the fact that they will grow most organisms. Examples of nutritive media include tryptic soy agar, nutrient agar, and blood agar.
2. **Differential medium** types are those that distinguish microorganisms from one another based on growth characteristics evident when grown on specific medium types. Organisms with differing growth characteristics typically show visible differences in growth when placed on differential media. Examples include blood agar, Eosin Methylene Blue (EMB) agar, Mannitol Salt agar, and MacConkey agar.
3. **Selective medium** types are formulated to support the growth of one group of organisms, but inhibit the growth of another. These media contain antimicrobials, dyes, or alcohol to inhibit the growth of the organisms not targeted for study. Selective medium types include EMB agar, Mannitol Salt agar, MacConkey agar, and Phenylethyl Alcohol (PEA) agar.
4. Some media may possess both selective and differential properties, allowing them to grow certain groups of organisms of interest and give the investigator a way to discern differences in the group based on a visible reaction with the media. These media can be powerful diagnostic tools in both medical and environmental settings.

Example:

1. MacConkey media:
   MacConkey agar is a selective and differential culture medium for bacteria designed to selectively isolate Gram-negative and enteric (normally found in the intestinal tract) bacilli and differentiate them based on lactose fermentation.
   MacConkey agar is recommended for the detection and isolation of coliforms and intestinal pathogens from stool, urine, water and other material. MacConkey media can be used for *Campylobacter, Enterobacter, Enterobacteriaceae, Enterococcus, Escherichia coli and Coliforms, Proteus, Salmonella, Shigella,* and *Staphylococcus.*

High yield!

Sorbitol can be used as a replacement sugar in MacConkey agar to assist in the isolation and differentiation of enteropathogenic *E. coli* serotypes such as *E. coli* O157:H7 by the presence of white circular colonies that are non-sorbitol fermenting.

Other media:

- Eosin methylene blue agar
  - Selective for gram negative organisms
  - Differential for lactose fermentation.
- Mannitol salt agar
  - Selective for staphylococci
  - Differential with respect to mannitol fermentation.
- Blood agar:
  - Is a nutrient media with differential properties with respect to hemolysis
  - Complete breakdown is known as beta hemolysis
  - Partial hemolysis is termed as alpha hemolysis
  - No change in hemolysis and no change in the medium is known as gamma hemolysis.

Note: A colicin is a type of bacteriocin produced by and toxic to some strains of Escherichia coli. Colicins bind to outer membrane receptors, using them to translocate to the cytoplasm or cytoplasmic membrane, where they exert their cytotoxic effect, including depolarization of the cytoplasmic membrane, DNase activity, RNase activity, or inhibition of murein synthesis. These substances do not play role in growth of *E. coli* on MacConkey culture media

4. Which of the following will grow on chocolate agar?

a. Neisseria meningitidis
b. Haemophilus influenzae
c. Vibrio cholerae
d. Listeria monocytogenes
e. Staphylococcus aureus

Ans. a,b,d

Option a	True	
Option b	True	
Option c	False	Alkaline peptone water (APW) is recommended as an enrichment broth, and thiosulfate citrate bile salts sucrose (TCBS) agar is the selective agar medium of choice for isolating V. cholerae O1
Option d	True	
Option e	False	Grows in rich media with aeration (e.g. Brain Heart Infusion Agar)

Is a non-selective enriched growth media used for isolation of pathogenic bacteria

- It is a variant of the blood agar plate, containing red blood cells that have been lysed by slowly heating to 80°C. Chocolate agar is used for growing fastidious respiratory bacteria, such as Haemophilus influenzae and Neisseria meningitidis.
- Thayer martin is selective media for Neisseria organism.
- Heated blood (chocolate) agar enriched with growth factors V (nicotinamide adenine dinucleotide [NAD]) and × (hematin) — selective media for H. Influenza.

5. Influenza, incorrect is:

a. HA activation > 60% efficacy
b. HA activation < 60% efficacy
c. Most common strain H3N2
d. Belongs to family orthomyxoviridae
e. 4 types of influenza virus cause human infections: A, B, C and D

Ans. b,e

Option a	True	Yes correct
Option b	False	Not correct
Option c	True	Yes, both H1N1 and H3N2 are most prevalent strains and included in the annual flu shot vaccines. H3N2 is however, slightly more prevalent compared to other Influenza viruses
Option d	True	Yes, correct
Option e	False	No, influenza virus is of three serotypes A,B,C which cause infections in humans. The influenza D strain cause influenza infection in cattle and other animals.

There are four types of influenza viruses: A, B, C and D. Human influenza A and B viruses cause seasonal epidemics. Influenza D viruses primarily affect cattle and are not known to infect or cause illness in people.

Vaccine for influenza:

- An A/Michigan/45/2015 (H1N1) pdm 09-like virus (updated)
- An A/Hong Kong/4801/2014 (H3N2)-like virus
- A B/Brisbane/60/2008-like (B/Victoria lineage) virus

6. Streptococcus Agalactiae is:

a. Coagulates negative
b. Catalase negative
c. Bacitracin sensitive
d. CAMP test positive
e. Hippurate hydrolysis negative

Ans. a, b, d

Option a	True	Yes, correct. Coagulase test is used to differentiate *Staphylococcus aureus* (positive) from Coagulase Negative Staphylococcus (CONS)
Option b	True	Yes, correct. Catalase positivity is to differentiate between staphylococcus (catalase positive) from streptococcus (catalase negative)
Option c	False	No, There is no zone of inhibition on bacitracin test
Option d	True	Yes, correct.
Option e	False	No, not correct. S. Agalactiae hydrolyses Hippurate and is used to differentiate from other beta hemolytic streptococci.

Ref: Ananthanarayan's Textbook of Microbiology. Pg 204; Patterson MJ. Streptococcus. In: Baron S, (ed). Medical Microbiology (4th/ed). Galveston (TX): University of Texas Medical Branch at Galveston; 1996. Chapter 13; https://microbiologyinfo.com/tag/streptococcus-agalactiae/S. Agalactiae, a member of the Lancefield Group B streptococci.

Microbiological features

Strept. Agalactiae

- ❑ CAMP positive
- ❑ Capsule positive
- ❑ Catalase negative
- ❑ Coagulase negative
- ❑ Oxidase negative

Clinical relevance: *S agalactiae* may cause:

Neonates: meningitis, neonatal sepsis, pneumonia, LRTI adults: vaginitis, puerperal fever, urinary tract infection, skin infection, endocarditis.

It is a beta-hemolytic, catalase-negative, and facultative anaerobe. The CAMP test is also another important test for identification of GBS. The CAMP factor produced by GBS acts synergistically with the staphylococcal β-hemolysin inducing enhanced hemolysis of sheep or bovine erythrocytes.

CAMP test

CAMP is an acronym for the authors of this test (Christie, Atkinson, Munch, and Peterson) which was identified in 1944.

Uses

1. It is used to distinguish the species *Streptococcus agalactiae* from other species of beta-hemolytic *Streptococcus.*
2. It is used to identify *Listeria monocytogenes* which also produces a positive CAMP reaction. CAMP test—Principle, Uses, Procedure and Result Interpretation.

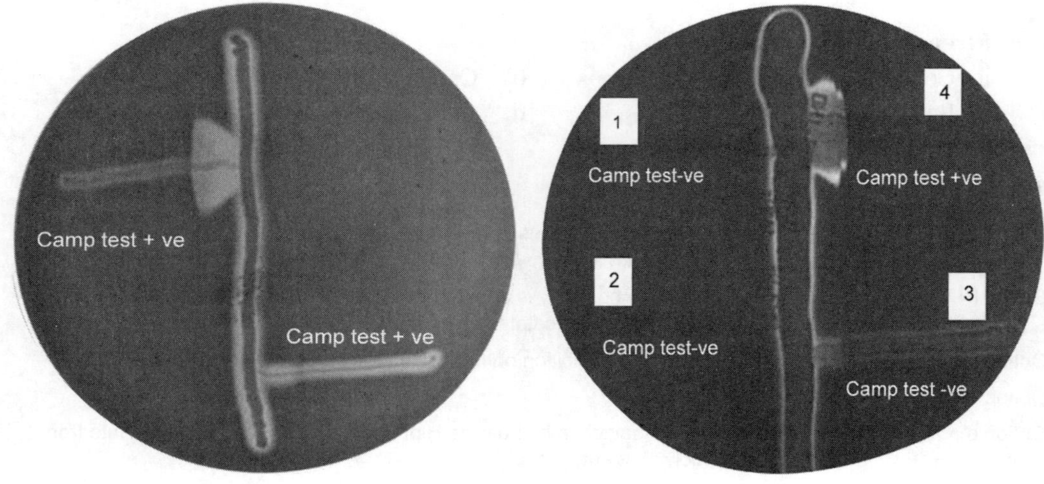

Positive: Enhanced hemolysis is indicated by an arrow head-shaped zone of beta-hemolysis at the junction of the two organisms.

Hippurate hydrolysis test

Hippurate is the glycine conjugate of benzoic acid. When hippurate is hydrolyzed by an organism glycine and benzoic acid are formed.

Uses:

1. Hippurate hydrolysis test is critical for separation of *Campylobacter jejuni* (hydrolyzes hippurate) and *Campylobacter coli* (negative) strains.
2. Aids in the differentiation of β-hemolytic *Streptococcus Agalactiae* from other β-hemolytic streptococci.

Organisms giving positive (+ve) test are:

- *Gardnerella vaginalis*
- *Campylobacter jejuni*
- *Listeria monocytogenes* and
- Group B streptococci (*Streptococcus agalactiae*)

Bacitracin test

The presumptive identification of beta hemolytic Group A streptococci from beta hemolytic non-Group A Streptococci is usually done by testing for sensitivity to bacitracin.

Streptococcus pyogenes is inhibited by the small amount of bacitracin in the disk; other beta-hemolytic streptococci usually or not.

Positive: (Bacitracin sensitive) Any zone of inhibition around the disk, Streptococcus pyogenes.

Negative: (Bacitracin resistant) No zone of inhibition, streptococcus Agalactiae.

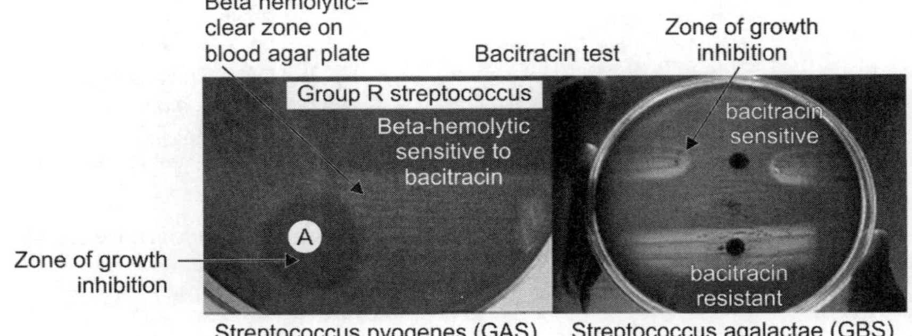

Coagulase test:

Coagulase test is used to differentiate *Staphylococcus aureus* (positive) from Coagulase Negative Staphylococcus (CONS). Coagulase is an enzyme produced by *S. aureus* that converts (soluble) fibrinogen in plasma to (insoluble) fibrin. *Staphylococcus aureus* produces two forms of coagulase, bound and free.

1. Slide coagulase test is done to detect bound coagulase or clumping factor.
2. Tube coagulase test is done to detect free coagulase.

Feature differentiation between STAPH and STREPT

	Staphylococcus	Streptococcus
Shape	Gram positive cocci in clusters (grape-like) because cell division occurs in various directions on multiple axes. Gram positive cocci in pairs, tetrads, short chains also seen.	Gram Positive cocci in pairs or short chains (cell division occurs in single axis)
Catalase Test (Most important test to differentiate Staph from Strep)	Positive (presence of catalase enzyme)	Negative
Growth requirement	Not fastidious (does not need enriched media)	Fastidious (needs enriched media).
Hemolysis	No hemolysis or beta hemolysis	Either alpha, or beta or gamma hemolysis (Hemolysis can be helpful to differentiate species of *Streptococcus*)
Common habitat	Mostly skin, anterior nares	Mainly mouth and respiratory tract
Common diseases	Pneumonia, meningitis, osteomyelitis, acute endocarditis, septic arthritis, surgical site infection, wound infection etc.	Pneumonia, sore throat, wound infection, necrotizing fasciitis, Scarlet fever, Rheumatic fever, Acute post-streptococcal glomerulonephritis
Most pathogenic species	*Staphylococcus aureus* *Staphylococcus saprophyticus* (in female)	*Streptococcus pneumoniae* *Streptococcus pyogenes* *Streptococcus agalactiae*
Useful diagnostic tests	Catalase test coagulase test Novobiocin sensitivity test	Catalase test Bacitracin sensitivity test (*S. pyogenes)* Optochin sensitivity test *(S. pneumoniae)* Bile solubility test *(S. pneumoniae)* CAMPT test *(S. agalactiae)*

7. Pig tapeworm may cause dangerous disease than beef tapeworm because:

a. Invasion of deep mucosa
b. CNS involvement
c. Larger size
d. Armed scolex
e. Eggs not infective to humans

Ans. b,d

Option a	False	No, not of major relevance
Option b	True	Yes, Tenia solium may lead to CNS space occupying lesions
Option c	False	No, size is almost same for both tenia, however, T. saginata may be as long as 25 m in certain patients.
Option d	True	Yes, correct
Option e	False	No, Pig tapeworm (T. solium) eggs are infective to humans

Microbiological relevance:

Properties	Tenia solium	Tenia saginata
Common Name	(Pork tapeworm)	(Best tapeworm)
Definitive host	Human	Human
Intermediate host	Pig	Cow/Cattle
Disease	Taeniasis and Cysticercosis	Taeniasis only
Transmission	**Eating raw or insufficiently cooked measly pork** containing the cysticerci.	**Eating of undercooked beef containing the cysticerci** ("measly" beef)
Size	Size of adult worm: 2-7 m	Size of adult worm: 5 m or less (sometime up to 25 m)
Scolex	• The scolex head is globular in outline and has four circular suckers.	• The scolex ("head") is quadrate in outline and has four circular suckers.
	• The head is provided with the rostellum armed with double row of alternating large and small hooklets. The rostellar hooklets are shaped like daggers or Arbian poniards (**armed scolex**)	• Rostellum and hooklets are absent (i.e. **unarmed scolex**)
Proglottids	• The total number of proglottids (segments) is an average of 1000. • The gravid uterus consists of a median longitudinal stem with **5–13 compound lateral branches** on each side • The gravid segments are expelled passively, in chains of 5-6 at a time, and not singly. • *T. solium* may produce 50,000 eggs per proglottid.	• The number of proglottids varies from 1000–2000. • The gravid uterus consists of a central longitudinal stem with **15-30 lateral branches on each side**; these in turn sub-branch leaving practically no space in between. • The gravid segments are expelled singly • *T. saginata* may produce up to 100,000 eggs per proglottid.

Contd…

Contd...

Properties	Tenia solium	Tenia saginata
Eggs	• Eggs of *Tenia solium* and *Tenia saginata* are morphologically indistinguishable. • The **eggs are not floated** in the saturated solution of NaCl.	
Eggs (Infectious nature)	Infectious to humans	Eggs of *Tenia saginata* are not infectious to humans. They are infective to cattle only

Clinical Relevance

Tenia solium

1. Intestinal tapeworm
   - Ingestion of encysted larvae (cysticerci) in undercooked pork.
2. Cysticercosis
   - Ingestion of eggs
   - Eggs hatch and larvae migrate throughout the body
   - Larvae penetrate tissue and encyst there, forming cysticerci.
3. Neurocysticercosis
   - As above, except larvae encyst in the brain causing "*Swiss cheese*" lesions
   - Neurocysticercosis is a common cause of adult-onset seizures.

Cysticercosis features

1. Cysticercosis features—depends on the site and number of cysticerci that develop.
2. The scolex of T. Solium has anterior circle of sharply spined hooks arranged in a double row. These are under muscular control and work with the four suckers to adhere to the gut wall higher intestinal disturbance. These hooked scolex cause more inflammation and distress to Gut mucosa.
3. M/c site is CNS—(most commonly space occupying lesion of the brain or globe of eye).
4. May lead to hydrocephalus (involvement of ventricles and cisternae).

5. Infection in specific sites may lead to epilepsy, mental disturbances, or a meningeal syndromes.
6. Most of the damage or the features of cysticercosis—occur due the severe inflammatory response occurring after the death and disruption of the parasite.

Intestinal tapeworm

1. Ingestion of encysted larvae (cysticerci) in undercooked beef
2. Humans do NOT develop cysticercosis after ingesting eggs from T. Saginata.

Diagnosis

1. ELISA
2. CT—sensitive and specific for diagnosis
3. Biopsy examination of a subcutaneous nodule containing cysticerci
4. X-ray of skull and soft tissue may reveal calcified cysticerci
5. Eosinophilia may occur in the invasive stage
6. A positive indirect hemagglutination test using antigen from pig's cysticerci
7. Intestinal tapeworms—diagnosed by stool examination.

8. HPV features

a. RNA virus
b. Cancer is caused by 16, 18 serotypes
c. Divided in five genera
d. Recently phase 3 trial has been approved for nonavalent vaccine
e. Henital warts are most common by HPV 1 and HPV 4

Ans. b,d *Ref: Lange 13th/ed p673*

Option a	False	No, it is a DNA virus
Option b	True	Yes, correct
Option c	False	No it has over 100 types of HPV virus
Option d	True	Yes, correct
Option e	False	No, genital warts are common by HPV 6 and HPV 11

- ❑ Human papilloma virus may lead to benign tumors of squamous cells.
- ❑ HPV are non enveloped virus with double stranded DNA and icosahedral nucleocapsid
- ❑ Inactivation of p53 and RB proteins is important step in pathogenesis of cancer
- ❑ There are 100 types of papilloma viruses classified on the basis of DNA fragment analysis

HPV related diseases:

- ❑ Genital warts are the most common sexually transmitted diseases
- ❑ Skin and plantar warts - HPV 1-4
- ❑ Genital warts (condylomata acuminate) by HPV 6 and HPV 11
- ❑ Carcinoma cervix, penis, anus and other premalignant lesions (intraepithelial neoplasia) associated with HPV 16 and HPV 18

Diagnosis:

- PCR to detect presence of DNA

Treatment

- Podophyllin, liquid nitrogen, salicylic acid
- Surgical removal of warts
- Alpha interferon

Vaccines:

1. Gardasil – four types of HPV (6,11,16,18)
2. Cervarix – recombinant vaccine with 16,18 type HPV
3. Gardasil 9 – nonavalent vaccine wth HPV 6, 11, 16, 18, 31, 33, 45, 52, and 58

Circumcision reduces the risk of infection by HPV

9. Which disease may be caused by spirochetes species:

a. Syphilis
b. Leptospirosis
c. Pinta
d. Legionella
e. Lyme Disease

Ans. a,b,c,e *Ref: Ananthnaryan paniker, 7th/ed 377; Lange 13th/ed 442*

Option a	True	Yes, correct
Option b	True	Yes, correct
Option c	True	Yes, correct
Option d	False	No, it is not part of spirochete species
Option e	True	Yes, correct

Three genera of spirochetes cause human infections:

1. Treponema
2. Borrelia
3. Leptospira

- Spirochetes are thin walled, flexible, motile, spiral rods
- Seen by dark field microscopy, silver impregnation or immunofluorescence

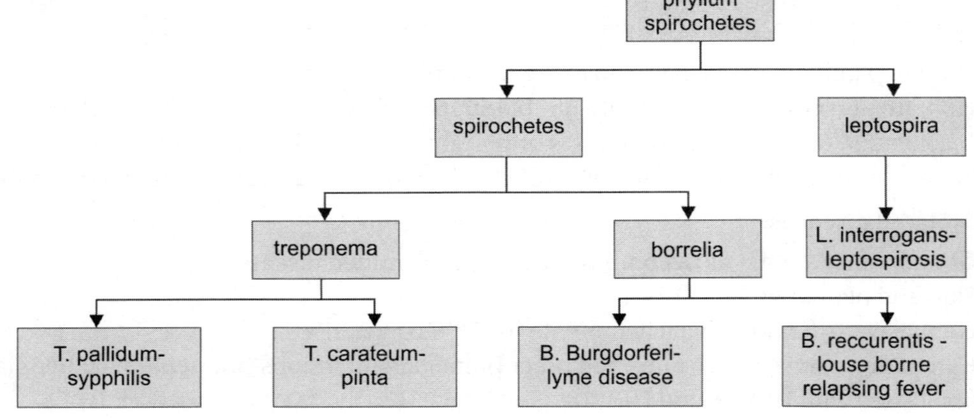

Species	Disease	Mode of Transmission	Diagnosis	Morphology	Growth in Bacte-riologic Media	Treatment
Treponema pallidum	Syphilis	Intimate (sexual) contact; across the placenta	Microscopy; serologic tests	Thin, tight, spirals, seen by dark field illumination, silver impregnation, or immunofluorescent stain	–	Penicillin g
Borrelia burgdorferi	Lyme disease	Tick bite	Clinical observations; microscopy	Large, loosely coiled; stain with Giema stain	+	Tetracycline or amoxicillin for acute; penicilling G for chronicle
Borrelia recurrentis	Relapsing fever	Louse bite	Clinical observations; microscopy	Large, loosely coiled; stain with Giemsa stain	+	Tetracycline
Leptospira interrogans	Leptospirosis	Food or drink contaminated by urine of infected animals (rats, dogs, pigs, cows)	Serologic tests	Thin, tight spirals, seen by dark field illumination	+	Penicillin G

Microbiology

1. Which of the following are true about rotavirus infection?

a. Most commonly seen in adult of > 30 year age group
b. Person to person transmission may occur
c. Severity of disease decreases with each repeat infection
d. Commonest cause of diarrhea in infants and children
e. Single infection provide lifelong immunity against reinfection

Ans. b, c, d

Option a	False	Causes moderate-to-severe diarrhea in infants and children
Option b	True	
Option c	True	The reduced severity of rotavirus disease in older children and adults is due primarily to the immunity induced by previous rotavirus infections
Option d	True	
Option e	False	Reinfections are common among children

Explanation

- *Rotavirus and Escherichia coli (EPEC)* are the two most common etiological agents of moderate-to-severe diarrhea in infants and children in low-income countries. Other pathogens such as cryptosporidium and shigella species may also be important.
- *Mode of transmission:* The primary mode of transmission is the fecal-oral route, usually through close contact between people. Because the virus is stable in the environment, transmission also can occur through ingestion of contaminated water or food and contact with contaminated surfaces or objects.
- *Clinical manifestation*
  - Incubation period: 1–3 days.
  - Typical symptoms include watery diarrhea, fever, abdominal pain, and vomiting, leading to dehydration.
  - Rota viruses have been divided into 3 groups (A, B and C) on the basis of their epidemiology.
    Group A: Single most important cause of endemic severe diarrheal illness in infants and young children worldwide (in cooler months in temperate climates).
    Group B: Outbreaks of diarrheal illness in adults and children in China and SE Asia.
    Group C: Sporadic cases and occasional outbreaks of diarrheal illness in children.
- *Rotaviruses* are ubiquitous. By age 3 years, 90% of children have serum antibodies to one or more types. This high prevalence of rotavirus antibodies is maintained in adults, suggesting subclinical reinfections by the virus. Rotavirus reinfections are common; it has been shown that young children can suffer up to five reinfections by 2 years of age. The reduced severity of rotavirus disease in older children and adults is due primarily to the immunity induced by previous rotavirus infections.
- *Pathogenicity:* Rotaviruses infect cells in the villi of the small intestine (gastric and colonic mucosa are spared). They multiply in the cytoplasm of enterocytes and damage their

transport mechanisms. Diarrhea caused by rotaviruses may also be due to impaired sodium and glucose absorption as damaged cells on villi are replaced by nonabsorbing immature crypt cells.

- *Laboratory diagnosis:* Demonstration of virus in stool collected early in the illness by ELISA or Immunoelectron microscopy. PCR is the most sensitive detection method. Rise in antibody titer by ELISA (seroprevalence purpose).
- *Prevention:* Rotarix® (RV1) Live attenuated vaccine containing serotype G1-4 and G9. It is given in 2 doses at ages ***2 months and 4 months.***

2. True about ZIKA virus:

a. Belong to flavivirus
b. First case detected in 1953 in Nigeria
c. RT PCR is useful in diagnosis
d. Causes macrocephaly
e. May presents with conjunctivitis

Ans. a, c, e *Ref: https://www.cdc.gov/zika/index.html; http://www.who.int/mediacentre/factsheets/zika/en/*

Option a	True	
Option b	False	First identified in Uganda in 1947 in monkeys
Option c	True	
Option d	False	Causes microcephaly
Option e	True	

- *Introduction:* Zika virus disease is caused by a virus transmitted primarily by Aedes mosquitoes. Zika virus is a mosquito-borne flavivirus that was first identified in Uganda in 1947 in monkeys through a network that monitored yellow fever. It was later identified in humans in 1952 in Uganda and the United Republic of Tanzania. Outbreaks of Zika virus disease have been recorded in Africa, the Americas, Asia and the Pacific. From the 1960s to 1980s, human infections were found across Africa and Asia, typically accompanied by mild illness. The first large outbreak of disease caused by Zika infection was reported from the Island of Yap (Federated States of Micronesia) in 2007. In July 2015 Brazil reported an association between Zika virus infection and Guillain-Barré syndrome. In October 2015 Brazil reported an association between Zika virus infection and microcephaly.
- *Clinical manifestation:* Zika virus disease can have symptoms including mild fever, skin rash, conjunctivitis, muscle and joint pain, malaise or headache. These symptoms normally last for 2–7 days. There is scientific consensus that Zika virus is a cause of microcephaly and Guillain-Barré syndrome. Links to other neurological complications are also being investigated. Infection with Zika virus may be suspected based on symptoms and recent history of travel (e.g. residence in or travel to an area with active Zika virus transmission).
- *Laboratory diagnosis:* The FDA has issued Emergency Use Authorization (EUA) for several diagnostic tools for Zika virus, including the Trioplex Real-Time RT-PCR (rRT-PCR) assay (should be performed on serum collected during the first two weeks after symptom onset and on urine samples collected less than 14 days after symptom onset) and the Zika MAC-ELISA (qualitative detection of Zika virus IgM Abs in serum or CSF).

- *Prevention and treatment:*
  - No vaccine exists to prevent Zika.
  - Prevent Zika by avoiding mosquito bites.
  - There is no specific medicine or vaccine for Zika virus.

3. Parasite which infects through ingestion of aquatic vegetation:

a. Fasciola hepatica
b. Fasciolopsis buski
c. Paragonimus westermani
d. Watsonius watsoni
e. Gastrodiscoides hominis

Ans. a, b, d, e

Option a	True	
Option b	True	
Option c	False	Infection occur after a person eats raw or undercooked infected crab or crayfish
Option d	True	
Option e	True	

- *Trematodes* (Flukes) include the helminths that are unsegmented, flat (flatworm) and leaf like.
  Classification based on the habitat:
  - Blood flukes: Schistosoma haematobium, S. mansoni, S. japonicum.
  - Hepatic flukes: Fasciola hepatica, Fasciola gigantica, Clonorchis species, Opisthorchis species.
  - Lung flukes: Paragonimus westermani
  - Intestinal flukes: Fasciolopsis buski, Heterophyes species, Metagonimus species, Watsonius species and Gastrodiscoides species.
- *Life cycle:* Trematodes complete their life cycle in 3 different hosts, one definitive host (man) AND two intermediate hosts.
  - 1st intermediate host: fresh water snail or mollusk.
  - 2nd intermediate host: either aquatic plant or fish or crab.
  - Mode of transmission: by eating aquatic plants, fishes or crabs harboring infective form (metacercariae) or by the penetration of free living cercariae (Schistosoma).
- Except Paragonimus westermani (crab or crab fish), all are infecting human by ingestion of aquatic vegetation containing metacercariae.

4. Which of the following dyads of vector with disease is/are correctly matched?

a. Rat flea—Endemic typhus
b. Sand flea—Oriental sore
c. Black fly—Kala-azar
d. Cyclops—Dracunculiasis
e. Louse—Chagas disease

Ans. a, d

Option a	True	
Option b	False	Caused by sandfly
Option c	False	Caused by sandfly
Option d	True	
Option e	False	Spread by kissing bugs

- Endemic typhus is caused by Rickettsia typhi by rat flea (Xenopsylla cheopis) or rarely by cat flea (Ctenocephalides).
- Oriental sore (cutaneous leishmaniasis) is caused by L. tropica complex. This condition also known as Delhi boil, Aleppo boil AND Baghdad button. Leishmania completes its life cycle in 2 hosts, vertebrate host (man, dog, rodents) and insect vector Phlebotomus (female sandfly).
- Visceral leishmaniasis (kala-azar—Hindi for black fever) is caused by L. donovani.
- Dracunculiasis, also called Guinea-worm disease (GWD), is an infection by the Guinea worm.
  - Life cycle: Definitive host (man) and Intermediate host (Cyclops/Copepods).
  - A person becomes infected when they drink water that contains cyclops infected with guinea worm L3 larvae (infective form).
- Chagas disease, or American trypanosomiasis, is caused by the parasite Trypanosoma cruzi. Infection is most commonly acquired through contact with the feces of an infected triatomine bug (or "kissing bug"), a blood-sucking insect that feeds on humans and animals.

5. All are feature of scrub typhus except:

a. Black eschar
b. Maculo-papular rash
c. More common in rural areas
d. Ciprofloxacin is drug of choice
e. Tick borne disease

Ans. d, e

Option a	True	The punched-out ulcer covered with a blackened scab that indicates the location of the mite bite
Option b	True	Common presentation
Option c	True	Most cases of scrub typhus occur in rural areas of Southeast Asia, Indonesia, China, Japan, India, and northern Australia
Option d	False	Doxycycline is DOC, given daily orally and continued for 3–4 days after defervescence
Option e	False	Transmitted by mite

- ***Black eschar***
  - Cutaneous anthrax generally occurs on exposed surfaces of the arms or hands followed in frequency by the face and neck. A pruritic papule develops 1-7 days after entry of the organisms or spores through a scratch. Initially, it resembles an insect bite. The papule rapidly changes into a vesicle or small ring of vesicles that coalesce, and a necrotic ulcer develops. The lesions typically are 1-3 cm in diameter and have a characteristic central black eschar. Marked edema occurs.
  - Rickettsialpox (Rickettsia akari) is a mild disease with a vesicular rash resembling that of varicella. About 1 week before onset of fever, a firm red papule appears at the site of the mite bite and develops into a deep-seated vesicle that in turn forms a black eschar.
- ***Scrub typhus/Chiggerosis/Bush typhus***
  - It is caused by *Orientia tsutsugamushi.*
  - Rickettsia are pleomorphic coccobacilli that are obligate intracellular pathogens similar to gram-negative bacteria but they do not stain with Gram stain.

- *Vector:* It is transmitted by the bite of infected trombiculid mites chiggers larva (Leptotrombidium deliensis in India and L. akamushi in Japan).
- *Clinical manifestation:* This disease resembles epidemic typhus clinically. One feature is the *eschar*, the punched-out ulcer covered with a blackened scab that indicates the location of the mite bite. Generalized lymphadenopathy, maculopapular rashes and lymphocytosis are common. Illness can be severe with associated cardiac and cerebral involvement leading to death in about 30% of patients.
- *Laboratory diagnosis:* Weil Felix test (OX K Abs detection), Specific Abs detection by ELISA, Real-time PCR.
- *Treatment:* Tetracyclines, preferably doxycycline, are effective, provided treatment is started early. Doxycycline is given daily orally and continued for 3–4 days after defervescence. In severely ill patients, the initial doses can be given intravenously. Chloramphenicol also can be effective.
- *Prevention:* No vaccine is available to prevent scrub typhus. Reduce your risk of getting scrub typhus by avoiding contact with infected chiggers. When traveling to areas where scrub typhus is common, avoid areas with lots of vegetation and brush where chiggers may be found.

6. Which of the following is/are caused by dermatophytes?

a. Madura foot
b. Athlete's foot
c. Kerion
d. Favus
e. Cradle cap

Ans. b, c, d

Option a	False	Caused by eumycetoma
Option b	True	
Option c	True	
Option d	True	
Option e	False	Caused by Malassezia furfur, non-dermatophyte fungus

- ❑ An actinomycetoma is a mycetoma caused by an actinomycete; a eumycetoma (maduromycosis, Madura foot) is a Mycetoma caused by a fungus. The fungal agents of mycetoma include, among others, Pseudallescheria boydii (anamorph, Scedosporium apiospermum), Madurella mycetomatis, Madurella grisea, E. jeanselmei, and Acremonium falciforme. Draining mycetomas are often superinfected with staphylococci and streptococci.
- ❑ Dermatophytes
  - Cutaneous mycoses are caused by fungi that infect only the keratinized tissue (skin, hair, and nails). The most important of these are the dermatophytes, a group of about 40 related fungi that belong to three genera: Microsporum, Trichophyton, and Epidermophyton.
  - In skin they are diagnosed by the presence of hyaline, septate, branching hyphae, or chains of arthroconidia.
  - Clinical manifestation: Kerion, Favus, Ectothrix, Endothrix, Tinea corporis, T. pedis (athlete foot), T. cruris, T. barbae, T. faciei, T. imbricate, T. unguium, T. manuum.

Skin disease	Location of lesions	Clinical appearance	Fungi most frequently responsible
Tinea corporis (ringworm)	Non-hairy smooth skin	Circular patches with advancing red, vesiculated border and central scaling. Pruritic	*Microsporum canis, Trichophyton mentagrophytes.*
Tinea pedist (athlete's foot)	Interdigital spaces on feet of persons wearing shoes.	Acute: Itching, red, vesicular. Chronic: itching, scaling, fissures.	*Trichophyton rubrum, T mentagrophytes, Epidermophyton floccosum.*
Tinea cruris (jock itch)	Groin	Erythematous scaling lesion in intertriginous area. Pruritic.	*T rubrum, T mentagrophytes, E floccosum.*
Tinea capitis	Scalp hair. Endothrix: fungus in side hair shaft. Ectothrix: fungus on surface of hair	Circular bald patches with short hair stubs or broken hair within hair follicles. Kerion rare. Microsporum infected hairs fluoresce	*Microsporum canis, Trichophyton tonsurans.*
Tinea barbae	Beard hair.	Edematous, erythematous lesion.	*T rubrum, T mentagrophytes.*
Tinea unguium (onychomycosis)	Nail	Nails thickened or crumbling distally, discolored, lusterless. Usually associated with tinea pedis	*T rubrum, T mentagrophytes, E floccosum.*
Dermatophytid (id reaction)	Usually sides and flexor aspects of fingers. Palm. Any site on body	Pruritic vesicular to bullous lesions. Most commonly associated with tinea pedis	No fungi present in lesion. May become secondarily infected with bacteria.

- ❑ Cradle cap (infantile seborrheic dermatitis) is caused by Malassezia furfur.

7. Which of the following has least minimum infective dose (MID) required for causing infection?

a. Salmonella typhi
b. Campylobacter jejuni
c. Shigella dysentery
d. Vibrio cholera
e. E. coli

Ans. c

Option a	False	Very large >105 organisms
Option b	False	Low (500 organisms)
Option c	True	Shigella's infectious dose is very less (10–100 bacilli)
Option d	False	Relatively large (10^4–10^6 organisms)
Option e	False	Very large (10^6–10^8 organisms)

1. Minimum lethal dose (MLD) is the minimum number of the organism required to produce death in animal under standard conditions and minimum infecting dose (MID) is the minimum number of the organism required to produce clinical infection in a susceptible animal under standard condition.

2. The lethal dose 50% (LD50) is the number of organism required to kill 50% of the animal tested and the infectious dose 50% (ID50) is the number of organism required for 50% of the population to show sign of infection. Pathogens having the lowest LD50 and ID50 values are the most virulent.
3. Shigella's infectious dose is very less (10-100 bacilli) so LD50 also will be less.

Infectious doses for some known microorganisms

- *Escherichia coli:* Very large (10^6 – 10^8 organisms)
- *Salmonella:* Quite large in order to definitely establish infection (e.g. >10^5 organisms) but infection may also be established by lower numbers (e.g. 10s of organisms)
- *Vibrio cholerae:* Relatively large (10^4 – 10^6 organisms)
- *Bacillus anthracis:* Relatively large (10^4 spores)
- *Campylobacter jejuni:* Low (500 organisms)
- *Francisella tularensis:* Very low (10 – 50 organisms)
- *Shigella:* Very low (10s of organisms)
- *Cryptosporidium parvum:* Very low (10 to 30 oocysts)
- *Escherichia coli O157:H7:* Very low (< 10 organisms)
- *Mycobacterium tuberculosis:* Very low (< 10 organisms)
- *Entamoeba coli:* Extremely low (from 1 cyst).

8. All are true about H1N1 influenza except:

a. Zanamivir commonly given through IV route
b. Fatality more in some high risk group
c. RT-PCR is used for investigation
d. WHO latest trivalent influenza vaccine contains two influenza A subtypes (H3N2 and H1N1) and tow influenza B component
e. CDC latest quadrivalent influenza vaccine contains two influenza A subtypes (H3N2 and H1N1) and tow influenza B component

Ans. a, d *Ref: https://www.cdc.gov/flu/protect/vaccine/vaccines.htm*

Option a	False	Given through inhalational route
Option b	True	
Option c	True	
Option d	False	WHO latest trivalent influenza vaccine contains two influenza A subtypes (H3N2 and H1N1) and one influenza B component
Option e	True	Quadrivalent vaccines will include an additional vaccine virus strain, a B/Phuket/3073/2013–like virus (Yamagata lineage)

- *Treatment* (A/H1N1 2009 flu)
  - DOC is neuraminidase inhibitors: Oseltamivir (Tamiflu) tablet and Zanamivir (inhalational forms).
- *High risk groups:* the following are at increased risk of complications associated with influenza virus infection.
  - Age: children (< 2 years) and old age (> 65 years) and Pregnancy.
  - Underlying chronic lung, cardiac, renal, hepatic and CNS conditions.
  - Low immunity.
- *Laboratory diagnosis*

- *Sample: Nasopharyngeal swab, kept at 4 °C.*
- Isolation of virus: Embryonated eggs and primary monkey kidney cell lines. Growth detected by hemabsorption and hemagglutination tests.
- Viral Ag detection by direct IF test.
- Abs detection by hemagglutination inhibition test, neutralization test and ELISA.
- Molecular tests: RT PCR detects viral RNA and Real time PCR quantifies viral RNA.

❑ *Vaccines*

- 2016–17 U.S. trivalent influenza vaccines will contain an A/California/7/2009 (H1N1)-like virus, an A/Hong Kong/4801/2014 (H3N2)-like virus and a B/Brisbane/60/2008-like virus (Victoria lineage). Quadrivalent vaccines will include an additional vaccine virus strain, a B/Phuket/3073/2013-like virus (Yamagata lineage).

9. Which of the following mechanism is/are used by bacteria to escape host defense mechanism?

a. Mycobacterium tuberculosis prevent intracellular killing by inhibiting phagolysosome formation
b. Streptococcus pyogenes by M protein
c. Neisseria meningitides by capsular polysaccharide
d. Staphylococcus aureus by iron-regulated outer membrane proteins
e. Polysaccharide capsules of H. influenza

Ans. a, b, c

Option a	True	
Option b	True	
Option c	True	
Option d	False	
Option e	False	The polyribose phosphate capsule of type b H influenzae is the major virulence factor

1. Survival of M. tuberculosis inside the macrophages: this is due to bacterial cell wall LAM which impairs phagosome-lysosome fusion by inhibiting increase in intracellular Ca^{2+} and phosphatidylinositol 3 phosphates.
2. M protein of Strep pyogenes is acid and heat stable, but trypsin labile. This substance is a major virulence factor of S. pyogenes. M protein is a filamentous structure anchored to the cell membrane that penetrates and projects from the streptococcal cell wall. When M protein is present, the streptococci are virulent, and in the absence of M type-specific antibodies, they are able to resist phagocytosis by polymorphonuclear leukocytes by inhibiting activation of the alternate complement pathway. S pyogenes that lack M protein are not virulent. Immunity to infection with group A streptococci is related to the presence of type-specific antibodies to M protein. Because there are more than 150 types of M protein, a person can have repeated infections with S pyogenes of different M types. Both groups C and G streptococci have genes homologous to the genes for M protein of group A, and M proteins similar to those of group A have been found on groups C and G streptococci.
3. Capsular polysaccharide of Meningococcus is the principle virulence factor by protecting bacteria from complements mediated phagocytosis.
4. Virulence factors of Staph. aureus.

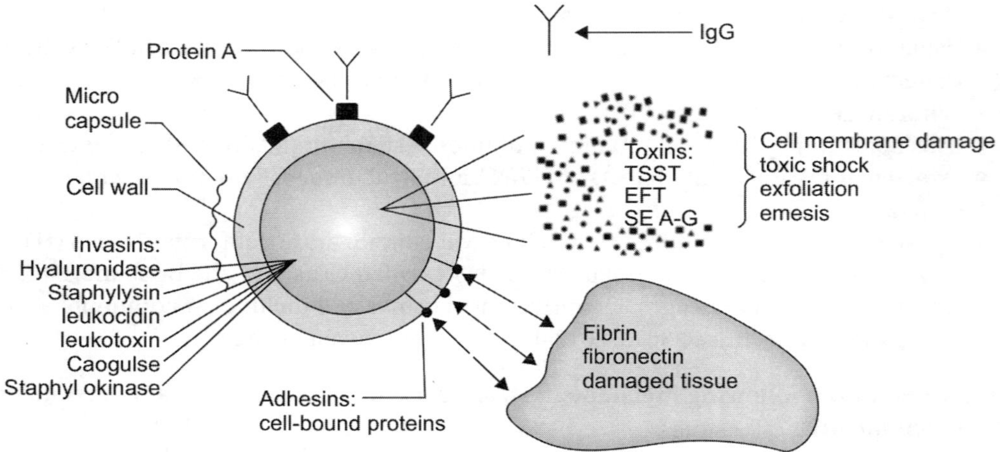

5. H. influenzae produces no exotoxin. The nonencapsulated organism is a regular member of the normal respiratory microbiota of humans. The capsule is antiphagocytic in the absence of specific anticapsular antibodies. The polyribose phosphate capsule of type b H. influenzae is the major virulence factor.

10. Dengue virus:

a. Flaviviridae
b. Type 4 most common in India
c. Positive tourniquet test > 10/sq inch
d. 2nd infection with another type IgG > IgM
e. Raised hematocrit by 20%

Ans. a, d, e

Option a	True	
Option b	False	DEN-1 and DEN-2 are widespread
Option c	False	Positive tourniquet test (> 20 petechial spots per square inch area in cubital fossa)
Option d	True	
Option e	True	

- Dengue virus belongs to family Flaviviridae. It is the most common arbovirus found in India. It has four serotypes (DEN-1 to DEN-4). Recently the fifth serotype (DEN-5) was discovered in 2013 from Bangkok.
- All four serotype have been isolated from India. Serotypes prevalence varies between seasons and places but DEN-1 and DEN-2 are widespread. DEN-5 has not been reported yet.
- Dengue hemorrhagic fever (DHF) is characterized by:
  - High grade fever
  - Hepatomegaly
  - Thrombocytopenia (platelet count < 1 lakh/mm^3)
  - Raised hematocrit (packed cell volume) by 20%
  - Positive tourniquet test (>20 petechial spots per square inch area in cubital fossa)
  - Spontaneous bleeding from skin, nose, mouth and gums.

- In secondary infection IgG Ab titers rise rapidly. IgG is often cross reactive with many flaviviruses and may give false positive result after recent infection or vaccination with yellow fever virus or JE.

11. True about pseudomonas aeruginosa:

a. Not lysine decarboxylase positive
b. Oxidase positive
c. Produce pyocyanin pigment
d. Gram positive aerobic
e. Has 6–12 flagella

Ans. a, b, c

Option a	True	
Option b	True	
Option c	True	
Option d	False	Gram negative aerobic bacilli
Option e	False	Single polar flagellum

1. P. aeruginosa is an oxidase positive, pigment producing, non-fermenting gram negative aerobic bacilli and motile via a single polar flagellum.
2. Pigments: Pyocyanin, Pyoverdin, Pyomelanin, Pyorubin.
3. It is a major pathogen among the hospitalized patients and in patients with cystic fibrosis.

12. All of the following may survive in absence of environmental oxygen except:

a. Obligate aerobe
b. Facultative anaerobes
c. Microaerophilic
d. Obligate anaerobes
e. Facultative aerobes

Ans. a, c

Option a	False	No, Oxygen is required by them
Option b	True	
Option c	False	No, Oxygen is required by them in low concentrations
Option d	True	
Option e	True	

	a. Obligate Aerobes	b. Facultative Anaerobes	c. Obligate Anaerobes	d. Aerotolerant Anaerobes	e. Micro-aerophiles
Effect of Oxygen on Growth	Only aerobic growth; oxygen required.	Both aerobic and anaerobic growth; greater growth in presence of oxygen.	Only anaerobic growth; ceases in presence of oxygen.	Only anaerobic growth; but continues in presence of oxygen.	Only aerobic growth; oxygen required in low concentration.

Contd...

Contd...

	a. Obligate Aerobes	b. Facultative Anaerobes	c. Obligate Anaerobes	d. Aerotolerant Anaerobes	e. Micro-aerophiles
Bacterial Growth in Tube of Solid Growth Medium					
Explanation of Growth Patterns	Growth occurs only where high concentrations of oxygen have diffused into the medium.	Growth is best where most oxygen is present, but occurs throughout tube.	Growth occurs only where there is no oxygen.	Growth occurs evenly; oxygen has no effect.	Growth occurs only where a low concentration of oxygen has diffused into medium
Explanation of Oxygen's effects	Presence of enzymes catalase and superoxide dismutase (SOD) allows toxic forms of oxygen to be neutralized; can use oxygen.	Presence of enzymes catalase and SOD allows toxic forms of oxygen to be neutralized; can use oxygen	Lacks enzymes to neutralize harmful forms of oxygen; cannot tolerate oxygen.	Presence of one enzyme, SOD, allows harmful forms of oxygen to be partially neutralized; tolerates oxygen.	Produce lethal amounts of toxic forms of oxygen if exposed to normal atmospheric oxygen.

13. True about serum marker of inactive carrier phase of chronic hepatitis B:

a. HBsAg positive
b. HBeAg positive
c. Anti-HBe antibody positive
d. Anti-HBcAb positive
e. Anti-HBsAb positive

Ans. a, c, d

Option a	True	
Option b	False	HBeAg negative
Option c	True	
Option d	True	
Option e	False	Anti HBsAb negative

1. Viral and immune markers are detectable in blood, and characteristic antigen antibody patterns evolve over time. The first detectable viral marker is HBsAg, followed by hepatitis B e antigen (HBeAg) and HBV DNA. Titers may be high during the incubation period, but HBV DNA and HBeAg levels begin to fall at the onset of illness and may be undetectable at the time of peak clinical illness. Core antigen does not appear in blood, but antibody to this antigen (anti-HBc) is detectable with the onset of clinical symptoms.
2. The IgM fraction is used in an important diagnostic assay for acute hepatitis B infection. Before current molecular assays were available, it was the only marker detectable in the

window period, the time between the disappearance of HBsAg and the appearance of anti-HBs. Patients who clear the virus lose HBsAg and develop anti-HBsAb, a long-lasting antibody associated with immunity. The presence of anti-HBsAb and anti-HBcAb (IgG) indicates recovery and immunity in a previously infected person, whereas a successful vaccination response produces antibody only to HBsAg.

3. HBeAg is another viral marker detectable in blood. It correlates with active viral replication and therefore high viral load and infectivity.

	HBsAg	HBeAg	Anti-HBc	Anti-HBe	Anti-HBs	HBV DNA
Acute infection	+/–*	+	+	–	–	+
Past infection	–	–	+	+/–	+	–
Occult HBV	–	–	+	–	–	+†
Chronic hepatitis B	+	+	+	–	–	+
Pre-core mutant	+	–	+	+	–	+
Healthy carrier	+	–	+	+	–	–

*May be negative in acute infections where HBsAg is below the limit of detection.
†HBV DNA may only be detectable with sensitive PCR methods.

14. DNA viruses are:

a. Hepedna virus
b. Orthomyxovirus
c. Parvovirus
d. Herpes virus
e. Pox virus

Ans. a, c, d, e

Option a	True	
Option b	False	They are RNA viruses
Option c	True	
Option d	True	
Option e	True	

1. Hepadnaviridae family: HBV is the only DNA virus among hepatitis viruses. This family also includes viruses of lower animals.
2. Orthomyxoviridae family: Influenza viruses are the member of this family. They are RNA viruses.
3. Parvoviridae: They are the simplest animal virus (non-enveloped DNA virus) infecting human, responsible for a common childhood exanthema called as erythema infectiosum (fifth disease).
4. Herpesviridae family: DNA viruses

Classification of human herpesviruses

Subfamily	*Growth cycle*	*Cytopathology*	*Site of latent infection*	*Official name*	*Common name*
Alpha-herpesvirinae	Short (12-18 hrs)	Cytolytic	Neurons	HHV1 HHV2 HHV3	HSV1 HSV2 Varicella-zoster virus

Contd...

Contd...

Subfamily	*Growth cycle*	*Cytopathology*	*Site of latent infection*	*Official name*	*Common name*
Beta-herpesvirinae	Long (>24 hrs)	Cytomegalic	Glands, kidneys	HHV5	CMV
		Lymphoproliferative	Lymphoid tissue (T-cells)	HHV6 HHV7	HHV6 HHV7
Gamma herpesviridae	Variable	Lymphoproliferative	Lymphoid tissue (B-cells)	HHV4 HHV8	EBV Kaposi's sarcoma associated herpes virus

5. Poxviridae family: Poxviruses are brick or oval-shaped viruses with large double-stranded DNA genomes. Poxviruses exist throughout the world and cause disease in humans and many other types of animals. Poxvirus infections typically result in the formation of lesions, skin nodules, or disseminated rash. Infection in humans usually occurs due to contact with contaminated animals, people, or materials. While some poxviruses, such as smallpox (variola virus), no longer exist in nature, other poxviruses can still cause disease. These include monkeypox virus, orf virus, molluscum contagiosum, and others.

15. Unlike nocardia, Actinomycosis is:

a. Facultative anaerobes
b. Not acid fast
c. Endogenous cause of disease
d. Environmental saprophyte
e. Grow at wide range of temperature range

Ans. a, b, c, d

Option a	True	Except for A. meyeri and A. israelii, as both are obligate anaerobe
Option b	True	
Option c	True	
Option d	True	Actinomyces are found in soil, their presence is important in the formation of compost
Option e	False	

Actinomyces israelii

Actinomyces is a genus of the Actinobacteria class of bacteria. They are all gram-positive and non-acid fast. Actinomyces species are facultatively anaerobic (except A. meyeri and A. israelii both obligate anaerobe), and they grow best under anaerobic conditions. Actinomyces species may form endospores, and, while individual bacteria are rod-shaped, Actinomyces colonies form fungus-like branched networks of hyphae. Actinomyces species are ubiquitous, occurring in soil and in the microbiota of animals, including the human microbiota. They are known for the important role to play in soil ecology; they produce a number of enzymes that help degrade organic plant material, lignin, and chitin. Thus their presence is important in the formation of compost.

Disease: *A. israelii* causes actinomycosis.

- **Important properties and pathogenesis:** *A. israelii* is an **anaerobe** that forms part of the **normal flora of the oral cavity**. After local trauma such as a broken jaw or dental extraction, it may invade tissues, forming filaments surrounded by areas of inflammation.

- **Clinical findings:** The typical lesion of actinomycosis appears as a hard, non-tender swelling that develops slowly and eventually drains pus through **sinus tracts**. Hard, yellow granules (**sulfur granules**) composed of a mass of filaments are formed in pus. In about 50% of cases, the initial lesion involves the face and neck; in the rest, the chest or abdomen is the site.Pelvic actinomycosis can occur in women who have retained an intrauterine device for a long period of time.
  - *A. Israelii* and *Arachnia* species are the most common causes of actinomycosis in humans. The disease is not communicable.
- **Laboratory diagnosis:** Diagnosis in the laboratory is made by (1) seeing gram positive branching rods, especially in the presence of sulfur granules; and (2) seeing growth when pus or tissue specimens are cultured in thioglycollate broth (Fluffy balls like growth at the bottom of the tube) under anaerobic conditions at 37 °C. Organisms can be identified by immunofluorescence. There are no serologic tests.
- **Treatment:** Treatment consists of prolonged administration of penicillin G, coupled with surgical drainage. There is no significant resistance to penicillin G.

16. Misfolded protein associated diseases is/are:

a. CJD
b. Alzheimer's
c. Huntington's
d. Kuru
e. None

Ans. a, d *Ref: Jawetz's Medical Microbiology, 27th/ed, 2016, McGraw-Hill Education; HARRISON'S Infectious Diseases, 1st/ed 2010, McGraw-Hill Education; Review of medical microbiology and immunology, 12th/ed, 2012, McGraw-Hill Education*

Option a	True	
Option b	False	
Option c	False	
Option d	True	
Option e	False	

1. Transmissible spongiform encephalopathies (Prion diseases)
   Degenerative central nervous system diseases—Kuru, Creutzfeldt-Jakob Disease (CJD), Gerstmann-Sträussler-Scheinker syndrome, fatal familial insomnia of humans, scrapie of sheep, transmissible encephalopathy of mink, bovine spongiform encephalopathy (BSE) of cattle, and chronic wasting disease of deer—have similar pathologic features. These diseases are described as transmissible spongiform encephalopathies. The causative agents are not conventional viruses; infectivity is associated with proteinaceous material devoid of detectable amounts of nucleic acid. The term "prion" is used to designate this novel class of agents.
2. Alzheimer's disease: There are some neuropathologic similarities between CJD and Alzheimer's disease, including the appearance of amyloid plaques. However, the disease has not been transmitted experimentally to primates or rodents, and the amyloid material in the brains of Alzheimer patients does not contain PrPSc protein.
3. Huntington's disease (HD) is typically inherited from a person's parents, with 10% of cases due to a new mutation. The disease is caused by an autosomal dominant mutation in either of an individual's two copies of a gene called Huntingtin.

17. True about leptospirosis is/are:

a. Penicillin is drug of choice
b. Zoonotic disease
c. Direct contact with skin
d. Incubation period is 2–3 months
e. Arboviral disease

Ans. a, b, c

Option a	True	
Option b	True	
Option c	True	
Option d	False	IP is 1-2 weeks
Option e	False	Zoonotic disease

1. **Treatment:**
   Mild leptospirosis: Oral doxycycline (100 mg twice a day for 7 days) or Amoxicillin (Alternative drug).
   Severe leptospirosis: Penicillin (DOC—1.5 million units IM, 4 times a day for 7 days) or Ceftriaxone/Cefotaxime (Alternative drug).
2. **Mode of transmission:** It is a zoonotic disease.
   The leptospirosis are essentially animal infections; human infection is only accidental, occurring after contact with water or other materials contaminated with the excreta of animal hosts. Rats, mice, wild rodents, dogs, swine, and cattle are the principal sources of human infection. They excrete leptospirae in urine both during the active illness and during the asymptomatic carrier state.
   3R's: The three important epidemiological determinants for leptospirosis (also known as Weil's disease) include exposure to rodents, rainfall and rice field.
3. Human infection usually results from leptospires, often in bodies of water, entering the body through breaks in the skin (cuts and abrasions) and mucous membranes (mouth, nose, conjunctivae). Ingestion is considered to be less important.
4. Incubation period of 1–2 weeks.
5. It is not a viral disease.

18. If purge rate in cholera is 500–1000 mL, it is known as:

a. Granules
b. Major
c. Mitus
d. Dumdum
e. Gravis

Ans. e

Option a	False	
Option b	False	
Option c	False	
Option d	False	
Option e	True	

- Cholera gravis, the most severe form of the disease, results when purging rate of 500–1000 mL/hr occur. This purging leads to dehydration manifested by decreased urine output, a sunken fontanel (in infants), sunken eyes, absence of tears, dry oral mucosa, shriveled hands and feet (washerwoman's hands), poor skin turgor, thready pulse, tachycardia, hypotension and vascular collapse.

- Most Vibrio cholerae infections are asymptomatic, and mild to moderate diarrhea due to V. cholerae infection may not be clinically distinguishable from other causes of gastroenteritis. An estimated 2% of infected patients will develop cholera gravis. The mortality rate in the 2% with C. gravis is 50% to 75%, giving an overall mortality in infected persons of 1–1.5%.

Ref: Nelson Textbook of Pediatrics: 20th/ed, p 1401, Elsevier Health Sciences 2011.
Disaster Medicine: 3rd/ed, p 635, Mosby Elsevier 2006.

19. Ninevalent HPV includes

a. 6, 11
b. 16, 18
c. 31, 33
d. 35, 58
e. 45, 55

Ans. a, b, c *Ref: https://www.cdc.gov/mmwr/preview/mmwrhtml/mm6411a3.htm*

Option a	True
Option b	True
Option c	True
Option d	False
Option e	False

- HPV is associated with cervical, vulvar, and vaginal cancer in females, penile cancer in males, and anal cancer and oropharyngeal cancer in both females and males.
- Similar to quadrivalent HPV vaccine (4vHPV), 9vHPV contains HPV 6, 11, 16, and 18 VLPs. In addition, 9vHPV contains HPV 31, 33, 45, 52, and 58 VLPs (virus-like particle).
- **Recommendations for use of HPV vaccines:** *ACIP (Advisory Committee on Immunization Practices)* recommends that routine HPV vaccination be initiated at age 11 or 12 years. The vaccination series can be started beginning at age 9 years. Vaccination is also recommended for females aged 13 through 26 years and for males aged 13 through 21 years who have not been vaccinated previously or who have not completed the 3-dose series. Males aged 22 through 26 years may be vaccinated.
    - Vaccination of females is recommended with 2vHPV, 4vHPV (as long as this formulation is available), or 9vHPV. Vaccination of males is recommended with 4vHPV (as long as this formulation is available) or 9vHPV.
    - 2vHPV, 4vHPV, and 9vHPV all protect against HPV 16 and 18, types that cause about 66% of cervical cancers and the majority of other HPV-attributable cancers. 9vHPV targets five additional cancer causing types, which account for about 15% of cervical cancers. 4vHPV and 9vHPV also protect against HPV 6 and 11, types that cause anogenital warts.

20. True about human papilloma virus is/are:

a. Papovavirus
b. DNA virus
c. Affects only skin in humans
d. Affects moist mucus tissue (mucous membranes)
e. Causes virus induced carcinoma

Ans. a, b, d, e

Option a	True
Option b	True

Option c	False	Mucous membranes are also affected
Option d	True	
Option e	True	

1. Formerly the papillomaviruses and polyomaviruses were together grouped under Papovaviridae family, but now they are separated as 2 different families (Papillomaviridae and Polymaviridae).
2. HPV are non-enveloped, icosahedral capsids and contains a double-stranded circular DNA.
3. Papillomaviruses are highly tropic for epithelial cells of the skin and mucous membranes.
4. HPV have oncogenic potential.

21. True about incubation period is/are:

a. Measles: 10–14 days
b. Hepatitis A: 10–12 days
c. Chickenpox: 20–30 days
d. Leptospirosis:10–14 days
e. Bubonic plague: 2–7 days

Ans. a, d, e

Option a	True	
Option b	False	
Option c	False	
Option d	True	
Option e	True	

1. HAV: incubation period is 15–45 days.
2. Chickenpox: incubation period is 10–21 days.

22. Which of the following is a dimorphic fungus?

a. Histoplasmosis
b. Sporothrix
c. Cryptococcus
d. Aspergillus
e. Malassezia furfur

Ans. a, b

Option a	True	
Option b	True	
Option c	False	True yeast
Option d	False	Mold
Option e	False	Mold, non-dermatophyte

- ❑ Dimorphic fungi are those fungi that can exist in two different morphological forms under two different environmental conditions. These fungi exist as molds in their natural habitat and in vitro at room temperature and as yeasts in vivo or in vitro at 37 °C. Most of the dimorphic fungi are responsible for systemic or deep mycoses. For definitive identification of the fungus, yeast to mold conversion should be demonstrated. All dimorphic Isolates known to cause systemic mycoses must be handled with caution in a biological safety cabinet.

- The dimorphic fungi are Histoplasma capsulatum, Blastomyces dermatitidis, Coccidioides immitis, Coccidioides posadasii, Paracoccidioides brasiliensis, Penicillium marneffei and Sporothrix schenckii.

- Cryptococcus is true yeast.
- Aspergillus is mold.
- Malassezia furfur: It is mold and the primary causative agent of Pityriasis versicolor.

23. DOC for strongyloides is/are:

a. Mebendazole
b. Albendazole
c. Ivermectin
d. DEC
e. Levamisole

Ans. b, c

Option a	False	
Option b	True	Alternative therapy
Option c	True	First line therapy
Option d	False	
Option e	False	

Treatment: Acute and chronic strongyloidiasis

First line therapy: Ivermectin, in a single dose, 200 μg/kg orally for 1–2 days.

Relative contraindications:

- Confirmed or suspected concomitant Loa loa infection
- Persons weighing less than 15 kg
- Pregnant or lactating women
- Oral ivermectin is available for human use in the United States.

Alternative: Albendazole, 400 mg orally two times a day for 7 days.

Relative contraindications:

- Hypersensitivity to benzimidazole compounds or any component of product.
- Use should be avoided in the 1st trimester of pregnancy.

24. Barrel-shaped eggs are seen in:

a. Hookworm
b. Pin worm
c. Strongyloides
d. Whipworm
e. Round worm (ascaris)

Ans. d

Option a	False	Hook or S shaped eggs
Option b	False	Elongate-oval in shape
Option c	False	Small oval thin-shelled bodies
Option d	True	Barrel shaped and brown
Option e	False	Oval to round in shape

1. The nematode (roundworm) Trichuris trichiura, also called the human whipworm. Whipworm is a soil-transmitted helminth (STH) and is the third most common roundworm of humans. Whipworm causes an infection called trichuriasis and often occurs in areas

where human feces are used as fertilizer or where defecation onto soil happens. The worms are spread from person to person by fecal-oral transmission or through feces-contaminated food.

2. The standard method for diagnosing the presence of whipworm is by microscopically identifying whipworm eggs (Barrel shaped with mucous plugs at poles) in a stool sample. Because eggs may be difficult to find in light infections, a concentration procedure is recommended.

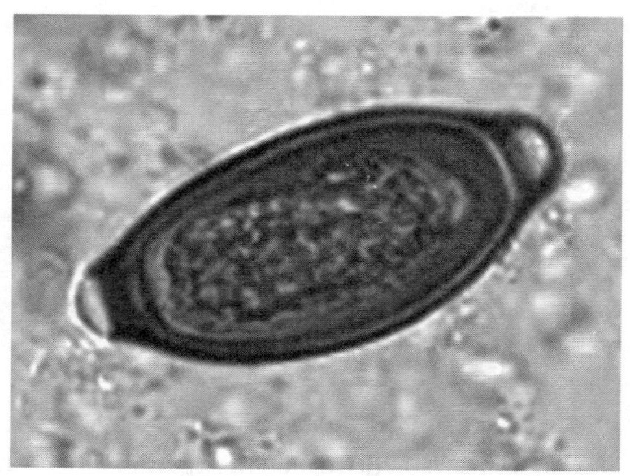

25. True about actinomyces is/are:

a. Not acid fast
b. Most common variety is craniofacial
c. Sulphur granules seen
d. Caused by Madurella madurai
e. Microaerophilic

Ans. a, c

Option a	True	
Option b	False	Cervicofacial is most common clinical manifestation
Option c	True	
Option d	False	It is fungus that causes Mycetoma
Option e	False	Facultatively anaerobic (except A. meyeri and A. israelii both obligate anaerobe)

1 Actinomycetes are diverse group of Gram-positive, catalase-positive, non-capsulated, non-motile bacilli arranged in chains or branching filaments. They are considered to be transitional forms between bacteria and fungi.

2. Important genera include: Actinomyces, Nocardia, Actinomadura, Streptomyces, Micropolyspora and Thermoactinomyces.

3. Some Actinomycetes are weak acid fast Nocardia, Rhodococcus.

4. Actinomyces: It is anaerobes not microaerophilic, most common clinical manifestation is Cervicofacial and pus discharge contains gritty, white or yellowish sulfur granules.

5. Madurella madurai: Mycetoma (Madura foot or Maduromycosis) is caused by fungus Madurella.

Forensic Medicine and Toxicology

1. Salicylate poisoning:

a. Alkaline diuresis is done
b. Presents with nausea, abdominal pain and tinnitus
c. Activated charcoal is not useful
d. Metabolic alkalosis is a late feature
e. Polyethylene glycol is used as antidote

Ans. a,b *Ref: Pareek, 6th/ed p11.2; Dixit Toxicology, p668*

Option a	True	Yes, correct. Alkalization of the urine enhances elimination of salicylates through ion trapping in the renal tubules
Option b	True	Yes, correct
Option c	False	No, activated charcoal is used in case of mild toxicity
Option d	False	No, metabolic acidosis is late feature
Option e	False	No, Polyethylene glycol is laxative and not antidote

Salicylate poisoning features:

1. Phase 1
   a. Hyperventilation resulting from direct respiratory center stimulation
   b. Respiratory alkalosis and compensatory alkaluria
   c. Potassium and sodium bicarbonate are excreted in the urine.
   d. Duration up to 12 hours.
2. Phase 2
   a. Paradoxical aciduria in the presence of continued respiratory alkalosis occurs when sufficient potassium has been lost from the kidneys
   b. Duration: 12-24 hours.
3. Phase 3 includes
   a. Dehydration, hypokalemia, and progressive metabolic acidosis
   b. Variable time of onset and duration. May vary from 4-6 hours to 24 hours.

Note:

Early features:

Nausea vomiting

Tinnitus (fairly indicating salicylate ingestion), diaphoresis

Hyperthermia is found in severe intoxication cases.

The therapeutic range of salicylate is 15-30 mg/dL. Patients are often symptomatic at salicylate concentrations higher than 40-50 mg/dL. Patients with salicylate concentrations approaching or exceeding 100 mg/dL usually have serious or life-threatening toxicity.

Blood level of 50 mg% are toxic whereas of 100 mg% are fatal to life.

Fatal dose – 15–30 gm

Fatal period – few minutes to several hours death rate is 7–8%.

Causes of Death

i. Uremia leading to circulatory failure (ii) Respiratory failure

Management principles

Principles of treatment include stabilizing the ABCs as necessary, limiting absorption, enhancing elimination, correcting metabolic abnormalities, and providing supportive care. No specific antidote is available for salicylates.

- Initial treatment should include the use of oral activated charcoal, especially, if the patient presents within 1 hour of ingestion
- Whole bowel irrigation (WBI) with polyethylene glycol was found to be more effective than single-dose activated charcoal in reducing absorption of enteric-coated acetylsalicylic acid
- Polyethylene glycol is a laxative with strong electrolyte and osmotic effects that has cathartic actions in the GI tract
- Sodium bicarbonate is used as a gastric, systemic, and urinary alkalinizer and has been administered in the treatment of acidosis resulting from metabolic and respiratory causes. Indications for hemodialysis include the following:
- Serum salicylate level greater than 120 mg/dL acutely or greater than 100 mg/dL 6 h post-ingestion
- Refractory acidosis
- Coma or seizures
- Noncardiogenic pulmonary edema
- Volume overload
- Renal failure.

Preparation	Poisonous substance	Symptoms and signs	Management
Moth balls	Naphthalene	Nausea, vomiting, pain abdomen, albuminuria and hematuria, pulmonary edema and coma	Stomach wash, soda bicarbonate, iv fluids. Oxygen and artificial respiration
Baby powder	Boric acid	Nausea, vomiting, diarrhea, convulsions, respiratory depression	Stomach wash, oxygen and artificial respiration
Insecticide spray	DDT/ organophosphorus compounds	Nausea, vomiting, tremors, convulsions, coma	Stomach wash, paraldehyde, oxygen and artificial respiration
Chalk	Arsenic, copper and lead in colored chalks	Nausea, vomiting, pain abdomen, symptoms of metallic poisoning	Stomach wash and treatment of metallic poisoning
Fireworks	Arsenic, mercury, lead and phosphorus	Burns	Burns to be treated

Contd...

Contd...

Preparation	Poisonous substance	Symptoms and signs	Management
Cosmetics (nail enamel, and thinners)	Potassium hydroxide, barium sulphate, acetone, methyl salicylates and denatured spirit	Nausea, vomiting, burning in stomach	Stomach wash
Baking powder	Tartaric acid	Nausea, vomiting, burning pain abdomen	Immediate soda bicarb to neutralize the acid
Baking soda	Sodium carbonate	Nausea, vomiting, abdominal distension	Vinegar
Crockery washing substance	Sodium and sodium polyphosphates	Variable symptoms depending on the substance	Symptomatic treatment
Match box and sticks	Silicates, antimony, phosphorus and potassium chlorate	Antimony and phosphorus poisoning	Treat symptoms of poisoning
Rat poison	Zinc phosphide	Nausea, hematuria	Stomach wash, inj. vitamin K i.m.,
Grain preservative	Aluminum phosphide	Bleeding	Oxygen and artificial respiration

2. **Supreme court verdict on rape in married female:**
   a. Consent for marriage, age is 16 years
   b. Intercourse with consent in married female, but age < 15 years is known as rape
   c. Married female age > 15 years, with consent is not rape
   d. Sexual intercourse by man with his wife, age > 18 years, without consent, is rape
   e. Minimum age of child under the child marriage restraint act 1929 is > 18 years

Ans. b,d,e *Ref: Writ Petition (Civil) No. 382 of 2013, Court of Madan B Lokur J*

Option a	False	No, consent for marriage is > 18 years
Option b	True	Yes, it is defined as rape
Option c	False	No, Married female age of consent for sexual intercourse is > 18 years
Option d	True	Yes correct
Option e	True	Yes, correct

Rape definition

Under the circumstances falling under any of the following seven descriptions:

- First—Against her will
- Secondly—Without her consent
- Thirdly—With her consent, when her consent has been obtained by putting her or any person in whom she is interested, in fear of death or of hurt.
- Fourthly—With her consent, when the man knows that he is not her husband and that her consent is given because she believes that he is another man to whom she is or believes herself to be lawfully married.

- ❑ Fifthly—With her consent when, at the time of giving such consent, by reason of unsoundness of mind or intoxication or the administration by him personally or through another of any stupefying or unwholesome substance, she is unable to understand the nature and consequences of that to which she gives consent.
- ❑ Sixthly—With or without her consent, when she is under eighteen years of age.
- ❑ Seventhly—When she is unable to communicate consent.

3. Gustafson's method:

a. Age determination from teeth in living persons
b. Age determination from teeth in dead persons
c. Dentine arrangement with age
d. Secondary dentition with age
e. Root transparency with age

Ans. b,d,e *Ref: Dixit Textbook of Forensic, p68*

Option a	False	No, it is for dead individuals
Option b	True	Yes correct
Option c	False	No, it for age determination using changes in a tooth and not dentition arrangement
Option d	True	Yes correct
Option e	True	Yes, correct

This method is used for estimation of age in the adults by studying the progressive changes in an individual tooth.

The age of a person is found by:

- ❑ By eruption of deciduous and permanent teeth
- ❑ Gustafson's criteria:
- ❑ Occlusion attrition of the tip of the tooth
- ❑ Secondary dentine deposition in the apex of pulp cavity
- ❑ Apical migration of attachment of periodontal membrane
- ❑ Increase in root transparency—Is best single criterion
- ❑ Root resorption.

Accumulation of cementum around the root. This method was later modified by Johanson; age can be calculated within + 5 years.

- ❑ Comparative identification from the teeth by charting.

Gustafson's Method

Pathological conditions can alter each of the factors separately:

- ❑ *Attrition:* It is wearing and tearing on the opposing mastication surface of the teeth of the upper and lower gums due to continuous friction.
- ❑ *Periodontosis:* loosening of the teeth, exposure of length of root and deposition of stony hard debris over a long period.
- ❑ *Secondary dentine:* With advanced age there is deposition of secondary dentine tissue in pulp cavity. The process progress until whole of pulp cavity is replenished and the size of cavity decreases.

- *Root resorption*: It is another decaying change involving both cementum and dentine that shows grooves.
- *Cementum apposition*: Cementum deposition increases due to change in the surface of tooth near the end of roof and forms incremental lines.
- *Root transparency*: It occurs in the root from below upwards in the lower jaw and above downwards in the upper jaw due to rarefaction of dentine tissue.

  R0—No transparency noticed anywhere

  R1—Transparency noticeable mostly over apical region

  R2—Transparency up to 1/3rd from the apical region

  R3—Transparency noticeable up to 2/3rd of the length of the root from apex

  Root transparency is the most reliable method.

  The anterior are most suitable as they erupt early and the changes are present in earlier

Point formula as given by Gustafson is An+Pn+Rn+Cn+Tn+Sn = Total points indicates the Age in years.

4. Criminal ground under psychiatric disorder:

a. Delusion b. Illusion
c. Hallucination d. OCD
e. Conduct disorder

Ans. a,b,c,d *Ref: Matthew T Huss, Forensic Psychology. John Wiley and Sons, 2008, p162; Dixit Textbook of Forensic Medicine, p501*

Option a	True	Yes, correct
Option b	True	Yes, correct
Option c	True	Yes, correct
Option d	True	Yes, correct
Option e	False	No, not correct

Totally deprived of his understanding and memory and doth not know what he is doing, no more than an infant, than a brute, or a wild beast.'

In forensic psychiatry, the 'insanity defense' is sometimes the case, which however is very difficult to prove in the court.

The diseases or mental conditions applied under insanity defense and the person is not held responsible for his deeds are as follows:

1. Psychosis/Neurosis
2. Delirium—delirium tremens, Korsakoff's psychosis
3. Delusion
4. Hallucination
5. Illusion
6. Obsession
7. Impulse
8. Lucid interval (after or with insanity).

Conduct disorder (CD) is a mental **disorder** diagnosed in childhood or adolescence that presents itself through a repetitive and persistent pattern of behavior in which the basic rights of others or major age-appropriate norms are violated. These behaviors are often referred to as "antisocial behaviors.

5. Unnatural sexual offence—sodomy:

a. IPC 377 b. IPC 375
c. IPC 497 d. IPC 498
e. IPC 376

Ans. a

Option a	True	Yes, correct
Option b	False	No, it is for rape
Option c	False	No, it deals with adultery
Option d	False	No, it deals with dowry (remember dowry death is 304b)
Option e	False	No, it deals with rape punishment

Central Government Act

Section 377 in the Indian Penal Code

377. Unnatural offences—Whoever voluntarily has carnal intercourse against the order of nature with any man, woman or animal, shall be punished with 1 (imprisonment for life), or with imprisonment of either description for a term which may extend to ten years, and shall also be liable to fine.

Explanation—Penetration is sufficient to constitute the carnal intercourse necessary to the offence described in this section.

The types of several offences as penile/anus penetration, penile/oral penetration, finger/anile penetration, finger/vaginal penetration or object/vaginal penetration are serious sexual offences of unnatural nature and are to be covered under Section 377 which provides stringent punishment.

IPC's of Importance

300	Murder (Sufficient to cause death)/Infanticide	324	Dangerous weapons/Poisons/Corrosives
302	Punishment for murder/Infanticide	325	Punishment for Grievous Injury
303	When a life imprisonment prisoner kills another prisoner (removed from IPC now)	326	Dangerous Weapons/Poisons/Corrosives
304	Punishment for culpable homicide	328	Poisons
304A	Criminal Negligence/Rash & Negligent Act	331	Assault
304B	Dowry death	351	Assault Definition
306	Abetment of suicide	354	Punishment for Indecent Assault
309	Attempt for suicide	375	Rape
312	Medical negligence/Causing miscarriage	376	Punishment for Rape
313	Causing miscarriage without the consent of the female	376A	Man with his wife during separation
314	Death by an act done for miscarriage	376B	Public servant with women in custody
315	Act to prevent child birth or to cause it die	376C	Superintendent of Jail, Remand Home
316	Death of quick unborn child/Criminal Abortion	376D	Member of the management or staff of a hospital with any women in that hospital

317	Abandoning Infant	377	Unnatural Offences/Lesbianism/Male to male/ Anal/Oral sex
318	Concealment of Birth/Punishment for Abandonment	493	Cohabitation by deceitfully inducing to a belief of lawful marriage
319	Hurt	497	Adultery/Artificial Insemination
320	Grievous Injury	498A	Dowry death—Relatives
323	Punishment for Hurt		

6. Magnan syndrome:

a. Associated with cannabis
b. Associated with cocaine
c. Experience of paraesthesia
d. Olfactory hallucination is characteristic
e. Delusional parasitosis

Ans. b,c,e *Ref: Steven B Karch, Karch's Pathology of Drug Abuse, Fifth Edition, p145; Dixit Textbook of Forensic, p601*

Option a	False	No, it is associated with cocaine psychosis
Option b	True	Yes correct
Option c	True	Yes correct
Option d	False	No, tactile hallucination is typical
Option e	True	Yes, correct

Delusional parasitosis – is most characteristic feature of cocaine abuse.

Cocaine abuse may also be associated with few other psychiatric manifestations as:

- Schizophrenia
- Organic mental disorders
- Dementia
- Behavioral and psychological.

Pathology and related effects

1. Brain/cognition
   - Increased rate of glucose uptake by brain, especially in basal ganglia and orbitofrontal cortex
   - Decreased cerebral flow
   - Cerebral vasculitis—especially with levamisole adulteration—associated with neurological excitement (also responsible for tactile hallucination and skin changes)
   - SAH and interventricular bleed
   - Impaired cognition, movement disorders
   - Cocaine related vasoconstriction
2. Cocaine related kidney disease
3. Increased thrombosis
4. Suppression of HPA axis
5. Cocaine induces immune-suppression
6. Cocaine induced hepatic injury—production of cocaethylene by esterification of cocaine.

7. Cannabis withdrawal features:

a. Depressed mood
b. Increased appetite
c. Tachycardia
d. Cannabis use disorder is use > 1 month
e. Weight loss

Ans. a,c,e *Ref: Dixit Forensic Medicine and Toxicology, p599; Gorelick DA, Levin KH, Copersino ML, et al. Diagnostic Criteria for Cannabis Withdrawal Syndrome. Drug and Alcohol Dependence. 2012;123(1-3):141-7. doi:10.1016/j.drugalcdep.2011.11.007; Roffman R, Robert S Stephens. Cannabis Dependence: its Nature, Consequences and Treatment, p60; Morrison J Dsm-5 Made Easy: The Clinician's Guide to Diagnosis. Guilford Publications, 2017 p424*

Option a	True	Yes, correct
Option b	False	No, it is decreased appetite and weight loss
Option c	True	Yes, correct
Option d	False	No, it is prolonged and heavy use of more than 3 months
Option e	True	Yes, correct

Cannabis withdrawal syndrome (DSM 5):

- Cessation of cannabis use that has been heavy and prolonged (i.e., usually daily or almost daily use over a period of at least a few months).
- Three or more of the following signs and symptoms develop within approximately 1 week after cessation of heavy, prolonged use:
  - Irritability, anger or aggression
  - Nervousness or anxiety
  - Sleep difficulty (i.e., insomnia, disturbing dreams)
  - Decreased appetite or weight loss
  - Restlessness
  - Depressed mood
  - At least one of the following physical symptoms causing significant discomfort: abdominal pain, shakiness/tremors, sweating, fever, chills, or headache.
- The signs or symptoms cause clinically significant distress or impairment in social, occupational, or other important areas of functioning.
- The signs or symptoms are not attributable to another medical condition and are not better explained by another mental disorder, including intoxication or withdrawal from another substance.

Cannabis use disorder:

- In early remission—After full criteria for cannabis use disorder were previously met, none of the criteria for cannabis use disorder has been met for at least 3 months but for less than 12 months (with an exception provided for craving).
- In sustained remission—After full criteria for cannabis use disorder were previously met, none of the criteria for cannabis use disorder has been met at any time during a period of 12 months or longer (with an exception provided for craving).

  Cannabis intoxication delirium—include attention and cognition defects

  Cannabis induced psychotic disorder—delusions and/or hallucinations

  Cannabis induced anxiety disorder—panic attacks.

Forensic Medicine and Toxicology

1. Which is the correct statement regarding OPC poisoning—delayed neuropathy?

a. After 2–4 months of OPC toxicity
b. Both motor and sensory neurons affected
c. Due to inhibition of other enzymes
d. Recovery complete
e. Damage to the pyramidal tracts

Ans. b, e *Ref: Review of FMT, Gautam Biswas, 3rd/ed p600 and 601*
CDC—Agency for toxic substance and disease registry

Option a	False	Occurs 1–5 weeks after severe toxicity
Option b	True	
Option c	False	Due to severe cholinesterase inhibitor toxicity only
Option d	False	Recovery is incomplete with motor neurons being permanently damaged
Option e	True	

Neurological manifestations are the most important sequelae of OPC compound poisoning. Organophosphate induced delayed polyneuropathy (OPIDP)—is a rare, delayed neurotoxic effect, which occurs 1–5 weeks after severe toxicity from some cholinesterase inhibitors. There is symmetrical sensory-motor axonal degeneration of the peripheral nerves and spinal cord.

Paralysis types in OPC toxicity	Termed as	Appears after	Presenting features
Type I Paralysis	Acute paralysis or cholinergic crisis occurs due to excessive stimulation of muscarinic receptors by Ach due to blockade of acetylcholinesterase by an OP agent.	24 to 48 hours	Sharp, cramp-like pains in the calves
Type II Paralysis	Intermediate syndrome, occurs due to dysfunction of neuromuscular junction caused by downregulation of presynaptic and postsynaptic Nicotinic receptors due to release of excessive Ach and Ca^{2+} respectively.	24 to 96 hours	Muscular weakness affecting predominantly the proximal muscles and neck flexors
Type III Paralysis	Delayed neurotoxicity/polyneuropathy, pure motor or predominantly motor axonal neuropathy	1 to 5 weeks	Weakness which appears initially in distal leg muscles ("stocking-glove" distribution) followed by small muscles of the hands and later it may extend proximally

Following are the salient features of Type III OPC poisoning-induced delayed neuropathy:

1. Both sensory and motor neurons are involved. Motor alterations such as slowed conduction and, eventually, bilateral and symmetrical weakness progressing to flaccidity of the distal skeletal muscles of the lower and upper extremities occur.
2. Spasticity, hypertonicity, hyperreflexia, clonus, and abnormal reflexes, indicative of damage to the pyramidal tracts and a permanent upper motor neuron syndrome occurs at later stage.
3. In severe cases, ataxia and Paralysis (motor symptoms) remain permanently, hence, recovery is not complete.
4. Patients with mild cases recover over several months; those with more serious polyneuropathies have persistent effects.
5. Sensory symptoms resolve over 1 to 2 months. Hence, recovery affects only sensory nerves, while motor neurons may permanently lose function.

2. Which of the following is/are true regarding Perjury?

a. Willfully giving false statement under oath
b. Section 190 IPC deals with perjury
c. Voluntarily giving false evidence under oath
d. The witness is liable to be prosecuted for perjury
e. Abortion > 20 weeks of gestation

Ans. a, c, d *Ref: Medical Jurisprudence and Toxicology MODI 24th/ed; Chapter 4, p68-70 and Review of FMT, Gautam Biswas, 3rd/ed; p 51*

Option a	True	True, lying under oath
Option b	False	Section 191 IPC and Sec 344 CrPC deal with perjury
Option c	True	True, willfully giving false statement or evidence
Option d	True	Imprisonment up to 7 years and fine
Option e	False	Does not involve any element of false statement/evidence under oath. Taken care by MTP act

Oath (Sec 51 IPC): Witness is required to swear by Almighty God that he will tell the truth, the whole truth and nothing but the truth.

Perjury: A witness after taking oath willfully makes a false statement which he knows or believes to be false. It is defined under Sec 191 IPC and Sec 344 CrPC.

Section 191 of Indian Penal Code declares that when a person, who is under legal obligation, either on oath or under any provision of law, to state the truth, to declare upon any subject, knowingly makes false statement, the statement which he believes that it is false or he believes that it is not true, commits the offence under this section.

Prosecution/Punishment for perjury: Provided under Section **193 IPC,** according to which imprisonment which may extend to Seven years, and will also be fined. (Imprisonment up to 7 years and fine).

Sec. 190 IPC: Deals with imprisonment for giving threat of injury to any person for the purpose to refrain from making a legal application for protection against any injury to public servant.

3. Bite mark may aid in:

a. Collection of DNA sample
b. Identification of accused
c. Assessment of height
d. Assessment of type of teeth
e. Assessment of age

Ans. b, d, e *Ref: Review of FMT, Gautam Biswas, 3rd/ed p94*

Option a	False	Nucleic acid degrading enzymes of saliva degrade DNA
Option b	True	By pattern of teeth and occlusal surfaces of teeth
Option c	False	
Option d	True	
Option e	True	

- The science of bite mark identification can be used to link a suspect to a crime.
- Bite mark analysis can elucidate the kind of violence and the elapsed time between its production and examination.
- It can show if the bite mark was produced intravitam or post mortem and in case of several bite marks, identify the sequence of them.
- It can be extremely useful in establishing a link between the bitten person and the biter or excluding the innocent.
- The pattern of teeth, occlusal surfaces of teeth are helpful in identification of the accused.
- The saliva contains cells like squames which can yield DNA sample to be matched with the accused. However, presence of nucleic acid degrading enzymes (nucleases) within saliva can readily degrade DNA, especially if it is on a living victim, as the skin's ambient temperature accelerates the process.
- Several terms used to describe the type of bite mark:
  - Abrasion—a scrape on the skin
  - Artifact—when a piece of the body, such as an ear lobe, is removed through biting
  - Avulsion—a bite resulting in the removal of skin
  - Contusion—a bruise
  - Hemorrhage—a profusely bleeding bite
  - Incision—a clean, neat wound
  - Laceration—a puncture wound
- Though a person's teeth may look the same, they are different in size, shape, arrangement, wear and tear, damage, age, quality and quantity and habits of the individual.

4. True about corpus delicti:

a. Medical negligence
b. Body of offence
c. It includes body of the victim and other facts which are conclusive of death by foul play
d. The essence of crime
e. Murder investigation

Ans. b, c, d, e *Ref: Review of FMT, Gautam Biswas, 3rd/ed p56*

Option a	False	
Option b	True	
Option c	True	
Option d	True	
Option e	True	

- Corpus delicti, means the "*body of the crime.*"
- Important concept in *murder investigation*.
- Every type of crime has its own corpus delicti.
- The term details the elements that need to exist in order for an act to be legally defined as a crime.
- There are five elements required before an act can legally be defined as a crime.
- Two of those elements, *actus reus* and *mens rea*, are of more importance in establishing the precise corpus delicti, while the remaining three are of more general application.
- The "corpus delicti rule" requires the prosecution to present independent evidence—more than a confession—of the corpus delicti.
- Term *Corpus delicti* refers to the principle that—it must be proven that the crime has actually occurred before a person is convicted of committing the crime.
- For example in charge of homicide it includes positive identification of the victim's dead body, photographs showing fatal injuries, bullet or clothing showing marks of weapon.

5. For a female to take divorce from her husband, the valid grounds is/are:

a. Infertility of female
b. Unemployment of male partner
c. Extramarital affair of male partner
d. Impotence of male partner
e. If she was married before the age of fifteen and she wants to renounce the marriage before she attains eighteen years of age

Ans. c, d *Ref: Hindu marriage act 1955 (Sec 5, 11, 12 and 13) and Review of FMT, Gautam Biswas, 3rd/ed p363*

Option a	False	
Option b	False	
Option c	True	
Option d	True	
Option e	False	

Grounds of divorce under Hindu Marriage Act, 1955:

1. Any marriage solemnized, whether before or after the commencement of this Act, may be dissolved by a decree of divorce on the ground that the other party:
   i. Is living in adultery; or
   ii. Has ceased to be a Hindu by conversion to another religion; or
   iii. Has been incurably of unsound mind for a continuous period of not less than three years immediately preceding the presentation of the petition; or
   iv. Has, for a period of not less than three years immediately preceding the presentation of the petition, been suffering from a virulent and incurable form of leprosy; or
   v. Had, for a period of not less than three years immediately preceding the presentation of the petition, been suffering from venereal disease in a communicable form (syphilis, AIDS); or
   vi. Has renounced the world by entering any religious order; or
   vii. Has not been heard of as being alive for a period of seven years or more by those persons who would naturally have heard of it, had that party been alive; or

viii. Has not resumed cohabitation for a space of two years or upwards after the passing of a decree for judicial separation against that party; or
ix. Has failed to comply with a decree for restitution of conjugal rights for a period of two years or upwards after the passing of the decree.

2. A wife may also present a petition for the dissolution of her marriage by a decree of divorce on the ground:
   i. In the case of any marriage solemnized before the commencement of this Act, that the husband had married again before such commencement or that any other wife of the husband married before such commencement was alive at the time of the solemnization of the marriage of the petitioner:
   Provided that in either case the other wife is alive at the time of the presentation of the petition; or
   ii. That the husband has, since the solemnization of the marriage, been guilty of rape, sodomy or bestiality.

The following are not considered as ground for divorce:

- Infertility/sterility of a female is not a ground of divorce.
- Unemployment is also not the ground for divorce
- The marriage done before the age of 18 years (for female) and 21 years (for male) are **void-ab-initio**, i.e. under Sec 5 of Hindu Marriage Act any marriage where the male is < 21 years and female < 18 years will be considered as "***null and void***".

6. Feature of gunshot injury is/are:
   a. Gutter injury
   b. Grease collar
   c. Radiating wound
   d. Tissue opening on opposite end
   e. Density of tissue does not affect nature of the wound

Ans. a, b, c, d, e *Ref: Review of FMT, Gautam Biswas, 3rd/ed p220-223*

Option a	True	Produce key-hole defects
Option b	True	Seen in entry wound
Option c	True	Seen in contact shot
Option d	True	
Option e	True	Tissue characteristics strongly affect the nature of the wound

- **Gutter injury**: Tangential entry of a bullet may produce key-hole defects with entrance and exit side-by-side.
- **Grease collar**: Seen surrounding the entry wound (the greasy dirt and impurities of the barrel are brought by bullet with it over the surface).
- **Radiating wound**: Here the '*radiating wound*' may be considered as Stellate wound seen in contact shot. Muzzle imprint and back spatter are also the findings in contact shot wound.
- **Exit wounds:** These are everted and puckered.
- Tissue characteristics (elasticity, density, anatomic relationships) strongly affect the nature of the wound.

7. Which of the following is seen in strangulation and not hanging?

a. Fracture of trachea and larynx
b. Contusion at margins of ligature
c. Pale face
d. Petechiae
e. No signs of struggle

Ans. a, b, d *Ref: Parikh's textbook of FMT, 7th/ed*

Option a	True	Fracture of trachea and larynx is rare in hanging
Option b	True	Contusions and abrasions around ligature are rare in hanging
Option c	False	Pale face is seen in hanging only
Option d	True	Pronounced petechiae in strangulation
Option e	False	Strangulation shows signs of struggle

❑ Differences between hanging and strangulation:

	Hanging	Strangulation
1.	Suicidal usually	Homicidal usually
2.	No signs of struggle	Signs of struggle
3.	Ligature found in position, above thyroid cartilage, mark incomplete, directed obliquely upward with a gap indicating position of the knot with no damage to the skin in the gap	Ligature may not be with the body but when found, usually completely encircles the neck horizontally below thyroid cartilage. There may be more than one turn of ligature and there is always some damage to skin underneath
4.	Abrasions and bruises around ligature mark rate	Abrasions and bruises around ligature mark common
5.	Dissection of ligature mark reveals a dry and glistening white band of subcutaneous tissue	Dissection of ligature mark reveals ecchymosed subcutaneous tissue
6.	Neck usually stretched	Neck not stretched
7.	Fracture of hyoid rare	Fracture of hyoid not rare in throttling cases (in the aged)
8.	Fracture of laryngeal cartilages and tracheal rings rare	Fracture of laryngeal cartilages and tracheal rings common
9.	Injury to carotid arteries in cases with a long drop	Injury to carotid arteries common
10.	Injury to muscles of neck rare	Injury to muscles of neck common
11.	Fracture dislocation of cervical vertebrae common in judicial hanging	Fracture dislocation of cervical vertebrae rare
12.	Saliva running out of the angle of the mouth vertically down along the neck and front of chest and abdomen	Saliva may not have escaped from mouth but if so, usually blood tinged and may not be vertically down
13.	External signs of asphyxia may not be well marked when death is due to any cause other than asphyxia	External signs of asphyxia usually well marked because of considerable violence that is commonly employed
14.	Face usually pale	Face congested and with pronounced petechiae
15.	Bleeding from nose and mouth very rare	Bleeding from nose and mouth common

8. What is a dangerous injury?

a. Type of grievous injury
b. Dislocation/Loss of 2 teeth
c. Spinal injury causing emasculation
d. No treatment given
e. May lead to death

Ans. a, e *Ref: Parikh's Textbook of FMT, 7th/ed*

Option a	True	Variety of grievous injury
Option b	False	Does not pose threat to life
Option c	False	Account towards grievous injury
Option d	False	If no treatment is given, it can lead to death
Option e	True	

Dangerous injury:

- Dangerous injury is a variety of grievous injury.
- It is an injury which possesses an immediate danger to life.
- It is either extensive or serious in relation to the organ or part wounded.
- The injury is fatal and may lead to death in the absence of surgical aid.
- Common examples are:
  - Gun shot wounds
  - Compound fractures of the skull
  - Trauma to a large or important blood vessel
  - Rupture of some internal organ, e.g. Spleen.

Grievous injury*:

- Emasculation (cutting of penis, castration, or causing loss of power of erection due to spinal cord injury).
- Permanent privation of sight of either eye.
- Permanent privation of hearing of either ear.
- Privation of any member (part, organ, limb) or joint.
- Destruction or permanent impairing of powers of any member or joint.
- Permanent disfiguration of head or face.
- Fracture or dislocation of bone or tooth.

  **Any hurt which endangers life, or which causes the sufferer to be , during the space of twenty days, in severe bodily pain or unable to follow his daily routine.*

9. Which of the following is found in drowning?

a. Edema aquosum
b. Emphysema aquosum
c. Paultof's hemorrhage
d. Gagging
e. Cutis anserina

Ans. a, b, c, e *Ref: Parikh's Textbook of FMT, 7th/ed*

Option a	True	Seen in submersion of unconscious person
Option b	True	
Option c	True	
Option d	False	Means to effect choking by prevention of air entering through mouth or nose
Option e	True	

Drowning

Death from asphyxia caused by a liquid entering the lungs and preventing the absorption of oxygen leading to cerebral hypoxia and cardiac arrest.

SIGNS OF IMMERSION

- The skin becomes somewhat opaque and wrinkled.
- Known as 'washerwoman's fingers,' develop after a few hours in cold water.

- After a few days, this macerated skin will begin to separate and, usually within 1–2 weeks the skin will peel off the hands and feet.
- Another early sign of immersion is cutis anserina or 'gooseflesh', due to contraction of the arrector pili muscles.
- However, this is partly due to cold (and may be seen in refrigerated bodies) and partly due to rigor mortis.
- Cutis anserina is not a specific sign of immersion.
- In average temperate conditions a body immersed in water will decompose at about half the speed of one left in air.
- After about a week, the body will be bloated and the face, abdomen and genitals will be distended with gas.

Typical drowning—(wet drowning)

Atypical drowning:

- Dry drowning—sustained laryngeal spasm upon entry on water into nasopharynx or larynx.
- Immersion syndrome—vagal inhibition.
- Submersion of unconscious—e.g. if a person is epileptic, or had myocardial ischemia, drunk, etc. during the fall into water. Edema aquosum is seen in such cases.
- Near drowning syndrome—if drowning is survived. Death occurs hours to days after resuscitation due to cerebral hypoxia, pulmonary edema, aspiration pneumonitis, electrolyte disturbances, etc.

Signs of antemortem drowning:

- *Fine froth* from the nose and mouth can be seen. This froth is not seen in dry drowning.
- In the respiratory tract, the typical changes are ballooning of lungs or *emphysema aquosum.*
- *Tardieu spots* are seen, the vascular bed being compressed by water filled alveoli.
- *Gettler's test* can be used to estimate the chloride content of blood from both sides of the heart.
- *Paltauf's hemorrhages in dry drowning:* The alveolar walls may rupture due to increased pressure during forced expiration and produce hemorrhages which when present sub-pleurally are called Paltauf's hemorrhages. Paltauf's hemorrhages are shining, pale bluish red and usually present in lower lobes of lungs.
- *Diatom's test.*

10. True about dying declaration is/are:

a. Need not be exhaustive
b. If two dying declarations have been given, they should be read separately.
c. Should be taken by a magistrate
d. If incomplete, it carries no value
e. Can be taken by doctor and police

Ans. a, b, c, d, e *Ref: Parikh's textbook of FMT, 7th/ed*

Option a	True	Recorded as narrated by the victim
Option b	True	All declarations to be read separately
Option c	True	First preference is magistrate
Option d	True	Dying declaration must be complete

Option e	True	Police can record the dying declaration but the investigating police officer is not allowed to remain present while the dying declaration is being recorded

Dying declaration:

- It is a statement—verbal or written, made by a person since deceased narrating the cause of his condition or circumstances leading to his impending death.
- If time permits, attending doctor should arrange for a magistrate to record the dying declaration of a person who is likely to die as a result of criminal violence.
- If the patient's condition is so grave that death or unconsciousness may supervene before the arrival of magistrate, the doctor should record the statement himself bearing in mind the following things.
  - The doctor has to issue two certificates: (i) initially, he has to certify that the patient is in a sound mental condition (compos mentis) to make the declaration, and (ii) when the declaration is concluded, he should certify that is was made while the declarant was compos mentis, it was read over to him, and that he accepted it as having been correctly recorded.
  - The declaration may be made orally but the person receiving it should commit it to writing at that time.
  - It should be recorded in the vernacular of the declarant in the presence of two disinterested witnesses. The questions put to him and his answers to them must be written down in full details and in identical words.
  - Nothing should be suggested to the victim nor should any attempt be made to elicit information by leading questions.
  - In cases of extreme weakness or cut throat injuries where the victim is unable to speak but able to make signs in answer to questions, these should be recorded in the form of questions and signs.
  - The declaration, when concluded, should be read over to the victim who should affix his signature or left thumb impression to it. It should also be signed by the doctor recording it as well as by the witnesses. If the statement is written by the patient himself, it should be signed by him, the doctor, and the witnesses.
  - If the declarant dies or becomes unconscious whilst the declaration is being recorded, the doctor should record as much information as he has obtained, and sign it himself.
  - The declaration should then be forwarded in a sealed cover to the appropriate magistrate.
  - The investigating police officer should not be allowed to remain present while the dying declaration is being recorded.

  The dying declaration forms an important evidence in criminal trial in the event of the victim's death. If the victim survives, it ceases to have any legal value. The declarant must then come to the court to give oral evidence and be cross examined for it. However, under section 157 IEA, the declaration may still be relied upon to corroborate the statement of the complainant at the time of oral examination.

11. Tests for blood stains is/are:

a. Acid phosphatase
b. Barberio
c. Takayama
d. Florence
e. Kastle-Meyer test

Ans. c, e *Ref: Parikh's Textbook of FMT, 7th/ed*

Option a	False	Enzyme produced by prostate gland
Option b	False	Used to detect spermine in semen stains
Option c	True	Confirmatory test
Option d	False	Used to detect semen
Option e	True	Presumptive test on blood

Tests for Blood stains are:

1. Phenolphthalein test (also known as the Kastle-Meyer test)—A Phenolphthalein solution is used to show the possible presence of blood based upon a peroxidase reaction of hemoglobin which produces a pink color.
2. Luminol test—A chemical compound, Luminol, is used in solution or sprayed onto suspected surfaces. This compound gives a strong blue fluorescence when viewed with a UV light. The Luminol reacts with hematin and produces a luminescence which is best observed in the dark.
3. Takayama test (hemochromogen test)—Through the application of Takayama reagent, hemochromogen crystals form by treating a small amount of blood or a stain fragment. The crystals are observable under a microscope and look like salmon-pink rhomboid crystals. This test does not require heating, and can be used on older samples.
4. Teichmann test (hemin crystal test)—Hemoglobin of the blood stain is converted to hemin, which in the presence of halogen, is converted to salt and forms brown rhombic crystals.

Chemical examination of Semen

- *Florence test: (Choline per Iodide crystals)*
  - A drop of Florence solution (Potassium iodine, iodine and water) is allowed to run under the cover slip.
  - If semen is present, dark-brown crystals of choline iodide appear immediately.
- *Barberio test:*
  - In Barberio's test, presence of spermine in semen is detected.
  - Spermine picrate crystals are seen.
- *Acid phosphatase test:*
  - Secreted by prostate gland.
  - Seminal fluid contains high amount of acid phosphatase.

12. Naltrexone is indicated in dependence for:

a. Alcohol
b. Cocaine
c. Cannabis
d. Opioids
e. Heroin

Ans. a, d, e *Ref: Parikh's Textbook of FMT, 7th/ed*

Option a	True	
Option b	False	Benzodiazepines are used to reverse cocaine toxicity
Option c	False	Can actually increase the cannabis abuse
Option d	True	
Option e	True	

- Naltrexone hydrochloride is an opioid antagonist.
- It completely blocks, reversibly, the subjective effects of intravenously administered opioids.
- When co-administered with morphine, on a chronic basis, naltrexone blocks the physical dependence to morphine, heroin and other opioids.
- This medication is also used to treat alcohol abuse. It can help people drink less alcohol or stop drinking altogether. It also decreases the desire to drink alcohol when used with a treatment program that includes counseling, support, and lifestyle.
- Naltrexone has not been seen to be effective as treatment for cannabis dependence, and might actually increase the abuse liability of cannabis.

13. Saturated salt solution can not be used in which of the following poisonings?

a. Aconite
b. Alcohol
c. Phenol
d. Heavy metals
e. Vegetable poisons

Ans. a, d, e *Ref: Parikh's Textbook of FMT, 7th/ed*

Option a	True	
Option b	False	Saturated salt solution can be used in alcohol intoxication
Option c	False	Saturated salt solution can be used in phenol ingestion
Option d	True	
Option e	True	

- Saturated solution of common salt should not be used in suspected cases of poisoning by:
  - Aconite
  - Heavy metals like corrosive sublimate
  - Vegetable poisons
  - Corrosive acids
- Rectified spirit should not be used in suspected cases of poisoning by:
  - Alcohol
  - Acetic acid
  - Carbolic acid
  - Kerosene
  - Paraldehyde
  - Phosphorus.

Orthopedics

1. 8-year-old fall on outstretched elbow leading to a supracondylar fracture (type II). The late complications would be:

a. Volkmann ischemia
b. Malunion
c. No union
d. Ulnar nerve palsy
e. Brachial nerve palsy

Ans. a,b,d *Ref: James H Beaty, James R Kasser Rockwood and Wilkins' Fractures in Children, Volume 3,. Lippincott Williams & Wilkins, 2010, p528; Mercer Rang, Rang's Children's Fractures; Lippincott Williams & Wilkins, 2005 pg 109.*

Option a	True	Yes, correct
Option b	True	Yes, correct
Option c	False	No, malunion is a late feature (not non-union)
Option d	True	Yes, correct
Option e	False	No, median, ulnar and radial nerves may be damaged. Brachial nerves injury occurs in shoulder joint trauma as accidents, prolonged labor, major trauma

Supracondylar fractures (SCF):

90% are seen in children younger than 10 years of age, with a peak age of 5-7 years

Classification of supracondylar fractures:

- Type I: Undisplaced
- Type II: Displaced with intact posterior cortex
- Type III: Complete displacement.

Radiological signs pointing to fracture:

- Anterior fat pad sign (sail sign): the anterior fat pad is elevated by a joint effusion and appears as a lucent triangle on the lateral projection
- Posterior fat pad sign
- Anterior humeral line should intersect the middle third of the capitellum in most children

Note: In children less than 4 years, the anterior humeral line line may pass through the anterior third without injury

- Obvious fracture line visible.

Complications include:

1. **Malunion**: Resulting in cubitus varus (varus deformity of the elbow, also known as gunstock deformity).
2. **Ischemic contracture** (Volkmann contracture) due to damage/occlusion to the brachial artery and resulting in volar compartment syndrome.
3. **Damage to the ulnar nerve** (most common) (tardy ulnar nerve palsy), median nerve, or radial nerve.

The principal complication of supracondylar fractures is injury to the brachial artery, which runs in close apposition to the site of this fracture. Damage to the artery can result in edema in the forearm with compartment syndrome developing.

Volkmann's ischemic contracture is contracture following circulatory occlusion of any kind. Most commonly, it is a complication of untreated compartment syndrome or a result of arterial injury. Ischemia results in muscle necrosis and later, muscle fibrosis and shortening.

Fibrosis in the flexor compartment pulls the fingers into flexion and the wrist into flexion and pronation.

Treatment:

- ❑ Flexor release operation
- ❑ Nerve grafting.

Treatment for SCF

- ❑ Type I: Cast immobilization
- ❑ Type II: Percutaneous pinning (CRIF) and cast immobilization with less than 90 degrees flexion
- ❑ Type III: Open reduction or closed reduction with percutaneous pinning.

Cubitus varus is often referred to as "Gunstock deformity", due to the crooked nature of the healing.

2. Patellar dislocation factors:

a. Genu varum
b. Loose quadriceps femoris
c. Ligamental laxity
d. Femoral torsion with anteversion
e. Lateral femoral condyle is shallow and hypoplastic

Ans. b,c,d,e *Ref: www.orthobullets.com; Brian D Coley. Caffey's Pediatric Diagnostic Imaging. Ed12. Elsevier Health Sciences, 2013. p1604; Alexander Meininger. Understanding the Patellofemoral Joint: From Instability to Arthroplasty; Volume 33, Elsevier Health Sciences, 2014. p537*

Option a	False	No, it is genu valgum (and not genu varum)
Option b	True	No, it is due to dysplastic vastus medialis oblique
Option c	True	Yes, correct
Option d	True	Yes, correct
Option e	True	Yes correct

Risk Factors Include

General Factors

1. Ligamentous laxity (Ehlers-Danlos syndrome)
2. Previous patellar instability event
3. "Miserable malalignment syndrome" a term named for the 3 anatomic characteristics that lead to an increased ***Q angle***:
   a. Femoral anteversion
   b. Genu valgum
   c. External tibial torsion/pronated feet.

Anatomical factors

4. Osseous:
    a. Patella alta: causes patella to not articulate with sulcus, losing its constraint effects
    b. Trochlear dysplasia
    c. Excessive lateral patellar tilt (measured in extension)
    d. Lateral femoral condyle hypoplasia.
5. Muscle:
    a. Dysplastic vastus medialis oblique (VMO) muscle.
6. Over pull of lateral structures:
    a. Iliotibial band
    b. Vastus lateralis.

Pathophysiology

1. Usually on noncontact twisting injury with the knee extended and foot externally rotated:
    a. Patient will usually reflexively contract quadriceps thereby reducing the patella
    b. Osteochondral fractures occur most often as the patella relocates.
2. Direct blow:
    a. Less common
    b. Ex. knee to knee collision in basketball, or football helmet to side of knee.

Presentation

- Acute dislocation: with large hemarthrosis
- Medial tenderness over the MPFL (medial patella femoral ligament)

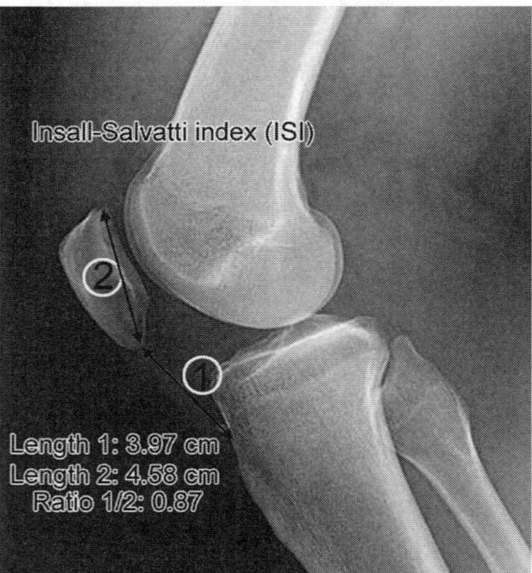

- Increase in passive patellar tension
- Patellar apprehension
- Increased Q angle
- J sign (patella subluxes laterally in active terminal extension).

3. Kienbocks:

a. AVN of scaphoid
b. Wrist pain increases with activity
c. Decreased grip strength
d. Earliest changes can be identified on CT scan
e. Sclerosis of lunate bone starts to occur in stage four of the disease

Ans. b,c *Ref: David E Brown, Randall D Neumann. Orthopedic Secrets p202; Grant Cooper. Blueprints Orthopedics p52*

Option a	False	No, It is AVN of the lunate
Option b	True	Yes, correct
Option c	True	Yes, correct
Option d	False	No, earliest changes are visible on MRI rather than a CT Scan
Option e	False	No, sclerosis of the lunate bone starts in the second stage of the disease.

- Avascular necrosis of the lunate leading to abnormal carpal motion.

Lichtman Classification		
Stage	**Description**	**Treatment**
Stage I	No visible changes on X-ray, changes seen on MRI	**Immobilization and NSAIDS**
Stage II	Sclerosis of lunate	**Joint leveling procedure** (ulnar negative patients) **Radial wedge osteotomy or STT fusion** (ulnar neutral patients) **Distal radius core decompression** **Revascularization procedures**
Stage IIIA	Lunate collapse, no scaphoid rotation	Same as Stage II above
Stage IIIB	Lunate collapse, fixed scaphoid rotation	**Proximal row carpectomy, STT fusion, or SC fusion**
Stage IV	Degenerated adjacent intercarpal joints	**Wrist fusion, proximal row carpectomy, or limited intercarpal fusion**

Imaging

CT

- Most useful once lunate collapse has already occurred
- Best for showing
- Extent of necrosis
- Trabecular destruction
- Lunate geometry.

MRI

- Best for diagnosing **early disease**. It is the most sensitive and specific investigation
- Rule out ulnar impaction syndrome (major DD).

Findings

- Decreased T1 signal intensity
- Reduced vascularity of lunate.

Signs/symptoms

- Typical complaint is aching of wrist and fingers.
- Decreased hand grip
- Decreased range of motion.

4. Tumor located on metaphysis

a. Osteochondroma
b. Osteoid osteoma
c. Chondroblastoma
d. Fibrous dysplasia
e. Tuberculosis

Ans. a,d

Option a	True	Yes, correct
Option b	False	No, it is diaphyseal
Option c	False	No, it is epiphyseal
Option d	True	Yes, correct
Option e	False	No, it is diaphyseal

Location of bone tumors/Lesions

Epiphyseal: (GC)

- Giant cell tumor
- Chondroblastoma.

Meptahyseal (SOFA-O)

- Simple bone cyst
- Osteosarcoma
- Fibrous dysplasia
- Aneurysmal bone cyst
- Osteochondroma.

Diaphyseal: (MALE-NOT)

- Multiple myeloma
- Adamantinoma
- Leukemia
- Ewings sarcoma
- Nonossifying fibroma
- Osteoid osteoma
- Tuberculosis.

5. True about osteoarthritis is/are:

a. In knee common than hip
b. Decreased thickness of subchondral bone
c. Characterized by increased water content
d. Decrease in metalloproteinases, gelatinase quantity
e. It is a non-inflammatory arthritis

Ans. a,d,e *Ref: Miller's Orthopaedics. 3rd/ed p55; Maheshwari 5th/ed p295*

Option a	True	Yes, correct
Option b	False	No, subchondral bone thickness is increased in osteoarthritis
Option c	True	Yes, correct
Option d	False	No, these are increased
Option e	True	Yes, correct

Osteoarthritis

- Degenerative disease of synovial joints that causes progressive loss of articular cartilage
- Knee OA is 2 times more common than hip OA

Primary OA: This occurs in a joint de novo. It occurs in old age, mainly in the weight bearing joints (knee and hip).

Secondary OA: It is secondary to an underlying disease, which may manifest even many years of start of the disease process.

The changes observed in articular cartilage affected by osteoarthritis include: increased water content (as a result of the disruption in architecture of the matrix molecules), decreased quantity of proteoglycans, decreased quantity of collagen with decreases in cross-linking and stiffness associated with degradation, increased thickness of subchondral bone, and increased chondrocyte activity and proliferation of chondrocytes.

Metalloproteinases, collagenases, gelatinases are increased in OA cartilage.

Causes of secondary OA

Avascular necrosis

- Idiopathic
- Post-traumatic, e.g. fracture of femoral neck
- Alcoholism
- Post-partum osteonecrosis
- Chronic liver failure
- Patient on steroids
- Patient on dialysis
- Sickle cell anemia.

Coxa vara

Congenital dislocation of hip (CDH)

Old septic arthritis of the hip

Malunited fractures

Fractures of the acetabulum

Risk Factors Include

- Age, genetic
- Female > males
- Articular trauma
- Heavy physical work
- Muscle weakness:
    - Pain at rest, stiffness, limping, restricted range of motion
    - Instability, locking or catching sensation.

OA Stages

Stage I: Early phase of OA

- Mild inflammatory changes in synovium.

Stage II: Middle phase of OA

- Moderate inflammatory changes of synovium
- Synovium becomes hypervascular.

Stage III: Late phases of OA

- Synovium becomes increasingly thick and vascular
- Subchondral bone attempts to remodel forming lytic lesion with sclerotic edges (different than bone cysts in RA)
- Bone cysts form in late stages.

X-ray Findings

- Joint space narrowing
- Osteophytes
- Subchondral sclerosis
- Subchondral cysts.

Treatment

- Weight restriction
- NSAIDS are the mainstay
- Surgical—Only indicated in advanced stages:
  - Arthroscopic debridement
  - Femoral osteotomy (for hip OA)
  - High tibial osteotomy (for knee OA)
  - Total hip replacement (THR)
  - Total knee replacement (TKR).

High yield

Joint Fluid Analysis			
Types of arthritis	**White blood cells**	**Polymorphonuclear leuckocytes (%)**	**Other characteristics**
Noninflammatory	200	25	Joint aspirate glucose and protein equal to serum values
Inflammatory	2000-75,000	50	↓ Joint aspirate glucose
Infectious	>80,000	>75	Thick cloudy fluid + Gram stain + Cultures ↓ Joint aspirate glucose, ↑ Joint aspirate protein

6. Regarding POP cast techniques, which of the following statement is true?

a. POP should be just dipped and taken out immediately after immersion into water
b. Leg casts moulds in 48-60 hours
c. Using hot water takes more time to mould
d. POP should be dipper vertically rather than horizontally
e. Compartment syndrome is immediate complication

Ans. b,d,e *Ref: Appley's System of Orthopaedics and Fractures, 9th/ed p698-700; Pocketbook of Orthopaedics and fractures 2nd/ed p55-67; Maheshwari Essentials of Orthopaedics 5th/ed p17-20*

Option a	False	No, POP should be dipped (vertically) completely in water and held there till the bubbling stops
Option b	True	Yes, correct
Option c	False	No, using cold water maximizes the moulding time
Option d	True	Yes, correct
Option e	True	Yes, correct

- Padding is placed from distal to proximal with a 50% overlap and minimum of two layers
- Cold water will maximize the moulding time
- Moulded with palms and not fingers
- Joints should be mobilized in the functional position
- Dip POP vertically till bubbles cease to come
- POP slab is applied distal to proximal
- Unpadded plaster is recommended in:
  - Colle's fracture
  - Scaphoid fracture
  - Bennett fracture.

Average setting time: 3–10 minutes

Drying time (time taken for the POP to convert from crystalline form to anhydrous form):

- Arm cast — 24-36 hrs
- Leg cast — 48-60 hrs
- Hip spica — up to 7 days

Average and recommended width of the POP cast:

- Arm/forearm — 6"
- Wrist 4"
- Thumb fingers — 3"
- Thigh and leg — 8"
- Ankle and foot — 6"

Orthopedics

1. Hyperphosphatemia is seen in:
   a. Vitamin D intoxication
   b. Renal failure
   c. Fanconi's anemia
   d. Tumor lysis syndrome
   e. Renal tubular damage

Ans. a, b, d *Ref: Apley's, 9/e; Maheshwari, 5/e*

Option a	True	
Option b	True	
Option c	False	Causes hypophosphatemia
Option d	True	Rare cause of hyperphosphatemia
Option e	False	Causes hypophosphatemia due to hypokalemia

Hyperphosphatemia, even of a quite severe degree, is largely a clinically asymptomatic condition.

Hyperphosphatemia can result from:
- Increased phosphate intake,
- Decreased phosphate excretion, or
- A disorder that shifts intracellular phosphate to extracellular space.

Increased intake can result from the following:
- Excessive oral or rectal use of an oral phosphate-saline laxative (phospho-soda)
- Excessive parenteral administration of phosphate
- Milk-alkali syndrome
- Vitamin D intoxication.

Decreased excretion can result from the following:
- Renal failure, acute or chronic
- Hypoparathyroidism
- Pseudohypoparathyroidism
- Severe hypomagnesemia
- Tumoral calcinosis
- Bisphosphonate therapy.

Shift of phosphate from intracellular to extracellular space can result from the following:
- Rhabdomyolysis
- Tumor lysis
- Acute hemolysis
- Acute metabolic or respiratory acidosis.

2. **True about Ewing's sarcoma:**
   a. Metaphysis of long bone is commonly involved
   b. Most common malignant tumor in children < 10 years of age
   c. Most of cases metastasize to lungs
   d. It is vascular in origin
   e. Surgery is definite treatment

Ans. b, c *Ref: Apley's, 9/e; Maheshwari, 5/e*

Option a	False	Diaphysis of long bones is involved
Option b	True	Occurs commonly in the age group of 5–15 years
Option c	True	
Option d	False	Ewing's sarcoma arises from endothelial elements in the marrow
Option e	False	Treatment is by radiotherapy and chemotherapy

Ewing's sarcoma:

- It is a rare tumor of bone occuring in diaphysis of long bones in children, with febrile attacks.
- Most common occurrence is in tibia, humerus, femur, fibula, and clavicle in order of frequency.
- Tumor begins in the medullary cavity at the middle of the shaft (this feature distinguishes it from osteosarcoma and giant-cell tumor).
- Areas of necrosis, hemorrhage and cyst formation occur. This may turn the tumor mass to red jelly.
- The lamellae in relation to tumor mass are destroyed.
- From the medulla, it extends through the haversian canal to the under surface of periosteum, leading to elevation of periosteum and deposition of new bone formation. These shells of new bone laid, parallel to shaft, are called as "onion layers".

Spread:

- *Direct spread*: Tumor spreads to cortex and through the haversian canals, it spreads to subperiosteal region. Tumor emboli can be seen in the tumor vessels and lymphatics.
- *Blood spread*: The most common site to which Ewing's sarcoma spreads, or metastasizes, is the lungs. Rarely liver may also be involved. Skull is almost always involved.
  - *Most important feature of tumor is its tendency to metastasize in other bones.*
- *Lymphatic spread*: Regional lymph nodes are often enlarged.

Symptoms:

- History of trauma is almost always present, followed by pain.
- Appearance of slow growing tumor in the middle of shaft of any one long bone and is a palpable mass.
- Back pain may indicate a paraspinal, retroperitoneal, or deep pelvic tumor.
- Systemic symptoms of fever and weight loss can also occur and indicate metastatic disease.

Investigation:

- X-ray shows diffuse rarefaction in diaphysis of bone, "onion layers", metastatic involvement of other bones, lung metastasis.

- MRI of the region can help in determining the extent of disease.
- Metastatic evaluation includes chest CT, radioisotopic bone scan, and bilateral bone marrow aspirate and biopsy.

Treatment:

- Consists of 6–9 months.
- *Radiotherapy:* Main treatment of this tumor.
- *Chemotherapy:* Combined with radiotherapy, is the accepted treatment.
- *Surgery:* Not used unless radiotherapy fails or there is unhealed pathological fracture.

3. Pirani scoring for CTEV includes:

a. Curvature of the lateral border of foot
b. Medial crease severity
c. Position of the lateral part of the head of the talus
d. Empty heel
e. Severity of the posterior crease

Ans. a, b, c, d, e *Ref: Apley's, 9/e; Maheshwari, 5/e*

Option a	True	
Option b	True	
Option c	True	
Option d	True	
Option e	True	

Pirani scoring

The Pirani score is a simple, easy to use tool for assessing the severity of each of the components of a congenital talipes equinovarus (CTEV).

Each component may score 0, 0.5 or 1

- Hind foot contracture score (HCFS):
  - Posterior crease
  - Empty heel
  - Rigid equinus
- Mid foot contracture score (MFCS):
  - Medial crease
  - Curvature of lateral border
  - Position of head of talus
- The least (best) total score for all categories combined is 0, and the maximum (worst) score is 6.
- A Pirani scoring of 4 or more is likely to require at least four casts, while a scoring less than 4 will require three or fewer.
- A foot with a hindfoot score of 2.5 or 3 has a 72% chance of requiring a tenotomy.
- The Pirani scoring system is reliable, quick, and easy to use, and provides a good forecast about the likely treatment for an individual foot, but a low score does not exclude the possibility that a tenotomy may be required.

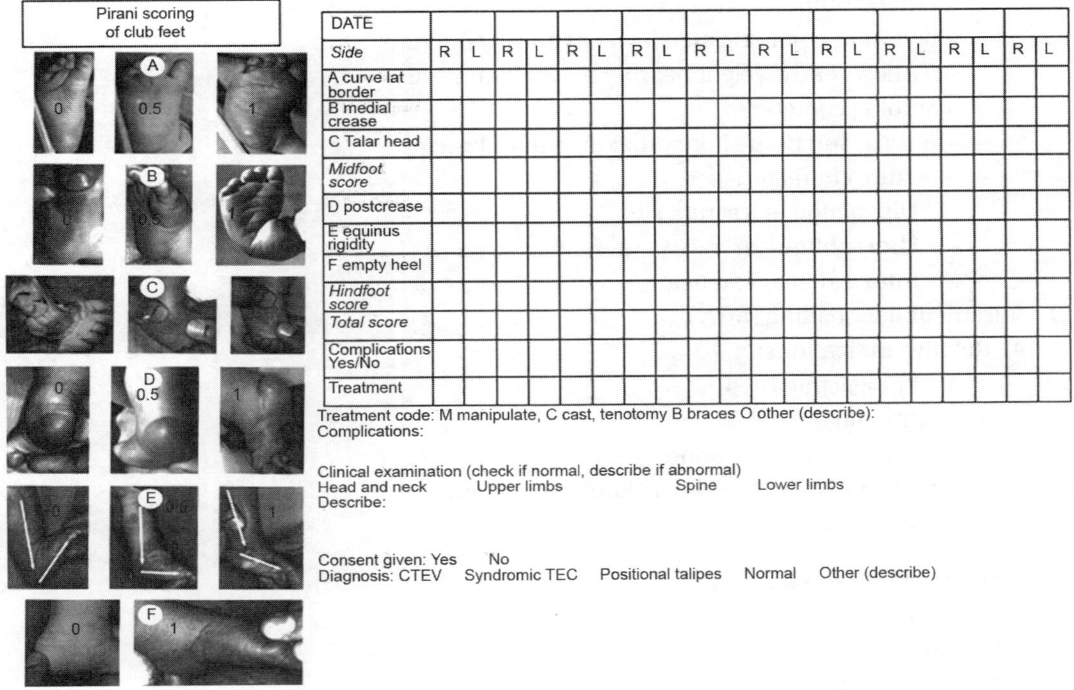

DATE																				
Side	R	L	R	L	R	L	R	L	R	L	R	L	R	L	R	L	R	L	R	L
A curve lat border																				
B medial crease																				
C Talar head																				
Midfoot score																				
D postcrease																				
E equinus rigidity																				
F empty heel																				
Hindfoot score																				
Total score																				
Complications Yes/No																				
Treatment																				

Treatment code: M manipulate, C cast, tenotomy B braces O other (describe):
Complications:

Clinical examination (check if normal, describe if abnormal)
Head and neck Upper limbs Spine Lower limbs
Describe:

Consent given: Yes No
Diagnosis: CTEV Syndromic TEC Positional talipes Normal Other (describe)

Fig. 8.1: Pirani scoring for CTEV.

4. Indication for surgical management of fracture of shaft of humerus includes:

a. Old age fracture
b. Brachial plexus injury
c. Multiple fractures
d. Pathological fractures
e. Vascular injury

Ans. b, c, d, e *Ref: Apley's, 9/e; Maheshwari, 5/e*

Option a	False
Option b	True
Option c	True
Option d	True
Option e	True

Operative management of fractured shaft of humerus includes:

- ❑ Open reduction and internal fixation
  - Absolute indications:
    - Open fracture
    - Vascular injury requiring repair
    - Brachial plexus injury
    - Ipsilateral forearm fracture (floating elbow)
    - Compartment syndrome

- Relative indications:
  - Bilateral humerus fracture
  - Polytrauma or associated lower extremity fracture
    - Allows early weight bearing through humerus
  - Pathologic fractures
  - Burns or soft tissue injury that precludes bracing
  - Fracture characteristics:
    - Distraction at fracture site
    - Short oblique or transverse fracture pattern
    - Intra articular extension

❑ Intramedullary nailing (IMN)

- Relative indications:
  - Pathologic fractures
  - Segmental fractures
  - Severe osteoporotic bone
  - Overlying skin compromise limits open approach
  - Polytrauma

5. Spur sign is seen in:

a. Supracondylar fracture of humerus
b. Radial head fracture
c. Fibula fracture
d. Talus fracture
e. Acetabular fractures

Ans. e *Ref: Apley's, 9/e; Maheshwari, 5/e*

Option a	False	
Option b	False	
Option c	False	
Option d	False	
Option e	True	

Spur sign is seen in acetabular fractures.

❑ The spur sign is the radiographic projection of the most distal (stable) part of the iliac wing, which remains attached to the axial skeleton through the sacroiliac joint.

❑ It represents posterior displacement of the sciatic buttress of the iliac wing fracture, which essentially disconnects the roof of the acetabulum from the axial skeleton.

❑ When this occurs, weight from the torso and upper body can no longer be supported by the acetabulum.

❑ On radiographs and CT, the spur sign appears as a shard of bone extending posteriorly at the level of the superior acetabulum.

❑ Evaluation of sequential CT images shows the fracture, which separates the sciatic buttress from the acetabular roof.

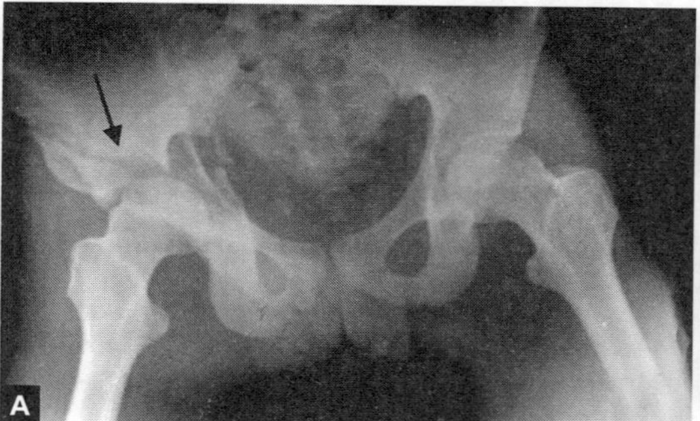

Fig. 8.2A: X-ray AP views of both column fracture in an 18M. Apart from disruption of both anterior and posterior column lines, no part of weight-bearing dome (arrow) remains attached to sciatic buttress, thus distinguishing it from T-shaped.

Fig. 8.2B: Obturator oblique view shows pathognomonic "Spur" sign (arrow), representing the intact portion of Iliac crest still attached to sacrolliac joint.

6. True about giant cell tumor (GCT):

a. Most commonly seen in 20–40 year age group
b. Proximal femur is affected most commonly
c. May involve sacrum
d. Occur as multiple lesions
e. Pulmonary metastasis occur rarely

Ans. a, c, e *Ref: Apley's, 9/e; Maheshwari, 5/e; S Das, 9/e*

Option	Answer	Explanation
Option a	True	
Option b	False	
Option c	True	
Option d	False	Typically occur as single lesion
Option e	True	

- Also known as osteoclastomas, relatively common bone tumors, usually arising from metaphysis and typically extending into the epiphysis of the long bones.
- 1/3rd are entirely benign, 1/3rd invade nearby tissues, 1/3rd metastasize.
- Tumor usually occurs between ages of 20–40 years.
- Develops in epiphyseal region soon after epiphyseal growth has ceased.
- Common sites are lower end of femur, upper end of tibia and lower end of radius.
- Microscopically they are characterized by prominent and diffuse osteoclastic giant cells and mononuclear cells (round, oval, or polygonal and may resemble normal histiocytes).
- Approximately 5–10% of GCTs are malignant. Sarcomatous transformation is seen, especially in radiotherapy treated inoperable tumors.
- Although rare (<5%), lung metastases are possible.
- They typically occur as single lesions.
- The most common involved sites are:
  - *Around the knee:* distal femur and proximal tibia
  - Distal radius
  - Sacrum
  - Vertebral body

Sign and symptoms:

- Vague discomfort and swelling near the end of the long bone.
- Pathological fractures.
- Joint may get stiff when the tumor invades articular cartilage.
- On pressing the swelling, "egg shell crackling" may be elicited.
- Local temperature of tumor usually normal.

Treatment:

- *Curettage:* If the tumor is entirely benign.
- *Wide excision:* Treatment of choice where site permits.
- *Radiotherapy:* Used for inaccessible tumor, or where excision not possible.
- *Amputation:* In cases of persistent recurrence or when malignancy has been confirmed by biopsy.

7. Cause (s) of avascular necrosis of femoral head:

a. Fracture of femoral neck due to trauma
b. Prolonged steroid use
c. Chronic alcohol use
d. Caisson disease
e. Sickle cell disease

Ans. a, b, c, d, e *Ref: Apley's, 9/e; Maheshwari, 5/e*

Option a	True	
Option b	True	
Option c	True	
Option d	True	Decompression sickness
Option e	True	Chronic progressive disability in sickle cell disease

- Most cases of AVN are *atraumatic* and include the following:
  - Excessive ***corticosteroid usage*** and ***alcohol abuse***.
  - Intravascular coagulation. Coagulation may occur secondary to extravascular compression (e.g., marrow fat enlargement), vessel wall injury (e.g., chemotherapy, radiation), or a thromboembolic event (e.g., fat emboli).
  - Ischemic insult to the femoral head results in infarcted subchondral bone.
  - Radiation avascular necrosis.
  - ***Decompression sickness—Caisson disease.***
  - ***Sickle cell disease—common occurrence.***
  - Gaucher's disease
  - Diabetes mellitus
  - HIV/AIDS
  - Pancreatitis
- *Traumatic* causes of femoral head AVN include the following:
  - ***Femoral neck fractures***
  - Hip dislocation
  - Slipped capital femoral epiphysis

Ref: Song HK, Choi HJ, Yang KH. Risk factors of avascular necrosis of the femoral head and fixation failure in patients with valgus angulated femoral neck fractures over the age of 50 years. Injury. 2016 Oct 19.

- ❑ Magnetic resonance imaging **(MRI)** is the study of choice in patients who demonstrate signs and symptoms that are suggestive of avascular necrosis but whose radiographs are normal.
- ❑ Surgical treatment of AVN can be done for either prophylactic measures (to retard progression) or reconstruction procedures (after femoral head collapse).

8. Gurd's criteria for fat embolism includes:

a. Hypoxemia $PaO_2 < 60$ mm Hg, $FiO_2 = 0.4$
b. Tachycardia < 110 bpm
c. Central nervous system depression disproportionate to hypoxemia
d. Axillary or subconjunctival petechiae
e. Deep vein thrombosis

Ans. a, c, d *Ref: Apley's, 9/e; Maheshwari, 5/e; Gurd AR, Wilson RI. The fat embolism syndrome. J Bone Joint Surg Br. 1974 Aug;56B(3):408-16*

Option a	True	
Option b	False	Tachycardia > 110 bpm
Option c	True	
Option d	True	
Option e	False	A sudden drop in hematocrit or platelet values

Fat embolism syndrome is a condition characterized by hypoxia, bilateral pulmonary infiltrates, and mental status change.

Gurd's and Wilson's criteria

- ❑ Major criteria:
  - Axillary or subconjunctival petechiae
  - Hypoxemia ($PaO_2 < 60$ mm Hg; $FiO_2 = 0.4$)
  - Central nervous system depression disproportionate to hypoxemia
  - Pulmonary edema
- ❑ Minor criteria:
  - Tachycardia >110 bpm
  - Pyrexia >38.5°C
  - Emboli present in the retina on fundoscopy
  - Fat present in urine
  - A sudden inexplicable drop in hematocrit or platelet values
  - Increasing ESR
  - Fat globules present in the sputum

For the diagnosis of fat embolism syndrome, at least one major and four minor criteria must be present.

Schonfeld's criteria

- ❑ Score:
  - Petechiae (5 points)
  - X-ray chest diffuse infiltrates (4 points)
  - Hypoxemia (3 points)
  - Fever (1 point)

- Tachycardia (1 point)
- Tachypnea (1 point)
- Confusion (1 point)

In this criteria, a score > 5 is diagnostic of fat embolism syndrome.

9. True about spinal tuberculosis is/are:

a. Middle path regimen is used in management
b. Cervical spine is most commonly affected
c. Commonly spread by hematogenous route from lung
d. Acute onset early paraplegia has good prognosis
e. Lower thoracic vertebra is most commonly involved

Ans. a, c, d, e *Ref: Maheshwari, 9/e; Campbell's Operative Orthopaedics, 13/e*

Option a	True	
Option b	False	Spinal TB is most common in the lower thoracic region or thoracolumbar junctional region
Option c	True	Blood-borne infection is the common route
Option d	True	Early onset type-I paraplegia resolves almost completely within 6 months of starting the treatment
Option e	True	Most common involvement

Spinal TB, also called as Pott's spine, is a very dangerous type of skeletal TB as it can be associated with neurologic deficit due to compression of adjacent neural structures and significant spinal deformity. Therefore, early diagnosis and management of spinal TB has special importance in preventing these serious complications.

Spinal TB is most common in the lower thoracic region or thoracolumbar junctional region.

This region is more susceptible because of:

- Presence of relatively large amount of spongy tissue in vertebral bodies of this region.
- Greater range of mobility.
- Maximum amount of weight bearing due to junction of two curvatures.
- Proximity of maximum number of abdominal lymph nodes to this region.
- Blood—borne infection is the common route. Lymph borne infection can also be seen.

Pathological process:

- A cold abscess can occur, if the infection extends to adjacent ligaments and soft tissues:
  - It may be collected under the anterior longitudinal ligament in front of vertebral bodies.
  - It may pass backwards and invade the vertebral canal, giving rise to Pott's paraplegia.
  - More commonly, abscesses in the lumbar region may descend down the sheath of the psoas to the femoral trigone region and eventually erode into the skin.
  - Anteriorly, it may bulge into pharynx or esophagus.
  - It may track into axilla following the course of brachial plexus and axillary vessels.

Pott's Paraplegia:

- Occurs due to compression of spinal cord.
- *Early onset paraplegia*: Occurs in active phase of disease and is complete. It is further of 2 types:

- *Type I:* Paraplegia caused by compression from soft material as cold abscess or caseous mass. It usually recovers completely within 6 months of starting the treatment.
- *Type II:* Usually caused by compression from hard solid material as sequestrated disc or a bone spike. Recovery is late and incomplete.

❑ *Late onset paraplegia*: Paralysis occurs late in the healing stage or even years after the active disease:
- Deformity and motor deficit are the most serious consequences of Pott disease.
- Backpain is the earliest and most common symptom.

Difference between tubercular and pyogenic spine	
Tubercular	***Pyogenic***
• Long standing history of months to years	• History of days to months
• Presence of active pulmonary tuberculosis—60%	• Not present
• Most common location thoracic spine followed by thoracolumbar region	• Most common location lumbar spine
• > 3 contiguous vertebral body involvement common—42%	• 19% only. Mostly involves 1 spinal segment—2 vertebrae and intervening disc.
• Vertebral collapse—67%	• 21% only

10. True about anterior cruciate ligament is/are:
a. Mostly occurs as a result of twisting force
b. May occur secondary to tibial fracture
c. Almost always associated with meniscal injury
d. Lachman test is highly sensitive test for tear
e. Immediate surgery needs to be done

Ans. a, b, c, d *Ref: Campbell's Operative Orthopaedics, 13/e*

Option a	True	
Option b	True	Occurs due to over-stretching or tearing of the anterior cruciate ligament
Option c	True	Lateral meniscal injury is more common than injury to the medial meniscus
Option d	True	
Option e	False	Surgical intervention should be delayed at least 3 weeks following injury

The anterior cruciate ligament (ACL) is the most commonly disrupted ligament of the knee, especially in athletes who participate in sports that involve rapid starting, stopping, and pivoting (e.g. soccer, basketball, tennis, netball and snow skiing).

Symptoms of an acute ACL injury may include the following:

❑ Feeling or hearing a "pop" sound in the knee
❑ Pain and inability to continue activity
❑ Swelling and instability of the knee
❑ Development of a large hemarthrosis

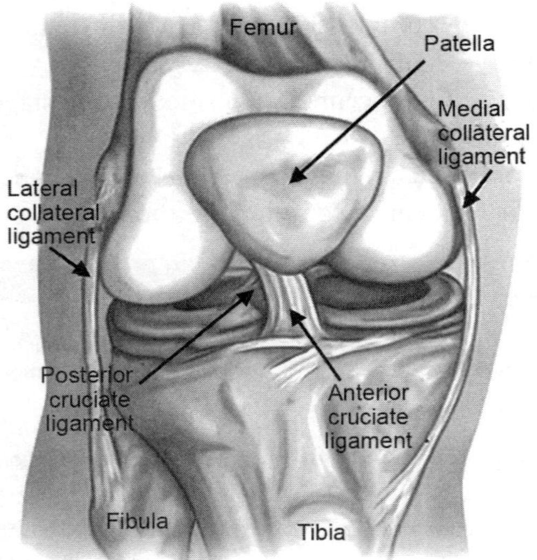

Fig. 8.3: Normal knee anatomy, front view.

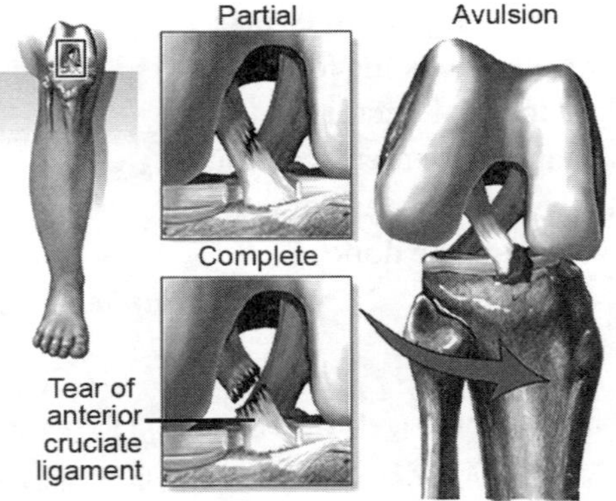

Fig. 8.4: Anterior cruciate ligament tear.

Associated with O'donoghue unhappy triad or terrible triad. It consists of:

- Anterior cruciate ligament (ACL) tear
- Medial collateral ligament (MCL) tear/sprain
- Medial meniscal tear (lateral compartment bone bruise)—lateral meniscal injury is more common than injury to the medial meniscus.

Diagnosis:

- ***The Lachman test*** is the *most sensitive test* for acute ACL rupture. It is performed with the knee in 30° of flexion, with the patient lying supine. The amount of displacement (in mm) and the quality of endpoint are assessed (e.g., firm, marginal, soft). Asymmetry in side-to-side laxity or a soft endpoint is indicative of an ACL tear. Although difficult to measure, a side-to-side difference of greater than 3 mm is considered abnormal.

- ***Pivot shift test*** is performed by extending an ACL-deficient knee, which results in a small amount of anterior translation of the tibia in relation to the femur. During flexion, the translation reduces, resulting in the "shifting or pivoting" of the tibia into its proper alignment on the femur. It is performed with the leg extended and the foot in internal rotation, and a valgus stress is applied to the tibia.
- ***Anterior drawer test*** is performed with the knee at 90° flexion, with the patient lying supine. There is an attempt to displace the tibia forward from the femur. If there is more than 6 mm of tibial displacement, an ACL tear is suggested. This test is not very sensitive and has been found to be positive in only 77% of patients with complete ACL rupture.
- ***MRI*** has a sensitivity of 90–98% for ACL tears.

Treatment:

Before any treatment, strengthening of the quadriceps and hamstrings, as well as ROM (Range of Motion) exercises are recommended.

Surgical intervention should be delayed at least 3 weeks following injury to prevent the complication of arthrofibrosis. The methods of surgical repair may be categorized into 3 groups: primary repair, extra-articular repair, and intra-articular repair.

Intra-articular reconstruction of the ACL has become the criterion standard for treating ACL tears.

Nonoperative treatment may be considered in elderly patients or in less active athletes who may not be participating in any pivoting type of sports (e.g., running, cycling). The goal is to obtain a full ROM and strength compared with the uninjured knee.

11. Features of L5,S1 disc prolapse include:

a. Lower back pain
b. Pain radiation to leg
c. Sensory loss in medial calf muscle
d. Knee jerk is lost
e. Bowel and bladder incontinence

Ans. a, b, e *Ref: Maheshwari, 9/e; Campbell's Operative Orthopaedics, 13/e*

Option a	True	
Option b	True	Also known as sciatica
Option c	False	Sensory loss in lateral calf muscles is seen
Option d	False	Ankle jerk sluggish or absent in L5/S1 prolapse
Option e	True	

- L5/S1 most common level for disc herniation
- Peak incidence is seen in 4th and 5th decades
- Only ~5% become symptomatic
- 3:1; male:female ratio
- Symptoms can affect the lower back, buttocks, thigh, anal/genital region (via the perineal nerve), and may radiate into the foot and/or toe
- Lower back pain (lumbago) is most common symptom
- Leg pain, commonly referred to as sciatica
- Lumbar disc herniation occurs 15 times more than cervical disc herniation, and is an important cause of lower back pain.

Pathoanatomy: Recurrent torsional strain leads to tears of outer annulus which leads to herniation of nucleus pulposis.

Clinical features:

- Can present with symptoms of axial back pain (low back pain): this may be discogenic or mechanical in nature.
- Radicular pain (buttock and leg pain)—often worse with sitting, improves with standing:
  - Symptoms worsened by coughing, valsalva, sneezing.
- Neurological symptoms:
  - Paraesthesias, most often described as 'pins and needles' corresponding to the dermatome of the affected nerve root.
  - Numbness in the leg or foot and weakness of the muscles.
  - Cauda equina syndrome (present in 1–10%). In cases with large disc material compressing the theca and roots, presents as:
    - Bilateral leg pain
    - Saddle anesthesia
    - Bowel/bladder incontinence.

Neurological deficit in disc prolapse

Level	*Nerve root affected*	*Motor weakness*	*Sensory loss*	*Reflexes*
L_5–S_1	S_1 root	Weakness of plantar flexors of the foot	Over lateral side of the foot	Ankle jerk sluggish or absent
L_4–L_5	L_5 root	Weakness of EHL* and dorsiflexors of the foot	Over dorsum of the foot and lateral side of the leg	Ankle jerk normal
L_3–L_4	L_4 root	Weakness of extensors of the knee	Over great toe and medial side of the leg	Knee jerk sluggish or absent

*EHL: Extensor hallucis longus.

Prognosis:

- 90% of patients will have improvement of symptoms within 3 months with nonoperative care.
- Size of herniation decreases over time (reabsorbed):
  - Sequestered disc herniations show the greatest degree of spontaneous reabsorption
  - Macrophage phagocytosis is mechanism of reabsorption.

Investigations:

- MRI is investigation of choice.

Treatment:

- Rest with Anti-inflammatory medications
- Indications for surgery:
  - Bladder and bowel involvement
  - Increasing neurological deficit
  - Failure of conservative treatment (6 weeks).

12. True about fractures of vertebrae is/are:

a. Wedge compression causes flexion injury

b. anterior longitudinal ligament runs along the posterior surface of the vertebral bodies

c. Vertical compression force does not extend to cervical spine

d. Chance fracture occurs due to flexion-distraction injury
e. Fracture dislocation is common in flexion rotation injury

Ans. a, d, e *Ref: Maheshwari, 9/e; Campbell's Operative Orthopaedics, 13/e*

Option a	True	
Option b	False	Anterior longitudinal ligament runs along the anterior surface of the vertebral bodies
Option c	False	In the cervical spine, this force results in a burst fracture
Option d	True	
Option e	True	

Spinal injuries are classified on the basis of mechanism of injury into the following types:

- Flexion injury—commonest spinal injury:
  - Can result in compression fracture of the vertebral body, C5 to C7;
  - In the dorsolumbar spine, this force can result in the wedge compression of a vertebra (L1 commonest, followed by L2 and D12).
  - Comparatively stable injury, if compression of the vertebra is less than 50% of its posterior height.
- Flexion-rotation injury—worst type of spinal injury because it leaves a highly unstable spine, and is associated with a high incidence of neurological damage. In the cervical spine this force can result in:
  - Dislocation of the facet joints on one or both sides; and
  - *Fracture-dislocation* of the cervical vertebra.

  In the dorsolumbar spine, this force can result in a *fracture-dislocation of the spine.*
- Vertical compression injury—common spinal injury. In the cervical spine, this force results in a *burst fracture*. It is an *unstable* injury.
- Extension injury—commonly seen in the cervical spine. This injury results in a *chip fracture* of the anterior rim of a vertebra. Sometimes, these injuries may be *unstable.*
- Flexion-distraction injury—recently described spinal injury due to seat belt use:
  - It commonly results in a horizontal fracture extending into the posterior elements and involving a part of the body.
  - It is termed as a '*Chance fracture*'.
  - It is an *unstable injury*.
- Direct injury—rare type of spinal injury. Any part of the vertebra may be smashed by a bullet, but, a lathi blow generally causes a fracture of the spinous processes only.
- Indirect injury due to violent muscle contraction—rare injury. It results in fractures of the transverse processes of multiple lumbar vertebrae.

Essential features of different types of spinal injuries

Mechanism	*Type of injury*	*Common site*	*Column failure*	*X-ray features*	*Stability*
Flexion injury e.g., Fall on buttock/head, Heavy object falling on flexed spine	Compression fracture	$L_1 > L_2 > D_{12}$ C_5-C_7	Only anterior column failure	Diminished anterior height of vertebra, posterior part remains intact	Stale

Contd...

Contd...

Mechanism	Type of injury	Common site	Column failure	X-ray features	Stability
Flexion-rotation injury e.g., Fall on one side, Blow on the side	Fracture dislocation	L_1, D_{12} C_5-C_7	All the three columns failure	Direct evidence (subluxation/ dislocation): • Posterior arch fracture • Broken facets • Vertebral body offset anteriorly *Indirect evidence:* • Broken ribs • Broken transverse processes • Increased disc height • Increased interspinous distance	Unstable
Vertical compression injury e.g., Object falling on head	Burst fracture	C_5-C_6	Anterior and middle columns failure	Diminished anterior and posterior heights of vertebra CT scan may be of help in demonstrating compromise of the spinal canal by bony fragments	May be unstable
Extension injury e.g., Motor vehicle accident, Shallow water diving	Avulsion fracture of anterior lip of vertebra	C_5–C_6, lumbar spine	Only anterior column failure	Small chip from margin of vertebra, CT scan of no help	Stable
Flexion-distraction injury e.g., Car seat belt injury	Chance fracture	Dorsal spine	Middle and posterior column failure	Horizontal fracture line through posterior arch and posterior part of body of the vertebra	May be unstable
Direct injury e.g., Bullet injury, Muscle contraction	Fracture of spinous or transverse processes	Any region	Any/All columns failure	Variable	Variable

13. True about avascular necrosis of femur is/are:

a. Putting weight on the affected side helps in early stages
b. Early changes can not be seen on X-ray
c. Bisphosphonates worsen the area of necrosis
d. Always unilateral
e. Total joint replacement is rarely done these days

Ans. b, c *Ref: Maheshwari, 9/e; Campbell's Operative Orthopaedics, 13/e; Appley's, 9/e*

Option a	False	Early stages are protected by reduced weight bearing
Option b	True	
Option c	True	Very rarely, bisphosphonates can cause/worsen the condition
Option d	False	Often bilateral
Option e	False	One of the very commonly done procedure

Causes of avascular necrosis of femoral head

- Idiopathic—commonest
- Alcoholism
- Steroid therapy
- Sickle cell disease
- Patient on renal dialysis
- Patient on anticancer drugs
- Postpartum necrosis
- Gaucher's disease
- Caisson's disease

- The disease is often bilateral (75%). Patient complains of pain in the groin or in front of the thigh.
- Limitation of abduction and internal rotation.
- X-rays may be normal in early stage; if suspicion is strong, a bone scan may be done.
- In later stage, an osteolytic lesion can be seen in superolateral part of the head.
- MRI (Investigation of Choice)—shows double line sign.

Treatment:

- Early stages are protected by **reduced weight bearing**. If the condition is diagnosed early, reduced weight bearing can be helpful in removing weight from the affected joint, and thus greatly lessen the risk for microfractures in weight-bearing surfaces. This may involve the use of crutches or the limitation of certain activities.
- **Core decompression**—Core decompression is a surgery in which the inner layer of bone is removed, theoretically allowing for better blood flow to the area of concern. This surgery is most effective for people in the earliest stages of the disease.
- **Osteotomy**—This surgery reshapes either the affected bone or surrounding bones in order to decrease stress on the afflicted area. The surgery is most effective for patients with advanced forms of the disease and for when avascular necrosis affects a large area of bone.
- **Muscle pedicle graft**—Quadratus femoris/Tensor fascia lata graft can be fixed in femoral head to augment vascularity.
- **Arthroplasty/total joint replacement**—This treatment is used in late-stage avascular necrosis and when the joint is destroyed. Total hip replacement one of the very commonly done procedure as most patients present at stage of arthritis.

14. True about osteomalacia:

a. Serum phosphate is low, Ca is low
b. Serum ALP is high
c. Looser's zone seen on radiology
d. Osteopenic area below cartilage
e. 25 and 1-25 dicholecalciferol levels are low

Ans. a, b, c, e *Ref: Maheshwari, 9/e; Campbell's Operative Orthopaedics, 13/e*

Option a	True	
Option b	True	
Option c	True	Also called pseudofractures
Option d	False	Bone content is demineralized
Option e	True	

Osteomalacia, means softening of bones, is the adult counterpart of rickets. It is primarily due to deficiency of vitamin d. This results in failure to replace the turnover of calcium and phosphorus in the organic matrix of bone. Hence, the bone content is demineralized and the bony substance is replaced by soft osteoid tissue.

Following presentations may be seen:

- *Bone pains:* Skeletal discomfort ranging from backache to diffuse bone pains may occur. Bone tenderness is common.
- *Muscular weakness:* The patient feels very weak. He may have difficulty in climbing up and down the stairs. A waddling gait is not unusual. Tetany may manifest as carpopedal spasm and facial twitching.
- Spontaneous fractures occur usually in spine, and may result in kyphosis.

Following investigations may be carried out:

- *Radiological examination:* Plain X-rays appear to be of 'poor quality', i.e. not sharp and well defined. It may show:
  - Diffuse rarefaction of bones.
  - *Looser's zone (pseudofractures):* These are radiolucent zones occurring at sites of stress. Common sites are the pubic rami, axillary border of scapula, ribs and the medial cortex of the neck of the femur. These are caused by rapid resorption and slow mineralization and may be surrounded by a collar of callus.
  - Triradiate pelvis in females.
  - Protrusio-acetabuli, i.e. the acetabulum protruding into the pelvis.
- *Bone biopsy:* A bone biopsy from the iliac crest usually confirms the diagnosis. The characteristic histological finding is excessive uncalcified osteoid.
- *Serum:* The serum **calcium level is low**, the **phosphates are low** and **alkaline phosphatase high**.

15. Test of anterior cruciate ligament is:

a. Lachman's
b. Pivot's
c. Reverse pivot
d. KT-1000
e. Appley's grinding

Ans. a, b, d *Ref: Maheshwari, 9/e; Campbell's Operative Orthopaedics, 13/e*

Option a	True	
Option b	True	
Option c	False	Positive reverse pivot shows PCL injury
Option d	True	
Option e	False	Used for meniscal injury

There are four main ligaments in the knee:

- The medial collateral ligament (MCL),
- Lateral collateral ligament (LCL),
- Anterior cruciate ligament (ACL)
- Posterior cruciate ligament (PCL).

Integrity of these can be tested by various tests.

Anterior cruciate ligament is the most commonly injured ligament. Following tests can be done to confirm the injury:

- ***The Lachman test*** is the *most sensitive test* for acute ACL rupture. It is performed with the knee in 30° of flexion, with the patient lying supine. The amount of displacement (in mm) and the quality of endpoint are assessed (e.g., firm, marginal, soft). Asymmetry in side-to-side laxity or a soft endpoint is indicative of an ACL tear. Although difficult to measure, a side-to-side difference of greater than 3 mm is considered abnormal.
- ***Pivot shift test*** is performed by extending an ACL-deficient knee, which results in a small amount of anterior translation of the tibia in relation to the femur. During flexion, the translation reduces, resulting in the "shifting or pivoting" of the tibia into its proper alignment on the femur. It is performed with the leg extended and the foot in internal rotation, and a valgus stress is applied to the tibia.
- ***Anterior drawer test*** is performed with the knee at 90° flexion, with the patient lying supine. There is an attempt to displace the tibia forward from the femur. If there is more than 6 mm of tibial displacement, an ACL tear is suggested. This test is not very sensitive and has been found to be positive in only 77% of patients with complete ACL rupture.

KT-1000 is a device that is used to check the laxity of leg incases of ACL tear. In addition to helping diagnose an ACL tear, the KT-1000 test can also be useful to determine the results of one's ACL reconstruction.

16. Most anterior to interspinous tibial plateau is:

a. Anterior cruciate ligament
b. Patellar tendon
c. Posterior cruciate ligament
d. Medial meniscus
e. Lateral meniscus

Ans. d *Ref: Maheshwari, 9/e; Campbell's Operative Orthopaedics, 13/e*

Option a	False
Option b	False
Option c	False
Option d	True
Option e	False

There are two knee menisci in each joint: medial and lateral. The menisci are described as having a central body with anterior and posterior horns. In cross-section, they have a triangular (bow-tie) shape, being thicker peripherally and thinning to a free-edge centrally. Each meniscus has a differing shape, size and attachments:

Medial meniscus:

- C-shape or semilunar
- Larger
- More open and wider; semicircular in shape

Lateral meniscus:

- Semicircular-like an incomplete circle, i.e. anterior and posterior tibial roots are very close to each other
- Smaller

Attachments

Medial meniscus:

- *The anterior horn of the medial meniscus attaches immediately anterior to the tibial attachment of the anterior cruciate ligament (ACL) in the intercondylar area.*
- Lateral aspect attached to the deep (third) layer of the medial collateral ligament.
- Posterior horn is attached to the posterior intercondylar area of the tibial plateau, between PCL insertion posteriorly and posterior root attachment of lateral meniscus, anteriorly.

Lateral meniscus

- The anterior horn of the lateral meniscus attaches immediately lateral to the tibial attachment of the ACL on the intercondylar area.
- No attachment to the lateral collateral ligament except anterior horn and posterior most portion of posterior horn; this is due to the passage of the intra-articular portion of the popliteus tendon.
- Posterior horn of the lateral meniscus attaches to the posterior intercondylar area of the tibial plateau anterior to the medial meniscus and posterior to ACL.

17. True about wrist ganglion is:

a. More common in females
b. Originate from external retinaculum
c. Excised by tourniquet
d. Dorsum of wrists involved
e. Related to luna trapezius joint

Ans. a, d *Ref: Maheshwari, 9/e; Campbell's Operative Orthopaedics, 13/e*

Option a	True	More common in 20–40 year females
Option b	False	Results from mucoid degeneration of the tendon sheath or the joint capsule
Option c	False	
Option d	True	
Option e	False	

- It is the commonest cystic swelling on the dorsum of the wrist.
- It results from mucoid degeneration of the tendon sheath or the joint capsule. A common site of occurrence is along the *extensor carpi radialis brevis,* as it passes over the dorsum of the wrist joint.
- Ordinarily, there are no symptoms other than the swelling itself.
- Sometimes, a mild discomfort or pain is experienced.
- The cyst may sometimes be so tense as to resemble a solid tumor of the tendon sheath.
- Often the cyst is multiloculated.
- Aspiration of the cyst is performed and an injection of hylase given.
- If the cyst recurs, excision may be required.

18. A child presents with CTEV, the last deformity to be corrected by Ponseti method is:

a. Equinus
b. Cavus
c. Varus
d. Talipes
e. All simultaneously

Ans. a *Ref: Maheshwari, 9/e; Campbell's Operative Orthopaedics, 13/e*

Option a	True	Last one to get corrected
Option b	False	First one to get corrected
Option c	False	
Option d	False	
Option e	False	

Ponseti's philosophy: This philosophy is based on better understanding of the pathoanatomy of the deformed foot:

- According to Ponseti, the calcaneocuboid-navicular complex is internally rotated (adducted) under the plantar flexed talus.
- Hence, the deformity can be corrected by bringing the complex back under the talus by gradually stretching the tight structures. This is done by putting thumb pressure over the talus head (and not over calcaneocuboid joint as in Kite's method).
- By doing this, the calcaneocuboid—navicular complex is externally rotated under the talar head.
- Treatment is started within 1st week of life.
- The *cavus aspect of the deformity is corrected first*, followed by the *adduction*, then *varus* and *lastly equinus*.
- After every manipulation, an above-knee PoP cast is applied, which is changed every 5–7 days.
- It is usually possible to correct all components of the deformity within 6 weeks.
- The equines deformity often remains undercorrected, and can be treated by percutaneous tenotomy of tendoachilles. The cut tendoachilles regenerates spontaneously.

19. True about fracture healing is/are:

a. Micromovement promotes healing
b. In primary healing, cartilage involvement is there
c. Woven bone is formed in primary fractures
d. In secondary healing, cartilage involvement is there.
e. Immobilization is golden rule for all fractures

Ans. a, b *Ref: Maheshwari, 9/e; Campbell's Operative Orthopaedics, 13/e*

Option a	True	Micromovement at fracture sites is known to promote callus formation and bridging of the bony fragments
Option b	True	
Option c	False	It forms initially in a new bone and later gets replaced by lamellar bone.
Option d	False	It is there in primary healing
Option e	False	It is not necessary to immobilize all fractures (e.g., fracture ribs, scapula, etc)

A fracture begins to heal soon after it occurs, through a continuous series of stages described below.

Stages of fracture healing (Frost, 1989)		
Stage of healing	***Approximate time***	***Essential features***
Stage of hematoma	Less than 7 days	Fracture end necrosis occurs. Sensitization of precursor cells.
Stage of granulation tissue	Up to 2–3 weeks	Proliferation and differentiation of daughter cells into vessels, fibroblasts, osteoblasts, etc. Fracture still *mobile*.
Stage of callus	4–12 weeks	Mineralization of granulation tissue. *Callus* radiologically visible. Fracture clinically united, *no more mobile*.
Stage of remodeling	1–2 years	Lamellar bone formation by multicellular unit based remodeling of callus. Outline of callus becomes dense and sharply defined.
Stage of modeling	Many years	Modeling of endosteal and periosteal surfaces, so that the fracture site becomes indistinguishable from the parent bone.

- **Primary fracture healing** occurs where fracture hematoma has been disturbed, as in fractures treated operatively. The bone heals directly, without callus formation, and it is therefore difficult to evaluate union on X-rays. Its first stage is characterized by the filling of the fracture gap by primary bone formation (connective tissue or fibrocartilage).
- **Secondary fracture healing** occurs in fractures where fracture hematoma is not disturbed, as in cases treated nonoperatively. There is healing, with callus formation, and can be evaluated on X-rays.

Factors affecting fracture healing:

- Age of the patient: Fractures unite faster in children.
- Type of bone: Flat and cancellous bones unite faster than tubular and cortical bones.
- Pattern of fracture: Spiral fractures unite faster than oblique fractures, which in turn unite faster than transverse fractures. Comminuted fractures heal slower.
- Disturbed pathoanatomy. These are:
  - Soft tissue interposition; and
  - Ischemic fracture ends.
- Type of reduction: Good apposition of the fracture results in faster union.
- Immobilization: It is not necessary to immobilize all fractures (e.g., fracture ribs, scapula, etc).

- They heal anyway. Some fractures need strict immobilization (e.g., fracture of the neck of the femur), and may still not heal.
- Micromovement at fracture sites is known to promote callus formation and bridging of the bony fragments, hence aising in fracture healing.

- Open fractures: Open fractures often go into delayed union and nonunion.
- Compression at fracture site: Compression enhances the rate of union in cancellous bone. In cortical bones, compression at the fracture site enhances rigidity of fixation, and possibly results in primary bone healing.

Woven bone: Woven bone is characterized by haphazard organization of collagen fibers and is mechanically weak.

- It is produced when osteoblasts produce osteoid rapidly. It is present in:
  - All fetal bones initially when the bone is laid down. Later it gets replaced by lamellar bone.
  - After fractures, the initial bone that unites the fracture is woven bone. It too gets replaced by lamellar bone.
  - Paget's disease.

Woven bone is weaker, with a smaller number of randomly oriented collagen fibers, but forms quickly.

20. Regarding pectus excavatum true is:

a. More common in females
b. Seen in Marfan's
c. Aggravated at puberty
d. Respiratory insufficiency
e. Sternum moves to the right

Ans. b, c, d

Option a	False	Male-to-female ratio of 3:1
Option b	True	
Option c	True	
Option d	True	
Option e	False	Posterior displacement of sternum

- Pectus excavatum is the most common type of congenital chest wall abnormality (90%), followed by pectus carinatum (5–7%).
- Occurrence is in an estimated 1 in 300–400 births, with male predominance (male-to-female ratio of 3:1).
- The condition is typically noticed at birth, and more than 90% of cases are diagnosed within the first year of life.
- Typically, the lower third of the sternum is more involved, and the upper third may appear fairly normal.
- Worsening of the chest's appearance and the onset of symptoms are usually reported during rapid bone growth in the early teenage years.
- The condition is associated with Marfan syndrome and Poland syndrome.
- Posterior displacement of the sternum in pectus excavatum can produce a heart deformity, with anterior indentation of the right ventricle.
- In lungs, restrictive or obstructive defect may be seen in older patients with marked chest wall defect.
- There are decreased pulmonary volumes.

Ophthalmology

1. Fundus examination using direct ophthalmoscopy:

a. Image seen is erect and vertical
b. Patient's left eye is seen by the doctor's right eye
c. Blurry margin on the temporal part of optic disc is normal
d. Is preferably done while the patient is in supine position
e. Has 15 times magnification.

Ans. a,e

Option a	True	Yes, correct
Option b	False	No, not correct. The physician should stand/sit slightly over the eye to be examined
Option c	False	No, not correct, the margins are blurred in case of papilledema, papilitis, post neuritic optic atrophy
Option d	False	No, the patient should be seated with doctor whether standing or sitting beside
Option e	True	Yes, correct

Fundus Examination—Features

- Media: Normally media is transparent
  - Causes of opacity: corneal opacity, lenticular opacity, hemorrhage, degeneration
- Optic disc:
  - Size: Rough size is 1,5 cm
  - Circular in shape
  - Well defined margins. Blurred margins indicate retinal pathology as papilledema, papillitis
  - Color – Normal is pink color
    - Hyperemia is seen in case of papilledema, papillitis
    - Palor disc in case of optic atrophy
    - Chalky white in case of optic atrophy
    - Yellow waxy in case of secondary or consecutive optic atrophy
  - Cup disc ratio – normal is 0.3
    - Large cup: Physiological or glaucoma
    - Cup fullness in case of papilledema, papillitis
  - Splinter hemorrhage: On the disc seen in case of open angle glaucoma and papilledema
  - Neovascularization: Diabetic retinopathy and sickle cell retinopathy
  - Kesten baum index: Large blood vessel versus the small blood vessel. Normal ratio is 4:16. The ratio is decreased in optic atrophy
- Macula
  - Macular hemorrhages, macular edema, macular hole
  - Hard exudates
  - Cherry red spots (CRAO)

- Retinal blood vessels
  - Narrowing, tortuosity, vascular pulsations
- General background
  - Superficial/deep retinal hemorrhage
  - Soft/hard exudates
  - Tumor of fundus
  - Peripheral retinal degenerations

Direct vs Indirect ophthalmoscopy

Table 9.1: Direct versus indirect ophthalmoscopy

	Feature	Direct ophthalmoscopy	Indirect ophthalmoscopy
1	Condensing lens	Not required	Required
2	Examination distance	As close to patient's eye as possible	At an arm's length
3	Image	Virtual Erect	Real Inverted
4	Magnification	About 15 times	4–5 times
5	Illumination	Not so bright, so not useful in hazy media	Bright, so useful for hazy media
6	Area of field in focus	About 2 disc diopters	About 8 disc diopter
7	Stereopsis	Absent	Present
8	Accessible fundus view	Slightly beyond equator	Up to oraserrata
9	Examination through hazy media	Not possible	Possible

2. Sensitivity of cornea, true is:

a. Low in viral infections
b. Low in acanthemeba
c. High in atopic conjunctivitis
d. Decreased in herpes
e. Maximum in the periphery

Ans. a, d *Ref: External Disease and Cornea, Section 8. Basic and Clinical Science Course, AAO, 2010, Parsons 21th/ed p118*

Option a	True	Yes, correct
Option b	False	No, not correct
Option c	False	No, it is
Option d	True	Yes, correct. It is low in herpes infection
Option e	False	No, not correct

The corneal sensitivity is one of the sensitive reflex in body.
The cornea is not innervated with the special receptors but may transmit pain or light touch.

Corneal Sensation

- Greatest in the central cornea except in elderly patients where it is more sensitive in the periphery
- Drops rapidly as distance increases from the limbus

- Falls with increasing age and is not affected by iris color
- More sensitive in the temporal limbus than the inferior limbus
- Reduction has been reported in Diabetes Type 1 and 2.

Corneal Sensitivity Decrease

- Dry eye
- Herpes simplex keratitis
- Herpes zoster ophthalmicus
- Surgical trauma (PK, LASIK, large limbal incisions, ablation of the trigeminal ganglion)
- Topical medications (anesthetics, NSAIDs, β-blockers, and carbonic anhydrase inhibitors)
- Cocaine abuse
- Cerebrovascular events
- Aneurysms
- Tumors (acoustic neuroma, neurofibroma, or angioma)
- Multiple sclerosis
- Leprosy
- Hereditary causes - Familial dysautonomia (Riley-Day syndrome)

Cochet Bonnet Esthesiometer

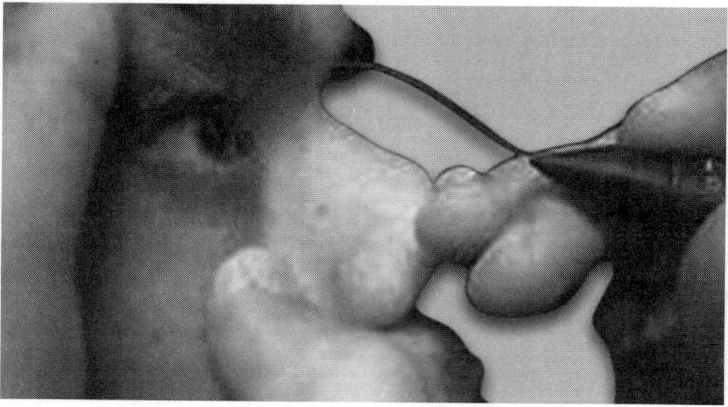

3. Dislocation of lens is not a typical feature of:

a. Duschene muscular dystrophy
b. Sulfatase deficiency
c. Galacatosemia
d. Marfan's
e. Homocystinssuria

Ans. a,c *Ref: Khurana, 4th/ed p202*

Option a	False	No, it is not reported to be typically associated
Option b	True	Yes, it is associated
Option c	False	No, it is not reported to be typically associated
Option d	True	Yes, it is associated
Option e	True	Yes, it is associated

Causes of Ectopia Lentis

Overall trauma is the leading cause of ectopia lentis.

Various ocular diseases associated with ectopia lentis are:

- Simple ectopia lentis may occur as a congenital disorder.
  - ADAMTSL 4 gene on chromosome 1 (AR Pattern)
  - FBN1 gene on chromosome 15 (AD pattern)

Most common is bilateral, symmetrical and supertemoral dislocation.

- **Ectopia lentis et pulillae:** Asymmetric eccentric pupils which are displaced in the opposite directions of lens dislocation. The pupils are characteristically oval, ectopic and dilate incompletely.

Other Ocular Diseases

- Aniridia
- Congenital glaucoma
- Pseudoexfoliation syndrome
- Syphillis
- Retinitis pigmentosa
- Intraocular tumor
- Axenfeld-Rieger syndrome
- Megalocornea
- Hypermature cataract

Other systemic diseases associated with ectopia lentis

- Marfan's syndrome
  - Most common heritable cause of ectopia lentis
  - Autosomal dominant
  - Fibrillin-1 gene on chromosome 15
- Homocystinuria
  - Second most common cause of ectopia lentis
  - Cystathionine – b – synthetase deficiency, autosomal recessive disease
  - Mental retardation, osteoporosis, chest deformities and increased chance of thrombosis
  - Bilateral and infro-nasal quadrant
- Weill-Marchesani syndrome
  - Mental retardation, short stature, stubby fingers
  - Autosomal recessive mesodermal dysplasia
  - Spherophakia, forward subluxation of the lens
- Sulfite oxidase deficiency
  - Autosomal recessive disorder of sulphur metabolism
  - Mental retardation, progressive muscular rigidity and decerebrate posture
- Hyperlysinemia
- Ehlers-Danlos syndrome
- Sturge-Weber syndrome

- Mandibulofacial dysostosis
- Wildervanck syndrome
- Conradi syndrome
- Pfaundler syndrome
- Crouzon syndrome
- Pierre Robin syndrome
- Sprengel deformity

4. Features of fungal corneal ulcer are all except:

a. Hypopyon is usually absent
b. Satellite lesion
c. Feathery margin
d. Depressed lesion
e. Corneal vascularization is present

Ans. a,d,e *Ref: Khurana, 4ed, pg 100*

Option a	False	No, not correct. A big hypopyon is seen
Option b	True	Yes, correct
Option c	True	Yes, correct
Option d	False	No, not correct. It is an elevated ulcer with rolled out margins
Option e	False	No, not correct. It is absent

Fungal Ulcer

Causes

- Filamentous fungi - aspergillus, fusarium, cephalosporium
- Yeasts - candida and Cryptococcus

Features

- Dry looking, grayish white elevated rolled out margins
- Feathery, finger like projections into the stroma under intact epithelium
- Sterile immune ring (yellow line of demarcation) may be seen
- Small satellite lesions around the ulcer.

Good to Remember

Diagnosis

- History of injury to eye by some vegetative material.
- Confirmation: examination of wet KOH, Calcofluor white, Gram's and Giemsa-stained films for fungal hyphae and culture on Sabouraud's agar medium.

Treatment: Topical antifungals (nystatin 3.5–5%) is the main stay.

Ophthalmology

1. Which type of cataract is/are associated with myotonic dystrophy?

a. Posterior subcapsular
b. Anterior subcapsular
c. Nuclear cataract
d. Cortical cataract
e. Zonular cataract

Ans. a, b *Ref: Parson's Diseases of the Eye - 22/e*

Option a	True	
Option b	True	
Option c	False	Usually associated with ageing
Option d	False	Seen in diabetics
Option e	False	Congenital cataract

Cataracts in myotonic dystrophy:

Cataracts are most common ocular manifestations of myotonic dystrophy, and may take any of the following three forms:

- A characteristic iridescent crystalline dust or Christmas tree cataracts seen underneath the capsule both anteriorly and posteriorly, unique to myotonic dystrophy
- Less specific, small, white, snowball like opacities or
- Typical aging changes.

2. Advantage of continuous curvilinear capsulorrhexis over can opener technique:

a. Preferred method of anterior capsulotomy in phacoemulsification
b. More chances of posterior capsular opacification
c. Keeps the nucleus in place
d. Resists radial tears
e. Helps in stabilizing and centering the lens implant

Ans. a, b, c, d, e

Option a	True	
Option b	True	
Option c	True	
Option d	True	
Option e	True	

Techniques of anterior capsulotomy:

- Can opener technique
- Linear capsulotomy
- Continuous circular capsulorrhexis

Intraoperative advantages of continuous curvilinear capsulorrhexis:

- A continuous circular aperture limits the risk of tears or radial cracks which tend to extend towards the equator and posterior capsule

- Hydrodissection is safe and allows the surgeon to perform phacoemulsification
- Restricts intraoperative turbulence inside the capsule
- Intraoperative stress on zonules is minimal and is distributed evenly over the equator
- It allows easy aspiration of the cortex because it does not leave any gaping anterior capsular flaps that may occlude the aspiration orifice
- It permits IOL to be positioned safely and symmetrically in the bag.

Drawbacks:

- Difficult to perform
- Difficult to completely clean the posterior capsule below the entrance point
- Opacification of part of capsule over the optic disc
- Difficult to examine retinal periphery
- Possible capsular block
- Possible shrinkage effect.

3. True about fluorescein dye:

a. Leaks from normal retinal vasculature
b. Leaks from normal choroid plexus
c. 50% of fluorescein is plasma protein bound
d. Hypofluorescence is seen in retinal detachment
e. Hyperfluorescence is seen in macular hole

Ans. b, e *Ref: Yanoff ophthalmology*

Option a	False	Remains confined in the retinal vessels
Option b	True	
Option c	False	Fluorescein passes freely into extravascular spaces
Option d	False	
Option e	True	

Fluorescein angiography of the fundus is based on the detection of fluorescent light emitted by a dye in retinal and choroidal circulation.

- Once injected approximately 80% of sodium Fluorescein dye is bound to the plasma proteins (particularly albumin) in blood stream
- Retinal circular: It remains confined in the retinal vessels due to the blood retinal barrier, thus facilitates delineation of retinal vessels
- Choroidal circulation: Fluorescein passes freely across the endothelium of the capillaries to the extravascular spaces
- The dye cannot pass across Burch membrane and intact retinal pigment epithelium.

Causes of hypofluorescence:

- Retinal or ocular artery occlusion
- Vitreous opacification
- Subhyaloid hemorrhage
- Intraretinal pathological: hemorrhage, vein occlusion, edema
- Choroidal pathology: Nevis, melanoma.

Causes of hyperfluorescence:

Seen in leakage of dye from intravascular to extravascular space

- Geographic atrophy
- Bull's eye maculopathy
- Macular hole
- Druses
- Vascular tumor or cavernous hemangioma, angioma in retina
- Retinoblastoma
- Choroidal hemangioma
- Retinal pigment epithelium detachment.

4. Ophthalmic changes in diabetes mellitus include:

a. Dry eyes
b. Retinitis pigmentosa
c. Retinal detachment
d. Ischemic optic neuropathy
e. Papillopathy

Ans. c, d, e

Option a	False	
Option b	False	
Option c	True	
Option d	True	
Option e	True	

Ocular changes in diabetes include:

- Lids: Xanthelasma, recurrent style or hordeolum
- Conjunctiva: Telangiectasia, slugging of blood in conjunctival vessels, subconjuncival hemorrhage
- Cornea: Pigment dispersal at the back of cornea, decreased corneal sensations. Punctate keratopathy, Descemet's folds, infective corneal ulcers, delayed epithelial healing
- Iris: Rubeosis iridis (neovascularization)
- Lens: Snowflake cataract, posterior subcapsular cataract, early onset, early maturation senile cataracts
- Vitreous: Vitreous hemorrhage and fibrovascular proliferation secondary to diabetic retinopathy
- Retina: Diabetic retinopathy – proliferative or non proliferative, maculopathy and lipaemia retinalis
- Glaucoma
- Optic nerve: Optic neuritis, diabetic papillopathy, non-arteritic ischemic optic neuropathy
- Extraocular muscles: ophthalmoplegia due to diabetic neuropathy
- Refraction: Hypermetropic shift in hypoglycemia, myopic shift in hyperglycemia and decreases accommodation.

Advanced diabetic eye disease

End result of uncontrolled proliferative diabetic retinopathy marked by:

- Persistent vitreous hemorrhage

- ❑ Tractional retinal detachment
- ❑ Neovascular glaucoma.

5. True about inferior ophthalmic vein is/are:

a. Joins superior ophthalmic vein in the lateral part of superior ophthalmic fissure
b. Drains into cavernous sinus
c. Communicates with pterygoid plexus
d. Accompanies ophthalmic artery
e. Communicates with angular veins

Ans. a, b, c

Option a	True	
Option b	True	
Option c	True	
Option d	False	Superior ophthalmic vein accompanies ophthalmic artery
Option e	False	Superior ophthalmic vein communicates with angular veins

Ophthalmic veins

Superior ophthalmic vein:

- ❑ Large vein that accompanies ophthalmic artery
- ❑ Commences above the medial palpebral ligament and runs backwards above the optic nerve along with the ophthalmic artery
- ❑ Passes through superior orbital fissure to drain into cavernous sinus
- ❑ Communicates anteriorly at its commencement, with the supraorbital and angular veins.

Inferior ophthalmic vein:

- ❑ Runs below the optic nerve
- ❑ Ends either by joining the superior ophthalmic vein or drains directly into cavernous sinus
- ❑ Communicates with pterygoid venous plexus by small veins passing through the inferior orbital fissure.

6. True about corneal ulcer is:

a. Disruption of endothelium
b. Disruption of epithelium
c. Discontinuation of epithelium with underlying inflammation
d. Disruption of cornea leading to thinning
e. Characterized by cellular infiltration

Ans. c, e

Option a	False	
Option b	False	
Option c	True	
Option d	False	
Option e	True	

Corneal ulcer

Loss of epithelium with inflammation of the surrounding cornea is called a corneal ulcer.

—*Parsons*

Corneal ulcer may be defined as discontinuation of normal epithelial surface of cornea associated with necrosis of the surrounding corneal tissue. Pathologically it is characterized by edema and cellular infiltration.

—*Khurana*

7. True about nodular episcleritis:

a. Can be associated with SLE
b. Take longer time to resolve than diffuse variety
c. More symptomatic than diffuse type
d. Painless
e. Elevated hard nodule

Ans. a, b, c, e *Ref: Parsons and Khurana*

Option a	True	
Option b	True	
Option c	True	
Option d	False	Associated with pain
Option e	True	

Episcleritis

Benign inflammatory affection of the deep subconjunctival connective tissues, including the superficial sclera lamellae.

Two types seen clinically:

1. *Simple or diffuse episcleritis*: There is sectoral or diffuse redness of one or both eyes mostly due to engorgement of large episcleral vessels. There is mild to moderate tenderness over the area of episcleral injection.
2. *Nodular episcleritis*: A circumscribed nodule of dense leukocytic infiltration, (as large as a lentil) usually 2–3 mm from the limbus. It is hard, tender and immovable. Appears purple as it is traversed by the deeper vessels.
   Nodular episcleritis tends to be more symptomatic and takes longer to resolve.

Ocular associations of SLE

- Retinopathy occurs in 10% patients
- Keratoconjuncivitis
- Nodules on sclera and episcleral
- Anterior uveitis
- Butterfly skin eruption over face involving the lower lids.

8. What is the WHO criteria for defining blindness?

a. < 3/60 vision with available correction
b. < 6/60 vision with available correction
c. < 3/60 vision with best correction
d. < 6/60 vision with best correction
e. < 3/60 vision without correction

Ans. c *Ref: Parsons 22/e*

Option a	False	
Option b	False	
Option c	True	
Option d	False	
Option e	False	

WHO definition of blindness	
Category of visual impairment	***Best corrected visual acuity (BCVA) in the better eye***
0 'Normal'	6/6 to 6/18, i.e. can see 6/18 or better
1 'Visual impairment'	< 6/18 to 6/60, i.e. cannot see 6/18, can see 6/60
2 'Severe visual impairment'	< 6/60 to 3/60, i.e. cannot see 6/60, can see 3/60
3 'Blind'	< 3/60 to 1/60, i.e. cannot see 3/60, can see 1/60
4 'Blind'	< 1/60 to only light perception, i.e. cannot see 3/60, can see light
5 'Blind'	No light perception, i.e. cannot see light
9 'Undetermined or unspecified'	

9. True about acanthamoeba keratitis:

a. More in those wearing rigid gas permeable than soft contact lenses user
b. Can occur as opportunistic infection in patients with herpetic keratitis
c. Can be cultured on non-nutrient agar enriched with E. coli
d. Painful condition
e. Radial keratoneuritis occur

Ans. b, c, d, e

Option a	False	Associated with wearing of soft contact lenses
Option b	True	
Option c	True	
Option d	True	
Option e	True	

Acanthamoeba keratitis is often associated with wearing of soft contact lenses. The usual source of infection is the saline solution used to clean or store the lens.

In non-contact lens users it may be related to swimming or bathing in contaminated water.

It can also occur as an opportunistic infection in patients with herpetic keratitis, bacterial keratitis, bullous keratopathy and neuroparalytic keratitis.

Organism: *Acanthamoeba castellanii*

Symptoms:

- May be asymptomatic or
- Mild foreign body sensation or
- Severe pain out of proportion to the degree of inflammation
- Watering
- Photophobia
- Blepharospasm
- Blurred vision.

Signs:

Epithelial lesions:

- ❑ Epithelial roughening, ridges
- ❑ Pseudodendrites
- ❑ Epithelial and sub-epithelial curvilinear opacities.

Stromal lesions:

- ❑ Radial keratoneuritis - Seen in 50% cases, a pathognomonic early sign, responsible for severe pain associated with keratitis
- ❑ Patchy and satellite stromal infiltrates
- ❑ Ring infiltrates
- ❑ Ring abscess.

Limbal and sclera lesions:

- ❑ Limbitis
- ❑ Scleritis
- ❑ Rarely posterior scleritis with optic neuritis.

Diagnosis

Clinical diagnosis is difficult

Laboratory diagnosis:

- ❑ Microscopy
  - ■ Potassium hydroxide mount
  - ■ Calcofluor white stain
  - ■ Lactophenol cotton blue stain
- ❑ Culture in non-nutrient agar may show trophozoites within 48–50 hours which gradually turn into cysts
- ❑ PCR
- ❑ Corneal biopsy.

10. True about phthisis bulbi:

a. Size of eye decreases
b. Removed by enucleation operation especially if painful
c. IOP increases late stage
d. Calcification may occur in Bowman's layer of cornea
e. Thinned sclera

Ans. a, b, d, e

Option a	True	
Option b	True	
Option c	False	IOP is markedly lowered
Option d	True	
Option e	True	

Phthisis bulbi

It is the final stage end result of any form of chronic uveitis, in which the eye becomes soft, shrunken, and atrophic. Development of this condition can be divided into the following overlapping stages.

- Stage of atrophic bulbi without shrinkage
  - Initial stage of loss of function due to continued inflammation and loss of nutritional support
  - Shape of globe is maintained
  - Vision is completely lost
  - Lens becomes cataractus
  - Retina develops serous detachment and atrophic changes
  - IOP is raised due to inflammation.
- Stage of atrophic bulbi with shrinkage
  - Occurs due to continued ciliary body dysfunction
  - Corneal becomes edematous and vascularised
  - Anterior chamber is collapsed
  - Eyeball becomes smaller and square shaped (maintained by 4 recti).
- Atrophic bulbi with disorganisation
  - Final stage, also called phthisis bulbi
  - IOP is markedly lowered
  - Size of eyeball is markedly reduced
  - Cornea become sclera like.

Histopathology:

- Disorganisation of all the intraocular tissues
- Calcification of bowman's layer of cornea, lens or retina
- Intra ocular ossification
- Thickened sclera.

Management:

- Requires removal by enucleation, especially when painful.

11. True about blue sclera is/are:

a. Not seen in Ehler-Danlos Syndrome
b. Thinning of sclera leads to visualization of uvea
c. Seen in osteogenesis imperfecta
d. Seen in Marfan's
e. Seen in pseudoxanthoma elasticum

Ans. b, c, d, e

Option a	False	Seen in Ehler-Danlos Syndrome
Option b	True	
Option c	True	
Option d	True	
Option e	True	

Blue sclera

Anonymous asymptomatic condition characterised by marked bluish discolouration of sclera due to thinning of sclera and cornea. The uveal pigment shines through the thin sclera producing a blue colour.

Associated conditions:

- Osteogenesis imperfecta
- Marfan syndrome
- Ehlers-Danlos syndrome
- Pseudoxanthoma elasticum
- Buphthalmos
- High myopia, keratoconus, keratoglobus
- Healed scleritis.

12. True about central retinal artery obstruction is/are:

a. Involves ophthalmic artery occlusion
b. Occurs due to embolization
c. Painful sudden loss of vision
d. Cattle tracking is seen
e. Cherry red spot

Ans. b, d, e *Ref: Ophthalmology by Myron Yanoff, 4/e; Khurana*

Option a	False	
Option b	True	
Option c	False	Abrupt but painless loss of vision
Option d	True	
Option e	True	

Central retinal artery obstruction

Usually occurs just proximal to lamina cribrosa or at its level.

Presentation: Abrupt, painless, severe loss of vision.

Signs:

- Visual acuity is markedly reduced
- Direct pupillary reflex is absent and relative afferent pupillary defect is positive
- Fundus examination:
  - Marked narrowing of retinal arteries
  - Milky white retina
  - Cherry red spot in the centre of macula
  - Cattle tracking, i.e. segmentation of blood column is seen in retinal veins
  - Atrophic changes at 4–6 weeks.

Aetiologies:

- Emboli
  - Cholesterol emboli
  - Calcium emboli
  - Platelet fibrin emboli
- Atherosclerosis related thrombosis

- Retinal arteritis
  - Giant cell arteritis
  - Polyarteritis nodosa
  - SLE
  - Wegener's granulomatosis
  - Scleroderma
- Thrombophilic disorders - inherited and acquired
- Other rare causes
  - Retinal migraine
  - Hemoglobinopathies
  - Use of OC pills
  - Polycythemia.

Ophthalmic artery occlusion

Acute simultaneous obstruction of both retinal and choroidal circulations is referred to as an ophthalmic artery occlusion. There can be a single blockage in the ophthalmic artery or multiple blockage sites involving both circulations.

Ophthalmic artery obstruction can be differentiated from central retinal artery obstruction by the following features:

- Severe visual loss, bare or no light perception
- Intense retinal whitening that extends beyond the macular area
- Little or no cherry red spot
- Marked choroidal perfusion defects on fluorescein angiography
- Non-recordable electroretinogram
- Late retinal pigment epithelium alterations.

Thus central retinal artery obstruction does not involve ophthalmic artery obstruction, rather both the conditions should be differentiated clinically.

13. True about secondary cataract:

a. Also known as posterior capsular cataract
b. Caused by UV rays
c. Treated by Nd:YAG laser
d. Removal may cause cystoid macular edema
e. Ring of Soemmering is seen

Ans. a, c, d

Option a	True	
Option b	False	
Option c	True	
Option d	True	
Option e	False	

Posterior capsular opacification (PCO) or after cataract or secondary cataract

Opacity which follows extracapsular extraction of the lens. In ECCE lens nucleus and cortex are removed and the capsular bag (posterior capsule and part of anterior capsule) is left in situ. PCO results from migration and proliferation of residual lens epithelial cells onto central posterior capsule, leading to decrease in visual function.

The cubical cells lining the anterior capsule continue their function of forming new lens fibres. These fibres are disorganised, abortive and opaque. Sometimes these fibres, enclosed between the two layers of capsule for a dense ring behind the iris called the ring of Soemmering. At other times, the subcapsular cells proliferate, and instead of forming lens fibres, develop into large balloon like cells which fill the pupillary aperture (Elschnig Pearls).

Treatment

- Nd:YAG laser posterior capsulotomy.

Complication:

Cystoid macular edema (CME)

It is a late complication of cataract surgery. Approximately 20% of patients who undergo uncomplicated phacoemulsification or ECCE develop CME. However, a clinically significant decrease in visual acuity is seen only in about 1% of these eyes.

If cataract extraction is complicated by posterior capsular rupture and vitreous loss, severe iris trauma or vitreous traction at the wound, there is significantly higher incidence of clinically apparent CME.

Since management of PCO is posterior capsulotomy, there are high chances of CME post removal of PCO.

14. True about congenital ptosis:

a. Lid lag
b. Surgery of levator palpebral muscle
c. Lagophthalmos is a complication of corrective surgery
d. Absence of lid crease
e. Uncorrected may lead to amblyopia

Ans. a, b, c, d, e

Option a	True	
Option b	True	
Option c	True	
Option d	True	
Option e	True	

Ptosis

Abnormal drooping of eyelid is called ptosis. In this condition the upper eyelid covers more than one sixth of cornea (about 2 mm).

Two types: Congenital and acquired.

1. ***Congenital ptosis***

Congenital weakness of levator palpebrae superioris

Features:

- Drooping of one or both of upper lids
- Lid crease is either diminished or absent
- Lid lag on down gaze (ptotic is lid is higher than the normal) due to tethering effect of abnormal LPS muscle
- LPS function may be poor.

Treatment:

- Congenital ptosis almost always needs surgical correction
- If visual axis is covered a correction should be carried out as soon as possible to avoid sensory deprivation amblyopia
- If ptosis is partial, the correction is carried out at 3–5 years of age.

Surgeries:

- Fasanella Servat operation or Torso conjunctivo Mullerectomy—for mild ptosis with good levator function. The lid is everted and two curved haemostats are placed grasping the conjunctiva, levator palpebrae superioris, and Muller muscle.
- Levator resection—for moderate and severe grades of ptosis with a moderate levator action
- Frontalis sling operation (brow suspension): for severe ptosis with no levator function.

2. ***Lagophthalmos***

Incomplete closure of palpebrae fissure when an attempt is made to shut the eyes. Seen in contraction of lids from:

- Cicatrisation
- Congenital deformity
- Ectropion
- Symblepharon
- Paralysis of orbicularis oculi muscle
- Proptosis due to exophthalmos
- Orbital tumor
- Following over resection of levator muscle for correction of ptosis
- Comatosed patients.

ENT

1. True about fungal sinusitis

a. Rarely fungal hyphae in mucoid
b. Common in immunocompromised-t
c. Antifungal mainstay of treatment
d. Steroids are contraindicated
e. *Apophysomyces* is an emerging pathogen for chronic granulomatous invasive sinusitis

Ans. b

Ref: Dhingra PL for ENT. p196;
S. Rao et al. Sino-orbital mucormycosis due to Apophysomyces elegans in immunocompetent individuals—an increasing trend. Am J Otolaryngol. 2006 Sep-Oct;27(5):366-9; BS Tuli, ENT. p192

Option a	False	No, there is fungal invasion by hyphae of the mucosa, submucosa, blood vessels
Option b	True	Yes, correct
Option c	False	No, surgery is the mainstay
Option d	False	No, they may be given postoperative
Option e	False	No, it is implicated for acute invasive fungal sinusitis. (asp. Flavus causes chronic granulomatous invasive sinusitis)

Rhizopus, Rhizomucor, Absidia, Mucor, Cunninghamella, Mortierella, Saksenaea, and *Apophysomyces* species, cause acute invasive fungal sinusitis.

A fumigatus is the only fungus associated with chronic invasive fungal sinusitis

Aspergillus flavus exclusively has been associated with granulomatous invasive fungal sinusitis.

Acute Invasive Sinusitis

- Rapid spread through vascular invasion
- Common in diabetics

Chronic Invasive Fungal Sinusitis

- Slowly progressive fungal disease
- Usual in diabetics
- May be associated with orbital apex syndrome

Chronic Granulomatous Invasive Sinusitis

- Immunocompromised individuals
- Rare in India

Histopathologic studies in acute invasive fungal sinusitis reveal hyphal invasion of the mucosa, submucosa, and blood vessels, including the carotid arteries and cavernous sinuses; vasculitis with thrombosis; haemorrhage; and tissue infarction.

Necrosis of the mucosa, submucosa and the blood vessels with low grade inflammation is seen in chronic invasive fungal sinusitis

Treatment

1. Surgery – treatment of choice for all fungal sinusitis
2. Steroids maybe indicated postoperatively
3. Nasal salt water washes
4. Amphotericin B > ketoconazole may be tried post-operative for Chronic invasive fungal sinusitis

2. Which of the following is/are correct physiological pairs:

a. Vestibular apparatus—optokinetic nystagmus
b. SCC—linear acceleration
c. Utricle—rotational acceleration
d. Saccule—rotational acceleration
e. Otolith organ—rotational movement

Ans. a. *Ref: Dhingra PL, 6th/ed p44; BS Tuli, textbook of ENT, p38*

Option a	True	Yes, optokinetic nystagmus and vestibule-ocular reflex function together for involuntary fixation of moving objects.
Option b	False	No, it is for rotatory movements
Option c	False	No it is for linear horizontal movements
Option d	False	No, it is for linear vertical movements
Option e	False	No, these are for linear movements in the horizontal or the vertical planes

The Vestibular – Ocular Reflex and the Optokinetic Nystagmus

In Vestibular-ocular reflex the semicircular canals of the inner ear measure rotation of the head and provide a signal for the oculomotor nuclei of the brainstem, which innervate the eye muscles. The muscles counter-rotate the eyes in such a way that a rightward head rotation causes an equal leftward rotation of both eyes, with the result that gaze direction stays stationary.

Optokinetic nystagmus refers to the response to full-field visual motion; OKN can be used as a crude assessment of the visual system. If one visual cortex is damaged, optokinetic nystagmus will be lost when objects move toward the side of the cortex lesion.

VOR works in conjunction with the optokinetic reflex (OKR), which is a feedback mechanism that ensures that the eye moves in the same direction and at almost the same speed as an image.

Optokinetic Test

- Patient is asked to follow a series of vertical stripes on a drum moving from right to left and then from left to right.
- Normally it produces nystagmus with slow component in the direction of moving stripes and fast component in the opposite direction.

- Optokinetic abnormalities are seen in brainstem and cerebral hemisphere lesions.
- Thus this test is useful to diagnose a central lesion.

The peripheral vestibular apparatus consists of the saccule, utricle, and semi-circular canals.

Saccule

- Globular sac shaped
- Medial wall of vestibule
- It is connected anteriorly to the cochlear duct by the ductus reuniens and posteriorly to the endolymphatic duct via the utriculosaccular duct.
- The saccular macula is an elliptical thickened area of sensory epithelium that lies on the anterior vertical wall of the saccule.

Utricle

- Larger than saccule
- Lies post-superior to saccule (on medial wall recess)
- The utricle is larger than the saccule and lies postero-superiorly to it in the elliptical recess of the medial wall of the vestibule.
- It is connected anteriorly via the utriculosaccular duct to the endolymphatic duct. The 3 semicircular canals open into it by means of 5 openings; the posterior and the superior semicircular canals share one opening at the crus commune.

Motion Sensors

1. The otolith organs include the utricle and the saccule
   a. Utricle – horizontal plane (front/back, left right)
   b. Saccule – sagittal plane (up down or vertical movement)
2. Semicircular canals – angular accelerations (head rotations)

Semicircular Canals

The 3 semi-circular canals are small, ring like structures: lateral or horizontal, superior or anterior, and posterior or inferior. They are oriented at right angles to each other and are situated so that the superior and posterior canals are at 45° angles to the sagittal plane and the horizontal canal is 30° to the axial plane.

One end of the canal is dilated to form the ampulla. The ampulla contains a saddle shaped ridge termed as crista ampularis (the sensory epithelium lies in the crista ampularis)

Each canal is responsive to the angular motion in that plane.

3. Schwartz sign, correct is:

a. Is a contraindication for surgery?
b. Indicates reversed blood flow
c. Bluish hue behind the tympanic membrane
d. 10% of cases
e. Near oval window

Ans. a,d,e *Ref: PL Dhingra, 6th/ed p450; Chris de Souza, Marcos V. Goycoolea, Neil M. Sperling. Otosclerosis: Diagnosis, Evaluation, Pathology, Surgical Techniques, and Outcomes. Plural Publishing (2014) p49*

Option a	True	Yes, correct
Option b	False	No, it indicates increased blood flow
Option c	False	No, it is pink / reddish hue posterior to tympanic membrane
Option d	True	Yes, correct
Option e	True	Yes, correct

Schwartz sign is a pink reflex, seen through intact tympanic membrane, in the area of oval window.

It indicates active otosclerosis usually during pregnancy.

SYMPTOMS of Otosclerosis

1. **Hearing loss:** This is the presenting symptom and usually starts in twenties. It is painless and progressive with insidious onset. Often it is bilateral conductive type.
2. **Paracusis Willisii:** An otosclerosis patient hears better in noisy than in quiet surroundings. This is because a normal person will raise his voice in noisy surroundings.
3. **Tinnitus:** It is more commonly seen in cochlear otosclerosis and in active lesions.
4. **Vertigo:** It is an uncommon symptom.
5. **Speech:** Patient has a monotonous, well-modulated soft speech.

Signs

1. Tympanic membrane is quite normal and mobile.
2. *Schwartz sign*: reddish hue may be seen on the promontory through the tympanic membrane
3. This is indicative of active focus with increased vascularity.

Contraindications to Stapedotomy

1. Single ear hearing
2. Positive Schwartz sign
3. Pregnancy
4. Young children
5. High risk profession
6. Otitis externa, tympanic membrane perforation
7. Other medical co-morbid conditions making unfit for surgery

4. Cochlear implant contraindicated in:

a. CSOM
b. Cochlear nerve damage
c. Post-lingual deafness
d. Auditory neuropathy
e. Mondini deformity

Ans. a,b,e *Ref: PL Dhingra, 6th/ed p125; Oguz Kadir Egilmez. Cochlear implant: indications, contraindications and complications. Scripta Scientifica Medica. 2015;47(4):9-16; BS Tuli, textbook of ENT p121*

Option a	True	Yes, contraindicated
Option b	True	Yes, contraindicated
Option c	False	No, not contraindicated, **Post-lingual deafness** is a **deafness** which develops after the acquisition of speech and language, usually after the age of six – which is not contraindication
Option d	False	No, not contraindicated
Option e	True	No, not contraindicated

Indications of cochlear implant:

1. Audiometric indications - Profound SNHL (> 90 dB)
2. Tinnitus (severe)
3. Patient having damage to cochlea with intact VIIIth nerve such as traumatic, congenital, labyrinthitis, presbyacusis, Ménière's disease, and drug toxicity.

Contraindications for the cochlear implantation	
Absolute	**Relative**
Agenesia of Cochlea	Inappropriate medical conditions
Agenesia of Cochlear Nerve	(e.g. pulmonary, cardiac, hematologic)
Severe mental disease	Uncontrolled epilepsy
Acute/chronic otitis media and mastoiditis without eradiation of the disease	Not being available for postoperative rehabilitation
Mental retardation (to cooperate with speech training)	

Major and minor complications of cochlear implanation	
Major	**Minor**
Cerebrospinal fluid fistula	Pain
Device failure	Simple skin infection
Displacement / misplacement of electrode	Dizziness
	Imbalance
Facial nerve paralysis or damage	Temporary facial paresis
Facial stimulation	Otitis media
Flap infection or hematoma	Hematoma on scalp
Perilymph gusher	Tinnitus
Rejection of the implant	Vertigo
Displacement of the implant	Chorda tympani damage
Mastoiditis	Damage to the dura
Meningitis	
Retraction pockets or cholesteatoma	
Subdural hematoma	

Mondini deformity: Patients have sensorineural hearing loss, which is usually bilateral as the basal turn of the cochlea is intact, high-frequency hearing is generally preserved.

The abnormality is thought to result from a relatively late insult during the 7th week of embryological development when most of the inner ear has already formed

(**Note:** Defects earlier than 7 weeks may result in cochlear aplasia or hypoplasia)

Mondini deformity features:

1. Abnormal cochlea with only 1.5 turns (rather than 2.5 normal turns)
2. Enlarged vestibule with normal semicircular canal
3. Enlarged endolymphatic sac and dilated vestibular aqueduct

Mondini deformity is associated with:

1. **Pendred syndrome:** Bilateral sensorineural hearing loss and goitre
2. **CHARGE syndrome:** Coloboma, heart defects, choanal atresia, growth retardation, genital abnormalities, and ear abnormalities
3. Klippel-Feil syndrome:
   - Short, webbed neck
   - Decreased range of motion (ROM) in the cervical spine
   - Low hairline
4. DiGeorge syndrome
   a. Chromosome 22q 11.2
   b. Velocardiofacial syndrome
   c. Conotruncal anomaly face (CTAF) syndrome

Management of Mondini Deformity

- Surgery
- Cochlear implant

Important long term complication: oozing of CSF, increased risk of meningitis

5. True about epiglottis:

a. Oval shaped
b. Serous glands
c. Mucous gland
d. LN drainage from both sides
e. Omega in children

Ans. c,d,e *Ref: PL Dhingra, 6th/ed p282*

Option a	False	No, it is a leaf shaped flap
Option b	False	No, it is made of elastic cartilage, which may contain mucus glands
Option c	True	Yes correct, Epiglottic cartilage shows several pits which lodge the mucous glands
Option d	True	Yes, lymphatics drain into the deep cervical nodes and thoracic duct
Option e	True	Yes, correct

Epiglottis

It is a leaf-like, yellow, elastic cartilage forming anterior wall of laryngeal inlet. It is attached to the body of hyoid bone by hyoepiglottic ligament, which divides it into suprahyoid and infrahyoid epiglottis.

Pre-epiglottic space: The Anterior surface of epiglottis is separated from thyrohyoid membrane and upper part of thyroid cartilage by a fat filled space known as pre-epiglottic space. *Clinical significance*: may be invaded in carcinoma of supraglottic larynx or the base of tongue.

Glossoepiglottic folds: are the mucous membrane covering the upper anterior part of the epiglottis reflects off the sides of the epiglottis

Aryepiglottic folds are mucosal folds on the posterior surface of the epiglottis

Valleculae epiglottica: The depressions on either side of the median fold, between the root of the tongue and the epiglottis.

Epiglottic cartilage shows several pits which lodge the mucous glands

Points to Remember

1. Larynx extends from C3 to C6 level and it descends to C6 level at 14 years of age.
2. Cricoid cartilage is the only complete ring present in the air passages.
3. All the intrinsic muscles of larynx are supplied by recurrent laryngeal except for cricothyroid which is supplied by external laryngeal (branch of superior laryngeal).
4. Infant's larynx differs from adult as it is situated high up (C2-C4), is of equal size in both sexes, is funnel shaped with narrow subglottis, the cartilages are softer and the epiglottis is narrow and folded. Its area is 24 sq mm and width is 6 mm.
5. Glottis consists of vocal cords, supraglottis extends from hyoid (superiorly) to glottis (inferiorly), subglottis extends from lower border of glottis to inferior border of cricoid.
6. Vocal cords have practically no lymphatics except for a small delphian node which lies on cricothyroid membrane (lymphatic watershed of larynx).
7. Epiglottis is omega shaped in neonates and infants.

Lymphatics: Lymphatic vessels from the epiglottis enter the infrahyoid node in order to pass to the deep cervical nodes. Further which drain in to the jugular trunk and thoracic duct.

ENT

1. All of the following are true about foreign body impaction in ear *except*:

a. Objects located medial to isthmus of canal is difficult to remove
b. Syringing is used for removal of vegetative body
c. Patients are usually asymptomatic
d. Blunt hook is used to remove rounded foreign body
e. GA is preferred in children to remove foreign bodies

Ans. b *Ref : Surgery of the ear, Glasscock – Shambaugh, 6/e; Otolaryngology by Paparella and Shumrick.*

Option a	True	Yes, true
Option b	False	Vegetative foreign bodies tend to absorb water and swell hence should not be removed by syringing
Option c	True	Yes, it is sometimes an incidental finding
Option d	True	Smooth or rounded objects are best removed with use of a right-angled blunt hook
Option e	True	For the uncooperative child, removal under general anaesthesia is required

Children are frequently referred to otolaryngologists for the management of ear canal foreign bodies. Primary care physicians often discover the foreign body when evaluating a child for otitis or it may be found incidentally during a well child visit.

It is safest to remove foreign bodies under direct visualisation with cerulean loop, right angle pick, alligator type forceps, cures or hook. The idea is to pull the foreign body and not push it in toward the tympanic membrane. Irrigation or syringing may be useful in certain inanimate foreign bodies. However vegetative foreign bodies tend to absorb water and swell hence should not be removed by syringing. Attempt to remove objects medial to isthmus may cause trauma and bleeding. Canal wall skin over the isthmus is very thin and quite sensitive. Trauma and bleeding from skin of canal complicate removal. Therefore objects located medial to isthmus are difficult to remove and should be removed using otomicroscopy. For the uncooperative child, removal under general anaesthesia is required, given the risk of tympanic membrane and ossification chain injury that can result from sudden movement of the distressed patient.

2. True about secretory otitis media:

a. Type C tympanogram may be seen in early stage of otitis media with effusion
b. Flat tympanogram is present
c. Leads to conductive deafness
d. Presence of cleft palate reduces its chance
e. Most common cause is Eustachian tube dysfunction

Ans. b, c, e *Ref: Cummings otolaryngology 5/e;Diseases of ENT, Dhingra, 6/e*

Option a	False	Type C tympanogram may be present in early stages of otitis media without effusion

Option b	True	
Option c	True	Mild to moderate conductive hearing loss
Option d	False	No, not correct
Option e	True	

OME or otitis media with effusion is also called secretory otitis media.

In contrast to rapid onset of signs and symptoms of acute inflammation in acute otitis media, OME is defined by middle ear effusion without signs and symptoms of inflammation.

Pathophysiology and risk factors:

I. Eustachian tube (ET) dysfunction

The three physiologic functions of Eustachian tube are: 1. Pressure regulation of middle ear, 2. Protection and 3. Clearance of secretions from middle ear.

In ears epithelial normal Eustachian tube function, the tube is closed when at rest. This arrangement protects the middle ear from nasopharyngeal sound pressure and reflux of secretions from the nasopharynx.

Middle ear pressure is equilibrated to atmospheric pressure through active intermittent openings of Eustachian tube caused by contraction of tensor veli palatini during swallowing, jaw movements and yawning. If ET function is impaired, negative pressure will develop in the middle ear. Causes of ET malfunction:

- Adenoid hyperplasia
- Chronic rhinitis and sinusitis
- Chronic tonsillitis
- Benign and malignant tumors of nasopharynx
- Craniofacial abnormalities : cleft palate, palatal paralysis, other craniofacial abnormalities, Down syndrome - Otitis media is considered universal in infants younger than 2 years with unrepaired cleft palate. In children with Down syndrome, ET function is poor and has low resistance.
- ET of infants died children is shorter, wider and more horizontal which accounts for higher rate of otitis media in children and infants. By the age of 7 years the tube has a more adult configuration.

II. Allergy

III. Unresolved otitis media

IV. Viral infections

V. Gastroesophageal reflux (possible role)

VI. Some studies have shown possible associations between premature birth, low birth weight and history of NICU admissions with recurrent OME.

Epidemiology

True incidence of OME is difficult to determine because by definition OME is asymptomatic. Approximately 65% of OME episodes in children resolve within 1 month.

Clinical evaluation

i. Tympanometry

Types of tympanogram

A. Indicates normal middle ear pressure

A_D – Unusually high peak pressure. Indicates tympanic membrane or ossicular chain hypermobility caused by strophic tympanic membrane scar or ossicular chain discontinuity.

A_S– Peak pressure at 0. Indicates ossicular chain fixation which may be caused by stapedial otosclerosis.

B. Flat tympanogram

Seen in otitis media with effusion, space occupying lesions of tympanic cavity and tympanic membrane perforations.

C. Indicates ***negative middle ear pressure*** as seen in ET dysfunction. May also be present in early stages of otitis media without effusion.

D. Has a ***notch*** in pressure peak. Often seen with scarred eardrums or with normal hypermobile eardrums.

ii. Otoscopy

- A pink, gray, yellow, or blue retracted tympanic membrane/TM with reduced or no mobility is usually seen with OME. While a red TM that is full or bulging is often a sign of Acute otitis media.
- TM is dull opaque with loss of light reflex.
- Thin leash of blood vessels may be seen along the handle of malleus or at the periphery of the TM.
- Sometimes fluid level or bubbles may be seen across the TM.
- Mobility of TM is restricted.

iii. Audiometry: Middle ear effusion may lead to mild to moderate conductive hearing loss.

iv. X-ray mastoid: Clouding of air cells may be seen due to presence of fluid.

3. Which of the following causes red/white colouration of tongue?

a. Median rhomboid glossitis
b. Hairy leukoplakia
c. Lichen planus
d. Geographic tongue
e. Fordyce's spots

Ans. a, b, c, d, e *Ref: Cummings otolaryngology 5/e; Diseases of ENT, Dhingra, 6/e*

Option a	True	Red
Option b	True	White
Option c	True	White striaform
Option d	True	Red
Option e	True	Yellowish brown pigment

Red/White lesions on tongue

- Leukoedema: Greyish white
- Oral leukoplakia: White patch or plaque
- Oral hairy leukoplakia: White lesion
- Oral lichen planus: White striaform lesions

- ❑ Submucous fibrosis: Erythema (redness) followed by decreased oral opening and tongue mobility
- ❑ Verruciform xanthoma: Surface may be depressed, flat or elevated and variably granular in texture
- ❑ Candidiasis
- ❑ Chronic discoid lupus erythematosus
- ❑ Fordyce spots: Yellowish brown
- ❑ Geographic tongue: Erythematous areas
- ❑ Nicotine stomatitis
- ❑ Median rhomboid glossitis–red.

4. True about antrochoanal polyp is/are:

a. Mostly associated with cystic fibrosis
b. It is steroid responsive
c. Commonly presents as unilateral nasal obstruction
d. Through posterior aperture moves to the nasopharynx
e. Is associated with maxillary sinusitis

Ans. a, b, c, d, e *Ref: Cummings otolaryngology 5/e; Diseases of ENT, Dhingra, 6/e*

Option a	True	
Option b	True	
Option c	True	
Option d	True	
Option e	True	

Nasal polyps

Etiology: Polyps may arise in inflammatory conditions of nasal mucosa, disorders of ciliary motility or abnormal composition of nasal mucus.

- ❑ Chronic rhinosinusitis, antrochoanal polyp arises from the mucosa of Maxillary antrum and hence is associated with maxillary sinusitis.
- ❑ Asthma
- ❑ Aspirin intolerance
- ❑ Cystic fibrosis
- ❑ Allergic fungal sinusitis
- ❑ Kartagener syndrome
- ❑ Young syndrome
- ❑ Churg-Strauss syndrome
- ❑ Nasal mastocytosis.

Symptoms

- ❑ Nasal stuffiness leading to total nasal obstruction may be the presenting symptom.
- ❑ Later obstruction may be bilateral as the polyp grows into the nasopharynx and obstructs the opposite choana.
- ❑ Partial or total loss of sense of smell
- ❑ Headache sneezing and watery nasal discharge
- ❑ Mass protruding from nostril
- ❑ Voice may become hyponasal.

Clinical evaluation

- As antrochoanal polyp grows posteriorly it may be missed on anterior rhinoscopy
- If it is visualised, it appears smooth greyish covered with nasal discharge
- It is soft and can be moved up and down with a probe.

Management

- Medical Management - early polyploid also changes may revert with antihistamines or steroids. Steroids may also be used after surgery to prevent recurrence.
- Removal by avulsion
- Endoscopic sinus surgery
- Caldwell Luc surgery for recurrent cases.

5. True about ear wax:

a. Produced by ceruminous glands in the inner 1/3rd of the EAC
b. Syringing is done to remove impacted wax
c. Ceruminolytic agent is used if wax is hard
d. Syringing is done towards the lower wall of meatus
e. Cerumen causes allergic reactions in external ear

Ans. b, c *Ref: Cummings otolaryngology 5/e; Diseases of ENT, Dhingra, 6/e*

Option a	False	Ceruminous glands are present in the outer 1/3rd of the EAC
Option b	True	Yes, true
Option c	True	Yes, true
Option d	False	Syringing is done along postero-superior wall of the meatus
Option e	False	No, not true

The external ear canal (EAC) is about 2.5 cm long and is composed of lateral one third of cartilaginous (membranous) portion and medial two third of bony portion. The skin lining the membranous canal is thicker, more mobile and endowed with sebaceous and apocrine (ceruminous) glands and hair follicles. The bony portion of the canal is lined by thin, immobile skin that lacks hair and glands and is continuous with the epithelium of the tympanic membrane. The bony cartilaginous junction or the isthmus is the narrowest part of EAC.

Cerumen or Wax

Sebaceous and ceruminous gland open into the space of hair follicles. Secretions of both these glands mix with desquamated epithelial cells and the keratin shed from tympanic membrane to form wax. Wax has a protective function as it lubricates the ear canal and also entraps small foreign materials. It has acidic pH and is bacteriostatic and fungistatic.

Impacted wax: It is an extremely common problem and can cause discomfort, hearing loss, tinnitus, dizziness, and chronic cough. Chronic manipulation with cotton tipped applicators, narrow external canals, hair in lateral canal, hearing aids, and earplug use have been associated with increased incidence of cerumen impaction.

Management

- Removal by syringing

Technique: Pinna is pulled upwards and backwards and stream of water from the ear string is directed along posterosuperior wall of the meatus.

- Ceruminolytics: The use of ceruminolytics before irrigation may increase success of irrigation by 97%. Especially useful when wax is had and cannot be removed by syringing alone.
  Water based (hydrogen peroxide, sodium bicarbonate etc.), oil based (arachis oil, turpentine, paradichlorobenzene, non water non oil based (carbamide peroxide).
- Instrumental manipulation with cerumen hook, scoop or Jobson Horne probe. Avoid breaking the cerumen.

6. True regarding Epistaxis:

a. Kiesselbach's plexus is a common site of bleeding
b. Trotter's method is first aid
c. Recurrent bleed from septum may be managed by elevation of mucoperichondrial flap and submucous resection operation
d. Sphenopalatine artery ligation can be done endoscopically
e. Maxillary artery ligation is preferred over endoscopic sphenopalatine artery ligation

Ans. a, b, c, d *Ref: Cummings otolaryngology 5/e; Diseases of ENT, Dhingra, 6/e*

Option a	True	90% of epistaxis occur in Little's area
Option b	True	In Trotter's method, patient is made to sit, leaning a little forward over a basin to spit any blood, and breathe quietly from the mouth
Option c	True	Yes, correct
Option d	True	Yes, correct
Option e	False	Endoscopic sphenopalatine artery ligation is favoured over maxillary artery ligation

Epistaxis

Usual sites:

- Little's area - Kiesselbach's plexus: Situated in the anterior inferior part of nasal septum just above the vestibule. Four arteries - anterior ethmoidal, septal branch of superior labial, septal branch of sphenopalatine anastomose to form the plexus. Usual site of finger nail trauma and epistaxis in young children. 90% of epistaxis occurs here.
- Retrocolumellar vein - this vein runs vertically downwards just behind the columella, crosses the floor of nose and joins venous plexus on the lateral nasal wall. Common site of venous bleeding in young people.
- Above the level of middle turbinate—from anterior and posterior ethmoid all vessels (internal carotid system)
- Below the level of middle turbinate - from branches of sphenopalatine artery
- Posterior part of nasal cavity : Blood flows directly into the pharynx
- Diffuse: both from septal and lateral nasal walls. Seen in general etiologies
- Nasopharynx.

Causes

Local:

- Trauma - finger nail trauma, injury to nose, fractures, intranasal surgery, violent sneeze

- Infections
  - Acute: viral rhinitis, nasal diphtheria, acute sinusitis
  - Chronic: crust forming diseases, e.g. Atrophic rhinitis, rhinitis Sicca, tuberculosis, syphilis, septal perforation, granulosa touts lesion of the nose like rhinosporidiosis.
- Foreign body
- Neoplasms
  - Benign: hemangioma, papilloma
  - Malignant: carcinoma, sarcoma
- Atmospheric changes: High altitudes, sudden decompression (Caisson disease)
- Deviated nasal septum
- Nasopharyngeal causes
  - Adenoiditis
  - Juvenile angiofibroma
  - Malignant tumors
- General
  - Hypertension
  - Thrombocytopenia from various causes
  - Haemophiliac
  - Vitamin K deficiency, scurvy
  - Hereditary hemorrhagic telangiectasia
  - Chronic nephritis
  - Drugs: salicylate, anticoagulants
  - Mediastinal tumors -raised venous pressure in the nose
  - Acute general infection: viral infections like influenza, measles, infectious mononucleosis, chicken pox, dengue fever; bacterial like rheumatic fever, whooping cough, typhoid; parasitic like malaria
  - Vicarious menstruation : epistaxis occurring at the time of menstruation.

Management:

- First aid:
  - Pinch the nose with thumb and index finger for about 5 min.
  - In trotter's method patient is made to sit leaning a little forward over a basin to spit any blood and breathe quietly from mouth
  - Cold compresses may be used to cause reflex vasoconstriction.
- Cauterisation: in anterior epistaxis when bleeding point has been located it can be cauterised with a bead of silver nitrate or coagulated with electrocautery
- Nasal packing
- Endoscopic cauterisation
- Elevation of mucoperichondrial flap and submucous resection operation : in case of persistent recurrent bleeds from the septum
- Ligation of vessels:
  - External carotid: ligation of the external carotid above the origin of superior thyroid artery. Avoided in favour of ligation of more peripheral branches
  - Maxillary artery: in case of uncontrolled posterior epistaxis
  - Ethmoidal arteries: in anterosuperior bleeding above the middle turbinate not controlled by packing

- TESPAL: Transnasal endoscopic sphenopalatine artery ligation – A mucosal flap is lifted in posterior part of lateral nasal wall, sphenopalatine artery is located and closed with vascular clip. Flap is then reposited. This procedure has high success rate in refractory posterior bleed. Favoured over maxillary artery ligation.

7. Peritonsillar abscess:

a. Hot potato voice
b. Dysphagia even to saliva
c. Bilateral sore throat
d. Uvula pushed to one side
e. Associated with halitosis

Ans. a, b, d, e

Option a	True	
Option b	True	
Option c	False	Usually unilateral
Option d	True	
Option e	True	

Peritonsillar abscess

Collection of pus in the peritonsillar space – between the capsule of tonsil and the superior constrictor muscle.

Etiology

- Usually follows acute tonsillitis
- May arise de novo.

Pathogenesis

One of the tonsillitis crests usually crypta magna gets infected and sealed off -> forms intra-tonsillar abscess -> abscess bursts through tonsillar capsule to cause peritonsillitis and later peritonsillar abscess.

Clinical features

- Severe sore throat: Usually unilateral may be bilateral occasionally
- Odynophagia: It is so marked that the patient cannot even swallow his own saliva and it dribbles
- Thick speech or hot potato voice
- Halitosis
- Ipsilateral ear ache
- Trismus due to spasm of pterygoid muscle
- General symptoms of infection and septicemia like fever, chill, malaise, body aches, headache etc.

Clinical examination

- Congestion and swelling of the tonsil, pillars and soft palate on the affected side
- Tonsil may not appear large as it may get buried in the swelling of adjacent areas
- Bulging of soft palate and anterior pillar above the tonsil
- Uvula is edematous, swollen and pushed to one side
- Mucopus may be seen covering the tonsillar region

- Cervical lymphadenopathy involving jugulodigastric lymph nodes
- Torticollis.

8. True statement regarding cochlear implant:

a. Absence of cochlear nerve is a contraindication
b. CSOM is a contraindication
c. Labyrinthitis ossificans is a contraindication
d. Mondini dysplasia is a contraindication
e. Aplasia of the cochlea is a contraindication

Ans. a, e

Option a	True	
Option b	False	Not correct
Option c	False	Not a contraindication but surgical modification may be required
Option d	False	Mondini dysplasia is a congenital condition resulting in SNHL
Option e	True	

Cochlear implant

An electronic device that can provide useful hearing for patients who have bilateral sensorineural hearing loss (non functional cochlear hair cells) and cannot benefit from hearing aid.

Generally a patient is considered a candidate for cochlear implantation if the following criteria are met:

- Bilateral profound sensorineural hearing loss (SNHL) with an unaided three frequency pure tone average of 70dB hearing loss or poorer in the better year.
- Speech discrimination score of less than 50% in the ear to be implanted and less than 60% in the best aided binaural condition
- Appropriate motivation and realistic expectations
- No evidence of central or auditory lesion
- No evidence of contraindications to surgery or anaesthesia.

Contraindications

- Central auditory lesion
- Absence of auditory nerve
- Aplasia of the cochlea
- Active middle ear infection or disease
- Contraindications to surgery, anaesthesia
- Patient not willing to follow up.

A prior history of meningitis with cochlear ossification or labyrinthitis ossificans or fibrosis does not exclude the patient from implantation but may necessitate modification of the surgical technique.

Chronic suppurative otitis media was initially viewed as a contraindication to cochlear implant in young children. However selective retrospective studies have shown that the prevalence and severity of otitis media does not increase following implantation if the ear is dry at the time of implantation. Some surgeons advocate a two stage surgery. First operation involves a radical mastoidectomy, eustachian tube obliteration, mastoid cavity obliteration with sewing of the ear canal. Cochlear implantation is performed uses 2 to 6 months post obliteration.

Thus CSOM is not a contraindication.

Mondini dysplasia is a congenital condition resulting in SNHL. Management is by cochlear implantation.

9. True about Le Fort fracture:

a. Types are 1 to 4
b. Involves zygoma fracture
c. Associated with malocclusion of teeth
d. Complete when it extends to pterygoid plate
e. Associated with CSF rhinorrhea

Ans. b, c, d, e

Option a	False	Types are 1, 2 and 3
Option b	True	
Option c	True	
Option d	True	
Option e	True	

Fractures of maxilla

Le Fort 1 (transverse): Fracture runs above and parallel to palate. Crosses lower part of nasal septum, maxillary Antra and pterygoid plates.

Le Fort 2 (pyramidal): Fracture passes through the root of nose, lacrimal bone, floor of the orbit, upper part of maxillary sinus and pterygoid plates. This fracture has some features common with the zygomatic fractures

Le Fort 3 (complete craniofacial disjunction): There is complete separation of cranial bones from mother facial bones. This fracture occurs at the level of skull base separating zygomas from the temporal and frontal bones. The fracture line passes through the root of nose, ethmoid frontal junction, superior orbital fissure, lateral wall of orbit, frontozygomatic and temporozygomatic sutures and the upper part of pterygoid plates.

Clinical features

- Malocclusion of teeth
- Elongation of mid face
- Mobility of maxilla
- CSF rhinorrhoea. Cribriform plate is injured in Le Forte 2 and 3 fractures.

Diagnosis

- X-rays: Waters' view, posteroanterior view, lateral view
- CT scan.

Preventive and Social Medicine

1. Pre-exposure prophylaxis is given for:

a. Hep B
b. Hep C
c. Rabies
d. Hep A
e. Varicella zoster

Ans. a,c,d and e

Option		
Option a	True	Yes, routine pre-exposure prophylaxis is indicated for HBV infection high risk individuals
Option b	False	No vaccine for HCV
Option c	True	Yes, routine pre-exposure prophylaxis is indicated for rabies infection high risk individuals
Option d	True	Routine pre-exposure prophylaxis is indicated for HAV infection high risk individuals
Option e	True	Yes, we have varicella immunoglobulin and varicella vaccine for pre and post exposure prophylaxis

Since there is no vaccine for Hep C – primary prevention is the best modality for prevention.

Hepatitis B prevention:

HEPATITIS A

Vaccine

- Types:
  - Inactivated hepatitis A vaccine for > 1 year of age, I/M, 2 doses, 6–12 months apart
  - Live vaccine as subcutaneous injection, single dose
- Commonly for high risk-individuals, post outbreak of hep A infection, travelers

Hep A Human Immunoglobulin

HAV infection maybe protected with HIG. There is 80–90% protection following HIG administration within 14 hours of exposure

Dose: 0.02–0.06 ml/kg, best protection efficacy for 2–3 months.

HEPATITIS B

Hepatitis B Vaccine

- As monovalent formulation or part of the recent pentavalent vaccine
- Given as
  - Children: 0.5ml I/M at birth, 6,10,14 weeks on anterolateral thigh
  - Adults 10–20 mcg at 0, 1, 6 months I/M in deltoid
- In case of interruption of vaccine schedule — continue and administered the delayed vaccine ASAP
- Pregnancy or lactation is not a contraindication for the vaccine

Hepatitis B immunoglobulin

- For acute exposure to HBsAg positive blood – in health care providers
- HbIG given as soon as possible within 6 hours, preferably not later than 48 hours
- 0.05 – 0.07 ml/kg BW – two doses 30 days apart

Passive active immunization

- Better efficacy than alone HbIG or vaccination
- Ideal for: Post exposure prophylaxis and prevention of mother to child transmission
- HBV vaccine 1ml (20 mcg/ml) I/M within 7 days of exposure and 1 and 6 months

RABIES

Types of Vaccine

- Human diploid cell vaccine
- Vero cell vaccine
- Chick embryo vaccine

Vaccine at point 2 and 3 have been recently developed and shown to have similar efficacy to human diploid cell vaccine but are less expensive.

- Do not contain thiomersal as preservatives
- Shelf life is > 3 years (storage at 2–8 °C)
- After reconstitution use within 6–8 hours

Recommended post-exposure prophylaxis

Types of contact with a suspect or confirmed rabid domestic or wild animal or animal unavailable for observation	Recommendations
Cat 1: Touching or feeding of animals, Licks on intact skin	None, if reliable case history is available
Cat 2: Nibbling of uncovered skin; Minor scratches or abrasions without bleeding.	Administer vaccine immediately.
Cat 3: Single or multiple transdermal bites or scratches. Contamination of mucous membrane with saliva (I.e. licks on broken skin) or contact with bats	Administer rabies immunoglobulin and vaccine immediately. + Local treatment of wound

Schedules:

Post-exposure:

- Essen Schedule: 0, 3, 7, 14, 28 - 5 visits, 1 ml per dose I/M
- Zareb Schedule (2-1-1) 0, 7, 21 - 3 visits, 1 ml per dose, I/M
- Thai red cross schedule (2-2-2-2) 0, 3, 7, 28 - 4 visits 0.1 ml per dose, I/D

Post -exposure in pre-vaccinated:

Option 1: 2 visit, 0, 3 days – 0.1 ml ID

Option 2: Single visit, 4 site (2 thigh + 2 deltoid), 0.1 ml ID

Post-exposure in immunocompromised:

5 visit - 0, 3, 7, 14, 28 - 5 visits, 1 ml per dose i/m

Rabies Immunoglobulin

Human rabies immunoglobulin (HRIG) – 20 IU/Kg BW

Equine rabies immunoglobulin (ERIG) – 40 IU/Kg BW

70% in and around the wound site, 30% I/M (note: the data is controversial and different sources provide different opinion. However, for exam purpose, we can understand that most of the Immunoglobulins are administered in and around wound, while remaining as I/M injection at a distant site).

Pre-exposure prophylaxis

3 visit – 0, 7, 28 days, 0.1 ml ID

Special Considerations

- The only contraindication to PrEP is severe reaction to rabies vaccine (which is very rare)
- There is NO contraindication to post-exposure prophylaxis as rabies is fatal disease
- Pregnancy, malnutrition, HIV, immunocompromised, infants, children – do NOT form any contraindications to this vaccine
- Individuals on 'chloroquine treatment' for malaria or any other purpose will require intramuscular injections rather than Intradermal injection (due to reduced response of vaccine)

VARICELLA ZOSTER

- VZ (varicella Zoster) Immunoglobulin (VZIG).
  - Given within 72 hours of exposure, 12.5 U/Kg BW (max. 625 Units), repeated after 3 weeks
  - No therapeutic value in established disease
- Varicella vaccine (OKA strain)
  - 0.5 ml S/C, as 2 doses 3 months apart , for age > 1 year
  - NO contraindication for HIV positive, clinically stable children.

VZIG and varicella vaccine are not combined as the VZIG is believed to bind the varicella vaccine and reduce efficacy.

2. HIV in 5-month-old child is confirmed by:

a. p24 Antigen assay
b. HIV ELISA
c. HIV DNA PCR
d. Viral culture
e. NAT

Ans. c, e *Ref: Park 24th/ed p368; WHO Early infant diagnosis guidelines 2017; WHO Information note, July 2017*

Option a	Not correct	p24 is a reliable method for diagnosis, but the instruments and consumables used are not available as in a national program mode
Option b	Not correct	Not, it is sensitive for screening for HIV, not for confirmed diagnosis
Option c	Yes, correct	Yes, most widely used (2)
Option d	Not correct	No, it is primarily for assessment of response to the ART, for assessing the prognosis of the case
Option e	Yes, correct	Yes, as per recent WHO guidelines (3), it should be taken as stand-alone diagnostic modality for HIV infected infants

- HIV DNA PCR is the most widely used initial assay for early infant diagnosis in industrialized countries.
- HIV RNA PCR and other nucleic acid detection techniques have also proved accurate and reliable, and they provide additional information about virological status that can assist in clinical management.
- Both HIV DNA and HIV RNA technologies are becoming less expensive, more automated and faster in producing results.
- Ultrasensitive p24 antigen detection is a reliable method for detection of HIV infection in infants aged over 6 weeks but the required equipment and consumables are not yet available for purchase in ways suitable for use in achieving national programme coverage.
- As resource-limited settings are increasingly able to purchase HIV DNA and HIV RNA kits and equipment, their choice of technology should be guided by potential public health benefits.

HIV Diagnosis

Clinical criteria

For adults: 2 major + 1 minor sign

Major signs:

- Weight loss > 10% of body weight
- Chronic diarrhoea
- Persistent fever > 1 month

Minor signs

- Persistent cough > 1 month
- Generalized pruritic dermatitis
- History of herpes zoster
- Generalized lymphadenopathy

For children: 2 major + 2 minor signs

Major signs:

1. Weight loss > 10% of body weight, or abnormal slow growth
2. Chronic diarrhoea > 1 month
3. Persistent fever > 1 month

Minor signs:

1. General lymph node enlargement
2. Oropharyngeal candidiasis

3. Recurrent common infections
4. Persistent cough
5. Generalized rash

Laboratory criteria

- ELISA
  - Most sensitive test – screening
- Western blot
  - Detecting antibody to specific viral core protein (p24 Ag)
  - Most specific – diagnostic test
- CD 4 Lymphocyte count (normal is > 950 CD4 / micro Liter)
  - Most widely used predictor of HIV progression
  - High risk of opportunistic infections / malignancy at CD4 < 200
- CD4 percentage
  - Better than absolute CD4 count
  - CD4 percentage < 14% indicates high risk for infections/ malignancy
- Viral HIV loads
  - Measures the amount of actively replicating HIV.
  - Correlates to HIV disease progression and response to ART
- p24 Antigen
  - Indicates acute HIV replication

Treatment: Treat ALL strategy

- Post exposure prophylaxis: With heavy exposure from known HIV positive
- 28 day course for: Adults: Tenofovir (TDF) + Lamivudine (3TC) + Lopinavir / ritonavir (LPV/r)
- Children < 10 years Zidovudine (ZDV / AZT) + Lamivudine (3TC) + Lopinavir / ritonavir (LPV/r)
- HIV Testing is recommended after 3 months following exposure.

3. **According to the biomedical waste guidelines, 2016, the material for incineration should be discarded in which color bags?**

   a. Red
   b. Blue
   c. Black
   d. Yellow
   e. White

Ans. c,d

Option a	No	No, it contains rubber, plastic which should not be incinerated
Option b	No	No, it contains glass and metal implants
Option c	Yes	Incineration may be done
Option d	Yes	Incineration may be done
Option e	No	No, it contains waste sharps, which can not be incinerated

Table 2: Average composition of hospital waste in India	
Material	**Percentage**
Paper	15
Plastics	10
Rags	15
Metal (sharps etc.)	1
Infectious waste	1.5
Glass	4.0
General waste (food waste, sweepings from hospital premises etc.)	53.3

Category

Category	Waste type	Bag type	Treatment
Yellow	Anatomical/soiled waste	Non chlorinated bags	Incineration
	Chemical waste, discarded medicine	Non chlorinated bags	Incineration
	Chemical liquid		Pre-treated before mixing
	Biotechnology, microbiological waste	Autoclave safe plastic bags	Pre-treat and sterilize
Red	Contaminated waste	Red-non chlorinated bags	Autoclave, microwave with shredding and / or sterilization
White	Waste sharps including metals	Puncture proof bins	Autoclave, dry heat sterilization, shredding or mutilation
Blue	Glassware Metallic body implants	Cardboard boxes	Disinfection and recycling

SCHEDULE–III
LABEL FOR BIO-MEDICAL WASTE CONTAINERS/BAGS

BIOHAZARD SYMBOL

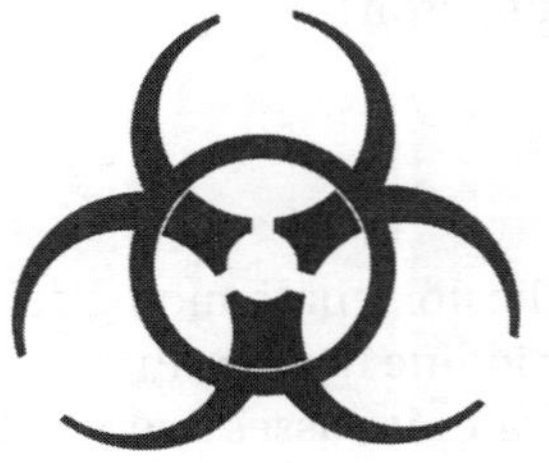

BIOHAZARD

CYTOTOXIC HAXZARD SYMBOL

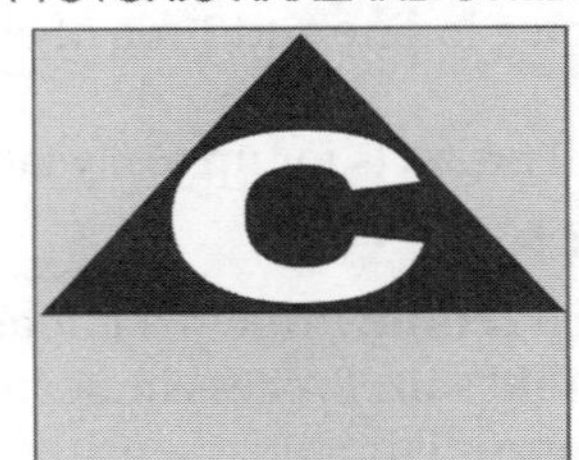

CYTOTOXIC

HANDLE WITH CARE

Note: Label shall be non-washable and prominently visible

4. **Iodine deficiency features:**
   a. Common in Himalayan belt region
   b. One time iodine injection used for life time treatment

c. Diagnosed by blood samples
d. Increased chances of spontaneous abortions and still births
e. Iodine monitoring at community level is achieved by iodine excretion determination

Ans. a,d,e

Option a	True	Yes, correct
Option b	False	No, it confers protection till 4 years
Option c	False	No, widely used parameter is urinary iodine excretion rate
Option d	True	Yes, correct
Option e	True	Yes, it is the principle indicator for assessment of Iodine deficiency disorders at community level

Ref: Park 24th/ed p662, 680

Iodine deficiency disorders consist of:

- Goiter
- Hypothyroidism
- Subnormal intelligence
- Delayed motor milestones
- Mental retardation
- Extrapyramidal symptoms as muscle weakness in limbs and spastic plegias
- Cretinism
- Spontaneous abortions / miscarriages

The iodine deficiency disorders have been found to be common in the Himalayan goiter belt. Most of the states of India are affected by iodine deficiency disorders.

Goiter Control:

- Iodization of salt:
  - 30 ppm at production level
  - 15 ppm at consumer level
- A new salt is known as double fortified salt which consists of iron and iodine as the constituents (40 mcg iodine and 1 mg of elemental iron)
- Iodized Oil
  - 1 ml iodized oil protects for up to 4 years

Indicators for NIDDCP

- **Urinary iodine excretion:** Principal impact indicator, epidemiological indicator
- **Iodine in household salt:** Process indicator for iodine monitoring
- **Neonatal hypothyroidism:** Most sensitive indicator for assessment of impact of NIDDCP
- **Goiter rate:** Chronic impact indicator

5. Which of the following statements are correct:

a. Screening of disease is a secondary prevention
b. Odds ratio is used to calculate association in case control studies
c. Sensitivity is proportion of test positive from the total diseased
d. Screening time is distance between the critical point of diagnosis and the usual point of diagnosis
e. False positive errors correspond to the beta errors

Ans. a,b,c,e

Option a	True	Yes, in context to screening of disease in apparently healthy individuals, comes as part of secondary prevention
Option b	True	Yes, correct
Option c	True	Yes, correct
Option d	False	No, not correct
Option e	True	Yes, it helps physician to decide the chances of an individual to have disease if the test shows a positive result. The test results alongside the clinical picture helps the physician to diagnose the disease in an individual.

	Disease +	Healthy –
Test +	True positive (TP)	False positive (FP)
Test -	False negative (FN)	True negative (TN)

- Sensitivity = TP / D+
- FNER = FN / D+
- Specificity = TN / D-
- FPER = FP / D-
- PPV = TP / T+
- NPV = TN / T-
- FNER = False negative error rate
- FPER = False positive error rate
- PPV = Positive predictive value
- NPV = Negative predictive value

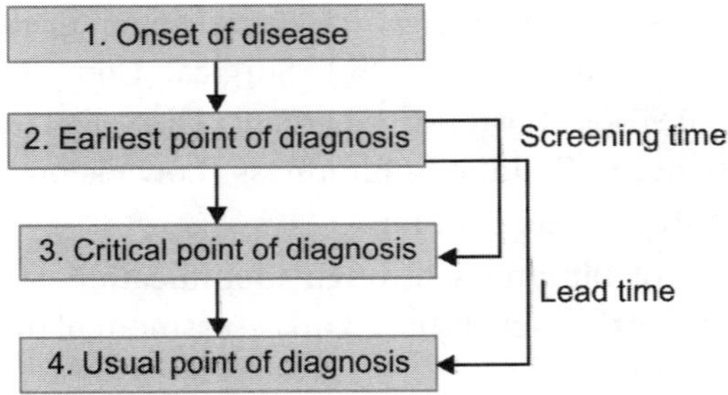

Points to remember:

- False positive error is more serious compared to False negative error
- False positive test is equivalent to the type 1 error or alpha error – False alarm
- False negative test is equivalent to the type 2 error or Beta error
- For screening tests, sensitivity of the test is important
- For diagnostic tests, specificity of the test is essential
- Higher false positive is due to
  - Low specificity
  - Low prevalence
  - High sensitivity

- Predictive values are maximum affected by the prevalence of the disease. Predicative values are not innate to the test and the prevalence has an effect over the PPV's
- Pre-test probability of the test is corresponding to the prevalence of the disease, whereas the positive post-test probability of the test is corresponding to the positive predictive value of the test
- If multiple tests are applied in series, the specificity of the complete testing panel increases

6. True about National Programme for Control of Blindness include:

a. Started in 1962
b. Eye camp method is used
c. Setting up of regional institute of ophthalmology for tertiary eye care
d. The target is to achieve blindness rate < 1% by 2020
e. All are true

Ans. b,c

Option a	False	No, started in 1976
Option b	True	Yes, correct – used for common eye diseases as cataract and refractive error corrections
Option c	True	Yes, correct
Option d	False	No, the target is to achieve blindness rate < 0.3% by 2020
Option e	False	Not applicable

National Programme for Control of Blindness was launched in the year 1976 as a 100% Centrally Sponsored scheme with the goal to reduce the prevalence of blindness from 1.4% to 0.3% by 2020.

Main causes of blindness are as follows: - Cataract (62.6%), Refractive Error (19.70%), Corneal Blindness (0.90%), Glaucoma (5.80%), Surgical Complication (1.20%) Posterior Capsular Opacification (0.90%), Posterior Segment Disorder (4.70%), Others (4.19%), Estimated National Prevalence of Childhood Blindness /Low Vision is 0.80 per thousand.

Goals and Objectives of NPCB in the XII Plan

- To reduce the backlog of blindness through identification and treatment of blind at primary, secondary and tertiary levels based on assessment of the overall burden of visual impairment in the country.
- Develop and strengthen the strategy of NPCB for "Eye Health" and prevention of visual impairment; through provision of comprehensive eye care services and quality service delivery.
- Strengthening and upgradation of RIOs to become centre of excellence in various sub-specialities of ophthalmology
- Strengthening the existing and developing additional human resources and infrastructure facilities for providing high quality comprehensive Eye Care in all Districts of the country;
- To enhance community awareness on eye care and lay stress on preventive measures;
- Increase and expand research for prevention of blindness and visual impairment
- To secure participation of Voluntary Organizations/Private Practitioners in eye Care

2017 update:

- The name has been changed to: National Program for Blindness and Visual Impairment
- The cut-off for blindness is visual acuity < 6/60 in the better eye with correction
- Screening of children for early identification of refractive errors and free spectacles under school eye program
- Include other diseases as glaucoma, refractive errors, age related macular degeneration, corneal blindness for active management and treatment under the program
- Promote eye donation

7. For the waste treatment, true statement is:

a. Aerobic sludge method is outdate method of sewage disposal
b. Sewage treatment plant has two primary chambers
c. Bio-aeration is unsatisfactory method
d. Trickling filters are bio-filtration method
e. Pyrolytic incineration is environment friendly

Ans. b, d, e

Option a	False	No, not correct, aerobic sludge method also known as the activated sludge method is the most modern method and satisfactory method for sewage treatment
Option b	True	Yes, correct
Option c	False	No, bio, aeration is synonymous with activated sludge method
Option d	True	Yes correct
Option e	True	Yes, it burns the waste at high degree and has pollution control devices. Thus the technology is environment friendly and is also called control air incineration

Incineration is burning under very high temperatures of 500–1000°C converting waste into bottom ash and fly ash.

Three types of incinerators:

- Double chamber pyrolytic incinerator
- Single chamber health care waste
- Rotary kilns

Double chamber pyrolytic incinerator:

- Ideal for infectious waste disposal
- Temperature between 900 — 1200°
- 50–250 Kg / hr of infectious waste is disposed off

Single chamber incinerator:

- Used for general health care waste disposal
- Carries risk of air pollution

Rotary Kiln incinerator:

- Rotating oven and post combustion chamber
- Specifically used for infectious and pathological hazardous waste
- Temperature is usually in range of 1200 – 1600°C

Other methods for biomedical waste disposal:

- **Chemical disinfection:** Involves treatment with bleaching powder, glutaraldehyde other ammonium / alcohol compounds

- Wet thermal treatment (autoclave) treatment with steam at specified temperature 121–149 °C) and pressure (15–50 psi) for specified time (60 mins)
- **Dry thermal treatment:** For sharps and other infectious waste for disposal. The matter is heated in rotating auger (drill rods) which causes weight and volume reduction of the waste
- **Deep burial:** Not recommended method for waste disposal, proper permission and record maintenance is required. Pit dimensions: 2 mts deep with 1.5 mt square
- **Plasma torch:** Uses plasma torch with temperature over 6000 deg C. All waste is converted to vapors and gas
- **Inertization:** Mixing of toxic or hazardous waste with cement, lime and water.
- **Hydroclave:** Advanced version of autoclave – to use steam / heat with even penetration
- **Microwave irradiation:** 30-40% volume reduction with minimal air pollution

8. Six sigma strategy:

a. Motorola established the concept
b. Low error or defects
c. Pertains to improve business process
d. Pertains to number needed to treat
e. Pertains to occupational health

Ans. a, b, c

Option a	True	Yes, correct
Option b	True	Yes, correct. This is the mainstay of the concept
Option c	True	Yes, correct. Better business is the desired goal
Option d	False	No, not correct
Option e	False	No, not correct

Pertains to improved

- Management methods
- Manufacturing quality
- Process control

Overall improved business

6σ (symbol of six sigma)

Features that set Six Sigma apart from previous quality-improvement initiatives include:

- A clear focus on achieving measurable and quantifiable financial returns from any Six Sigma project.
- An increased emphasis on strong and passionate management leadership and support.
- A clear commitment to making decisions on the basis of verifiable data and statistical methods, rather than assumptions and guesswork.

Preventive and Social Medicine

1. Vaccine to be given after 2 years:
   a. MMR vaccine
   b. Varicella/chickenpox
   c. Typhoid oral vaccine
   d. Pneumococcal vaccine
   e. IPV

Ans. c, d *Ref: https://www.cdc.gov/mmwr/preview/mmwrhtml/mm6411a3.htm; (Park/24) 108; 3. (Suryakanta/3rd) 280*

Option a	False	Given at 15–18 months of age
Option b	False	Given at > 1 year of age
Option c	True	
Option d	True	
Option e	False	Given at 14 weeks of age

❑ Types of vaccines

Live attenuated vaccine	Killed whole	Toxoid	Polysaccharide	Glycoconjugate	Recombinant
BCG	Typhoid	Diphtheria	Pneumococcus	Hib	HBV
OPV	Cholera	Tetanus	Meningococcus	Pneumococcus	HPV
Measles	Plague	Anthrax	HiB	Men ACYW	Cholera toxin B
Mumps	Pertussis	Acellular pertussis	Typhoid (Vi)		
Rubella	Influenza				
Typhoid	Typhus				
Varicella	IPV				
Cholera	JE				
Rotavirus	HAV				

❑ Related terminologies—frequently asked:
- Polyvalent vaccine
  - ***Nine-valent HPV***: 9vHPV is a noninfectious, virus-like particle (VLP) vaccine. Similar to quadrivalent HPV vaccine (4vHPV), 9vHPV contains HPV 6, 11, 16, and 18 VLPs, while in addition, it contains HPV 31, 33, 45, 52, and 58 VLPs. 9vHPV was approved by the Food and Drug Administration (FDA) on December 10, 2014, for use in females aged 9 through 26 years and males aged 9 through 15 years.
    Remember: 9vHPV and 4vHPV are licensed for use in females and males. Bivalent HPV vaccine (2vHPV), which contains HPV 16, 18 VLPs, is licensed for use in females only.
  - ***Pentavalent vaccine***: DPT, HepB, Hib (mixed vaccine)
  - ***Trivalent vaccine:*** OPV

- Freeze dried vaccine—powder form vaccine. These are mixed with diluents before administration.
  - BCG — Diluent - Normal saline
  - Measles — Diluent - Distilled water
  - MMR — Diluent - Sterile water

❑ Vaccine age of doses:

Vaccine	Schedule	Age at 1st dose	Maximum age	Diluent	Dose	Route site	Remarks
BCG	At birth	Birth	One year	Sodium chloride	0.05	ID, left upper arm	Except in symptomatic, untreated, severe immunocompromised HIV
OPV	At birth, 6, 10, 14 weeks 16–24 months	Birth	Five years	Nil	2 drops	Oral	Not recommended in severe immunocompromised HIV
Pentavalent	6,10,14 weeks	6 weeks	One year	Nil	0.5 mL	IM A/L thigh (left)	
Rota virus	6,10,14 weeks	6 weeks	One year				Not recommended > 2 years
IPV	14 weeks	14 weeks	One year	Nil	0.5 mL	IM A/L thigh (Right)	
DPT (B)	16–24 months, 5 years	-booster-	7 years		0.5 mL	IM A/L thigh (left)	
Measles	9–12 months, 16–24 months	9 months	5 years (1st dose until 2 years)	Sterile water	0.5 mL	SC right upper arm	Not recommended in— 1. HIV – symptomatic, 2. Severe immunocompromised 3. Pregnancy
JE	9 months, 16–24 months	9 months	15 years	Phosphate buffer	0.5 mL	SC, left upper arm	Launched in - UP, WB, Karnataka, Assam, Bihar – JE Endemic areas
Hep B	Birth	Birth	Within 24 hours				Not recommended in – Prematurity Low birth weight High risk group
TT	10 years 16 years						

❑ Special vaccines

Vaccine	Minimum age	Special considerations
Cholera (Dukoral)	> 2 years	
Cholera (Shanchol and mORCVAX)	> 1 years	

Contd...

Contd...

Vaccine	Minimum age	Special considerations
Typhoid (Vi PS)	> 2 years	
Typhoid (Ty21a)	> 5 Years	
Hib	6 weeks	Not recommended for age > 5 years Single dose if > 12 months age
Hep A	> 1 year	
Varicella	> 1 year	
HPV	> 9 years	2 dose schedule—9–13 years old 3 dose schedule—Pregnant females more than 15 years, HIV and immunocompromised
Dengue (CYD-TDV)	> 9 years	3 doses—six months apart

Injection site, type of needle and technique			
	Site	***Type of needle***	***Comments***
Intramuscular injections (needle should enter at a 90° angle)			
Preterms and neonates	Anterolateral thigh (junction of middle and lower third)	22–25 gauge, 5/8 inch	Skin should be stretched between thumb and forefinger
	Site	***Type of needle***	***Comments***
Infants (1 to < 12 months)	Anterolateral thigh	22–25 gauge, 1 inch	Bunch the skin subcutaneous tissue and muscle to prevent striking the bone
Toddlers and older children (12 months–10 years)	Deltoid or	22–25 gauge, 5/8 inch	Skin should be stretched between thumb and forefinger
	Anterolateral thigh	22–25 gauge, 1 inch	Bunch the skin, subcutaneous tissue and muscle
Adolescents and adults (11 years onwards)	Deltoid or anterolateral thigh	< 60 kg 1 inch < 60 kg 1.5 inch	
Intramuscular injections (needle should enter at a 45° to the skin)			
Infants	Thigh	22–25 G, 5/8 inch	
> 12 months	Outer triceps	22–25 G, 5/8 inch	
Intradermal injections			
All ages	Left deltoid	26/27 G, 0.5 inch	A 5 mm wheal should be raised

2. Cycle beads are associated with which of the following method of contraception?

a. Rhythm method
b. Symptothermal method
c. Coitus interruptus
d. Calendar method
e. Standard days method

Ans. e *Ref: Park, 24/e; Suryakanta, 3/e*

Option a	False
Option b	False

Option c	False
Option d	False
Option e	True

"Fertility Awareness" means that a woman learns how to tell when the fertile time of her menstrual cycle starts and ends. The fertile time is the time when she can get pregnant. The Standard Days Method involves identifying the fertile days during each menstrual cycle. Women with menstrual cycles ranging between 26 and 32 days can prevent pregnancy by avoiding unprotected sexual intercourse on days 8 to 19.

The Standard Days Method (SDM) is a new natural family planning method for women with menstrual cycles ranging between 26 and 32 days. This method involves identifying the fertile days during each menstrual cycle. Women with menstrual cycles ranging between 26 and 32 days can prevent pregnancy by avoiding unprotected sexual intercourse on days 8 to 19.

Most women using the SDM use a device called cycle beads—a string of color-coded beads that help women identify the days of their cycles when they can become pregnant and the days when pregnancy is very unlikely. The white beads, which represent the end of the cycle, indicate the time when the woman has a high probability of becoming pregnant if she has unprotected sexual intercourse.

How to use SDM

- On the day that your menstrual period starts, hold the Cycle Beads and move the rubber ring onto the first red bead.
- Each day, move the rubber ring onto the next bead, moving in the direction of the arrow.
- Avoid sexual intercourse or unprotected sexual intercourse on the days when the rubber ring is on any of the white beads.

Cycle beads

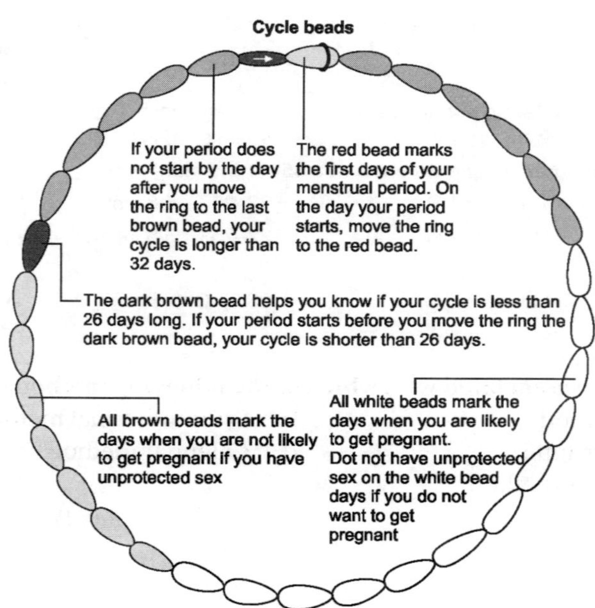

3. Importance of lepromin test are all *except*:
   a. Only has epidemiological significance
   b. Prognostic value
   c. Tells about immunity status of leprosy patients
   d. Differentiate between different type of leprosy
   e. Diagnostic value

Ans. a, c, e *Ref: Park, 24/e; Suryakanta, 3/e*

Option a	False	It is not appropriate to say epidemiological significance, as many cases would be classified as per the WHO clinical classification and lepromin test is not mandatory or diagnostic
Option b	True	Yes, we may say this Option as true. A patient of the Indeterminate type of leprosy with negative lepromin test has a grave prognosis since it is likely to turn into the lepromatous variety. Similarly a patient with 2+lepromin test belonging to the Maculo-anesthetic type or Borderline (BT) type has a favorable prognosis
Option c	False	Lepromin test will not tell about the immune status of an individual, rather it is indicative of the cell mediated immunity for classification of types of leprosy
Option d	True	Yes, lepromin test may classifiy the disease based on tuberculoid, lepromatous, intermediate type
Option e	False	It is obvious that Lepromin cannot be used as a diagnostic test since the very malignant form of the disease, namely the lepromatous type as well as some of the intermediate groups are negative

- **Tests for CMI**
  - Lepromin test
    - Early reaction (Fernandez rxn)
    - Late reaction (Mitsuda reaction)
  - LTT / LMIT (lymphocyte transformation test, leucocyte migration inhibition test) – for CMI
  - Tests for humoral response (antibody)
    - FLA ABS – almost 100% specific – best test
    - Monoclonal antibody – SACT (serum antibody competition test)
    - ELISA – based on phenolic glycolipid antigen (PGL)

Lepromin test:

Lepromin test detects cell mediated immunity. It simply measures the individual susceptibility or resistance. It does not indicate past or present infection. Lepromin positivity is associated with resistance to leprosy infection.

- Antigen used = Dharmendra antigen (1/16 conc.)
- After intradermal injection of 0.1 mL of lepromin antigen, two types of reactions can be seen.
- Fernandez reaction – early reaction
  - In 48 hours
  - Redness > 10 mm indicates positive test
  - Delayed type hypersentivity reaction

- Mitsuda reaction – Late reaction
  - In 21 days
  - Nodule > 5 mm indicates positive test
  - Indicates cell mediated immunity
  - May be false positive with BCG vaccine

The lepromin test may be used to classify the disease as follows:

Tuberculoid type (TT)	2+ to 3+
Maculoanesthetic type (MA)	1+ to 2+
Indeterminate type (I)	Neg. ± or +
Borderline type (BT)	1+ to 2+
Borderline borderline (BB)	± or +
Borderline lepromatous (BL)	Neg. or ±
Lepromatous type (LL)	Neg.

Tuberculoid (TT) type shows the highest host resistance, while the lepromatous type is "anergic" to the skin test and the Borderline group show varying degrees of positivity depending on their position in the immunological spectrum.

4. A leprosy person is presented with involvements of sural and radial nerve. Which type of regimen you will give:

a. Multibacillary treatment × 9 months
b. Multibacillary treatment × 12 months
c. Multibacillary treatment × 15 months
d. Paucibacillary treatment × 6 month
e. Single dose treatment of Rifampicin, Ofloxacin and Minocycline (ROM) is used for paucibacillary leprosy

Ans. b, d *Ref: Park, 24/e; Suryakanta, 3/e*

Option a	False	No, it is for 12 months
Option b	True	Yes, correct
Option c	False	No, it is for 12 months
Option d	True	Yes, correct
Option e	False	No, for paucibacillary, Multidrug therapy is given as per NLEP guidelines

National Leprosy Eradication Program (NLEP)

Diagnosis of leprosy

Diagnosis of leprosy under NLEP is based only on the presence of the characteristic lesions (supplemented by thickened peripheral nerve). Skin smears are not taken to reach a diagnosis. There are only two categories of patients.

- **Multibacillary** (MB) cases—Patients with 6 or more lesions with or without 2 or more peripheral nerve involvement.
- **Paucibacillary**(PB) cases—Patients with 5 or less lesion with or without 1 or no peripheral nerve involvement.

WHO-Recommended Multidrug Therapy (MDT) Regimens

Multibacillary leprosy (MB)

Day 1	Days 2–28
Rifampicin: 600 mg, supervised Dapsone: 100 mg, daily unsupervised Clofazimine: 300 mg. supervised	Dapsone: 100 mg, daily unsupervised Clofazimine: 50 mg, daily unsupervised

Note: 12 blister calendar packs (BCPs) to be finished by the patient (ideally in 12 months) before being declared as cured.

Paucibacillary leprosy (PB)

Day 1	Days 2–28
Rifampicin: 600 mg, supervised Dapsone: 100 mg, daily supervised	Dapsone: 100 mg, daily unsupervised

Note: 6 blister calendar packs (BCPs) to be finished by the patient (ideally in 6 months) before being declared as cured.

Adequate treatment:

- PB—six monthly doses within 9 months
- MB—12 monthly doses within 18 months
- Defaulter: not taken treatment for 12 months

Type of leprosy	Drugs used	Frequency of administration adults (children in bracket)	Dosage (adult) 15 years and above	Dosage (children 10–14 years)	Dosage children below 10 years	Criteria for RFT
MB leprosy	Rifampicin	Once monthly	600 mg	450 mg	300 mg	Completion of 12 monthly pulses in 18 consecutive months
	Clofazimine	Monthly	300 mg	150 mg	100 mg	
	Dapsone	Daily once	100 mg	50 mg	25 mg	
	Clofazimine	Daily for adults (every other day for children)	50 mg	50 mg (alternate day, not daily)	50 mg (weekly twice)	
PB leprosy	Rifampicin	Once monthly	600 mg	450 mg	300 mg	Completion of 6 monthly pulses 9 consecutive months
	Dapsone	Daily	100 mg	50 mg	25 mg daily or 50 mg alternate day	

MDT schedule:

- PB Adult: For people with PB leprosy and 15 years of age or more
- MB Adult: For people with MB leprosy and 15 years of age or more
- PB child: For people with PB leprosy and 10–14 years of age
- MB child: For people with MB leprosy and 10–14 years of age
- For children age < 10 years:
  - Rifampicin: 10 mg/ kg body weight, monthly once
  - Clofazimine: 1 mg /kg body weight daily and 6 mg/kg body weight, monthly once
  - Dapsone: 2 mg /kg body weight daily

Adverse Effects:

- DDS (dapsone) side effects (s/e): Hemolytic anemia, hepatitis, agranulocytosis
- CLF (clofazamine) dark red discoloration of skin, urine
- Other drugs: Minocylcine, clarithromycin, ethionamide

Core indicators of NLEP:

- Number of new cases detected per year
- Rate of new cases with grade two disability/100,000 population*
- Treatment completion
- Cure rate
- Child cases among new cases

Recently added indicator

5. Which of the following is true about data representation?

a. Histogram is used for presentation of discrete data
b. Scattered dots in scatter diagram indicate no correlation
c. Pictogram is represented by small pictures or symbols
d. Linear plot on regression graph indicate strong correlation
e. Pie chart is represented by quadrangular figures

Ans. b, c, d *Ref: Park, 24/e; Suryakanta, 3/e*

Option a	False	No, for continuous data
Option b	True	Yes, correct
Option c	True	Yes, correct
Option d	True	Yes, correct
Option e	False	No, it is sectoral presentation (in circle) of data with percentages

Data presentation:

- Quantitative variables:
  - Column charts - Histogram
  - Frequency polygon/curve
  - Ogive
  - Line diagram
  - Scatter plot
  - Box and whisker plot
- Qualitative variables:
  - Column charts - Bar chart
  - Pie chart
  - Pictogram
  - Spot maps
  - Venn diagrams
- Histogram
  - Is for continuous data
  - Joined column chart
  - Helps to have an approximate of central tendency (median, mode or mean) of the data

- Frequency polygon
  - Formed by joining the mid points of a histogram
- Ogive
  - Used for cumulative frequency
  - The curve is almost always uprising
- Line chart
  - Used to represent the time trends
  - Drawn between time and frequency of events/diseases
- Scatter plot
  - Used for correlation
  - Drawn between two variables
- Box and whisker
  - Used for graphical representation of the data distribution in quartiles (four partitions)
  - Box and whisker are useful in representing the data distribution for outliers, median and standard deviations (or range) of data
- Bar chart
  - Is for discrete data
  - Distantly placed column chart
- Pie chart
  - For sectoral presentation of data
  - Used in percentages and not absolute numbers
- Pictogram
  - Symbolic representation of data
- Spot maps
  - Geographical distribution of events, places, data
- Venn diagrams
  - Graphical presentation of qualitative data in circles with overlapping rings

6. True about HIV:

a. Progression is same in male and female
b. HIV 2—poor prognosis
c. HIV 1 is more common
d. Pneumocystis jeroveci is the most common opportunistic infection
e. Nevirapine prophylaxis is given for 6 months to an infant born to HIV female

Ans. a, c *Ref: Park, 24/e; Suryakanta, 3/e*

Option a	True	Yes, HIV prognosis is not gender based
Option b	False	No, HIV 2 is generally with lower mortality and lower HIV levels
Option c	True	Yes, correct, most common is HIV group M, subgroup C
Option d	False	No, pulmonary tuberculosis is considered to be the most common opportunistic infection in HIV
Option e	False	No, NVP prophylaxis is given for 6 weeks (and not six months)

- Recent data (India national data 2011 estimate, UNAIDS report 2013)
  - Prevalence of HIV in 15–49 is 0.27, incidence is 130 thousand per year
  - ART coverage as per WHO 2010 guidelines: 51% (2011 data)
- HIV-1 — Most common type, more virulent

- HIV-2 — Less frequent, less virulent
- HIV-1 three subgroups
  - M (major)
  - O (outlier)
  - N (neither M nor O)
- Group M (subtypes A to K)
  - Subtype B — most common in US, Europe
  - Subtype E — most common in Thailand, Bangkok, Vietnam
  - Subtype C (fastest-spreading type worldwide) — most common in India, Ethiopia, and Southern Africa.
- Most common cause of AIDS in India — HIV-1 group-M , Subtype-c. (Remember HIV 1 MC (most common))
  - Compared to HIV-1 infection, the clinical course of HIV-2 infection is generally characterized by a longer asymptomatic stage, lower plasma HIV-2 RNA levels, and lower mortality; however, progression to AIDS does occur.
  - Research have shown as lower transmission rates of HIV 2 compared to the HIV 1. The lower infectivity of HIV-2 is likely related to lower RNA levels
  - Slower progression to AIDS
    - HIV-2 infection is characterized by higher CD4 cell counts and lower viral RNA levels than that seen in HIV-1 infection
    - However, once advanced immunodeficiency develops, HIV-2–infected individuals have a high mortality

Center for Disease Control and Prevention (CDC) Recommendations for HIV-2 testing

- **Persons at risk for HIV-2 infection**
  - Sex partners of a person from a country where HIV-2 is endemic
  - Sex partners of a person known to be infected with HIV-2
  - People who received a blood transfusion or a non-sterile injection in a country where HIV-2 is endemic
  - People who shared needles with a person from a country where HIV-2 is endemic or with a person known to be infected with HIV-2
  - Children of women who have risk factors for HIV-2 infection or are known to be infected with HIV-2.
- **HIV-2 testing is also indicated for:**
- People with an illness that suggests HIV infection (such as an HIV-associated opportunistic infection) but whose HIV-1 test result is not positive
- People for whom HIV-1 Western blot exhibits the unusual indeterminate test band pattern of gag (p55, p24, or p17) plus pol (p66, p51, or p32) in the absence of env (gp160, gp120, or gp41).
- Potential initial treatment regimens for HIV-2 infection
- Initial therapy for treatment-naïve patients with HIV-2 infection should include a ritonavir-boosted protease inhibitor plus 2 nucleoside reverse transcriptase inhibitors unless drug resistance is detected or suspected. Therapy for drug-resistant HIV-2 infection must be individualized.

- HIV-2 is intrinsically resistant to non-nucleoside reverse transcriptase inhibitors and to enfuvirtide; thus, these drugs should not be included in an antiretroviral regimen for an HIV-2 infected patient.

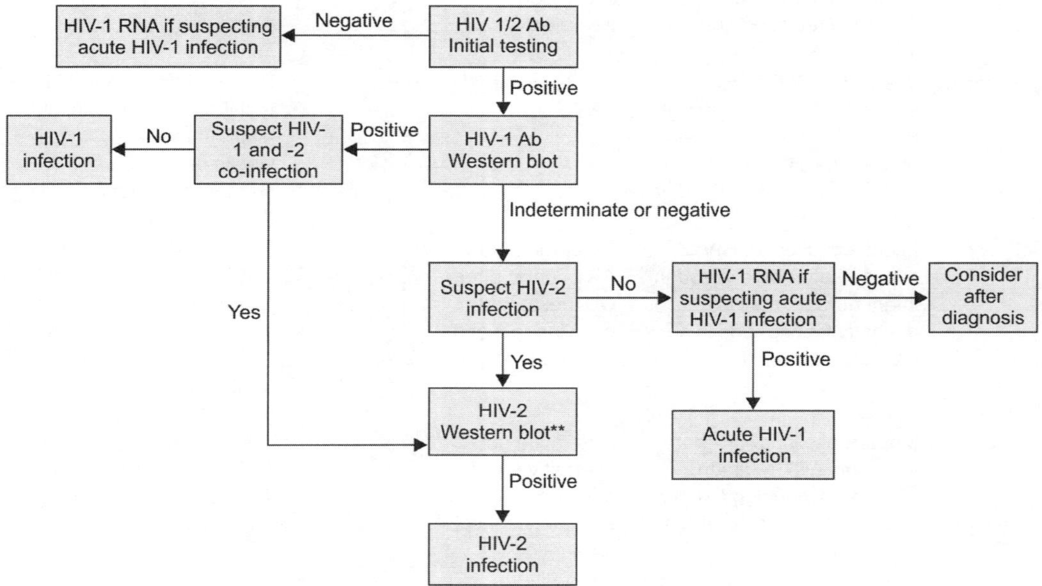

Ab: Antibody
**HIV-2 Ab Western blot testing is available commercially and in research laboratories (see test for details).

Ritonavir-boosted protease inhibitor	Nucleoside reverse transcriptase inhibitors
Lopinavir/ritonavir or Darunavir/ritonavir	Tenofovir + emtricitabine or lamivudine or Zidovudine + lamivudine (this combination may have more toxicity than tenofovir-based therapy)

Note: Adapted with permission from the following reference: British HIV Association guidelines for antiretroviral treatment of HIV-2-positive individuals 2010. HIV Med. 11:611-9.

Regarding nevirapine (NVP) prophylaxis:

Scenarios	Different clinical scenarios	Maternal antiretroviral therapy (ART)	Infant antiretroviral (ARV) prophylaxis	Duration of infant ARV prophylaxis
Scenario 1	Mother diagnosed with HIV during pregnancy	Initiate maternal ART	NVP	6 weeks
Scenario 2	Mother diagnosed with HIV during labor or immediately postpartum and plans to breastfeed	Initiate maternal ART	NVP	Extending NVP prophylaxis to 12 weeks

Contd...

Contd...

Scenario 3	Mother diagnosed with HIV during labor or immediately postpartum and plans exclusive replacement feeding (ERF)	Refer mother for HIV care and evaluation for treatment	NVP	6 weeks
Scenario 4	Infant identified as HIV exposed after birth [through infant (at 6 weeks or after) or maternal HIV antibody testing] and is breastfeeding	Initiate maternal ART	NVP	Perform infant DNA/PCR test if child is 6 weeks old or older. Immediately initiate 6 weeks or longer of NVP- strongly consider extending this to 12 weeks
Scenario 5	Infant identified as HIV exposed after birth (through infant or maternal HIV antibody testing) and is not breastfeeding	Refer mother to ART center after CD4 tests and baseline test and treatment	No NVP (No drugs)	Do HIV DNA/PCR test in accordance with national recommendations on early infant diagnosis; no infant ARV prophylaxis; initiate treatment if the infant is infected
Scenario 6	Mother receiving ART but interrupts ART regimen while breastfeeding (such as toxicity, stock-outs or refusal to continue)	Determine an alternative ART regimen or solution; counsel regarding continuing ART without interruption	NVP	Until 6 weeks after maternal ART is restarted or until 1 week after breastfeeding has ended

- Recent update:
  - Treat all HIV positive strategy
  - 90–90–90 HIV/AIDS
    - 90% diagnosed
    - 90% of diagnosed to receive ART
    - 90% of receiving ART to have viral suppresion

7. There is increased risk of which cancer in HIV patients:

a. Colon cancer b. Pancreatic cancer
c. Lymphoma d. Ca cervix
e. Liver cancer

Ans. a, c, d, e *Ref: Park, 24/e; Suryakanta, 3/e; Sigel K, Dubrow R, Silverberg M, Crothers K, Braithwaite S, and Justice A (2011). Cancer Screening in Patients Infected with HIV. Current HIV/AIDS Reports, 8(3), 142–152. http://doi.org/10.1007/s11904-011-0085-5*

Option a	True	Yes, it is common
Option b	False	No, not common
Option c	True	Yes, it is common
Option d	True	Yes, it is common
Option e	True	Yes, it is common

Infection with HIV weakens the immunity and may lead to carcinogenicity.

The following are the most important of the cancer-related viruses:

- Infection with most of these viruses is more common among people infected with HIV than among uninfected people.
- Human herpesvirus 8 (HHV-8), also known as Kaposi sarcoma-associated herpes virus (KSHV), is the cause of Kaposi sarcoma.
- Epstein Barr virus (EBV) causes some subtypes of non-Hodgkin and Hodgkin lymphoma.
- Human papillomavirus (HPV) causes cervical cancer and some types of anal, penile, vaginal, vulvar, and head and neck cancer.
- Hepatitis B virus (HBV) and hepatitis C virus (HCV) both can cause liver cancer.
- Anal cancer is clearly linked to infection with hrHPV. It is also suspected that immunosuppression augments the development of anal squamous cell dysplasia.
- Breast cancer is the most important cancer in females. The current recommendations are biennial mammography for early screening of the disease.
- Colorectal cancer is especially amenable to screening, as premalignant adenomas exhibit a slow progression to malignancy, and are often visibly identifiable and treatable via colonoscopy. Despite these advantages, half of colorectal cancers present at advanced stage, likely due to inadequate adherence to screening and barriers to health care utilization present in some populations. The recommended tests for colorectal cancer screening are:
  - Fecal occult blood testing
  - Sigmoidoscopy
  - Colonoscopy
- Other screening cancers are:
  - Hepatocellular cancer
  - Lung cancer
  - Prostate cancer
- Other, less common types of cancer that may develop in people with HIV/AIDS are Hodgkin's lymphoma, angiosarcoma, anal cancer, oral cancer, throat cancer, lung cancer, testicular cancer and multiple types of skin cancer including basal cell carcinoma, squamous cell carcinoma, and melanoma.

8. Correct pair is:

a. Chaga's disease—black fly
b. Epidemic typhus—rat flea
c. Oriental sore—sand fly
d. Dracunculosis—cyclops
e. Relapsing fever—soft tick

Ans. c, d, e *Ref: Park, 24/e; Suryakanta, 3/e*

Option a	False	No, Chagas disease is by reduviid bug, also known as 'chigger'
Option b	False	No, epidemic typhus is predominantly louse borne
Option c	True	Yes, correct
Option d	True	Yes, correct
Option e	True	Yes, correct

Diseases Transmitted

- ***Human lice:*** TREP—Trench fever, relapsing fever, epidemic typhus, pediculosis
- ***Rat flea:*** CHEP—Chiggerosis, hymenolepis deminuta, endemic typhus, plague (bubonic typhus)
- ***Sand fly:*** KOSO—Kala-azar, Oriental sore, sandfly fever, Oraya fever

- ***Black fly:*** Onchocerciasis
- ***Redviid bugs:*** Chaga's Disease
- ***Hard tick:*** TTT VV HH—Tick typhus, tick paralysis, tularemia, viral encephalitis, viral fever, hemorrhagic fever, human babesiosis.
- ***Soft tick***—Q fever, relapsing fever
- ***Itch mite:*** Scabies
- ***Trombiculid mite***—Scrub typhus, rickettsial-pox
- ***Cyclopes:*** Guinea worm disease, fish tapeworm (*Diphyllobothrium latum*)

Rickettsial diseases:

Organism	Disease	Arthropod vector	Vertebrate reservoir	Clinical severity	Geographic distribution
Spotted fevers[c]					
Rickettsia rickettsii	Rocky Mountain spotted fever	Tick[a]	Dogs, rodents	+	Rocky Mountain states, eastern USA
R. akari	Rickettsial pox	Mite[a]	Mice	–	Asia, Far east, Africa, USA
R. conorii	Mediterranean spotted fever	Tick	Dogs	+	Mediterranean
Typhus					
R. prowazekii	Epidemic typhus	Louse	Human[b]	++	Africa, South America
R. typhi	Endemic typhus	Flea	Rodents	–	Worldwide
Orientia tsutsugamushi	Scrub typhus	Mite[a]	Rodents	++	Far East
Others					
Coxiella bumetii	Q fever	None	Sheep, goats, cattle	+	Worldwide
Bartonella quintana	Trench fever	Louse	Human	+	Asia, Africa, Central and South America[d]
Ehrlichia chaffeensis[e]	Fever (ehrlichiosis)	Tick	White-tailed deer		USA, Japan *(E. sennetsu)*

[a]Vertically transmitted in arthropod.
[b]Non-human vertebrates are possibly also involved.
[c]Other rickettsiae cause similar tick-borne fevers in Africa, India, Australia.
[d]Multiply extracellulary; 1 million soldiers infected in the First World War.
[e]Isolated at Fort Chaffee, Arkansas; parasitizes lymphocytes, monocytes, neutrophils.

9. Correct pairs of definition is/are:

a.	Latent period	Time period between two outbreaks
b.	Serial interval	Difference between the primary case and secondary case
c.	Incubation period	Is the time period between the onset of pathogenesis and the appearance of signs and symptoms
d.	Generation time	Time period between the entry of agent and maximum infectivity
e.	Period of communicability	Duration of the longest incubation period and the convalescence period

Ans. b, c, d *Ref: Park, 24/e; Suryakanta, 3/e*

Option a	False	Time between onset of pathogenesis and appearance of signs of the non-communicable disease
Option b	True	

Option c	True	
Option d	True	
Option e	False	The time period for which the case is infectious to others

Explanation:

The correct definitions are as follows:

Latent period	Time between onset of pathogenesis and appearance of signs of the non-communicable disease
Serial interval	Difference between the primary case and secondary case
Incubation period	Is the time period between the onset of pathogenesis and the appearance of signs and symptoms
Generation time	Time period between the entry of agent and maximum infectivity
Period of communicability	The time period for which the case is infectious to others
Other definitions	
Primary case	First case of the community
Secondary case	Subsequent cases after the primary case (within the longest one incubation period)
Index case	The first observed case – may be the primary or may not be the primary case
Sporadic	Scattered cases
Endemic	Persistent presence of a disease in an area
Epidemic	An increase in number of cases (usually sudden) which is clearly in excess than the expected frequency, but at least should be more than +2 SD or more than 80% of the expected frequency
Pandemic	A disease crossing two large water bodies or two continents or two WHO regions

10. Disease control would be an appropriate term for:

a. Post elimination
b. Pre-eradication
c. The disease symptoms have shown decline
d. The disease is not community health problem
e. There are no new cases

Ans. b, c, d *Ref: Park, 24/e; Suryakanta, 3/e*

Option a	False	No, post elimination sequence, usually will be eradication level
Option b	True	Yes, pre-eradication will be control and elimination
Option c	True	Yes, control literally means – control progression of disease
Option d	True	Yes, correct
Option e	False	No, 'no new cases' essentially is term used for no transmission phase (elimination) or when the pathogen is exterminated (eradication)

	Definition	Disease
Control	It is a stage of low disease occurrence. The control phase is said to have been achieved when the disease transmission exists but at a low level, so that the disease is not a public health problem	Most diseases as tuberculosis, vector borne diseases, blindness

Contd...

Contd...

Elimination	It is the stage of disease control, wherein there is interruption of transmission thus leading to decline in the cases or mere absence of the disease from an area in a defined population. The point of concern is that there will be no new cases, but the pathogen (or the agent) will be existent in the environment.	Yaws, Trachoma (in children) Neonatal tetanus
Eradication	It is the ultimate achievement of the state of 'conquering' the disease. The pathogen(agent) is exterminated and is 'not' existent in the natural environment.	Small pox Wild polio Dracunculosis (from India)

11. Which of the following is/are true about tuberculosis in India:

a. India has approximately ¼ th of Global of TB
b. MDR-TB among notified new pulmonary TB patients is about 5%
c. 5% of TB patients estimated to be HIV positive
d. MDR-TB among retreatment cause is about 15%
e. Incidence is around 2 million new TB cause annually

Ans. a, c, d, e *Ref: Park, 24/e; Suryakanta, 3/e*

Option a	True	
Option b	False	No, MDR-TB in new TB cases 2–3% and 12–17% in re-treatment cases
Option c	True	
Option d	True	MDR-TB among retreatment cases is about 12–17%
Option e	True	As per estimates 2015, incidence if TB cases in India is 2.8 million

India accounts for one fourth of the global TB burden. In 2015, an estimated 28 lakh cases occurred and 4.8 lakh people died due to Tb. The table below shows the estimated figures for TB burden globally and for India reported in WHO Global TB Report for the year 2015.

Estimates of TB Burden (2015)	Global	India
Incidence TB cases	104 lakh	28 lakh
Mortality of TB	14 lakh	4.8 lakh
Incidence HIV TB	11.7 lakh	1.1 lakh
Mortality of HIV-TB	3.9 lakh	37,000
MDR-TB	4.8 lakh	1.3 lakh

India bears second highest number of estimated HIV associated TB in the world.

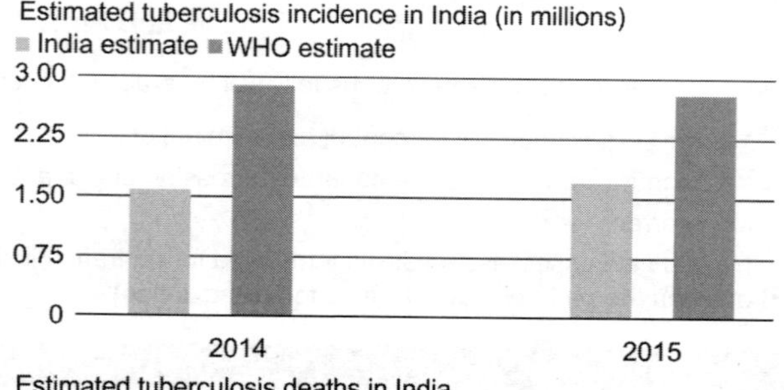

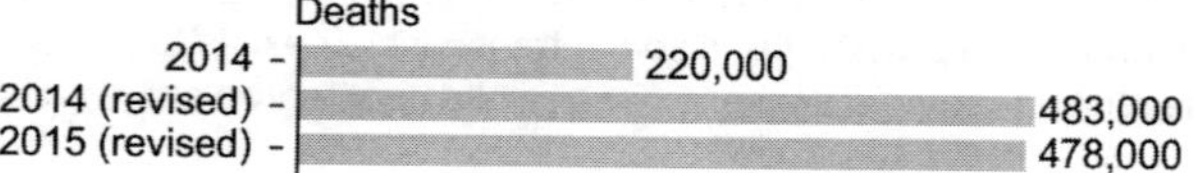

12. True about milk pasteurization is/are:

a. Phosphatase test
b. Nitric acid test
c. Coliform count
d. Methylene blue reductase test
e. Solid non-fat

Ans. a, c *Ref: Park, 24/e; Suryakanta, 3/e*

Option a	True	Yes, used to check for pasteurization
Option b	False	No, it is for checking for adultration of argemone Mexicana for mustard oil
Option c	True	Yes, used to check for pasteurization
Option d	False	No, it is done before pasteurization – to check for gross contamination of milk
Option e	False	No, it is done before pasteurization for assessment of quality of milk

Milk hygiene

In a milk processing plant, the first sequence is usually to check for the quality of the milk, based on which the further payments are made to the milk vendors.

- Milk quality assessed using
  - Lactometer
  - SNF testing – Solid non-fat testing – gives the proportion of the solid non-fat in milk (which might act as adulterant to increase the viscosity of the milk)
- Gross contamination of milk – using Methylene blue reductase test (MBRT)
- Pasteurization of milk

Methods of pasteurization:

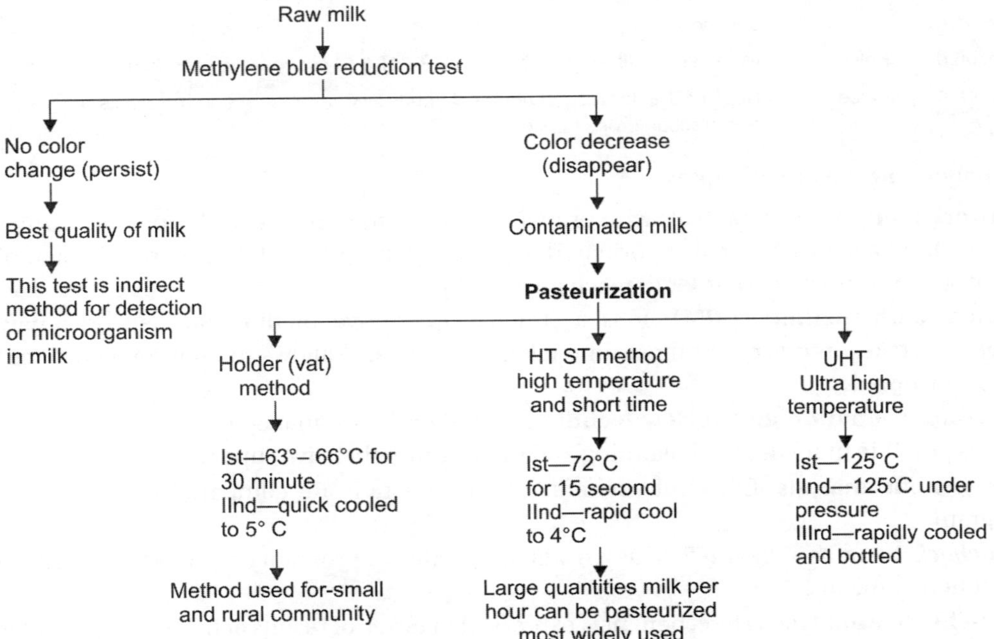

- Methods to assess for pasteurization
  - *Phosphatase test*: Phosphatase enzyme is destroyed by heating; hence the presence of phosphatase enzyme indicates a non-pasteurized milk

- *Coliform count*: Coliform in the milk should ideally be zero. Coliform counts >100 cfu/mL suggest poor milking practices, dirty equipment, contaminated water, dirty milking facilities, and/or cows with subclinical or clinical coliform mastitis.
- *Standard plate count (SPC)*: The SPC is used to monitor progress since consistent application of proper milking system cleaning practices, proper milking practices, udder hygiene and good mastitis prevention and control practices should allow dairy producers to produce milk with a low SPC, which is less than 5,000 colony forming units (cfu)of bacteria per milliliter.
- *Enzyme alkaline phosphatase (ALP) levels*: Should be less than 350 mIU/L. The presence of ALP activity above this level indicates a failure and may be due to either inadequate pasteurization or post pasteurization contamination with raw milk.

13. Regarding PERT and CPM, true statement is:

a. Repeated activities are best monitored by PERT
b. Small activities are divided into small milestones in PERT
c. CPM uses deterministic model rather than probabilistic model
d. Main objective is lowest time and cost in CPM
e. PERT is mainly used for non-research projects

Ans. b, c *Ref: Park, 24/e; Suryakanta, 3/e*

Option a	False	No, repeated activities are best monitored by CPM
Option b	True	Yes, correct
Option c	True	Yes, correct
Option d	False	No, cost and time optimization for PERT and cost optimization for CPM
Option e	False	No, PERT is for research projects and CPM for non-research projects as construction projects, etc.

Management: Basic principles

Network analysis: Branch deals with proper planning, drafting, testing, implementation and execution of a series of activities oriented towards a common goal. It is a graphic plan of all events to be completed in order to reach an end objective.

Critical path method (CPM): It is a strategic quantitive method for network analysis. ***Keyword***: takes into account most time taking activity and allows to analyze activity as per time consumed.

Program evaluation and review technique (PERT): It is a management technique which makes possible more detailed planning and more comprehensive supervision.

Cost-benefit analysis: Economic benefits of any program are compared with cost of that program.

Drawback: Benefits in health field as a result of a particular program can't always be expressed in monetary means.

Cost-effective analysis: Here, benefit is expressed in terms of results achieved, e.g. no. of lives saved and no. of days free from disease.

Planning programming budgeting system (PPBS): It calls for grouping of activities into programs related to each objective, so as to help decision makers to allocate resources efficiently.

Zero budget approach: Starting from a Zero Base of no funds for a program, every rupee is sanctioned, even for ongoing program.

The most important differences between PERT and CPM are provided below:

- PERT is a project management technique, whereby planning, scheduling, organizing, coordinating and controlling of uncertain activities is done. CPM is a statistical technique of project management in which planning, scheduling, organizing, coordination and control of well-defined activities takes place.
- PERT is a technique of planning and control of time. Unlike CPM, which is a method to control costs and time.
- While PERT is evolved as research and development project, CPM evolved as construction project.
- PERT is set according to events while CPM is aligned towards activities.
- A deterministic model is used in CPM. Conversely, PERT uses probabilistic model.
- PERT technique is best suited for a high precision time estimate, whereas CPM is appropriate for a reasonable time estimate.
- PERT deals with unpredictable activities, but CPM deals with predictable activities.
- PERT is used where the nature of the job is non-repetitive. In contrast to, CPM involves the job of repetitive nature.
- There is a demarcation between critical and non-critical activities in CPM, which is not in the case of PERT.
- PERT is best for research and development projects, but CPM is for non-research projects like construction projects.
- Crashing is a compression technique applied to CPM, to shorten the project duration, along with least additional cost. The crashing concept is not applicable to PERT.

Basis for comparison	PERT	CPM
Meaning	PERT is a project management technique, used to manage uncertain activities of a project.	CPM is a statistical technique of project management that manages well defined activities of project.
What is it?	A technique of planning and control of time.	A method to control cost and time.
Orientation	Event-oriented	Activity-oriented
Evolution	Evolved as Research and Development project	Evolved as construction project
Model	Probabilistic model	Deterministic model
Focuses on	Time	Time-cost trade-off
Estimates	Three time estimates	One time estimate
Appropriate for	High precision time estimate	Reasonable time estimate
Management of	Unpredictable activities	Predictable activities
Nature of jobs	Non-repetitive nature	Repetitive nature
Critical and non-critical activities	No differentiation	Differentiated

14. True statement for dengue is:

a. Dengue vector in India is *Aedes albopictus*
b. Recurrent infection IgG is found

c. The vaccine used is live virus vectored tetravalent vaccine
d. Dengue vaccine is approved for three dose schedule
e. Neutralization test will rule out other viral infections

Ans. a, b, c, e *Ref: Park, 24/e; Suryakanta, 3/e*

Option a	True	Yes correct
Option b	True	Yes correct
Option c	True	Yes correct
Option d	False	No, it is a three dose vaccine series
Option e	True	Yes correct

Recombinant subunit vaccine	P64K of *Neisseria meningitidis* as fusion protein
DNA vaccine	Tetravalent DNA vaccine
VLP vaccine	
Virus vectored vaccine (CYD/TDV)	Tetravalent chimeric EDIII fusion protein from a replication-deficient adenovirus vaccine vector

Dengue vector:

Aedes albopictus is a small, dark mosquito with a white dorsal stripe and banded legs.
- They are strongly attracted to bite humans, but will feed on cats, dogs, squirrels, deer and other mammals, as well as birds. They will bite any exposed skin surface. They bite outdoors and indoors, but are usually found outside.
- These mosquitoes can use natural locations or habitats (for example treeholes and plants) and artificial containers with water to lay their eggs.

Aedes aegypti is a small, dark mosquito with white lyre shaped markings and banded legs.
- They prefer to bite indoors and primarily bite humans.
- These mosquitoes can use natural locations or habitats (for example treeholes and plant axils) and artificial containers with water to lay their eggs. They lay eggs during the day in water containing organic material (e.g., decaying leaves, algae, etc.) in containers with wide openings and prefer dark-colored containers located in the shade.

Diagnosis of dengue:
- Isolation of the dengue virus from serum, plasma, leukocytes, or autopsy samples.
- Demonstration of a fourfold or greater change in reciprocal immunoglobulin G (IgG) or IgM antibody titers to 1 or more dengue virus antigens in paired serum samples.
  - IgM antibodies are produced first and tests for these are most effective when performed at least 7–10 days after exposure. Levels in the blood rise for a few weeks, then gradually decrease. After a few months, IgM antibodies fall below detectable levels.
  - IgG antibodies are produced more slowly in response to an infection. Typically, the level rises with an acute infection, stabilizes, and then persists long-term. Individuals who have been exposed to the virus prior to the current infection maintain a level of IgG antibodies in the blood that can affect the interpretation of diagnostic results.
- Demonstration of dengue virus antigen in autopsy tissue via immunohistochemistry or immunofluorescence or in serum samples via enzyme immunoassay (EIA).
- Detection of viral genomic sequences in autopsy tissue, serum, or cerebral spinal fluid (CSF) samples via polymerase chain reaction (PCR) assay.

Interpretation of antibody result

IgM Result	IgG Result	Possible interpretation
Positive	Negative	Current infection
Positive	Positive	Current infection
Low or negative or not tested	Four-fold increase in samples taken 2–4 weeks apart	Recent infection
Low or negative	Positive	Past infection
Negative	Negative	Too soon after initial exposure for antibodies to develop or symptoms due to another cause

Positive IgM and IgG tests for dengue antibodies detected in an initial blood sample mean that it is likely that the person became infected with dengue virus within recent weeks. IgM antibody tests can be positive if a person has been infected with a similar virus, such as chikungunya (called cross-reaction). If an initial IgM antibody test is positive, a second test called the Plaque Reduction Neutralization Test (PRNT) is used to confirm the presence of antibodies to dengue virus and to help rule out other viral infections.

Dengue vaccine:

The first dengue vaccine, Dengvaxia (CYD-TDV) by Sanofi Pasteur, was first registered in Mexico in December, 2015. CYD-TDV is a live recombinant tetravalent dengue vaccine that has been evaluated as a 3-dose series on a 0/6/12 month schedule in Phase III clinical studies. It has been registered for use in individuals 9-45 years of age living in endemic areas.

15. True about Vision 2020 is/are:

a. Opthalmia neonatorum is eliminated
b. Retinal surgery at tertiary center
c. Cataract surgery at primary center
d. Training centers are 100 in number
e. Corneal transplant is done at training centers

Ans. b, e *Ref: Park, 24/e; Suryakanta, 3/e*

Option a	False	No, it is still prevalent in few areas
Option b	True	Yes correct
Option c	False	No, basic eye care and refractive error correction at primary level
Option d	False	No, the training centers are proposed to be 200 in number in India.
Option e	True	Yes correct

- Ophthalmia neonatorum remains a significant cause of ocular morbidity, blindness and even death in underdeveloped countries.
- The organisms causing ophthalmia neonatorum are acquired mainly from the mother's birth canal during delivery and a small percentage of cases are acquired by other ways.
- *Chlamydia* and *Neisseria* are the most common pathogens responsible for the perinatal infection.
- Fortunately in most cases, laboratory studies can identify the causative organism and unlike other form of conjunctivitis, this perinatal ocular infection has to be treated with systemic antibiotics to prevent systemic colonization of the organism.

- Routine prophylaxis with 1% silver nitrate solution (Crédés method) has been discontinued in many developed nations for the fear of development of chemical conjunctivitis.
- Ophthalmia neonatorum is still a significant cause of ocular morbidity in both developing and underdeveloped countries.

Treatment for:

- Ophthalmia neonatorum due to *N. gonorrhoea*
  - Intravenous Penicillin G 100,000 Units /kg/day for 1 week
  - A single dose of ceftriaxone 50 mg/kg as s single dose (maximum 125 mg) is highly effective and recommended by WHO guidelines
- Ophthalmia neonatorum due to *Chlamydia trachomatis*
  - Oral erythromycin syrup, 50 mg/kg/day, in 4 divided doses for 14 days
  - Adjunct therapy: Topical erythromycin
- Ophthalmia neonatorum due to Herpes simplex
  - Low dose systemic acyclovir (30 mg/kg/day IV divided tid) for 2 weeks or
  - Vidarabine (30 mg/kg/day in divided doses IV) for at least 2 weeks

Diseases under India vision 2020:

- Cataract
- Refractive errors
- Diabetic retinopathy
- Age related macular degeneration
- Childhood blindness—nutritional blindness
- Trachoma
- Glaucoma
- Diabetic retinopathy

16. Which of the following can be autoclaved?

a. Plastic
b. Glass
c. Non-stainless steel
d. Fibroscope
e. Polyurethene

Ans. a, b, d *Ref: Suryakanta, p100, 3/e*

Option a	True	
Option b	True	
Option c	False	
Option d	True	
Option e	False	

- Autoclaves provide a physical method for disinfection and sterilization.
- They work with a combination of steam, pressure and time. Autoclaves operate at high temperature and pressure in order to kill microorganisms and spores.
- They are used to decontaminate certain biological waste and sterilize media, instruments and lab ware.
- Regulated medical waste that might contain bacteria, viruses and other biological material are recommended to be inactivated by autoclaving before disposal.

There are two basic techniques for sterilizing solutions: *Autoclaving* and *sterile filtration.*

Compatible/incompatible materials	
Autoclave: Compatible materials	***Autoclave: Incompatible materials***
• Tissue culture flasks • Surgical instruments • Glassware • Pipette tips • Media solutions • Animal food and bedding • Waste • Polypropylene (Secondary containers) • Stainless steel • Gloves	• Acids, bases and organic solvent • Chlorides, sulphates • Seawater • Chlorine, hypochlorite, bleach • Non-stainless steel • Polystyrene (PS) • Polyethylene (PE) • Low density (LDPE) and high density polyethylene (HDPE) • Polyurethane

Never autoclave:

- Flammable, reactive, corrosive, toxic or radioactive materials
- Household bleach
- Any liquid in a sealed container
- Any material contained in such a manner that it touches the interior surfaces of the autoclave
- Paraffin-embedded tissue.

17. Zika virus:

a. Ocular
b. Vertical transmission
c. Flavivirus
d. High mortality
e. Requires hospitalization

Ans. a, b, c *Ref: https://www.cdc.gov/zika*

Option		
Option a	True	Conjunctivitis
Option b	True	Yes, vertical transmission occurs
Option c	True	Yes, spread by Aedes mosquito
Option d	False	Mild infection in adults
Option e	False	Symptomatic management

- Zika virus (ZIKV) is a member of the virus family Flaviviridae.
- It is spread by daytime-active *Aedes* mosquitoes, such as a. aegypti and a. albopictus.
- Infection often causes no or only mild symptoms, similar to a very mild form of dengue fever. Patients can have symptoms including mild fever, skin rash, conjunctivitis, muscle and joint pain, malaise or headache. These symptoms normally last for 2–7 days.
- It can spread by vertical (or "mother-to-child") transmission, during pregnancy or at delivery, microcephaly +/– neurological complaints can be seen in the newborn.
- Can trigger Gullian-Barre syndrome
- Management—symptomatic. Paracetamol and rest may help with the symptoms.

18. Scrub typhus, true is:

a. Lice as vector
b. Truncal rash
c. Eschar
d. Ciprofloxacin
e. Incubation period is 2-7 days

Ans. b, c, e *Ref: Park, 24/e; Suryakanta, 3/e*

Option a	False	No, it is transmitted by mite
Option b	True	Yes, the macular rash is on trunk on 5–8th day
Option c	True	Yes, correct
Option d	False	No, tetracycline is the drug of choice
Option e	True	Yes, correct

Scrub typhus

- Scrub typhus is transmitted to humans and rodents by some species of trombiculid mites ("chiggers", Lepto-trombidium deliense and others).
- The mite is very small (0.2–0.4 mm) and can only be seen through a microscope or magnifying glass.
- Scrub typhus is an acute, febrile, infectious illness that is caused by *Orientia* (formerly *Rickettsia*) *tsutsugamushi.*
- The incubation period of scrub typhus is about 5 to 20 days (mean, 10–12 days) after the initial bite
- Bite—painless, usually on groin, genitalia or neck - leading to scab (eschar) formation.
- Headache, malaise, prostration and a macular rash appearing around the 5th day of illness. Generalized lymphadenopathy and lymphocytosis are common.
- A macular rash develops on the trunk during the 5th to 8th day of fever, often extending to the arms and legs. It may disappear rapidly or become maculopapular and intensely colored.
- Cough is present during the 1st week of fever, and pneumonitis may develop during the 2nd week.
- Weilfelix reaction is strongly positive with *Proteus* strain OXK.
- Tetracycline is the drug of choice. Dose 500 mg three times a day for 1 week.
- Vector control:
  - Insecticide—lindane
  - Mite repellent—diethyltoulamide
  - Miticial chemical—benzyl benzoate.

Bite of mite:

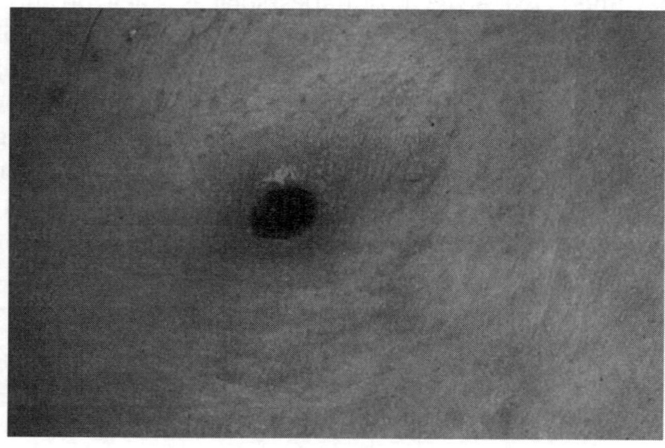

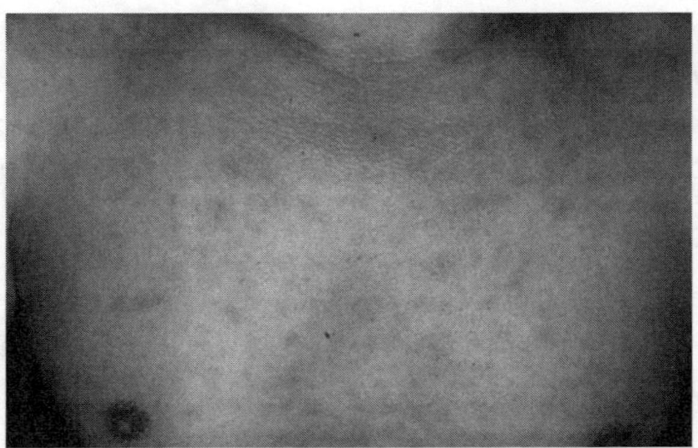

Courtesy: Yoshiki Taniguchi, Md. From Taniguchi, Y: Eschar, fever, and rash in a 43-year-old man. Dermatology Online Journal 3(2), 1997.

19. Which of the following spread through aquatic vegetation?

a. *Watsonius watsoni*
b. *Fascioli psisbuski*
c. *Schistosoma haematobium*
d. *Fasciola hepatica*
e. *Ascaris lumbricoides*

Ans. a, b, d *Ref: Park, 24/e; Suryakanta, 3/e*

Option a	True	Yes, correct.
Option b	True	Yes, correct.
Option c	False	No, it is spread by contact with water
Option d	True	Yes, correct.
Option e	False	No, it is spread by contact with infected faeces.

Discuss:

1. *Watsonius watsoni:* Infection occurs through ingestion of contaminated vegetables and raw meat, in which the viable infective metacercaria are deposited from snails, which are the intermediate hosts.
2. *Fascioli psisbuski:* The trematode *Fasciolopsis buski,* the largest intestinal fluke of humans. The mammalian hosts become infected by ingesting metacercariae (from snails) on the aquatic plants. After ingestion, the metacercariae excyst in the duodenum and attach to the intestinal wall, which later develop into adult flukes in 3 months.
3. *Schistosoma haematobium:* Human contact with water is thus necessary for infection by schistosomes. Various animals, such as dogs, cats, rodents, pigs, horse and goats, serve as reservoirs for *S. japonicum*, and dogs for *S. mekongi.*
4. *Fasciola hepatica:* In humans, maturation from **metacercariae** into **adult flukes** takes approximately 3 to 4 months. The adult flukes (*Fasciola hepatica*: up to 30 mm by 13 mm; *F. gigantica*: up to 75 mm) reside in the large biliary ducts of the mammalian host. *Fasciola hepatica* infect various animal species, mostly herbivores (plant-eating animals).
5. *Ascaris lumbricoides:* Most common helminthic infection. Man is the only reservoir. Feces containing the fertilized eggs is the infective material.

Extra Edge:

Life cycle of *Fasciola hepatica*

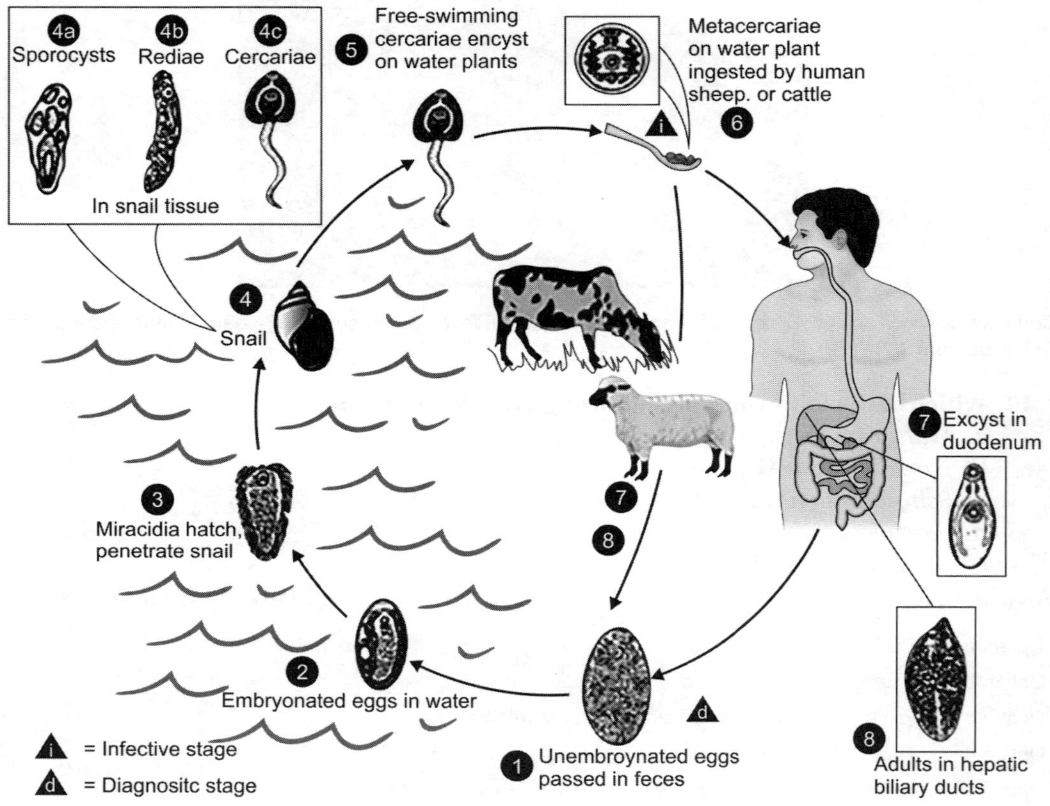

20. Which of the following content is/are more in human milk than cow's milk?

a. Protein
b. Iron
c. Carbohydrate
d. Fat
e. Vitamin C

Ans. c, e *Ref: Park, 24/e; Suryakanta, 3/e*

Option a	False	No, not correct
Option b	False	No, not correct
Option c	True	Yes, correct
Option d	False	No, not correct
Option e	True	Yes, correct

Nutritive value of various milk sources:

		Buffalo	Cow	Goat	Human
Fat	(g)	6.5	4.1	4.5	3.4
Protein	(g)	4.3	3.2	3.3	1.1

Contd...

Contd...

Lactose	(g)	5.1	4.4	4.6	7.4
Calcium	(mg)	210	120	170	28
Iron	(mg)	0.2	0.2	0.3	
Vitamin C	(mg)	1	2	1	3
Minerals	(g)	0.8	0.8	0.8	0.1
Water	(g)	81.0	87	86.8	88
Energy	(kcal)	117	67	72	65

Extra Edge:

Human milk:

- Higher amount of tryptophan and sulphur containing amino acids (cysteine)
- Higher amount of linolenic acid, oleic acid and docosahexaenoic acid (DHA)
- Good amount of vitamin A and vitamin D
- Higher amount of sugar (lactose)
- Higher amount of vitamin C

Toned milk:

It contains 1 part of water, 1 part of natural milk and 1/8 part of skimmed powder.

21. True about rabies is/are:

a. In category I wounds, treatment is given
b. In category II, immunoglobulins are given along with treatment of the wound.
c. In a previously immunized patient, immunoglobulins are not given.
d. If a person reports after 3 days of animal bite, immunoglobulins are not given
e. Modified Thai schedule is intradermal injections

Ans. c, e *Ref: Suryakanta, 496, 3/e; CDC guidelines; Park, 24/e*

Option a	False	No, no treatment required
Option b	False	No, no immunoglobulin required in category II bite
Option c	True	Yes, it is not required due to anamnestic response
Option d	False	No, rabies immunoglobulin (RIG) is given irrespective of time, in all cat III bites
Option e	True	Yes, correct

Administration of antirabies immunoglobulin	
Equine	***Human***
Dose: 40 IU/kg body weight max 3000 IU 1 mL contains 300 IU, i.e. max 10 mL	Dose: 20 IU/kg body weight max 1500 IU 1 mL contains 150 IU, i.e. max 10 mL
• After hypersensitivity testing as much as possible of the serum is administered locally, i.e. at the site of bite, rest of it IM in gluteal region • Given within 7 days of starting the vaccination • If patient is sensitive, 1st dose of vaccine is doubled. This is not a substitute for anti-rabies serum (ARS).	

Categories of contact and recommended post-exposure prophylaxis (PEP)	
Categories of contact with suspect rabid animal	***Post-exposure prophylaxis measures***
Category I—touching or feeding animals, licks on intact skin	None

Contd...

Contd...

Category II—nibbling of uncovered skin, minor scratches or abrasions without bleeding	Immediate vaccination and local treatment of the wound
Category III—single or multiple transdermal bites or scratches, licks on broken skin; contamination of mucous membrane with saliva from licks, contacts with bats	Immediate vaccination and administration of rabies immunoglobulin; local treatment of the wound

Rabies vaccine schedule

- Essen regimen: The 5-dose regimen prescribes 1 dose on each of days 0, 3, 7, 14, and 28; as shown below.

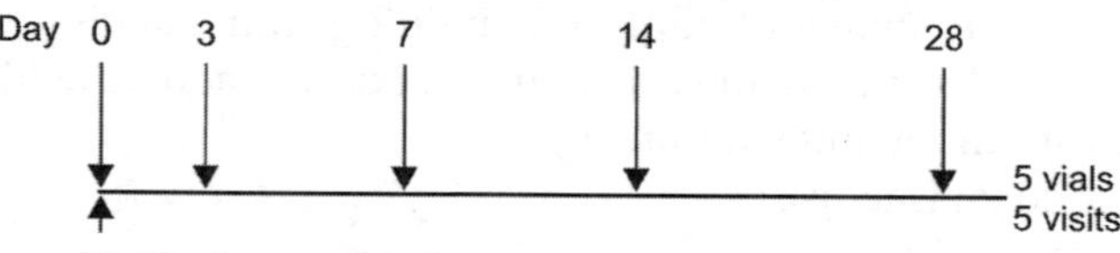

- Zagreb regimen: The 4-dose abbreviated multisite regimen prescribes 2 doses on day 0 (1 in each of the 2 deltoid or thigh sites) followed by 1 dose on each of days 7 and 21, as shown below.

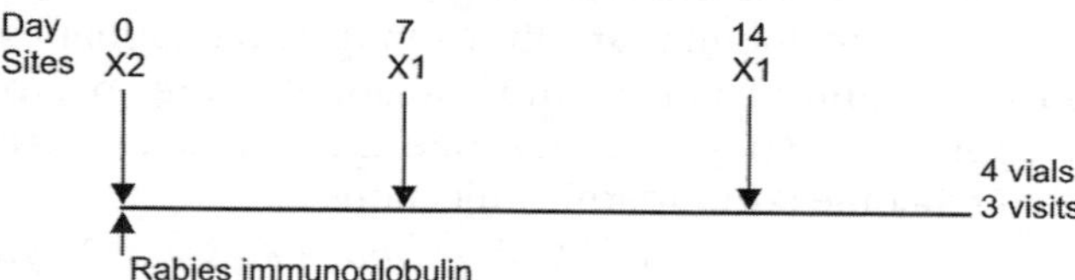

- Modified Thai red cross schedule

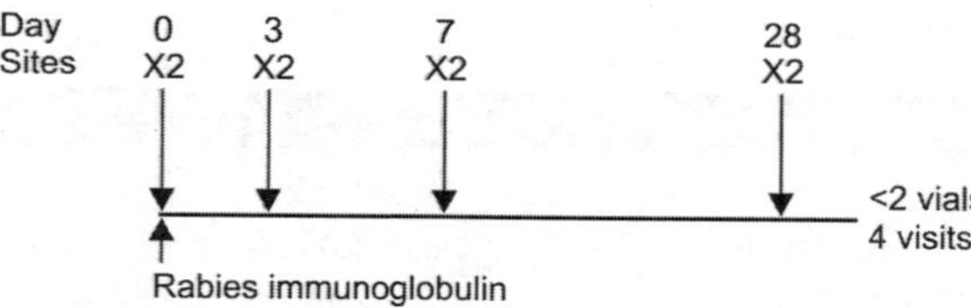

- Oxford intradermal schedule
  8 + 0 + 4 + 0 + 1 + 1

This is recommended with HDCV or PCEC—vaccine and not PVR- Vaccine.

- **Day 0**—eight doses, each of 0.1 mL given intradermal, at eight different sites, simultaneously, over both deltoid, both lateral thigh, both suprascapular region and both lower quadrant of the abdomen.
- **Day 3**—nil.
- **Day 7**—4 doses, each of 0.1 mL given intradermal, at four sites, over both deltoid and both thighs.

- ❑ **Day 14**: Nil
- ❑ **Day 28 and 30**: one dose, 0.1 mL is given intradermal, at one site over deltoid region. 4 visits ;<2 vials
- ❑ **Remember:** HDCV is the WHO Gold standard vaccine

There are two types of rabies immunoglobulin (RIG):

- ❑ Equine rabies immunoglobulin (ERIG)/ARS (Equine origin)
  - ▪ Dose 40 IU/kg body weight
- ❑ Human rabies immunoglobulin (hRIG) (Human origin)
  - ▪ Dose 20 IU/kg body weight

It is a usual practice to instil the RIG into the depth of wound and infiltrate near the wound. The remaining half should be given IM to gluteal region.

RIG/ARS is known to have local viricidal/neutralizing effect and prevents the virus from entering the susceptible nerve cells. The use of RIG is life saving and failure to use RIG amounts to dereliction of duty under Consumer Protection Act. Hence RIG should be given irrespective of the delay in seeking treatment.

However, in case of exposure to a vaccinated individual, the RIG is not required as it shows a anamnestic response.

Anamnestic response: The first contact with any antigen sensitize individual affected and promote the primary immune response. Next of the sensitized individuals with same antigen result in a more rapid and massive reaction, called the secondary immune response or a booster response" or the "anamnestic reaction".

22. True about ebola is/are:

a. Transmitted through aerosol
b. Hemorrhagic manifestations show poor prognosis
c. Cough and upper respiratory symptoms are common
d. Transmitted by fluids
e. Encephalitis is a feature

Ans. b, c, d *Ref: http://www.who.int/mediacentre/factsheets/fs103/en/;https://www.cdc.gov/vhf/ebola/about.html; Ref: Park, 24/e; Suryakanta, 3/e*

Option a	False	No, it is uncommon to be spread via air or droplet infections
Option b	True	Yes, correct
Option c	True	Yes, correct
Option d	True	Yes, correct
Option e	False	No, it is rare or may be associated with severe complicated Ebola infections

Ebola is an acute, serious illness which can be fatal, if untreated. Within the genus Ebolavirus, five species have been identified: Zaire, Bundibugyo, Sudan, Reston and Taï Forest

Ebola—Extra Edge

- ❑ **Mode of transmission**

  People get Ebola through direct contact (through broken skin or mucous membranes in, for example, the eyes, nose, or mouth) with

  - ▪ Blood or body fluids (including but not limited to urine, saliva, sweat, feces, vomit, breast milk, and semen) of a person who is sick with or has died from Ebola,

- Objects (like needles and syringes) that have been contaminated with body fluids from a person who is sick with Ebola or the body of a person who has died from Ebola,
- Infected fruit bats or primates (apes and monkeys), and
- Possibly from contact with semen from a man who has recovered from Ebola (for example, by having oral, vaginal, or anal sex).

❑ **Clinical picture**
- Incubation period 2–20 days
- The person is 'non-infective' during the incubation period
- General symptoms are earliest and most common - fever, myalgia, sore throat
- Followed by vomiting, diarrhea and rash
- Renal, hepatic impairment, hemorrhagic manifestations could be the sequel leading to fatality

❑ **Diagnostics:**
- Antibody-capture enzyme-linked immunosorbent assay (ELISA)
- Antigen-capture detection tests
- Serum neutralization test
- Reverse transcriptase polymerase chain reaction (RT-PCR) assay
- Electron microscopy
- Virus isolation by cell culture.

❑ **WHO recommended:**
- Nucleic acid test (NAT)
- Rapid antigen detection using ELISA
  Recommended sample:
- Whole blood in EDTA
- Oral fluid specimen

Treatment—symptomatic:

❑ **Prevention**
- Vaccine - rVSV-ZEBOV (trial vaccine)
- Risk reduction measures:
  - Wildlife to human transmission
  - Human to human transmission
  - Sexual transmission

23. PHC covers a population of:

a. 30,000 in plains
b. 30,000 in hilly area
c. 20,000 in hilly area
d. 20,000 in plains
e. 20,000 in tribal areas

Ans. a, c, e *Ref: Park, 24/e; Suryakanta, 3/e*

Option a	True	Yes, correct
Option b	False	No, it is incorrect
Option c	True	Yes, correct
Option d	False	No, it is incorrect
Option e	True	Yes, correct

The health care infrastructure in rural areas has been developed as a three tier system and is based on the following population norms:

Center	Population norms	
	Plain area	Hilly/tribal/difficult area
Sub-Center	5000	3000
Primary Health Center	30,000	20,000
Community Health Center	1,20,000	80,000

PHC is the first contact point between village community and the Medical Officer.

PHC—Extra edge

- The PHC Standards have been revised as follows:
  - PHC in hilly, tribal or difficult areas to be for 20,000 population
  - In plain areas, the PHC will be for 30,000 population
  - In urban areas, under the revised NHM plan, 1 (urban) PHC for 50,000 population.
  - Upgradation of block level PHC to a CHC
- PHC may further be of two types:
  - Type A PHC—PHC with < 20 deliveries per month
  - Type B PHC—PHC with more than 20 deliveries per month

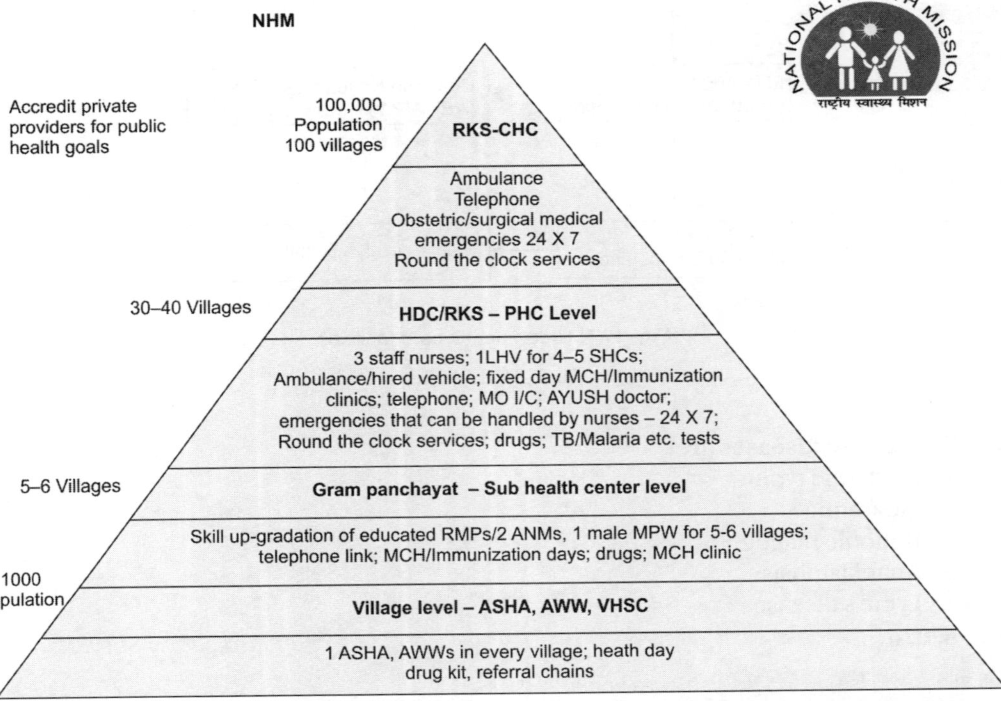

RKS: Rogi Kalyan Samiti; CHC: Community Health center; PHC: Primary Health center; SHC: Sub Health center; LHV: Lady Health Visitor; RMP: Rural/Registered Medical Practitioner; ASHA: Accredited social health activist; AWW: Anganwadi worker; AYUSH: Ayurveda, yoga and naturopathy, unani, siddha and homoeopathy; YHSC: Village Health and sanitation committee; MO(I/C): Medical officer In-charge; MPW: Multipurpose worker; MCH: Maternal and child health services; ANM: Auxiliary nurse midwife; HDC: Hospital development committee.

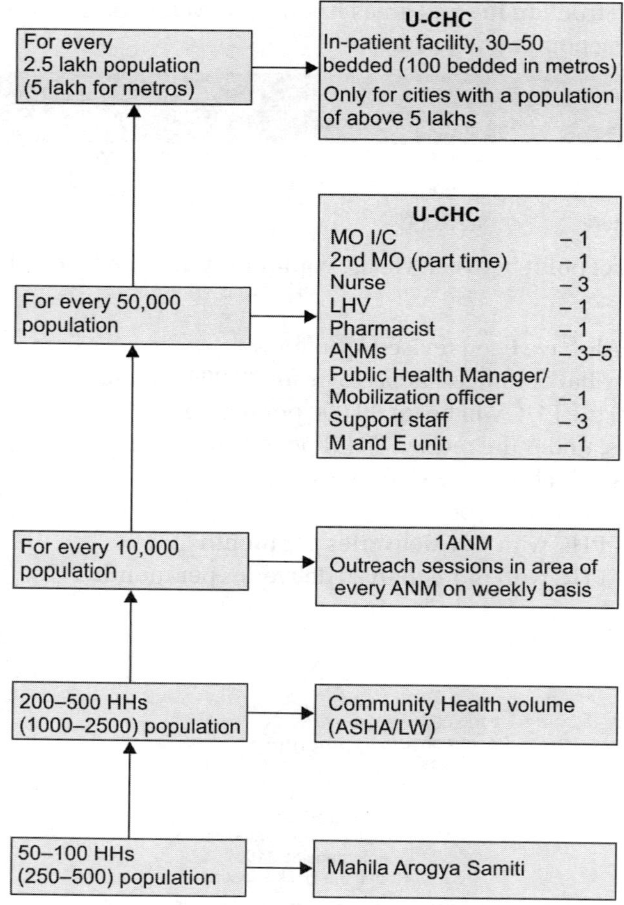

Fig. 11.4: Urban health care facilities.

HHS: Households

24. Tick borne diseases are:

a. Epidemic typhus
b. Tularemia
c. Bubonic plague
d. Anaplasmosis
e. Lyme's disease

Ans. b, d, e *Ref: Park, 24/e; Suryakanta, 3/e*

Option a	False	No, it is louse borne
Option b	True	Yes, correct
Option c	False	No, the vector is rat flea—Xenopsylla cheopis
Option d	True	Yes, correct
Option e	True	Yes, correct

Hard ticks	Soft ticks
• They belong to the family ixodidae.	• The belong to the family Argasidae.
• Capitulum is anterior in position.	• Capitulum is ventral in position.
• Scutum is present.	• Scutum is absent.
• Dorsally sexual dimorphism is well marked, i.e. scutum covers the entire dorsal surface in male and covers only a small portion in the female.	• Sexual dimorphism is absent dorsally.
• Spiracles exist behind the fourth pair of legs.	• Spiracles exist between the third and the fourth pair of legs.
• Festoons are present in some hard ticks.	• Festoons are absent.
• They cannot resist starvation. So they are always found on the body of the host (Day and night) (like lice).	• They can resist starvation for months. Therefore they are found on the body of the host only while feeding blood (i.e. only during night times) (like bedbugs).
• They require continuous blood meal.	• They require intermittent blod meal.
• They are always found on the body of their hosts.	• They are found in cracks and crevices during day time and on the body of the host during night times.
• Gravid female lays hundreds or thousands of eggs at one sitting.	• Eggs are laid in batches of 2–100 over a long period of time.
• Nymphal stage is one.	• Nymphal stages are five.
• Important species are *Dermacentor andersoni, Haemophysalis spinegera.*	• Important specimen is *Ornithodoros moubata.*
• Diseases transmitted are Tick typhus, (Africa) Tick paralysis, Tularemia, Viral encephalitis, Hemorrhagic fever (KFD), Human babesiosis. Rocky Mountain Spotted fever (USA), Q-fever (in US and Australia).	• Disease transmitted is Endemic Relapsing fever, caused by *Borrelia duttoni*, a spirochete.

Causative agent	Disease	Vector
Virus	Yellow fever, Dengue fever Dengue hemorrhagic fever Chickungunya, West-Nile fever Japanese encephalitis Phlebotomus fever Kyasanur Forest disease	Mosquito Mosquito Mosquito Mosquito Sandfly Hard tick
Rickettsiae	Epidemic typhus, trench fever Endemic (murine) typhus tick typhus Q-fever Rocky mountain spotted fever Rickettsial pox, scrub typhus	Louse Rat flea Tick Tick Mite
Bacteriae	Typhoid, cholera, Shigellosis, plague	Housefly Rat flea
Spirocheta	Relapsing fever	Louse
Protozoa	Malaria Leishmaniasis African trypanosomiasis Chaga's disease	Mosquito Sandfly Tsetse fly Reduviid bug
Nematoda	Filariasis Dracunculiasis Onchocerciasis	Mosquito Cyclops Black fly

Lyme disease is caused by the bacterium *Borrelia burgdorferi* and is transmitted to humans through the bite of infected blacklegged ticks.

Clinical picture:

- Typical symptoms include fever, headache, fatigue, and a characteristic skin rash called erythema migrans.
- If left untreated, infection can spread to joints, the heart, and the nervous system.

Anaplasmosis is a disease caused by the bacterium *Anaplasma phagocytophilum*. This pathogen is transmitted to humans by the bite of an infected tick.

Clinical picture:

- The first symptoms of anaplasmosis typically begin within 1–2 weeks after the bite of an infected tick
- Fever, myalgia, arthralgia, severe headache
- Severe clinical presentations may include difficulty breathing, hemorrhage, renal failure or neurological problems.

25. Period of communicability in measles is:

a. 2 days before and 7 days after the rash
b. 6 weeks after rash
c. 3 months after rash
d. 4 days before rash, 4 days after rash
e. 7 days after rash, 7 days after rash

Ans. d *Ref: Park, 24/e; Suryakanta, 3/e*

Option a	False	No, not correct
Option b	False	No, not correct
Option c	False	No, not correct
Option d	True	Yes, correct
Option e	False	No, not correct

Disease/ conditon	Signs/ symptoms	Incubation period	Mode of transmission	Period of communicability	Exclusion/ attendance	Prevention
Measles (R)	Fever, runny nose, cough, rash by 3rd day	10–14 days (varies 7–18 days)	Contact with respiratory droplets	4 days before rash onset to 4 days after rash onset	**Index case:** Excluded until 4 days after rash onset **Contacts:** Contacts who are not immunized excluded until 14 days after last case.	**Vaccine available:** 2 doses of measles containing vaccine (MMR)

Contd...

Contd...

Disease/ conditon	Signs/ symptoms	Incubation period	Mode of transmission	Period of communicability	Exclusion/ attendance	Prevention
Mumps R	Swelling and pain of the parotid gland, fever, mild URI symptoms	12–25 days Average of 18 days	Direct contact with saliva or respiratory droplets	2 days before through 9 days after the onset of parotitis	**Index case:** Exclude for 9 days following the onset of symptoms **Contacts:** Susceptible contacts shall be excluded from the 12–25 days from exposure.	**Vaccine available** 2 doses of mumps containing vaccine, (MMR)
Rubella (German Measles) R	Mild rash illness, significant risk to the fetus	14–17 days	Direct or droplet contact with nose and throat secretions if an infected person	7 days from the appearance of the rash through 4 days afterward	**Index case:** Excluded for 7 days after the onset of the rash **Susceptible contacts:** Students without proof of immunity shall be excluded until 23 days after last reported case	**Vaccine available:** 2 doses of a rubella containing vaccine (MMR)
Varicella R	Fever, fatigue, followed by rash illness that progresses into itchy, fluid-filled blisters	10–21 days	Contact with infectious respiratory secretions	2–5 days prior to the onset of the rash through the stage when the lesions have crusted over (usually 7 days)	**Index case:** Exclude until the vesicles become dry **Susceptible contacts:** Do not exclude	**Vaccine available:** 2 doses of age appropriate varicella vaccine. The vaccine is effective in preventing disease within 5 days of exposure; a varicella-zoster immunoglobin may be given within 3 days of exposure to lessen the severity of disease in those who can not safely receive the vaccine

Contd...

Contd...

Disease/ conditon	Signs/ symptoms	Incubation period	Mode of transmission	Period of communicability	Exclusion/ attendance	Prevention
Pertussis (R)	Initial cough, coryza, eye irritation, leading to a progressive cough that comes in bursts, may be followed by a 'whoop'	Usually 10 days, may vary from 6–20 days	Direct contact with infectious respiratory secretions.	From onset of cough and cold-like illness through 5 days of appropriate antibiotic therapy. If not on antibiotics, 21 days from the onset of the cough/cold-like illness.	**Symptomatic index case:** Exclude for 5 days while receiving appropriate antibiotic therapy. **Symptomatic contact of a confirmed case:** Exclude for 5 days while receiving antibiotic therapy. **Asymptomatic direct contacts:** Do not exclude asymptomatic contacts. They should receive prophylaxis.	**Vaccine available:** Age appropriate vaccination—DTaP, Tdap Antibiotic prophylaxis for direct contacts

Disease	Duration
Chicken pox, herpes zoster	6 days after rash onset, or till crusting develops
Measles	7 days after rash onset
Cholera	48 hours after antibiotic onset
Diphtheria	Till 2 consecutive throat swabs are negative
Salmonella/Shigella	Till 3 consecutive stool cultures are negative
Hepatitis A	3 weeks
Influenza	3 days
Polio	2 weeks in adults and 6 weeks in children
Pertussis	4 weeks
Mumps	Till swelling subsides

26. Due to increased risk of infection, which of the following vaccines is indicated in symptomatic HIV+ve?

a. MMR
b. HPV
c. HiB
d. Influenza
e. Varicella

Ans. b, d *(Ref: 1. https://www.cdc.gov/ncird/index.html; 2. http://www.immunize.org/catg.d/p4041.pdf; 3. Guidelines for Prevention and Management of Common Opportunistic Infections/Malignancies among HIV-Infected Adult and Adolescent. NACO 2007*

Option a	False	Not mandatory, may be given if benefit is more than the risk
Option b	True	Yes, recommended for PLHIV
Option c	False	Not mandatory, may be given if benefit is more than the risk
Option d	True	Yes, given to protect individual and further transmission of the disease
Option e	False	Not mandatory, may be given if benefit is more than the risk

Immunization and Vitamin A Supplementation

HIV-exposed/infected children should be immunized according to the following schedule:

- Live vaccines should be avoided in all severely immune compromised infants (CD4% < 25% or WHO stage 3 and 4).
- Vitamin A supplementation should be as per the national immunization schedule.
- National immunization schedule is as follows:

Immunization chart for children living with HIV

Age	*Vaccines*	*Age*	*Vaccines*
Birth	OPV	9 months	Measles
	BCG		
	Hepatitis B		
6 weeks	OPV	15 months	MMR
	DPT		
	Hepatitis B		
	Hib*		
10 weeks	OPV	18 months	OPV DPT Hib*
	DPT		
	Hepatitis B		
	Hib*		
14 weeks	OPV	4.5–5 years	OPV
	DPT		DPT
	Hepatitis B		
	Hib*		

*Available only at few states

Additional vaccines like varicella, MMR, IPV, Pneumococcal, Hepatitis A—as per IAP schedule. Live vaccines should be avoided in symptomatic children till such a time when there CD4 improves as a response to ART.

WHO currently recommends administering a single dose of BCG vaccine to all infants living in areas where tuberculosis is highly endemic as well as to infants and children at particular risk of exposure to tuberculosis in countries with low endemicity. BCG vaccine is contraindicated in people with impaired immunity, and WHO does not recommend BCG vaccination for children with symptomatic HIV infection.

For PLHIV, the following vaccines are recommended

In general, it is preferable to avoid live-virus vaccines if an alternative inactivated vaccine is available, as in the case of influenza. However, many vaccines are available only as live-virus vaccines, and there are concerns about administration of live, attenuated disease-causing organisms to HIV-infected patients with severe immune-compromised.

HIV +ve and CD4 > 200

- Influenza vaccine each year to protect against seasonal flu
- Tdap vaccine to protect against whooping cough and tetanus
- Pneumococcal vaccine to protect against pneumonia and other pneumococcal diseases
- Meningococcal conjugate vaccine series which protects against meningococcal disease
- Hepatitis B vaccine series to protect against hepatitis B
- HPV vaccine series to protect against human papillomavirus—up to age 26 years
- MMR vaccine to protect against measles, mumps, and rubella if not taken during childhood
- Varicella vaccine to protect against chickenpox if immunity is presumably absent.

HIV +ve and CD4 less than 200

- Influenza vaccine each year to protect against seasonal flu
- Tdap vaccine to protect against whooping cough and tetanus
- Pneumococcal vaccine to protect against pneumonia and other pneumococcal diseases
  - Adults and adolescents with CD4 counts ≤200 cells/mm^3 should be administered a single dose of 23-valent polysaccharide pneumococcal vaccine if they have not received it during the preceding five years.
  - Annual influenza vaccination may also help prevent superinfections.
- Meningococcal conjugate vaccine series which protects against meningococcal disease
- Hepatitis B vaccine series to protect against hepatitis B
- HPV vaccine series to protect against human papillomavirus—up to age 26 years.

27. True about sand fly is/are:

a. Smaller than mosquito
b. Found in overhead tanks
c. Causes chikungunya
d. Does not fly by choice
e. Male never bites

Ans. a, d, e *Ref: Park, 24/e; Suryakanta, 3/e*

Option a	True	Yes, correct
Option b	False	No, they are found in cracks or burrows or furrows
Option c	False	No, chikungunya is a viral disease with Aedes as vector
Option d	True	Yes, correct. It does not fly (by choice or not..!)
Option e	True	Yes, correct

Eggs:

- Breeding place—peridomestic soil
- Torpedo shaped, bigger than mosquito and flies

Larva:

- Live in soil
- Have stigmata—respiratory passage

Adults:

- Sand-fly have wings, but it hops
- Sand-fly are hairy insects and wings are not adapted to flight
- They are endophilic and stay in cracks and furrows in walls or cool damp places
- Predominant night time bitter
- Only females bite and the bite is painful and irritating
- The size is smaller than a mosquito and can pass through a mosquito net

Disease	Vector	Causal organism	Reservoir
	Sandfly borne diseases		
Leishmaniasis			
(a) Visceral (Kala-azar)	*Phlebotomus argentipes*	*Leishmania donovani*	Man/Man made
(b) Cutaneous (oriental sore)	*P. papatasi*	*L. tropica*	Man/Man made
(c) Espundia	*P. sergenti*	Virus	Man/Man made
(d) Sandfly fever	*P. sergenti/P. papatasi*	Virus	Man

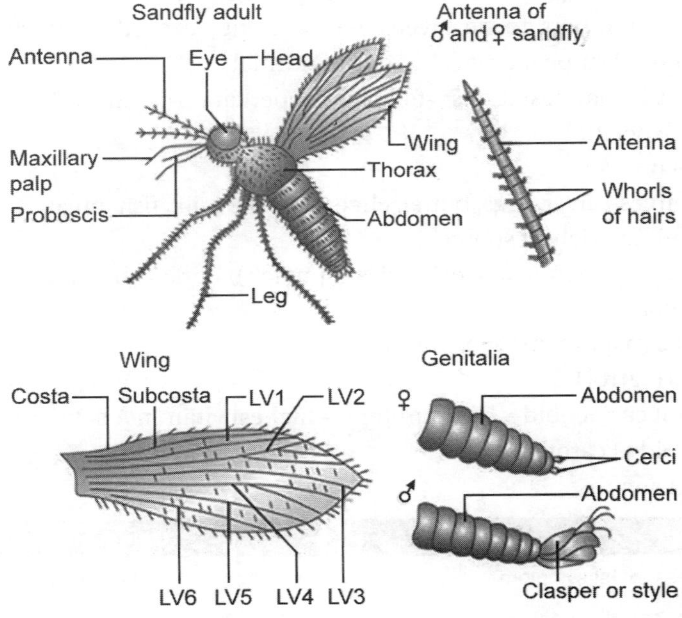

Fig. 11.5: Sandfly

Source: Ratnaswamy GK. A Handbook of Medical Entomology and Elementary Parasitology, 1/e, 1974.

28. Vitamin A toxicity:

a. Orange color skin
b. Palpable liver
c. Papilledema
d. Hypercalcemia
e. Poor vision

Ans. a, b, c, d, e *Ref: Park, 24/e; Suryakanta, 3/e*

Option a	True	Yes, correct
Option b	True	Yes, correct

Option c	True	Yes, correct
Option d	True	Yes, correct
Option e	True	Yes, correct

Recommended dietary allowance

- Requirement
  - Adult—600 mcg/day retinol, i.e. 4800 mcg β carotene, i.e. 2000 IU
  - Lactation—950 mcg per day of retinol, i.e. 7600 mcg β carotene, i.e. 3170 IU
  - Infant—350 mcg per day, i.e. 2800 mcg β carotene, i.e. 1170 IU
  - Pregnancy—800 mcg/day of retinol, i.e. 6400 mcg β carotene or 2666 IU
    - Antenatal mothers to be given vitamin A not exceeding 10,000 IU per day till symptoms disappear or levels come to normal
    - Extraocular manifestations—follicular hyperkeratosis, anorexia, growth retardation (all non-specific)
- Sources of vitamin A
  - Animal sources—liver, eggs, butter, cheese, whole milk, fish, meat
  - Fish liver oils are richest source
  - Plant sources—green leafy vegetables (spinach), darker the green leaves, higher the Vitamin A content
  - Yellow fruits (papaya, mango, pumpkin)
  - Some roots (carrot)
- Most important carotenoid—beta carotene—highest vitamin A activity
  - Rice is devoid of carotene
- Vitamin A deficiency:

Deficiency	Criteria of public health problem
• XN Night Blindness → 1st symptom	> 1%
• X1A Conjunctival. Xerosis → 1st clinical sign	
• X1B Bitot's spot	> 0.5%
• X2 Corneal xerosis	> 0.01%
• X3A Corneal ulcer	> 0.05%
• X3B Keratomalacia	
• XS Corneal scar/X F Fundal changes	
• Serum retinol: Less than 10 mcg/dL in > 5% population (normal value—20 mcg/dL)	

The acute toxic dose of vitamin A is 25,000 IU/kg, and the chronic toxic dose is 4000 IU/kg every day for 6–15 months.

- Symptoms of acute (short-term) toxicity
  - Nausea, headache, fatigue, loss of appetite, dizziness, dry skin, desquamation, and cerebral edema.

- Symptoms of chronic (longer-term) toxicity:
  - Dry itchy and cracking skin, desquamation, dry lips, scaling anorexia, headache, psychiatric changes, cerebral edema, bone and joint pain, osteoporosis, and hip fracture.
  - Papilledema
  - Skin color changes
  - Sleep disorders
- Severe toxicity can lead to eye damage, high levels of calcium, and liver damage.
- In children, signs of toxicity include irritability, drowsiness, dizziness, delirium, coma, vomiting, diarrhea, increased pressure in the brain with bulging fontanelles in infants, headache, swelling of the optic disk, bulging eyeballs, visual disturbances, and skin redness and peeling.
- People with liver disease and high alcohol intake may be at risk for liver toxicity from vitamin A supplementation. Vitamin A toxicity may lead to intrahepatic cholestasis.
- Vitamin A is highly teratogenic in pregnancy, especially in the first 8 weeks with daily intake more than 10,000 IU; however, it is also a cofactor in night vision and bone growth.

Complication after vitamin A toxicity include:

- Hypercalcemia
- Failure to thrive
- Renal failure (secondary to hypercalcemia)
- Hepatic failure

Adverse effects of isotretinoin

Birth defects (when taken during pregnancy), intracranial hypertension, depression, and suicidal ideation have been reported with isotretinoin.

29. True about iron plus initiative:

a. For children <12 years
b. For children >6 months
c. Weekly Fe-FA tablets to all children at Anganwadis
d. Weekly Fe-FA to all school going children
a. Biannual deworming

Ans. a, b, c, e *Ref: Park, 24/e; Suryakanta, 3/e*

Option a	True	Yes, correct
Option b	True	Yes, correct – it is given biweekly age 6–60 months
Option c	True	Yes, correct—biweekly throughout the period 6–60 months of age and de-worming for children 12 months and above.
Option d	False	No, not only to school going children
Option e	True	Yes correct. National deworming day on 10th Feb and 10th August every year

Reproductive, Maternal, Newborn, Child and Adolescent Health (RMNCH + A) guidelines:

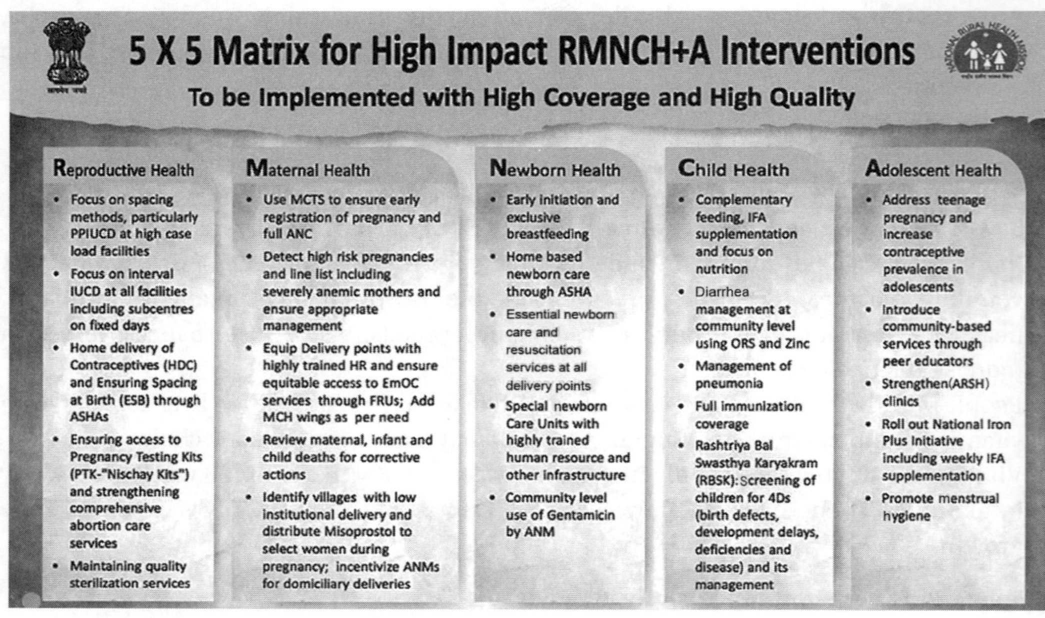

5 X 5 Matrix for High Impact RMNCH+A Interventions

To be Implemented with High Coverage and High Quality

Reproductive Health
- Focus on spacing methods, particularly PPIUCD at high case load facilities
- Focus on interval IUCD at all facilities including subcentres on fixed days
- Home delivery of Contraceptives (HDC) and Ensuring Spacing at Birth (ESB) through ASHAs
- Ensuring access to Pregnancy Testing Kits (PTK-"Nischay Kits") and strengthening comprehensive abortion care services
- Maintaining quality sterilization services

Maternal Health
- Use MCTS to ensure early registration of pregnancy and full ANC
- Detect high risk pregnancies and line list including severely anemic mothers and ensure appropriate management
- Equip Delivery points with highly trained HR and ensure equitable access to EmOC services through FRUs; Add MCH wings as per need
- Review maternal, infant and child deaths for corrective actions
- Identify villages with low institutional delivery and distribute Misoprostol to select women during pregnancy; incentivize ANMs for domiciliary deliveries

Newborn Health
- Early initiation and exclusive breastfeeding
- Home based newborn care through ASHA
- Essential newborn care and resuscitation services at all delivery points
- Special newborn Care Units with highly trained human resource and other infrastructure
- Community level use of Gentamicin by ANM

Child Health
- Complementary feeding, IFA supplementation and focus on nutrition
- Diarrhea management at community level using ORS and Zinc
- Management of pneumonia
- Full immunization coverage
- Rashtriya Bal Swasthya Karyakram (RBSK): Screening of children for 4Ds (birth defects, development delays, deficiencies and disease) and its management

Adolescent Health
- Address teenage pregnancy and increase contraceptive prevalence in adolescents
- Introduce community-based services through peer educators
- Strengthen(ARSH) clinics
- Roll out National Iron Plus Initiative including weekly IFA supplementation
- Promote menstrual hygiene

Targets of RMNCH+A (under NHM)

- Infant mortality rate (IMR) < 25 (By 2025)
- Maternal mortality ratio (MMR) < 100
- Stillbirth rate (SBR) < 10 (By 2035)
- Neonatal mortality rate (NNMR) < 10 (by 2035)
- Total fertility rate (TFR) < 2.1
- Couple protection rate (CPR) > 60%

Iron plus initiative

Under National Iron+ Initiative, the following age groups are covered for lifelong supplementation of Iron from the age of 6 months onwards:

6–60 months	1 mL of IFA syrup containing 20 mg of elemental iron and 100 mcg of folic acid	Biweekly throughout the period 6–60 months of age and de-worming for children age 12 months and above.
5–10 years	Tablets of 45 mg elemental iron and 400 mcg of folic acid	Weekly throughout the period 5–10 years of age and biannual de-worming
10–19 years	100 mg elemental iron and 500 mcg of folic acid	Weekly throughout the period 10–19 years of age and biannual de-worming
Pregnant and lactating female	100 mg elemental iron and 500 mcg of folic acid	One tab daily for 6 months before delivery and 6 months after delivery (2015 change in RMNCH+A)
Women of reproductive age (WRA) female	100 mg elemental iron and 500 mcg of folic acid	Weekly throughout the reproductive period

National deworming day:

- National deworming day on 10th February and 10th August
- Dose, schedule
  - 12–24 months—200 mg
  - 24–59 months—400 mg
  - Every months
  - Total—7 tablets (8 doses) to all under five children
- 6 Wash strategy
  - Wash utensils
  - Wash hands
  - Wash vegetables
  - Water (purified)
  - Wear footwear
  - Water closet (WC) (use toilets)

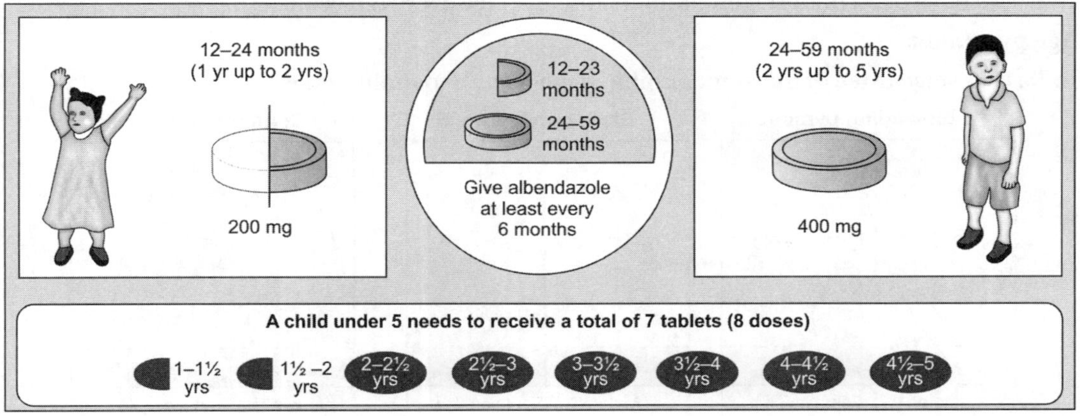

30. True about census:

a. Dependency ratio < 40
b. Year of big divide 1921
c. India is in low stationary phase
d. First census was conducted in 1881
e. Population pyramid is cylindrical

Ans. b, c, d *Ref: Park, 24/e; Suryakanta, 3/e*

Option a	False	No, the dependency ratio is 52
Option b	True	Yes, correct
Option c	True	Yes, correct
Option d	True	Yes, correct
Option e	False	No, the age pyramids are pyramid in shape and not cylindrical

Census data:

- Annual growth rate 1.19 (2015)
- Decadal growth rate 17.64 (2011)

- ❑ Crude birth rate 21.4
- ❑ Crude death rate 7.2
- ❑ Eligible couple 15–18 %
- ❑ Population < 15 years 30%
- ❑ Population < 5 years 13%
- ❑ Population > 60 years 08%
- ❑ Total fertility rate 2.4
- ❑ Couple protection rate 54%
- ❑ Literacy rate 74%
- ❑ Rural population 72%
- ❑ Attended deliveries 76%
- ❑ Life expectancy 67.5 years

The year of big divide - 1921

The Census of 1881 which was undertaken on 17th February, 1881 by WC Plowden, Census Commissioner of India was a great step towards a modern synchronous census. Since then, censuses have been undertaken uninterruptedly once every ten years.

Age pyramids:

India is in stage three of the demographic stage—late expanding stage

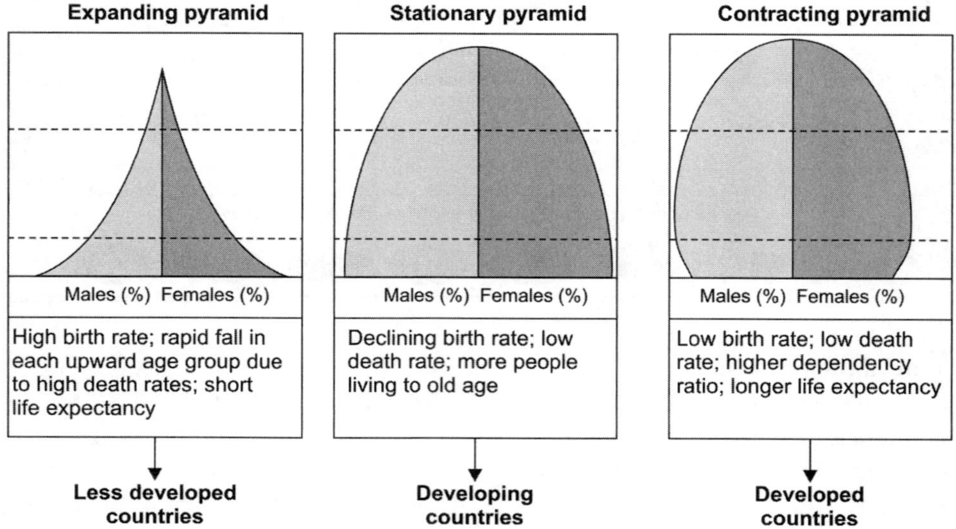

Expansive population pyramids show larger numbers or percentages of the population in the younger age groups. These types of pyramids are usually found in populations with very large fertility rates and lower than average life expectancies. The age-sex distributions of many Third World countries would probably display expansive population pyramids.

Constrictive population pyramids display lower numbers or percentages of younger people. The age-sex distributions of the United States fall into this type of pyramid.

Stationary or near-stationary population pyramids display somewhat equal numbers or percentages for almost all age groups. Of course, smaller figures are still to be expected at the oldest age groups. The age-sex distributions of some European countries, especially Scandinavian ones, will tend to fall into this category.

Age dependency ratio:

Age dependency ratio is the ratio of dependents—people younger than 15 or older than 64—to the working-age population—those ages 15-64.

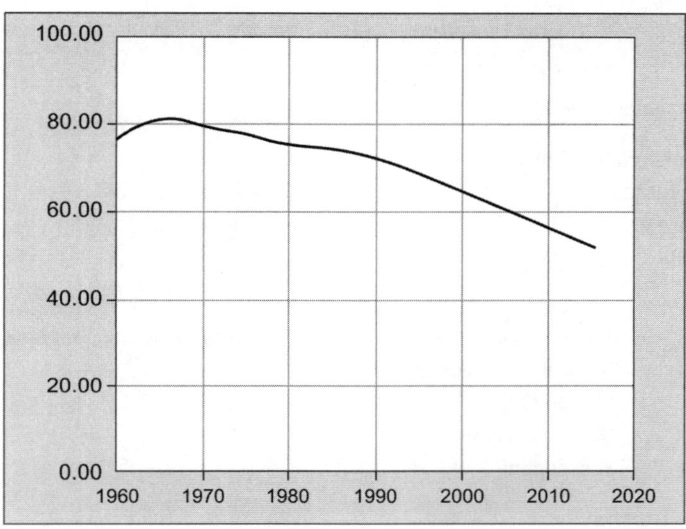

Dependency ratios over last 15 years

Year	Dependency ratio
2015	52.2
2010	56.3
2005	60.1
2000	64.3

Census data

Age group (years)	Census 2011@
0–4	9.3
5–9	10.5
10–14	11.0
15–59	60.3
60+	8.6

31. Drugs which can be used in treatment of rifampicin resistant leprosy?

a. Rifapentin
b. Clindamycin
c. Dapsone
d. Minocycline
e. Moxifloxacin

Ans. c, d, e *Ref: Park, 24/e; Suryakanta, 3/e*

Option a	False	No, resistance to one rifamycin derivative would lead to resistance to all rifamycin group of drugs
Option b	False	No, not used for leprosy
Option c	True	Yes, correct
Option d	True	Yes, correct (new drug use)
Option e	True	Yes, correct (new drug use)

For detail – refer to next question no 32

32. Leprosy is characterized by:
- a. Leonine facies
- b. Small ear lobules
- c. Saddle nose
- d. Micrognathia
- e. Madarosis

Ans. a, c, e *Ref: Park, 24/e; Suryakanta, 3/e*

Option a	True	Yes, correct. It is peculiar, deeply furrowed, lion like appearance of the face
Option b	False	No, it is elongation of ear lobules
Option c	True	Yes, correct
Option d	False	No, it is a square jaw
Option e	True	Yes, correct

Manifestations of leprosy:
- ❑ Macular lesions with sensation loss
- ❑ Madarosis (alopecia on lateral aspect of eyebrows)
- ❑ Nodular skin deformity (lepromas). The diffuse type results in the thickened skin appearance of a leonine facies (lion like facies)
- ❑ Nasal infiltration can cause a saddle-nose deformity and impaired olfaction. Hoarseness (leprous huskiness) and stridor are a result of laryngeal involvement
- ❑ Oral lepromas, usually located on the hard and soft palate, uvula, tongue (cobblestoning), lips, and gums, can progress to necrosis and ulceration
- ❑ Infiltration of the helix or megalobule (elongation and wrinkling of the earlobe) may occur.
- ❑ Lymphadenopathy and hepatomegaly can result from organ infiltration.
- ❑ Aseptic necrosis and osteomyelitis can occur with repeated trauma after joint invasion.
- ❑ Brawny edema of the lower extremities is a late finding.

If left untreated, the signs of advanced leprosy can include:
- ❑ Paralysis and crippling of hands and feet
- ❑ Shortening of toes and fingers due to reabsorption
- ❑ Chronic non-healing ulcers on the bottoms of the feet
- ❑ Blindness
- ❑ Loss of eyebrows
- ❑ Nose disfigurement

Other complications that may sometimes occur are:
- ❑ Painful or tender nerves
- ❑ Redness and pain around the affected area
- ❑ Burning sensation in the skin

Differential diagnosis of leonine facies:

- Acute complications of sarcoidosis
- Colloid milium
- Dermatologic manifestations of leprosy
- Granuloma annulare
- Morphea
- Nodular localized cutaneous amyloidosis
- Porphyria cutaneatarda
- Scleredema
- Xanthomas

33. RNTCP true statement is:

a. Two sputum samples collected
b. Category 1,2,3
c. Only DOTS are to be notified
d. All TB cases are referred to Integrated Counselling and Testing Centre (ICTC) for screening
e. Does not include MDR treatment

Ans. a, d *Ref: Park, 24/e; Suryakanta, 3/e*

Option a	True	Yes, two samples are collected – spot and morning sample
Option b	False	No, there are three categories – Cat 1, 2 and 4
Option c	False	No, all pulmonary TB, and extrapulmonary TB have to be notified
Option d	True	Yes, correct
Option e	False	No, it does take care of all MDR, XDR and TDR's

TB notification

- Who will notify: Every healthcare providers meaning clinical establishments run or managed by the Government (including local authorities), private or NGO sectors and/or individual practitioners.
- When to notify: On diagnosis or initiation of anti-TB treatment of a Tuberculosis case. Such reporting to the nodal public health authority to be done at least on monthly basis.
- Which cases to notify: All tuberculosis cases diagnosed and/or treated; whether under DOTS strategy or not. It includes both pulmonary and extrapulmonary TB cases.
- Definitions:
  - New TB case: Patient who has never been treated with anti-TB drugs or has been treated with anti-TB drugs for less than one month from any source.
  - Recurrent TB case: Patient who has been treated for tuberculosis in the past and been declared successfully treated (cured/treatment completed) at the end of their treatment regimen.
  - Treatment change: Patient returning after interruption, and patients put on a new treatment regimen and due to failure of the current treatment regimen.

The categories were re-organized as per below:

- Category 1 for the treatment of new patients
- Category 2 for previously treated patients

- Category 4 for patients requiring treatment for MDR TB
- Category 5 for patients requiring treatment for XDR TB

Tuberculosis—Extra Edge

TB Diagnosis:

Pulmonary TB

- Tuberculin skin test (TST) and interferon gamma release assay (IGRA):
  - TST and IGRA are not recommended for the diagnosis of active tuberculosis
  - Standardized TST may be used as a complimentary test in children
- Serological tests are banned and not recommended for diagnosing tuberculosis.
- Combination of sputum and CXR is the most sensitive tool and recommended for diagnosis of tuberculosis

Extrapulmonary suspected TB:

- For all patients (adults, adolescents and children) with presumptive extrapulmonary TB, appropriate specimens from the presumed sites of involvement must be obtained for microscopy/culture/cartridge-based nucleic acid amplification test (CBNAAT)/molecular test/histopathology examination and drug sensitivity testing (DST).

MDR suspects

MDR suspect criteria
Criteria A: • All failures of new TB cases • Smear +ve previously treated cases who remain smear +ve at 4th month onwards • ***All pulmonary TB cases*** who are contacts of known MDR TB case
Criteria B—in addition to Criteria A: • All smear +ve previously treated pulmonary TB cases at diagnosis • Any smear +ve follow up result in new or previously treated cases
Criteria C—in addition to Criteria B: • All smear –ve previously treated pulmonary TB cases at diagnosis • HIV TB co-infected cases at diagnosis

MDR diagnosis

MDR diagnostic technology	Choice
Molecular DST [e.g. line probe assay (LPA) DST]	First
Liquid culture isolation and LPA DST	Second
Solid culture isolation and LPA DST	Third
Liquid culture isolation and Liquid DST	Fourth
Solid culture isolation and DST	Fifth

MDR pre-treatment evaluation

- Detailed history (including screening for mental illness, drug/alcohol abuse etc.)
- Weight
- Height
- Complete blood count with platelets count
- Blood sugar to screen for diabetes mellitus

- Liver function tests
- Blood urea and S. creatinine to assess the kidney function
- TSH levels to assess the thyroid function
- Urine examination - routine and microscopic
- Pregnancy test (for all women in the child bearing age group)
- Chest X-ray

Grouping of anti-TB drugs	
Grouping	***Drugs***
Group 1: First-line oral anti-TB agents	Isoniazid (H); Rifampicin (R); Ethambutol (E); Pyrazinamide (Z)
Group 2: Injectable anti-TB agents	Streptomycin (S); Kanamycin (Km); Amikacin (Am); Capreomycin (Cm); Viomycin (Vm).
Group 3: Fluoroquinolones	Ciprofloxacin (Cfx); Ofloxacin (Ofx); Levofloxacin (Lvx); Moxifloxacin (Mfx); Gatifloxacin (Gfx)
Group 4: Oral second-lie anti-TB agents	Ethionamide (Eto); Prothionamide (Pto); Cyeloserine (Cs); Terizadone (Trd); *Para*-aminosalicylic acid (PAS)
Group 5: Agents with unclear efficacy (not recommended by WHO for routine use in MDR-TB patients)	Clofazimine (Cfz); Linezolid (Lzd); Amoxicillin/Clavulanate (Amx/Clv); Thioacetazone (Thz); Imipenem/cilastatin (Ipm/Cln); High-dose isoniazid (high-dose H); Clarithromycin (Clr)

RNTCP regimen for MDR TB:

6 (9) Km LvxEto Cs Z E

+

18 LvxEto Cs E

[Reserve/Substitute drugs: PAS, Mfx, Cm]

This regimen comprises of 6 drugs—Kanamycin, Levofloxacin, Ethionamide, Pyrazinamide, Ethambutol and Cycloserine during 6–9 months of the Intensive Phase and 4 drugs—Levofloxacin, Ethionamide, Ethambutol and Cycloserine during the 18 months of the Continuation Phase.

RNTCP regime for XDR

The **Intensive Phase** (6–12 months) will consist of 7 drugs—Capreomycin (Cm), PAS, Moxifloxacin (Mfx), High dose-INH, Clofazimine, Linezolid, and Amoxyclav.

The Continuation Phase (18 months) will consist of 6 drugs—PAS, Moxifloxacine (Mfx), High dose-INH, Clofazimine, Linezolid, and Amoxyclav.

RNTCP Regimen for XDR TB: 6–12 cm, PAS, Mfx, High dose-H, Cfz, Lzd, Amx/Clv/18 PAS, Mfx, High dose-H, Cfz, Lzd, Amx, Clv (Reserve/Substitute drugs: Clarithromycin, Thiacetazone)

34. DOC for mycoplasma non-gonococcal urethritis:

a. Azithromycin
b. Doxycycline
c. Penicillin
d. Ceftriaxone
e. cefixime

Ans. a, b *Ref: 1. Moi H, Blee K, Horner PJ. Management of non-gonococcal urethritis. BMC Infectious Diseases. 2015;15:294. doi:10.1186/s12879-015-1043-4; 2. http://naco.gov.in/sites/default/files/Syndromic%20Poster_REDUCEd.pdf; 3. http://www.iusti.org/regions/europe/pdf/2016/2016EuropeanNGUGuideline.pdf; 4. https://www.cdc.gov/std/treatment/2010/urethritis-and-cervicitis.htm*

Option a	True	Yes, it was the first line management of NGU
Option b	True	Yes, this is DOC, current guidelines (2016)
Option c	False	No, not correct
Option d	False	No, not correct
Option e	False	No, not correct

Urethritis may be:

- Gonococcal, when *Neisseria gonorrhoeae* is detected, or
- Non-gonococcal (NGU)
- Nonspecific urethritis (NSU) applies to non-gonococcal non-chlamydial urethritis

Non-gonococcal urethritis (NGU), or inflammation of the urethra, is the most common treatable sexually transmitted syndrome in men, with approximately 20–50% of cases being due to infection with *Chlamydia trachomatis* and 10–30% *Mycoplasma genitalium*. Other causes are *Ureaplasma urealyticum, Trichomonas vaginalis,* anaerobes, Herpes simplex virus (HSV) and adenovirus.

Urethritis is characterized by discharge, dysuria and/or urethral discomfort but may be asymptomatic.

- Symptoms
  - Urethral discharge
  - Dysuria
  - Penile tip irritation
  - Urethral discomfort and/or itch
- Signs
  - Urethral discharge
  - Penile tip erythema
  - Normal examination
- Complications
  - Epididymo-orchitis
  - Sexually acquired reactive arthritis—acute or chronic

The diagnosis of urethritis is confirmed by demonstrating an excess of polymorpho-nuclear leucocytes (PMNLs) in a stained smear. However, an excess of mononuclear leucocytes in the smear indicates a viral etiology.

Management:

- Recommended syndromic regimen: Doxycycline 100 mg twice daily for seven days.
  - Azithromycin 1 gram stat should not be used routinely because of the increased risk of inducing macrolide antimicrobial resistance with *Mycoplasma genitalium*
- If *M. genitalium*-positive: Azithromycin 500 mg stat, then 250 mg od for 4 days.
  - A test of cure 3–5 weeks after treatment in those who tested positive for *M. genitalium* should be performed.

Extra Edge:

Syndromic management—as part of 'suraksha clinics' under the National AIDS Control Organization (NACO).

Contents of the STI/RTI drug kits			
STI/RTI syndromic diagnosis	***Name of the kit prescribed***	***Colour coding of the kit***	***Contents of the kits (Name of the drugs)***
Urethral discharge (UD) Cervicitis (CD) Ano-rectal discharge (ARD) Painful scrotal swelling (PSS) Presumptive treatment (PT)	Kit-1	Gray	1 tablet of Azithromycin (1 gram)/2 tablets of Azithromycin (500 mg) and 1 tablet of cefixme (400 mg)
Vaginitis (VD)	Kit-2	Green	1 tablet of Secnidazole (2 gram)/2 tablets of Secnidazole (1 gram) and Fluconazole (150 mg)
Genital ulcer disease non herpetic (GUD-NH)	Kit-3	White	Injection Benzathine penicillin (2.4 MU) + 1 tablet Azithromycin (1 gram) + distilled water (10 mL)+
Genital ulcer disease non herpetic (GUD-NH)-for patients allergic to penicillin	Kit-4	Blue	28 tablets/capsules of Doxycycline (100 mg) and 1 tablet of Azithromycin (1 gram)/2 tablets of Azithromycin (500 mg)
Genital ulcer disease—herpetic (GUD-H)	Kit-5	Red	21 tablets of Acyclovir (400 mg)
Lower abdominal pain (PAP/PID)	Kit-6	Yellow	1 tablet of cefixime (400 mg) 28 tablets of Metronidazole (400 mg) 28 tablets of Doxycycline (100 mg)
Inguinal bubo (IB)	Kit-7	Black	42 tablets of Doxycyline (100 mg) and 1 tablet of Azithromycin (1 gram)

35. Which of following is true for malaria?

a. Not a public health problem
b. Chloroquine resistance not seen
c. Sexual phase in mosquito
d. Chemoprophylaxis is not done
e. Relapse do not occur

Ans. c *Ref: Park, p269, 24/e; https://www.cdc.gov/malaria/about/biology/*

Option a	False	No, Malaria is still a public health problem
Option b	False	No, Chloroquine resistance is seen in many malaria endemic areas
Option c	True	Yes, correct. Refer to explanation below
Option d	False	No, false. Chemoprophylaxis is done
Option e	False	Relapse does occur in Plasmodium vivax

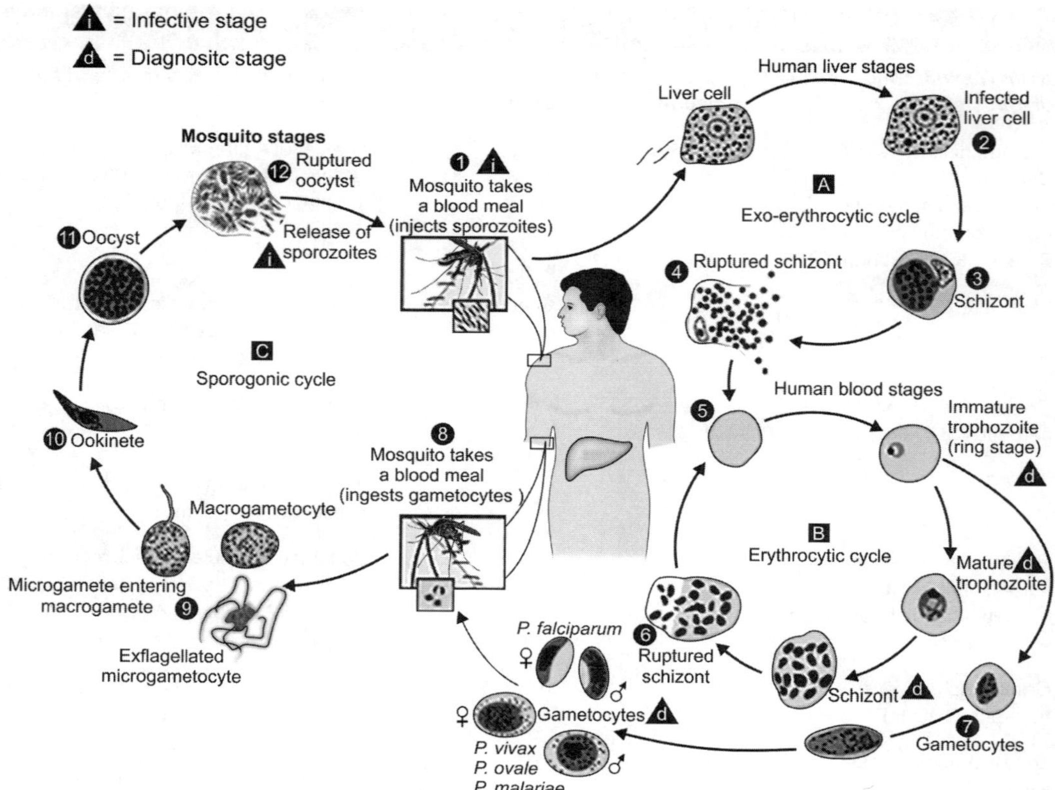

The malaria parasite life cycle involves two hosts. During a blood meal, a malaria-infected female *Anopheles* mosquito inoculates sporozoites into the human host 1. Sporozoites infect liver cells 2 and mature into schizonts 3, which rupture and release merozoites 4. (Of note, in *P. vivax* and *P. ovale* a dormant stage [hypnozoites] can persist in the liver and cause relapses by invading the bloodstream weeks, or even years later.) After this initial replication in the liver (exo-erythrocytic schizogony A), the parasites undergo asexual multiplication in the erythrocytes (erythrocytic schizogony B).

Merozoites infect red blood cells 5. The ring stage trophozoites mature into schizonts, which rupture releasing merozoites . Some parasites differentiate into sexual erythrocytic stages (gametocytes) 7.

Blood stage parasites are responsible for the clinical manifestations of the disease. The gametocytes, male (microgametocytes) and female (macrogametocytes), are ingested by an *Anopheles* mosquito during a blood meal 8. The parasites' multiplication in the mosquito is known as the sporogonic cycle C. While in the mosquito's stomach, the microgametes penetrate the macrogametes generating zygotes 9. The zygotes in turn become motile and elongated (ookinetes) 10,which invade the midgut wall of the mosquito where they develop into oocysts 11. The oocysts grow, rupture, and release sporozoites 12, which make their way to the mosquito's salivary glands. Inoculation of the sporozoites 1 into a new human host perpetuates the malaria life cycle.

The entire pre-erythrocytic phase lasts about 5–16 days depending on the parasite species on an average 5–6 days for *P. falciparum*, 8 days for *P. vivax*, 9 days for *P. ovale*, 13 days for *P. malariae* and 8–9 days for *P. knowlesi*.

Malaria Epidemiology:

- World: Most deaths occur among children living in Africa, where a child dies every minute from malaria.
- In India, about 50% of the infections are reported to be due to *P. falciparum* and 4–8% due to mixed infection and rest due to *P. vivax*.
- *P. ovale* is very rare and mostly confined to regions in Africa.

Malaria - host factors:

- Predominantly rural disease
- Male > females
- Persons with duffy negative RBC trait are 'resistant' to *P. vivax* malaria
- Infants born of immune mothers are generally protected during the first 3–5 months by maternal IgG antibody; infants born of semi-immune mothers are only partially protected. Active immunity is species-specific, that is, immunity against one strain does not protect against another.

Environmental factors:

- Maximum prevalence: July to November—seasonal disease
- Optimum temperature: 20–30°, relative humidity of 60% or higher
- Anophiline mosquito not found in altitude above 2000–2500 mts.

Vector factors:

- *An. culicifacies* — rural areas
- *An. stephensi* — urban areas
- *An. fluviatitlis* — foot hills, forest areas

Mode of transmission:

- Infected vector—may be infective during entire life time
- Direct—via blood or blood products
- Congenital malaria—may occur, but is rare

Relapse:

- It is usual for vivax and ovale malaria to relapse more than 3 years after the patient's first attack.
- Recurrences of falciparum malaria usually disappear within 1–2 years.
- *P. malariae* has a tendency to cause prolonged low-level, asymptomatic parasitaemia.

Incubation period:

- Falciparum malaria—9–14 days
- Vivax malaria—8–17 days
- Quartan malaria—18–40 days
- Ovale malaria—16–18 days

Clinical features:

- Cold stage—15 mins to 1 hr—parasites are demonstratable
- Hot stage—2–6 hours

- Sweating stage—2–4 hours
- *P. falciparum*—classical 48 hrs cycle
- *P. malariae*—72 hours cycle

Diagnosis:

- Microscopy
  - Thick film—parasite identification
  - Thin film—species identification
  - High sensitivity
- Serological test—used in epidemiological studies. Indicates current or past infection
- RDT—rapid diagnostic tests
  - High false negative results

Treatment of Malaria

P. vivax cases

- Cholorquine 25 mg/kg divided over 3 days (10,10,5 mg/kg on each day)
- Primaquine 0.25 mg/kg daily for 14 days

P. falciparum infection

- Artesunate (AS) for 3 days
- Sulphadoxine+pyrimethamine (SP) on day 1.
- Primaquine (PQ) 0.75 mg/kg on day 2

* in North-eastern states—artemether (20 mg) + lumefantrine (120 mg)

Dosage chart for treatment of falciparum malaria with ACT-SP

Age group (Years)	1st day		2nd day		3rd day AS
	AS	SP	AS	PQ	
0–1* Pink blister	1 (25 mg)	1 (250+ 12.5 mg)	1 (25 mg)	Nil	1 (25 mg)
1–4 Yellow blister	1 (50 mg)	1 (500 + 25 mg each)	1 (50 mg)	1 (7.5 mg base)	1 (50 mg)
5–8 Green blister	1 (100 mg)	1 (750 + 37.5 mg each)	1 (100 mg)	2 (7.5 mg base each)	1 (100 mg)
9–14 Red blister	1 (150 mg)	2 (500 + 25 mg each)	1 (150 mg)	4 (7.5 mg base each)	1 (150 mg)
15 and above White blister	1 (200 mg)	2 (750 + 37.5 mg each)	1 (200 mg)	6 (7.5 mg base each)	1 (200 mg)

*SP is not to be prescribed for children < 5 months of age and should be treated with alternate ACT

*ACT-AL is not to be prescribed for children weighing less than 5 kg

Treatment failure:

- Early treatment failure
  - Parasitemia on day 2 higher than day 0
  - Development of danger signs
- Late clinical failure
  - Presence of parasitemia between day 4 and day 28 with axillary temperature > 37.5°C
- Late parasitological failure
  - Presence of parasitemia on any day between 7 and 28 days of treatment initiation with axillary temperature < 37.5°C

Chemoprophylaxis

- Short-term (< 6 weeks)
  - Doxycycline started one day before arrival in risk area. Taken daily
  - Weekly chloroquine - started 1 week before arrival
- Long-term (>6 weeks)
  - Chloroquine (if CQ sensitive area)
  - Mefloquine

All drugs to be continued for at least 4 weeks after the last exposure to the parasite endemic area.

Indicators for malaria transmission

- API—annual parasitic index
  - Measure of malaria incidence in the community
- ABER—annual blood examination rate
  - Indicator if operational efficiency
  - Target—at least 10% of the population should be screened
- SPR—slide positivity rate
  - Indicator for impending outbreak

36. True regarding HDI is:

a. Life expectance range is 20-85 years
b. HDI range is 0–1
c. Literacy range is 0–10
d. Schooling years range from 0–15
e. GDP per capita ranges from $ 200 - $ 2000

Ans. a, b, d *Ref: http://hdr.undp.org/en/composite/HDI; http://hdr.undp.org/sites/default/files/hdr2016_technical_notes.pdf; Park, 24/e; Suryakanta, 3/e*

Option a	True	Yes, correct
Option b	True	Yes, correct
Option c	False	No, the expected years of schooling is 0–18 years
Option d	True	Yes, correct
Option e	False	No, income is ranging from 100–75000 $ PPP

Human Development Index (HDI): A composite index measuring average achievement in three basic dimensions of human development—a long and healthy life, knowledge and a decent standard of living.

Life expectancy at birth: Number of years a newborn infant could expect to live if prevailing patterns of age-specific mortality rates at the time of birth stay the same throughout the infant's life.

Expected years of schooling: Number of years of schooling that a child of school entrance age can expect to receive if prevailing patterns of age-specific enrolment rates persist throughout the child's life.

Mean years of schooling: Average number of years of education received by people ages 25 and older, converted from education attainment levels using official durations of each level.

Gross national income (GNI) per capita: Aggregate income of an economy generated by its production and its ownership of factors of production, less the incomes paid for the use of factors of production owned by the rest of the world, converted to international dollars using PPP rates, divided by midyear population.

GNI per capita rank minus HDI rank: Difference in ranking by GNI per capita and by HDI value. A negative value means that the country is better ranked by GNI than by HDI value.

Calculating HDI:

Dimension	Indicator	Minimum	Maximum
Health	Life expectancy (in years)	20	85
Education	Expected years of schooling (in years)	0	18
	Mean years of schooling (in years)	0	15
Standard of living	Gross national income per capita(2011 purchasing power parity $)	100	75000

	Human development index (HDI)	Life expectancy at birth	Expected years of schooling	Mean years of schooling	Gross national income (GNI) per capita	HDI rank
India	0.624	68.3	11.7	6.3	5663	131

Data source: http://hdr.undp.org/en/composite/HDI access date 10 Aug 2017

$$\text{Dimension index} = \frac{\text{Actual value} - \text{minimum value}}{\text{Maximum value} - \text{minimum value}}$$

The HDI is the geometric mean of the three dimension indices:

$$\text{HDI} = (I_{health} * I_{education} * I_{income})^{\frac{1}{3}}$$

Calculations for HDI, iHDI, mHPI is as follows:

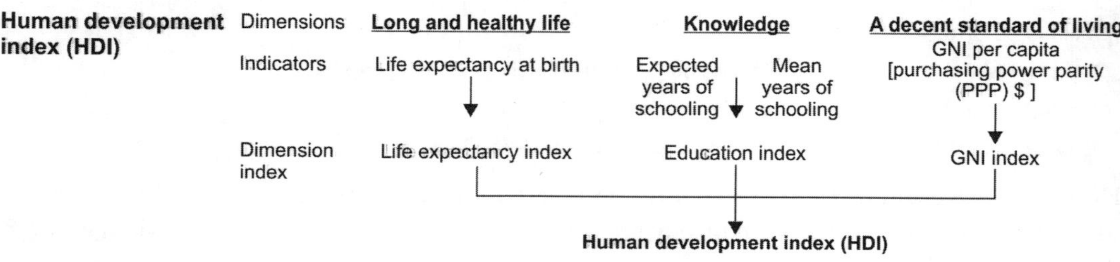

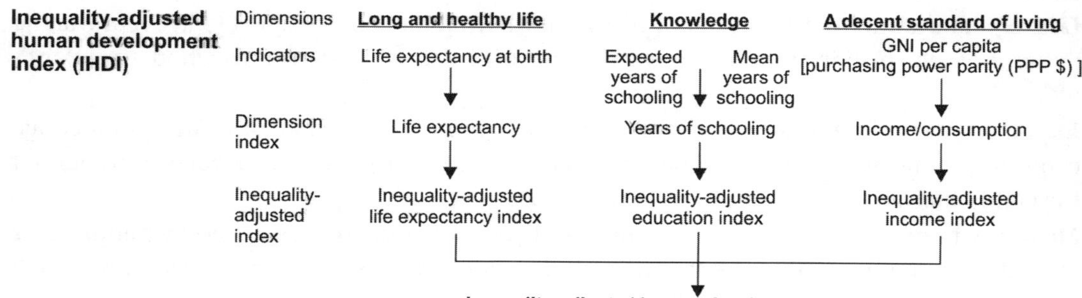

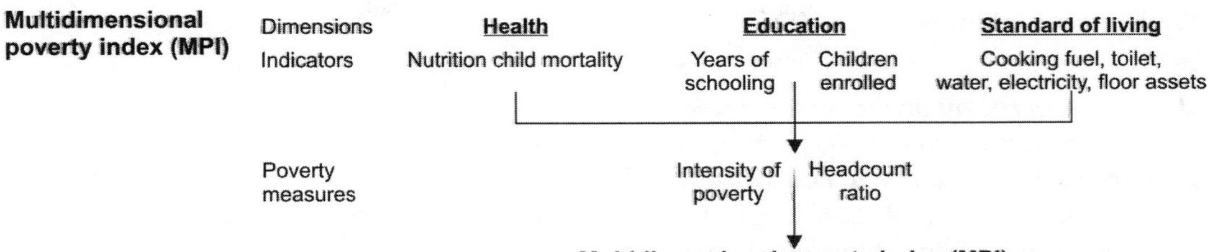

Comparing HDI, human poverty index (HPI) and physical quality life index (PQLI)	
Human development index	***Human poverty index***
Life expectancy at birth	Probability at birth of Not surviving till 40 years
Knowledge and education 1. Adult literacy rate 2. Gross enrollment ratio	Adult literacy rate
Standard of living GDP per capita at purchasing power of parity	Average population 1. Without access to drinking water 2. Children under weight for age

Physical quality of life index	
Infant mortality	Range from 0 to 100
Life expectancy at age 1	
Literacy	

37. OCP decreases all of the following *except*:

a. Migraine
b. Breakthrough bleeding
c. Dysmenorrhea
d. Menorrhagia
e. Mood changes

Ans. a *Ref: Park, 24/e; Suryakanta, 3/e*

Option a	False	No, OCPs would potentiate migraine or headaches. They are contraindicated in case of migraine with any neurological effects
Option b	True	Yes, they would decrease
Option c	True	Yes, they would decrease
Option d	True	Yes, they would decrease
Option e	True	Its doubtful, systematic reviews point towards a benefit in mood changes or no effect. However, some females may experience a deterioration of mood changes, especially in case of depression or previous history of mood changes.

Ref: Consortium of emergency contraception in India. WHO-CCR in human reproduction—AIIMS, Delhi; https://womensmentalhealth.org/posts/you-asked-do-oral-contraceptives-cause-mood-swings-or-depression/—MGH centre for women's health – reproductive psychiatry resource and information centre, Harvard medical school. USA; Effects of Oral Contraceptive Pills on Mood: Lessons Learned from Longitudinal Studies. Miller, Erin et al. Canadian Journal of Diabetes, Volume 39, Issue 6, 536. DOI:http://dx.doi.org/10.1016/j.jcjd.2015.09.041.

Birth or control for birth

OCP

- ***First generation oral contraceptives***
  - Products containing 50 μg or more of ethinylestradiol (EE).
- ***Second generation oral contraceptives***
  - Products containing 30–35 μg of EE and levonorgestrel (LNG) or norgestimate or other members of norethindrone family.
- ***Third generation oral contraceptives***
  - Products containing 20 or 30 μg EE and desogestrel or gestodene.

    Pills may also be categorized based on the amount of ethinylestradiol :
    - ***High dose*** oral contraceptives are pills containing 50 μg or more of Ee.
    - ***Low dose*** oral contraceptives include pills containing 30–50 μg of Ee.
    - ***Ultra low dose*** oral contraceptives are pills containing less then 30 μg of Ee.

Mechanism of action:

- Inhibit ovulation by inhibiting gonadotrophin secretion via an effect on both pituitary and hypothalamic centers. The progestational agents suppress LH and estrogens suppress FSH.
- In addition, the progestational agent also makes the endometrium unsuitable for implantation and thickens cervical mucus making it impervious to sperm.

Contraindications for Low Dose COCs

- ***Absolute contraindications:***
  - Breastfeeding mothers up to 6 months postpartum
  - Up to 3 weeks postpartum in non breastfeeding mothers
  - More than 35 years of age with risk factors for cardiovascular disease, e.g. hypertension, smoking, vascular disease, etc.
  - History of deep vein thrombosis/pulmonary embolism
  - Patient undergoing major surgery with prolonged immobilization
  - Current and past history of cardiovascular accident
  - Valvular heart disease with superimposed complications like pulmonary artery hypertension and atrial fibrillation.
  - History of migraine with focal neurological symptoms at any age
  - Current or past history of breast cancer
  - Diabetes mellitus with complications like neuropathy and retinopathy
  - Current gallbladder disease or history of jaundice related with use of combined oral contraceptives
  - Active liver disease or cirrhosis
  - Benign or malignant tumors of the ovary
  - Patients on drugs likely to affect metabolism of the COCs, e.g. Rifampicin, griseofulvin, phenytoin, barbiturates, etc.
- ***Relative contraindications:***

  Conditions when COCs can be prescribed under supervision include :
  - Breastfeeding women more than 6 months postpartum.
  - History of gestational diabetes, cholestasis in pregnancy or pregnancy-induced hypertension
  - Women under 35 years of age with risk factors for cardiovascular disease

- History of cholecystectomy
- Age > 40 years
- Superficial venous thrombophlebitis
- Uncomplicated valvular heart disease
- Unexplained vaginal bleeding
- Cervical intraepithelial neoplasia and cervical cancer awaiting treatment
- Diabetes mellitus (well controlled) with no vascular disease

Time of starting:

COCs can be started on any day within the first five days of menstrual bleeding, preferably on the first day.

Within three to six weeks after childbirth in non-lactating mothers.

Missed pill:

- If one white pill is missed, she should take that pill as soon as she remembers and the next pill on the usual time. No additional contraceptive method is required.
- If she misses 2 pills in the first two weeks, she should take two pills on each of the next two days and an additional method is to be used for next 7 days.
- If she misses two pills in the third week, or more than 2 active pills are missed at any time, then a new packet has to be started on the same day and an additional contraceptive method to be used for 7 days.
- If she misses one brown tablet then she should throw the missed pill and take rest of the tablets as usual.

Note: Even if no pills are missed, woman should be instructed to use a back-up method for 7 days after an episode of gastroenteritis.

38. Contraindications to Cu-IUD insertion include:

a. Cervicitis and vaginitis
b. Suspected pregnancy
c. Septic abortion within last one year
d. Ectopic abortion
e. Unknown cause of bleeding

Ans. a, b, c, e *Ref: Park, 24/e; Suryakanta, 3/e*

Option a	True	
Option b	True	
Option c	True	
Option d	False	Contraindication for hormonal IUD and not Cu-IUD
Option e	True	

IUD types:

- 1st Generation IUDs—inert IUDs
  - Lippes loop
  - Grafenberg's rings and devices
- 2nd Generation IUDs—CuTs

  Copper IUDs

  Copper wire or copper sleeves are put on the plastic frame (polyethylene frame). Examples include Copper T, CuT380 A, Multiload 375 etc.

The various types of Copper IUDs differ from each other by the amount of copper. The initial Copper IUDs were wound with 200–250 mm^2 wire (CopperT 200). The modern copper containing devices contain more copper and a part of copper in the form of solid tubal sleeves rather than wire. This increases the efficacy and life span (Cu T-380 A).

- ***CuT 380A:*** It is a T shaped device with a polyethylene frame holding 380 mm^2 of exposed surface area of copper. The IUD frame contains barium sulfate thus making it radio-opaque.
- ***CuT-380Ag:*** It is identical to 380 A except that the copper wire on the stem has a silver core to prevent fragmentation and extend the life span of the copper.
- ***CuT 380 slimline*:** It has copper sleeves flushed at the ends of horizontal arms to facilitate easier loading and insertion. The performance of CuT-380 Ag and the CuT-380 slimline is equal to that of CuT-380 A.
- ***Multiload 375:*** It has 375 mm^2 of copper wire wound around its stem. The flexible arms are designed to minimize expulsions. The multiload 375 and T Cu-380 A are similar in their efficacy and performance.
- ***Nova T*:** It is similar to the CuT-200, containing 200 mm^2 of copper. However, the Nova T has a silver core to the copper wire, flexible arms, and a large flexible loop at the bottom to prevent cervical perforation.

- 3rd Generation IUD—Hormonal IUDs
  - ***Progestasert:*** It is a T shaped IUD made of ethylene and vinyl acetate copolymer containing titanium dioxide. The vertical stem contains a reservoir of 38 mg progesterone together with barium sulfate dispersed in silicone fluid. The progesterone is released at the rate of 65 μg per day.
  - ***Levonorgestrel (LNG)—20 (Mirena):*** This T shape and device has a collar attached to vertical arm containing 52 mg of levonorgestrel dispersed in polydimethyl siloxane. It releases 15 μg of levonorgestrel per day in vivo and is effective for 7–10 years.

Time of insertion

- Within 10 days of start of menstruation (ideal within 7 days)
- With 48 hrs postpartum
- After 6 weeks postpartum (within 10 days of menstruation)
  - She can expect some cramping for a day or two after insertion, vaginal discharge for a few weeks after insertion and slightly heavier menstrual period with possible bleeding between the menstrual periods during first few months after insertion.
  - Follow-up visit after 3–6 weeks or after next menstrual period to ensure that IUD is in place and no infection has developed.
  - Information about kind of IUD and when to have her IUD removed or replaced.

Side effects:

- Cramping pain
- Vaginal discharge / spotting / slightly heavy bleeding

Complications:

- PID
- Expulsion (rare)
- Perforation (rare)
- Ectopic pregnancy (only with hormonal IUDs)

Emergency contraception:

- Most effective within 5 days of unprotected intercourse
- Best to use CuT 380 A

  Note: Hormonal IUDs are not indicated for emergency contraception

IUD indications:

- Contraception
- Emergency contraception
- Dysmenorrhea
- Menorrhagia
- Endometrial CA/ cervical CA

  For all ages, regardless of obstetrical history or risk of STI.

IUD use is safe in women with the following conditions:

- History of an ectopic pregnancy
- History of pelvic surgery
- Hypertension or other forms of heart disease
- History of deep venous thrombosis
- History of migraine headaches
- Anemia
- Diabetes
- Endometriosis
- Smoking

IUD contraindications:

- Uterine bleeding of unknown cause
- Active PID, septic abortion
- Pregnancy
- Copper allergy (for copper IUDs only)
- Significantly distorted uterine anatomy
- Unexplained vaginal bleeding concerning for pregnancy or pelvic malignancy
- Gestational trophoblastic disease with persistently elevated beta-human chorionic gonadotropin levels
- Active pelvic infection (e.g. pelvic inflammatory disease, untreated cervicitis, puerperal sepsis, immediate postabortion or postpartum infection, endomyometritis, pelvic tuberculosis)

Specific contraindications to Mirena

- Current deep vein thrombosis/pulmonary embolism
- Current or past history of ischemic heart disease
- Migraine with focal neurological symptoms (at any age)
- Current and past history of breast cancer
- Active viral hepatitis, cirrhosis of liver and benign or malignant liver tumors
- History of ectopic pregnancy/abortion.

Insertion of mirena:

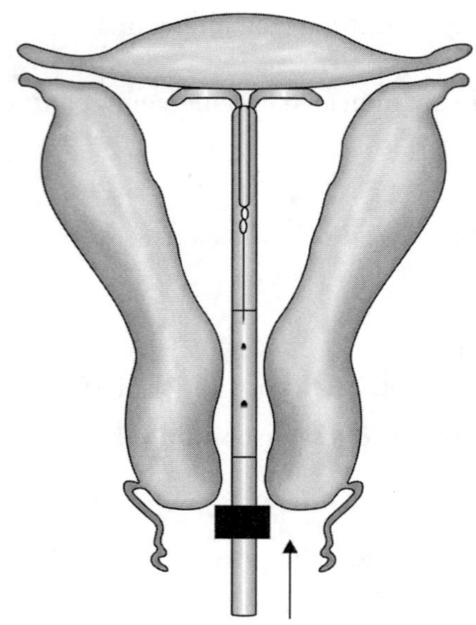

Insertion of CuT 380 A:

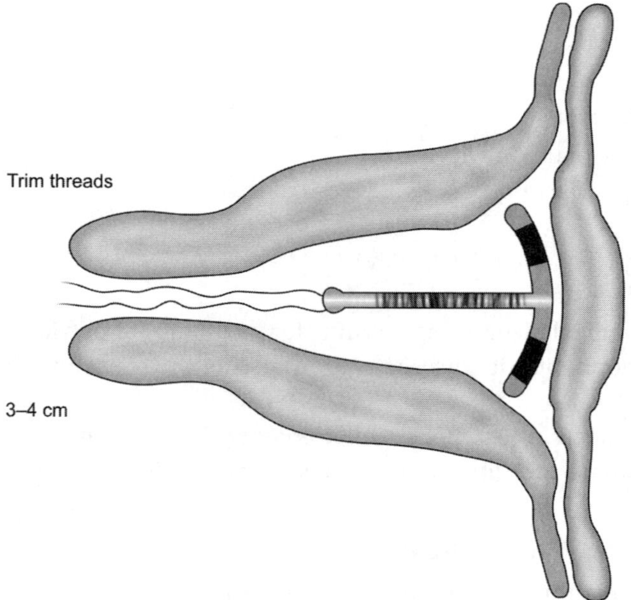

39. True about fractional inactivated polio vaccination is:

a. Given intramuscularly
b. Given intradermal
c. Dose given is 0.5 mL
d. Dose given is 0.1 mL
e. Dose is 6 week and 14 weeks

Ans. b, d, e *Ref: Park, 24/e; Suryakanta, 3/e*

Option a	False	No, it is given ID in upper arm (opposite to BCG arm)
Option b	True	Yes, correct
Option c	False	No, dose is 0.1 mL
Option d	True	Yes, correct
Option e	True	Yes correct

Difference between OPV and IPV		
	Oral Polio Vaccines (OPV)	*Inactivated Polio Vaccines (IPV)*
Types	Trivalent (tOPV): 1, 2, and 3 Bivalent (bOPV): 1 and 3 Monovalent (mOPV): 1, 2, or 3	Trivalent
Pros	Cheap; Easy to administer Good intestinal immunity. Excreted in feces; Confers passive immunity	No risk of vaccine associated paralytic poliomyelitis (VAPP). Humoral immunity. Highly effective. Immune response similar between industrialized and developing settings.
Cons	Associated with VAPP (extremely rare; approx. 1 per 2.7 million first doses of vaccine) and circulating vaccine derived polioviruses (cVDPVs). In tropical developing countries, lower immune response necessitates > 3 doses and additional booster doses. Interference from type 2 may lower immune response to types 1 and 3.	More costly than OPV. Cannot be administered by volunteers; requires injection. Does not confer passive immunity.

- A fractional dose is one-fifth (1/5, 0.1 mL) of a full dose of IPV, injected via the intradermal (ID) route
- fIPV is safe, effective and immunogenic
- fIPV can be given alone, or at the same time as any other vaccine
- In children also receiving oral polio vaccine (OPV), two doses of fIPV given at 6 and 14 weeks will help to "boost" their mucosal immunity against polioviruses
- fIPV can be used in all types of polio immunization activities: In routine immunization, in supplementary immunization activities (SIAs), and in outbreak response.

IPV is heat and freeze sensitive

- IPV loses potency when **exposed to heat** or **when frozen**
  - Store at +2°C to +8°C
- IPV is **freeze sensitive**
  - **Unlike OPV**, which can be frozen
  - The "shake test" is ineffective in determining whether IPV has been frozen
  - If you suspect that **IPV may have been frozen, the vial must be discarded**
- Do not use if vaccine has a cloudy appearance

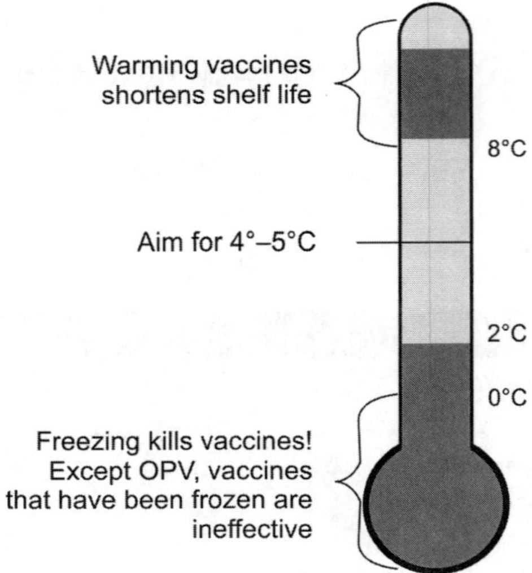

- IPV vial has a VVM on the vial label
- The VVM registers **cumulative heat exposure**, and changes from light to dark
- Check the VVM on each vaccine vial
- If inside square is the *same* color, or *darker* than the circle, **do not use** the vaccine

How to read a vaccine vial monitor?

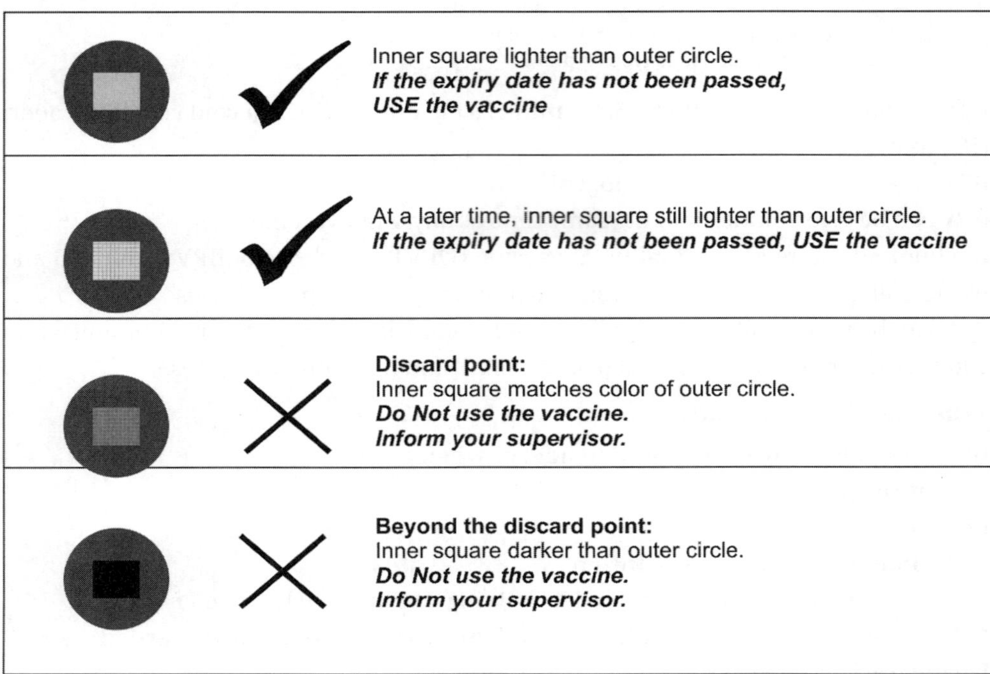

What is fractional dose IPV (fIPV)?

A fractional dose of IPV is a smaller dose of the same vaccine, equal to 1/5 of a standard dose. Studies show that **2 doses of fractional dose IPV** administered by intradermal injection produce an even stronger immune response than a single full IPV dose.

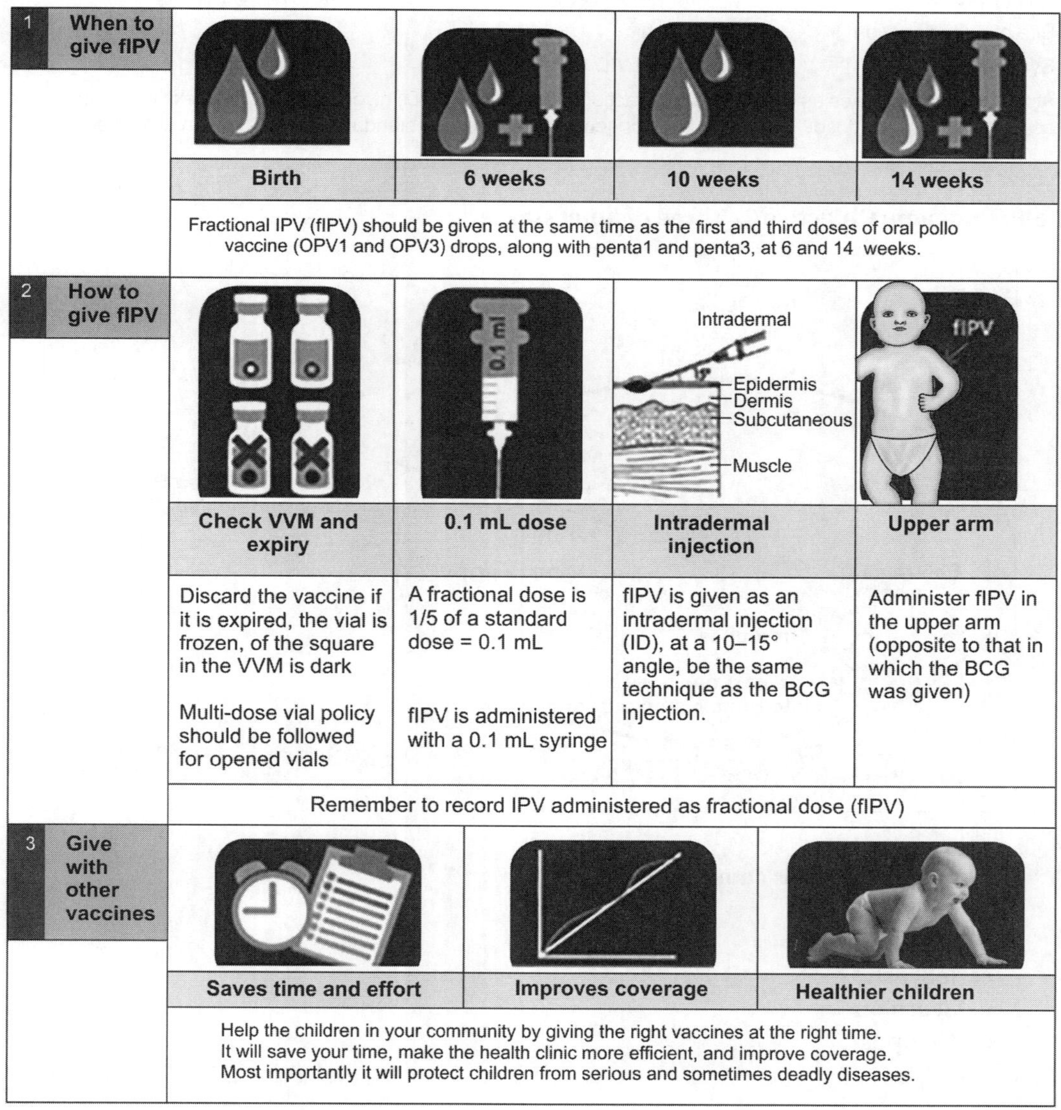

Studies have demonstrated that a single fractional dose of IPV (1/5 of the full dose) gives lower seroconversion rates than a single full dose but after 2 fractional doses the rates are similar to those after 2 full doses.

Furthermore, **2 fractional doses of IPV, given intradermally at 6 and 14 weeks provide higher seroconversion rates than a single full dose (intramuscular) given at 14 weeks.**

Comparing IPV and fIPV		
	IPV	*Fractional IPV (fIPV)*
Volume per dose	0.5 mL	0.1 mL
Schedule	1 dose: 14 weeks	2 doses: 6 and 14 weeks
Administration	Intramuscular (IM) injection	Intradermal (ID) injection
Site of administration	Thigh	Upper arm
Syringe	0.5 mL AD syringe	0.1 mL AD syringe
Are two fractional doses as effective as a single standard dose?	Two fractional doses of IPV (ID) given at 6 and 14 weeks produces better immunogenicity than a single standard dose (IM) given at 14 weeks	

Extra Edge:

Polio Endgame Objective 2 : Three distinct stages

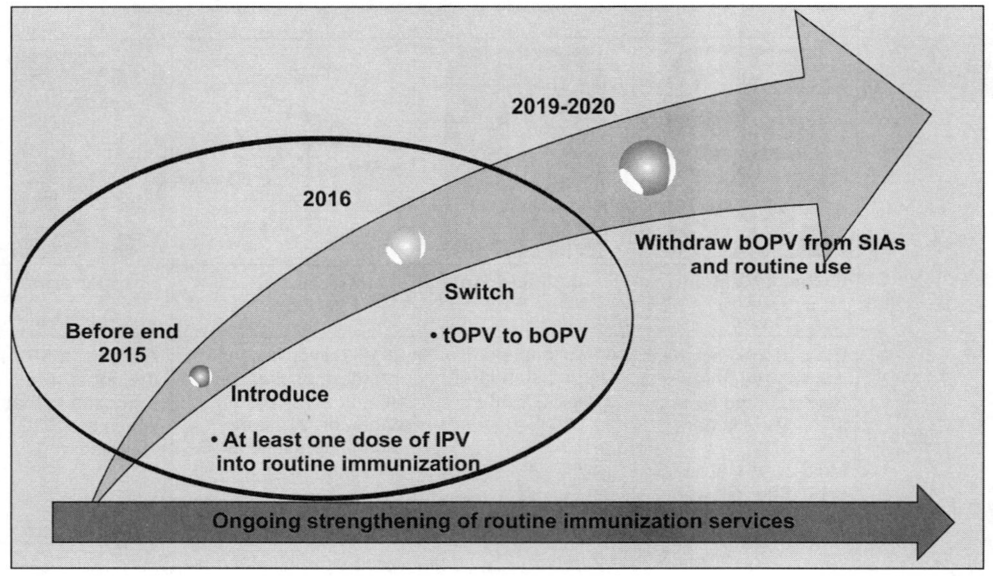

40. Neuroexcitation is caused by:
   a. Tick
   b. Mosquito
   c. Jellyfish
   d. Scorpion
   e. Octopus

Ans. a, c, d, e *Ref: Park, 24/e; Suryakanta, 3/e*

Option a	True	
Option b	False	
Option c	True	
Option d	True	
Option e	True	

Key venom effects*		
Venom component	***Clinical effects***	***Type of venomous animal***
Neurotoxin Paralytic	Flaccid paralysis	Some snakes, paralysis ticks, cone shells, blue-ringed octopus
Excitatory	Neuroexcitation: autonomic storm, cardiotoxicity, pulmonary edema	Some scorpions, spiders, jellyfish
Myotoxins	Systemic or local myolysis	Some snakes
Cardiotoxins	Direct or indirect cardiotoxicity; cardiac collapse shock	Some snakes, scorpions, spiders, and jellyfish
Hemostasis system toxins	Vary from rapid coagulopathy and bleeding to thrombosis, deep venous thrombosis and pulmonary emboli	Many snakes and a few scorpions Brazilian caterpillars
Nephrotoxins	Renal damage	Some snakes, multiple bee, wasp stings
Necrotoxins	Local tissue injury/necrosis, shock	Some snakes, a few scorpions, spiders, jellyfish and stingrays
Allergic toxins	Induce acute allergic response (direct and indirect)	Almost all venoms but particularly those of social insects (bees, wasps, ants)

*All venom components have lethal potential.

Venomous animals and human envenoming			
Phyla	***Principal venomous animal groups***	***Estimated number of human cases/year***	***Estimated number of human deaths/year***
Chordata	Snakes Spiny fish Stingrays	> 2.5 million ? > 100000 ? > 100000	> 100000 Close to 0 ? < 10
Arthropoda	Scorpions Spiders Paralysis ticks Insects	> 1 million ? > 100000 ? > 1000 ? > 1 million	? < 5000 ? < 100 ? < 10 ? > 1000*
Mollusca	Cone shells Blue-ringed octopus	? < 1000 ? < 100	? < 10 ? < 10
Coelenterata	Jellyfish	? > 1 million	? < 10

*Social insect stings cause death by anaphylaxis rather than primary venom toxicity, except for massive multiple sting attacks.

General systemic effects

By definition, these are non-specific. Shock is an important complication of major local envenoming by some snake species and, if inadequately treated, can prove lethal, especially in children.

Specific systemic effects

These are important in both diagnosis and treatment:

- *Neurotoxic flaccid paralysis* can develop very rapidly, progressing from mild weakness to full respiratory paralysis in less than 30 minutes (blue-ringed octopus bite, cone shell sting), or may develop far more slowly, over hours (some snakes) to days (paralysis tick). For neurotoxic snakes, the cranial nerves are usually involved first, with ptosis a common initial sign. From this, paralysis may extend to the limbs, with weakness and loss of deep tendon reflexes, then respiratory paralysis.

- *Excitatory neurotoxins* cause an 'autonomic storm', with profuse sweating, variable cardiac effects and cardiac failure, sometimes with pulmonary edema (notably Australian funnel web spider bite, some scorpions such as Indian red scorpion). This type of envenoming can be rapidly fatal (many scorpions, funnel web spiders), or may cause distressing symptoms but constitute a lesser risk of death (widow spiders, banana spiders).

Medicine

1. **Features of non-ST elevation MI (NSTEMI) include:**
   a. Increase in troponin levels and ST depression
   b. Aspirin, Clopidogrel and LMW are used for treatment
   c. STEMI has better outcome than NSTEMI
   d. Thrombolytics are not given
   e. Angiography should be done after 72 hrs

Ans. a,b,d

Option a	True	Correct
Option b	True	Correct
Option c	False	NSTEMI and unstable angina have better outcome than STEMI
Option d	True	Thrombolytics are beneficial in STEMI
Option e	False	Early angiography within 48 hours is done.

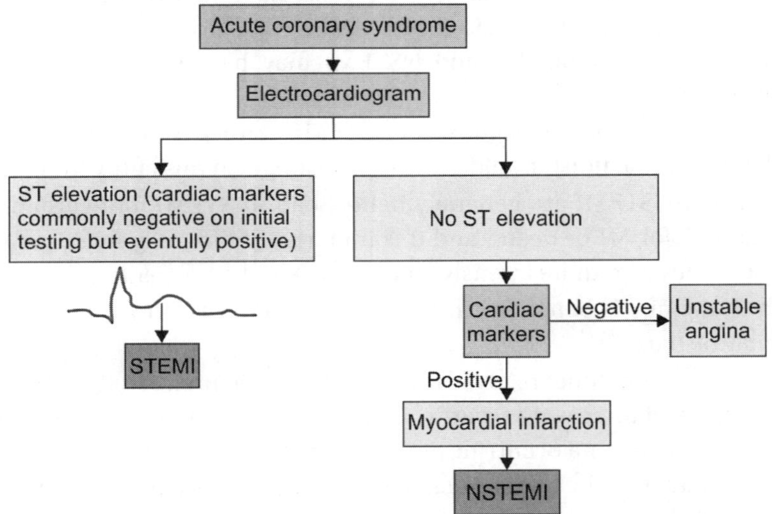

Summary of treatment differences between cardiac events			
	Stable angina	Unstable angina/non-ST elevation MI	ST elevation MI
Aspirin	Yes	Yes	Yes
Beta blockers	Yes	Yes	Yes
Nitrates	Yes	Yes	Yes
Heparin (enoxaparin)	No	Yes	Yes, but only after thrombolytics

Contd...

Contd...

	Stable angina	Unstable angina/non-St elevation MI	ST elevation MI
GPIIb/IIIa meds	No	Yes	No
Thrombolytics	No	No	Yes, but not as good as PCI
CCBs	No	No	No
Warfarin	No	No	No
Antiplatelet drug	No	Yes	Yes

Bottom Line

1. tPA (thrombolytics) are beneficial only with ST elevation MI.
2. Heparin is best for non-ST elevation MI.
3. GP IIb/IIIa inhibitors are best for non-ST elevation MI and those under going PCI and stenting.
   GPIIb/IIIa inhibitors are best with stenting.

- ❑ NSTEMI is more severe than UA, and is considered to have occurred if ischemia produces damage detectable by biochemical markers of myocardial injury (troponin I or CK-MB).
- ❑ If there are no detectable serum markers of myocardial injury 12–18 hours after symptom onset, the patient should be diagnosed with UA.
- ❑ At the time of presentation, UA and NSTEMI may be indistinguishable and can be identically managed.
- ❑ Thefefore, in establishing the diagnosis of NSTEMI, cardiac troponins (elevated enzymes show evidence of infraction) should be used to distinguish this entity from UA.

Outcomes in UA/NSTEMI are generally better than in STEMI, but certain UA/NSTEMI patients are high risk for MI or death, and it is important to identify these patients at initial screening because they ay require intensive monitoring and management.

Thrombolytic therapy is beneficial in patients with STEMI, but is not effective in UA or NSTEMI and may be harmful.

Unstable angina is sometimes referred to as 'crescendo' or 'preinfarction' angina. Typically, it is defined as angina of increasing severity, frequency, duration; angina showing increasing resistance to nitrates; or angina occurring at rest. Experts also regard *any new-onset angina* as unstable. Sudden change in the pattern of angina usually means a physical change within the coronary arteries, such as hemorrhage into an atherosclerotic plaque or rupture of a plaque with intermittent thrombus formation.

UA: Unstable Angina
STEMI: ST elevation Myocardial Infarction
NSTEMI: Non-ST Elevation Myocardial Infarction

2. Microsatellite abnormality is seen in:

a. Ataxia telangiectasia
b. Myotonic dystrophy
c. Huntington chorea
d. Spinocerebellar ataxia
e. Osler Weber Rendeu syndrome

Ans. b,c,d

Option a	False	No, it is autosomal recessive trait with mutation in the ATM gene (on 11q22-23)
Option b	True	Yes, correct
Option c	True	Yes, correct
Option d	True	Yes, correct
Option e	False	No, OWRD is commonly seen due to the defect in the endoglin gene (ENG) on chromosome 9. It is autosomal dominant disease

Table 1: Diseases with microsatellite abnormality

Disease range	Reiterated trinucleotide	Normal range of reiteration	Disease range of reiteration
Spinal and bulbar muscular atrophy, Kennedy's disease	CAG	11–33	40–62
Huntington's disease	CAG	11–34	42–100
Spinocerebelllar ataxia type 1	CAG	<29–36	43–>60
Fragile X	CGG	6–54	250–400
Myotonic dystrophy	CTG	5–30	>50

The microsatellite sequence in these diseases are linked to a coding gene, which is affected by the expansion of the trinucleotide sequence. These cases of microsatellite-dependent disease represent two classes. Fragile X and myotonic dystrophy have their trinucleotide sequence linked to the noncoding ends of the gene, while in the three diseases with CAG expansion, coding for polyglutamine, the microsatellite is located within the coding part of the gene.

Genetic permutation: An initial increase of the trinucleotide sequence functions as a premutational event. Above a critical number of repeats, the system becomes unstable and usually more sequences are added, eventually resulting in symptoms.

Genetic anticipation: A characteristic of these diseases is the fact that the symptoms tend to be more severe in subsequent generations because of amplification during gametogenesis or in the zygote, known as genetic anticipation.

Fragile X was the first recognized case of a genetic disease with an instability of trinucleotide repeats. It is a common neurological disease that causes mental retardation, which is inherited as an X-linked dominant trait. It is manifested by chromosome breakages at specific sites. The disease is associated with an expansion of a microsatellite repeat of CGG trinucleotides in the 5′ untranslated end of the gene FMRJ.

Ataxia-telangiectasia (A-T) is an autosomal recessive, complex, multisystem disorder characterized by progressive neurologi c impairment, cerebellar ataxia, variable immunodeficiency with susceptibility to upper and lower respiratory infections, impaired organ maturation, X-ray hypersensitivity, ocular and cutaneous telangiectasia and a predisposition to malignancy.

3. Pulse oximetry gives inaccurate reading in:

a. Dark skin
b. Co-poisoning
c. Patient on nasal oxygen
d. Ventilation through bag & mask
e. Hypovolemia

Ans. b, e *Ref: http://www.who.int/patientsafety/safesurgery/pulse_oximetry/en/index.html (Accessed on Jan 30, 2018)*

Option a	False	Not correct
Option b	True	Yes, correct
Option c	False	Not correct
Option d	False	Not correct
Option e	True	Yes, correct

There are TWO numerical values obtained from the pulse oximeter monitor:

1. The oxygen saturation of haemoglobin in arterial blood. Since the oximeter detects the saturation peripherally on a finger, toe or ear, the result is recorded as the peripheral oxygen saturation described as SpO_2.
2. The pulse rate in beats per minute, averaged over 5 to 20 seconds. The signal strength of the pulse oximeter falls if the circulation becomes inadequate.

Several factors can interfere with the correct function of a pulse oximeter including:

- **Light:** Bright light (such as the operating theatre light or sunlight) directly on the probe may affect the reading. Shielding the probe from direct light may assist in this.
- **Shivering:** Movement may make it difficult for the probe to pick up a signal.
- **Pulse volume:** The oximeter only detects pulsatile flow. When the blood pressure is low due to hypovolemic shock or the cardiac output is low or the patient has an arrhythmia, the pulse may be very weak and the oximeter may not be able to detect a signal
- Vasoconstriction reduces blood flow to the peripheries. The oximeter may fail to detect a signal if the patient is very cold and peripherally vasoconstricted.
- Carbon monoxide poisoning may give a falsely high saturation reading. Carbon monoxide binds very well to haemoglobin and displaces oxygen to form a bright red compound, carboxyhemoglobin. This is only an issue in patients following smoke inhalation from a fire.

4. Reliable markers of CPR include:

a. Increased cardiac output
b. Increased diastolic pressure
c. Reduced $ETCO_2$
d. Chest recoil of 2 cm should be done
e. Up to 60 chest compressions per minute

Ans. a,b

Option a	True	Yes, correct
Option b	True	Yes, correct. Effective CPR raises diastolic pressure to >20 mm Hg
Option c	False	No, $ETCO_2$ increases with effective CPR
Option d	False	No, not correct. Chest compression with recoil of 5 cms is indicative of a good CPR
Option e	False	100-120 chest compressions per minute

Cardiopulmonary resuscitation (CPR) consists of the use of chest compressions and artificial ventilation to maintain circulatory flow and oxygenation during cardiac arrest.

End-tidal carbon dioxide ($ETCO_2$) correlates with systemic blood flow and resuscitation rate during cardiopulmonary resuscitation (CPR) and may potentially direct chest compression performance.

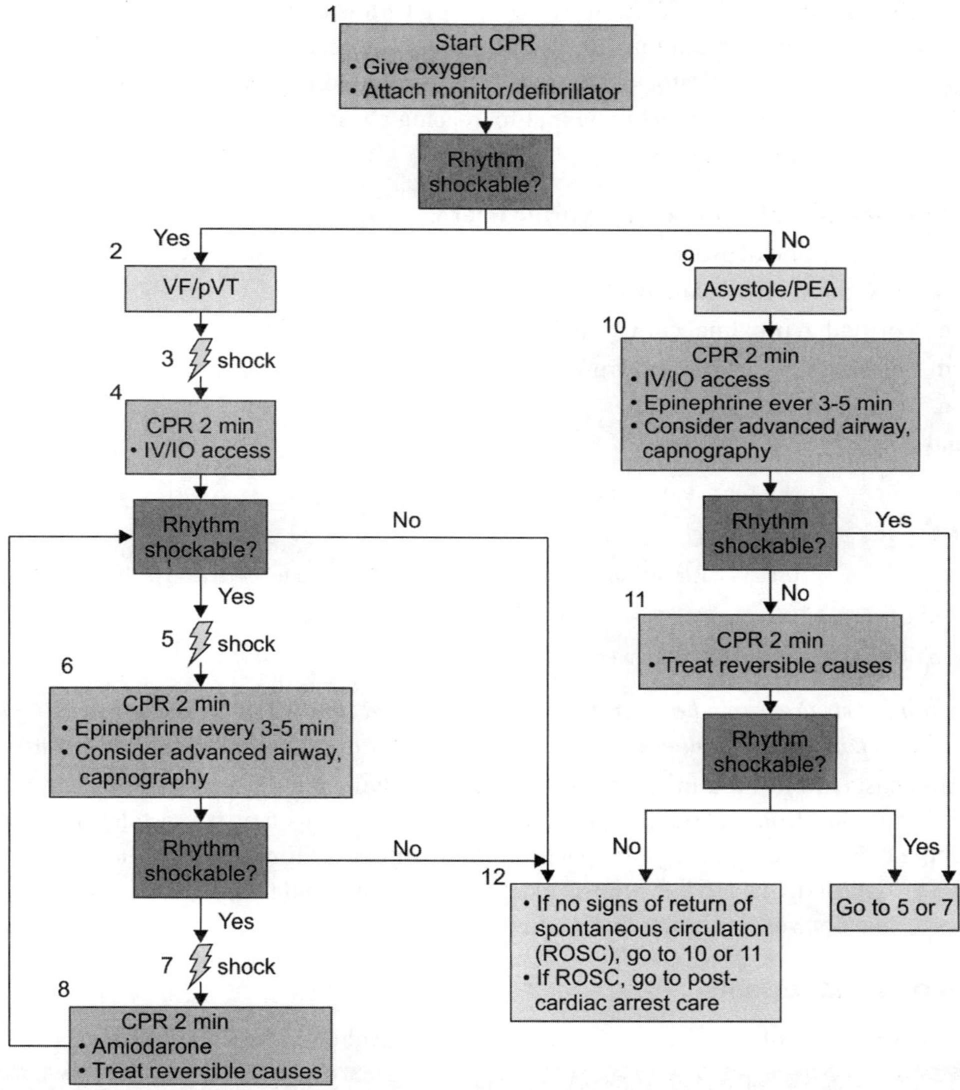

During cardiac arrest, high-quality CPR is essential to generate blood flow to vital organs and to achieve return of spontaneous circulation (ROSC).

$ETCO_2$ can be measured during CPR whether ventilating via bag-mask, laryngeal mask airway, or endotracheal tube.

$ETCO_2$ During CPR

CPR is a low cardiac output state during which $ETCO_2$ becomes less dependent on CO_2 production and ventilation and more linearly related to cardiac output. Flow of systemic venous blood to the pulmonary vasculature becomes rate limiting for the elimination of CO_2 and a surrogate for blood flow produced by chest compressions. After ventricular fibrillation, the $ETCO_2$ decreases to zero during the no-flow period and increases again with effective CPR. The inability to produce significant of $ETCO_2$ during CPR is a prognostic indicator for lack of return of spontaneous circulation (ROSC) in adults, whereas an abrupt increase in $ETCO_2$ during CPR can be an indicator of ROSC. $ETCO_2$ production during CPR has been used to compare CPR techniques and to show that increasing chest compression force, but not rate, increases blood flow production.

5. True about Sediments/casts in urine is/are:

a. Tamm-Horsfall protein is not seen
b. WBC are seen in acute pyelonephritis
c. Formed in proximal convoluted tubule
d. Hyaline casts are more common
e. Waxy casts are seen in obese individuals

Ans. b,d

Option a	False	No. These are commonly seen
Option b	True	Yes, correct
Option c	False	Urinary casts are formed only in the distal convoluted tubule (DCT) or the collecting duct
Option d	True	Yes, correct
Option e	False	Also called as renal failure casts

Urinary casts are formed only in the distal convoluted tubule (DCT) or the collecting duct. The proximal convoluted tubule (PCT) and loop of Henle are not locations for cast formation.

Urine casts are formed in the renal tubules, usually in the distal convoluted tubules or collecting tubules, from gelled protein which may include in its matrix crystals, fat, bacteria, cells or the residue thereof. The principal protein constituent of the gel is uromucoid or Tamm-Horsfall glycoprotein, which is synthesized and secreted by tubular epithelial cells probably in the ascending loops of Henle and distal convoluted tubules.

Types of Urinary Casts

Urinary casts can be divided into two main categories: Acellular and Cellular Casts.

Acellular casts	Cellular casts
Hyaline casts	Red blood cell casts
Granular casts	White blood cell casts
Waxy casts	Bacterial casts
Fatty casts	Epithelial cell casts

Hyaline casts are the most common type of casts which are composed of solidified Tamm-Horsfall mucoprotein.

Table 2: Types of urinary casts and associated conditions.

Casts	Composition	Associated conditions
Hyaline casts	Solidified Tamm-Horsfall mucoprotein	• Normal individuals • Dehydration • Heavy exercise
Granular casts	Various cell types (Degeneration of cellular casts, Aggregates of plasma proteins or immunoglobulin light chains)	• After strenuous exercise • Chronic renal diseases • Acute tubular necrosis
Waxy casts *(renal failure casts)*	Various cell types (Final stage of degeneration of cellular casts)	• Severe chronic renal disease • Renal amyloidosis
Fatty casts	Lipid droplets within the protein matrix of the cast	• Tubular degeneration • Nephrotic syndrome • Hypothyroidism
RBC casts	Red blood cells	• Pyelonephritis • Glomerulonephritis • Acute interstitial nephritis • Lupus nephritis
WBC casts	White blood cells	• Glomerulonephritis
Ephithelial cell casts	Renal tubular Epithelial cells	• Renal tubular necrosis • Viral diseases • Kidney transplant rejection
Bacterial cell casts	Bacterial cells	• Acute pyelonephritis • Intrinsic renal infection

6. True about Patent Ductus Arteriosus is/are:

a. Continuous machinery murmur is present
b. Seen in <5% of all congenital heart defects
c. Poor feeding
d. Left ventricular hypertrophy
e. Spontaneous closure after birth never occurs

Ans. a,c d

Option a	True	Yes, correct
Option b	False	No, it is seen in 5–10% of CHD's
Option c	True	Yes correct
Option d	True	Yes, correct
Option e	False	No, spontaneous closure may occur in very preterm infants

- Patent vessel between descending aorta and left pulmonary artery (normally, functional closure within first 15 hrs of life, anatomical closure within first days of life)
- **Epidemiology**
  - **5–10% of all congenital heart defects**
  - Delayed closure of ductus is common in premature infants (1/3 of infants <1,750 g); this is different from PDA in term infants
  - **Natural history:** Spontaneous closure common in premature infants, less common in term infants

- **Clinical presentation**
  - **History:** Asymptomatic, or have apneic or bradycardic spells, poor feeding, accessory muscle use, CHF Physical exam: Tachycardia, bounding pulses, hyperactive precordium, wide pulse pressure, continuous 'machinery' murmur best heard at left infraclavicular area Investigations
- **ECG:** May show left atrial enlargement, LVH, RVH
- **CXR:** Normal to mildly enlarged heart, increased pulmonary vasculature, prominent pulmonary artery
- **Echo:** Diagnostic
- Management
- **Indomethacin:** Antagonizes prostaglandin E2, which maintains ductus arteriosus patency; only effective in premature infants
- Catheter or surgical closure if PDA causes respiratory compromise, failure to thrive, or persists beyond 3rd month of life.

7. True about Atrial Septal Defect is/are:

a. S2 widely split and fixed
b. Crescendo-decrescendo systolic ejection murmur
c. Right Bundle Branch Block (RBBB)
d. Cyanotic lesion
e. Significant left atrial enlargement

Ans. a,b,c

Option a	True	Yes, correct
Option b	True	Yes correct
Option c	True	Yes correct
Option d	False	No, it is an acyanotic lesion
Option e	False	No, Left atrial enlargement is rare only if clinically significant mitral regurgitation.

Atrial Septal Defect

- **3 types:** Ostium primum (common in DS), ostium secundum (most common type, 50-70%), sinus venosus (defect located at entry of superior vena cava into right atrium)
- **Epidemiology:** 6-8% of congenital heart lesions
- Natural history
  - 80–100% spontaneous closure rate if ASD diameter <8 mm
  - If remains patent, CHF and pulmonary HTN can develop in adult life
- Clinical presentation
  - **History:** Often asymptomatic in childhood
  - **Physical exam:** Grade 2-3/6 pulmonic outflow murmur, widely split and fixed S2
  - Children with large ASDs may have signs of heart failure (tachypnea, failure to thrive, hepatomegaly, pulmonary rales/retractions)
- Investigations
  - **ECG:** Right Axis Deviation, mild RVH, RBBB

- **CXR:** Increased pulmonary vasculature, cardiac enlargement
- **Echocardiography:** Test of choice

❑ **Management:** Elective surgical or catheter closure between 2–5 year of age

8. True about Milk alkali syndrome:

a. Hyperglycemia
b. Hypercalcemia
c. Hyperkalemia
d. Hypokalemia
e. Nephrocalcinosis

Ans. b

Option a	False	No, not correct
Option b	True	Yes, correct
Option c	False	No, not correct
Option d	False	No, not correct
Option e	False	No, not correct

Milk-alkali syndrome is caused by the ingestion of large amounts of calcium and absorbable alkali, with resulting hypercalcemia.

Calcium-alkali syndrome is now more common in postmenopausal women with the use of over-the counter (OTC) calcium and vitamin D supplements.

Milk-alkali syndrome can have an acute course with rapid induction of hypercalcemia and acute renal failure soon (within a week) after excess calcium carbonate is begun. A more chronic course also is observed. In this form, irreversible renal failure may ensue, but many patients have partial recovery with a timely diagnosis.

Patients may have severe mental status changes that include obtundation and coma, especially as serum calcium levels rise higher than 15 mg/dL.

Hypercalcemia may produce EKG changes such as shortened QT/QTc interval and nonhypothermic J (or Osborn) waves.

Hypercalcemia

❑ **Mild:** Total Ca 10.5-11.9 mg/dL (2.5–3 mmol/L) or Ionized Ca 5.6–8 mg/dL (1.4–2 mmol/L)

❑ **Moderate:** Total Ca 12-13.9 mg/dL (3–3.5 mmol/L) or Ionized Ca 8–10 mg/dL (2–2.5 mmol/L)

❑ **Hypercalcemic crisis:** Total Ca 14–16 mg/dL (3.5–4 mmol/L) or Ionized Ca 10–12 mg/dL (2.5–3 mmol/L)

Common causes of hypercalcemia:

GRIEF MD

❑ **G**ranulomatous diseases (sarcoidosis)

❑ **R**enal failure (milk alkali syndrome)

❑ **I**mmobilization (prolonged)

❑ **E**ndocrine causes: Primary hyperparathyroidism (most common) — Solitary adenoma, generalized hyperplasia, multiple endocrine neoplasia type 1 or type 2A

❑ **F**amilial hypocalciuric hypercalcemia

Malignancy

Drugs - Vitamin **D**, thiazi**D**e

The signs and symptoms are those of hypercalcemia from any cause.

Clinical

- **Neurologic:** Hypercalcemia results in decreased mental activity such as lethargy and confusion.

GI

- Hypercalcemia results in decreased bowel activity such as constipation and anorexia but commonly gives nausea and vomiting as well.
- Pancreatitis occurs because of the precipitation of calcium in the pancreas. Severe pancreatitis, however, is associated with hypocalcaemia because of binding of calcium to malabsorbed fat in the intestine.
- Gastric and intestinal ulcers may be associated

Renal

- Hypercalcemia results in polyuria and polydipsia because of the induction of nephrogenic diabetes insipidus. Calcium also precipitates in the kidney, resulting in both kidney stones as well as nephrolithiasis.

Cardiovascular

- Hypertension occurs in 30–50% of patients with hypercalcemia.
- ECG: QT shortening

  Treatment: IV fluid rehydration followed by loop diuretics (furosemide)

9. Simple febrile seizure:

a. Seen in preschool children
b. Developmental delay seen in simple febrile seizure
c. Meningitis is usually the cause
d. Generalized tonic clonic seizure
e. Antiepileptic drugs are usually prescribed

Ans. a,d

Option a	True	Yes, correct
Option b	False	No, Children with simple febrile seizures are neurologically and developmentally healthy before and after the seizure.
Option c	False	Fever (and seizure) is not caused by meningitis, encephalitis, or any other illness affecting the brain
Option d	True	Yes, correct
Option e	False	Prophylaxis with antiepileptic drugs not recommended

Pediatric febrile seizures, which represent the most common childhood seizure disorder, exist only in association with an elevated temperature.

Division of febrile seizures into 3 groups, as follows:

- Simple febrile seizures
- Complex febrile seizures
- Symptomatic febrile seizures

Signs and Symptoms

Simple febrile seizure

- The setting is fever in a child aged 6 months to 5 years
- The single seizure is generalized and lasts less than 15 minutes
- The child is otherwise neurologically healthy and without neurologic abnormality by examination or by developmental history
- Fever (and seizure) is not caused by meningitis, encephalitis, or any other illness affecting the brain
- The seizure is described as either a generalized clonic or a generalized tonic-clonic seizure

Complex febrile seizure

- Age, neurologic status before the illness, and fever are the same as for simple febrile seizure
- This seizure is either focal or prolonged (i.e., >15 min), or multiple seizures occur in close succession

Symptomatic febrile seizure

- Age and fever are the same as for simple febrile seizure
- The child has a pre-existing neurologic abnormality or acute illness

Neither computed tomography (CT) nor magnetic resonance imaging (MRI) is indicated in patients with simple febrile seizures.

Workup

- **History:** Determine focus of fever, description of seizure, medications, trauma history, development, family history
- **Physical exam:** LOC, signs of meningitis, neurological exam, head circumference, focus of infection
- Septic workup including LP if suspecting meningitis (strongly consider if child <12 months; consider if child is 12–18 months; only if meningeal signs present if child >18 months)
- If typical febrile seizure, investigations only for determining focus of fever
- EEG/CT/MRI brain not warranted unless atypical febrile seizure or abnormal neurologic findings

Management

- Counsel and reassure patient and parents
  - Febrile seizures do not cause brain damage
  - Very small risk of developing epilepsy: 9% in child with multiple risk factors; 2% in child with typical febrile seizures compared to 1% in general population
  - 33% chance of recurrence (mostly within 1 year of first seizure and in children <1 year old)

- Antipyretics and fluids for comfort (though neither prevent seizure)
- Prophylaxis with antiepileptic drugs not recommended
- If high risk for recurrent or prolonged seizures, have rectal or sublingual lorazepam at home
- Treat underlying cause of fever

10. True about atrial tachyarrhythmia is/are:

a. QRS complexes preceded with P waves
b. Three different P wave forms can be seen
c. Most common cardiac rhythm disturbance
d. Narrow QRS complex
e. Beta blockers are drug of choice

Ans. a,b,d

Option a	True	Yes, correct
Option b	True	Yes, correct
Option c	False	Atrial fibrillation with very rapid rate >200 bpm is the most common condition causing cardiac rhythm disturbance
Option d	True	Yes, correct
Option e	False	β-blockers may be contraindicated because of severe pulmonary disease in the patients

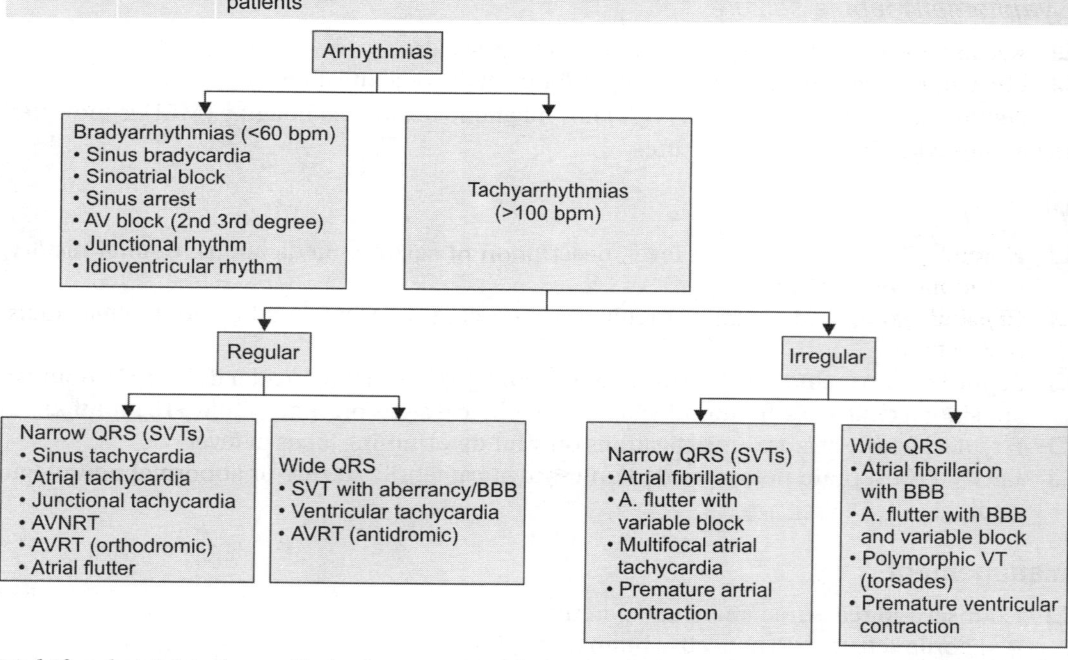

Multifocal atrial tachycardia is characterized by an irregular supraventricular rhythm, at rates 100–200 beats/min.

- The morphology of the P waves (at least 3 different P wave forms) varies from beat to beat, as does the PR interval. Each QRS complex, however, is preceded by a P wave.

- ❑ Generally seen in elderly patients or those with chronic lung disease who are experiencing respiratory failure
- ❑ Use diltiazem, verapamil, or digoxin; avoid beta blockers because of lung disease

11. Multiple sclerosis:

a. Relapse and remitting
b. Gene involved is HRA-B27
c. Neurologic deficits both in time and space
d. Diagnosis is made by MRI brain
e. Urinary retention never occurs

Ans. a,c,d

Option a	True	Relapsing remitting, or progressive neurologic symptoms due to inflammation, demyelination, and axonal degeneration
Option b	False	HLA-DRB1 gene has been demonstrated to be a genetically susceptible
Option c	True	Yes correct
Option d	True	Yes correct
Option e	False	Urinary urgency or retention are the most common initial presenting features

Definition

A chronic inflammatory disease of the CNS characterised by relapsing remitting or progressive neurologic dysfunction due to inflammation, demyelination and axonal degeneration

Clinical Patterns of MS

- ❑ Relapsing remitting (RRMS) 85%, primary progressive (PPMS) 10%, progressive relapsing (PRMS) 5%, secondary progressive (SPMS)
- ❑ Benign MS (BMS):retrospective diagnosis made after 15 years of mild disease, with no evidence of worsening (in functional ability and MRI)
- ❑ Most RRMS goes on to become SPMS

Genetic

- ❑ Polygenetic – HLA DRB1 gene
- ❑ MS is more common in areas high low vitamin D levels and low sun exposure levels
- ❑ F : M = 3:1, age of onset 2nd – 3rd decade

Features

- ❑ Numbness, visual disturbances
- ❑ Weakness or spasticity
- ❑ Diplopia
- ❑ **Lhermitte's sign:** Flexion of neck causes electric shock sensation down back into limbs indicating cervical cord lesion

- **Uhthoff's phenomenon:** Worsening of symptoms (classically optic neuritis) in heat
- **SPMS:** Classically weakness of legs in pyramidal distribution paired with cerebellar findings of arms (i.e. intention tremor)

Diagnosis for RRMS

- Demonstration of both dissemination in time and space based on the revised McDonald criteria (2010)
  - Dissemination in time: 2 or more attacks, simultaneous presence of asymptomatic gadolinium enhancing and non-enhancing MRI lesions at any time, or a new T2 and/or gadolinium-enhancing lesion(s) on follow-up MRI
  - Dissemination in space: >1 T2 lesions on MRI in at least 2 of the 4 CNS regions (periventricular, juxtacortical, infratentorial, or spinal cord) or developing a second attack that implicates a different CNS region.

Investigations

MRI

- Demyelinating plaques appear as hyperintense lesions on t_2 weighted MRI with active lesions showing enhancement with gadolinium
- **Dawson's fingers:** Periventricular lesions extending into the periventricular area

CSF

- Oligoclonal bands with increased IgG concentration

12. True about AIDS defining cancer:

a. Non-Hodgkins lymphoma
b. Kaposi's sarcoma
c. Anal carcinoma
d. Nasopharyngeal carcinoma
e. Adipose tissue carcinoma

Ans. a,b *Ref: Harrisons/19th, pg 1215; https://www.cdc.gov/mmwr/preview/mmwrhtml/rr5710a2.htm*

Option		
Option a	True	Yes, correct, it is also most common malignancy in HIV infected.
Option b	True	Yes, correct
Option c	False	No, it not AIDS defining malignancy
Option d	False	No, it not AIDS defining malignancy
Option e	False	No, it not AIDS defining malignancy

AIDS Defining Cancer

- Bacterial infections, multiple or recurrent*
- Candidiasis of bronchi, trachea, or lungs
- Candidiasis of esophagus†
- Cervical cancer, invasive§

- Coccidioidomycosis, disseminated or extrapulmonary
- Cryptococcosis, extrapulmonary
- Cryptosporidiosis, chronic intestinal (>1 moth's duration)
- Cytomegalovirus disease (other than liver, spleen, or nodes), onset at age >1 month
- Cytomegalovirus retinitis (with loss of vision)[†]
- Encephalopathy, HIV related
- Herpes simplex: Chronic ulcers (>1 month's duration) or bronchitis, pneumonitis, or esophagitis (onset at age >1 month)
- Histoplasmosis, disseminated or extrapulmonary
- Isosporiasis, chronic intestinal (>1 month's duration)
- Kaposi sarcoma[†]
- Lymphoid interstitial pneumonia or pulmonary lymphoid hyperplasia complex[*†]
- Lymphoid, Burkitt (or equivalent term)
- Lymphoid, immunoblastic (or equivalent term)
- Lymphoid, primary, of brain
- *Mycobacterium avium* complex or *Mycobacterium kanasasii*, disseminated or extrapulmonary[†]
- *Mycobacterium tuberculosis* of any site, pulmonary,[†§] disseminated,[†] or extrapulmonary[†]
- *Mycobacterium*, other species or unidentified species, disseminated or extraplumonary[†]
- *Pneumocystis jirovecii* pneumonia[†]
- Pneumonia, recurrent[†§]
- Progressive multifocal leukoencephalopathy
- *Salmonella* septicemia, recurrent
- Toxoplasmosis of brain, onset at age >1 month[†]
- Wasting syndrome attributed to HIV

The most prevalent of the HIV-related lymphomas is diffuse large B-cell non-Hodgkin's lymphoma, followed by Burkitt's lymphoma.

Non-AIDS Defining Maligancies

- Lung cancer – 3 times increased risk than HIV-uninfected
- Leukemia – 3 times increased risk than HIV-uninfected
- Anal Cnacer
- Hodgkin's disease
- Liver cancer – increased risk if HIV+ person has chronic Hep B or Hep C
- Testicular Cancer
- Melanoma
- Oropharyngeal cancer
- No increased incidence rate for colorectal or renal cancers
- Decreased incidence rate breast and prostate cancer

13. True about Brown-Sequard syndrome:

a. Posterior column defect
b. LMN lesion
c. 2 ipsilateral signs and 1 contralateral sign
d. Contralateral loss of pain and temperature sensation
e. Ipsilateral loss of pain and temperature sensation

Ans. c,d

Option a	False	No, it is Dorsal column defect
Option b	False	No, it is Upper motor neuron lesion
Option c	True	Yes, correct
Option d	True	Yes, correct
Option e	False	No, not correct

Brown-Séquard syndrome is an incomplete spinal cord lesion characterized by a clinical picture reflecting hemisection injury of the spinal cord, often in the cervical cord region.

Patients with Brown-Séquard syndrome suffer from ipsilateral upper motor neuron paralysis and loss of proprioception, as well as contralateral loss of pain and temperature sensation. A zone of partial preservation or segmental ipsilateral lower motor neuron weakness and analgesia may be noted. Loss of ipsilateral autonomic function can result in Horner syndrome.

Brown-Séquard Syndrome

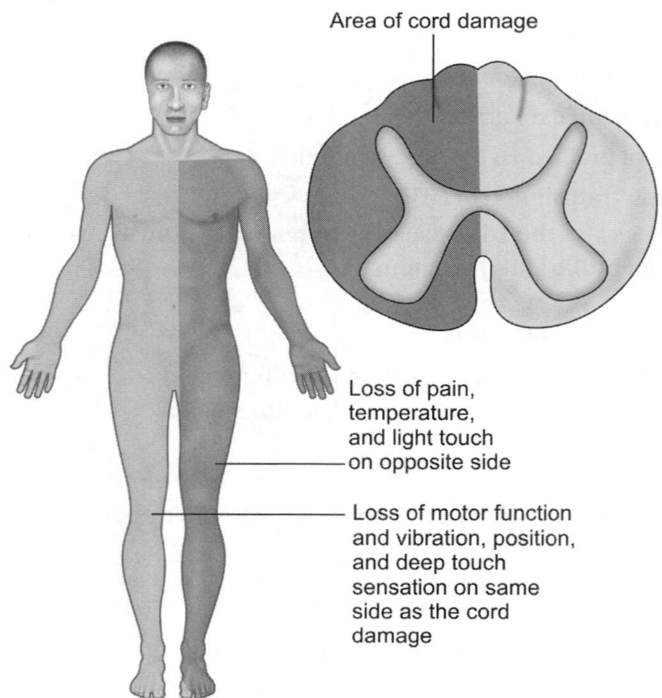

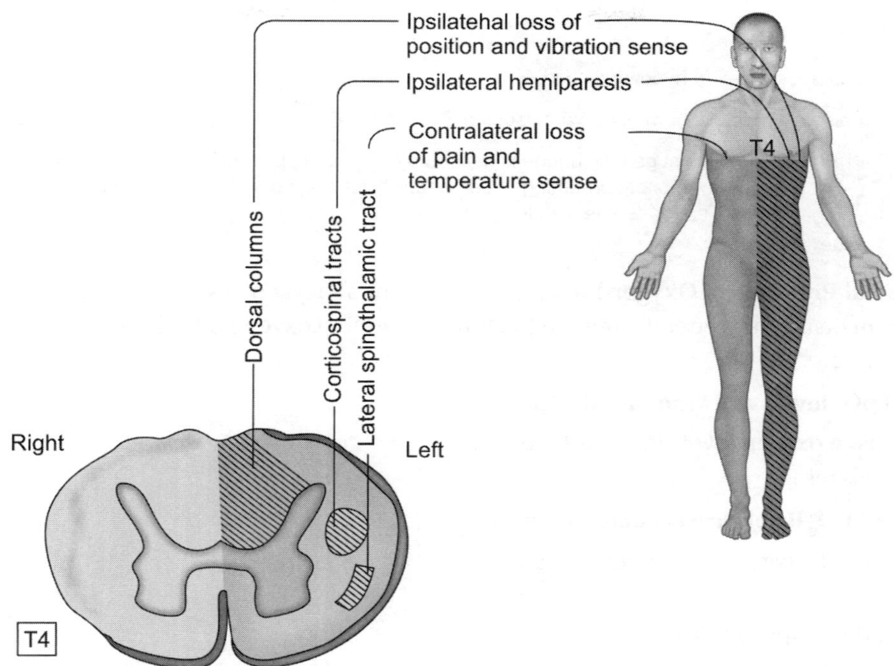

Hemisection of the cord results in a lesion of each of the 3 main neural systems:

1. The principal upper moto neuron pathway of the corticospinal tract
2. One or both dorsal columns
3. Spinothalamic tract.

The hallmark of a lesion to these 3 long tracts is presentation with 2 ipsilateral signs and 1 contralateral sign.

- Lesion of the corticospinal tract results in an ipsilateral spastic paresis below the level of the injury.
- Lesion to the fasciculus gracilis or cuneatus results in an ipsilateral loss of joint position sense, tactile discrimination, and vibratory sensations below the lesion.
- Lesion of the spinothalamic tract results in a contralateral loss of pain and temperature sensation starting 1 or 2 segments below the level of the lesion.

At the level of the lesion, there will be an ipsilateral loss of all sensation, including touch modalities as well as pain and temperature, and an ipsilateral flaccid paralysis in muscles supplied by the injured spinal cord segments.

14. Arterial pO_2 is low in:

a. Hyperventilation
b. CO Poisoning
c. Obstructive sleep apnea
d. COPD
e. Cystic fibrosis

Ans. c,d,e

Option a	False	Seen in hypoventilation
Option b	False	PaO_2 is normal in CO poisoning
Option c	True	Insufficient gas exchange is caused by alveolar hypoventilation (or breathing too little) with chest breathing. It can happen, for example, during sleep or during physical exercise for people with lung diseases.
Option d	True	
Option e	True	

PO_2 (Partial Pressure of Oxygen) reflects the amount of oxygen gas dissolved in the blood. It primarily measures the effectiveness of the lungs in pulling oxygen into the blood stream from the atmosphere.

Elevated pO_2 levels are associated with:

- ❑ Increased oxygen levels in the inhaled air
- ❑ Polycythaemia

Decreased PO_2 levels are associated with:

- ❑ Decreased oxygen levels in the inhaled air
- ❑ Anemia
- ❑ Heart decompensation
- ❑ Chronic obstructive pulmonary disease
- ❑ Restrictive pulmonary disease
- ❑ Hypoventilation

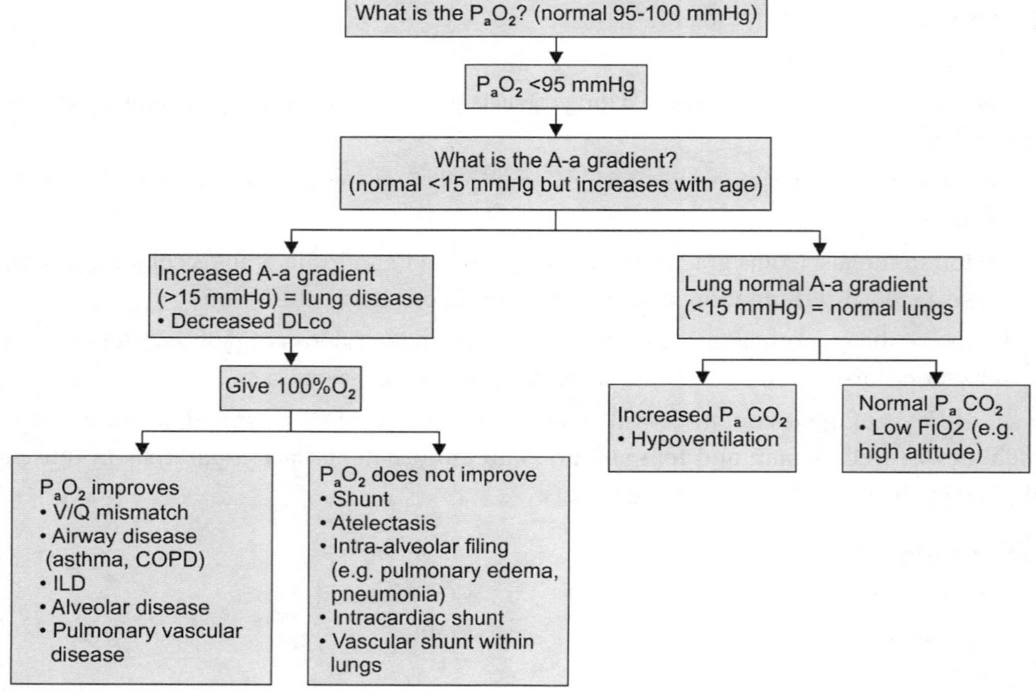

15. Capnography is used for:

a. Assesses ventilation
b. Confirming tube position
c. Pulmonary embolism
d. Assesses oxygenation
e. Wave form starts at the start of inspiration

Ans. a,b,c

Option a	True	Yes, correct
Option b	True	$ETCO_2$ in exhaled gas measured by capnography – a mandatory method for confirming the ETT is in the airway
Option c	True	Yes, correct
Option d	False	No, it assesses Ventilation
Option e	False	No, The waveform starts at the beginning of exhalation, and senses air from dead space in the upper airway and bronchi.

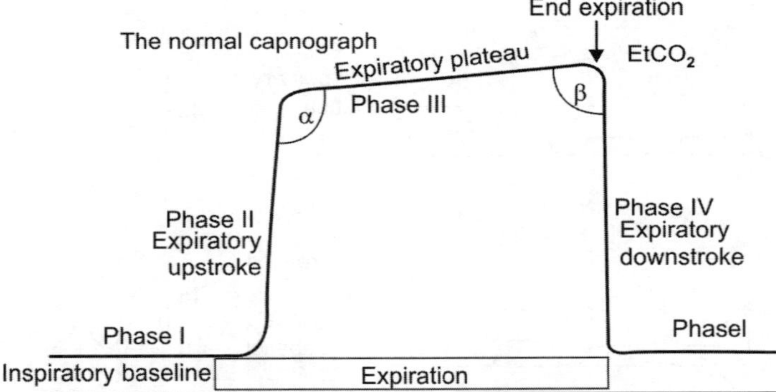

Waveform capnography represents the amount of carbon dioxide (CO_2) in exhaled air, which assesses ventilation. This measures **end-tidal CO_2 ($ETCO_2$)** which is **normally 35–45 mm Hg**.

Capnography also measures and displays respiratory rate. Changes in respiratory rate and tidal volume are displayed immediately as changes in the waveform and $ETCO_2$.

Capnography assesses ventilation, which is different from oxygenation. Ventilation is the air movement in and out of the lungs, while oxygenation is the amount of oxygen inhaled by the lungs that reaches the bloodstream. Pulse-oximetry assess oxygenation, and works by measuring the how much of each red blood cell is bound with oxygen. It is expressed as a per cent, or SPO_2. A normal SPO_2 is 92–96%.

If a patient has slow or shallow respirations, and a high $ETCO_2$ reading, this tells us that ventilation is not effectively eliminating CO_2 (**hypercarbia**), and that the brain is not responding appropriately to CO_2 changes. This may be caused by an overdose, head injury, or seizure.

Good to Know

Capnography waveforms

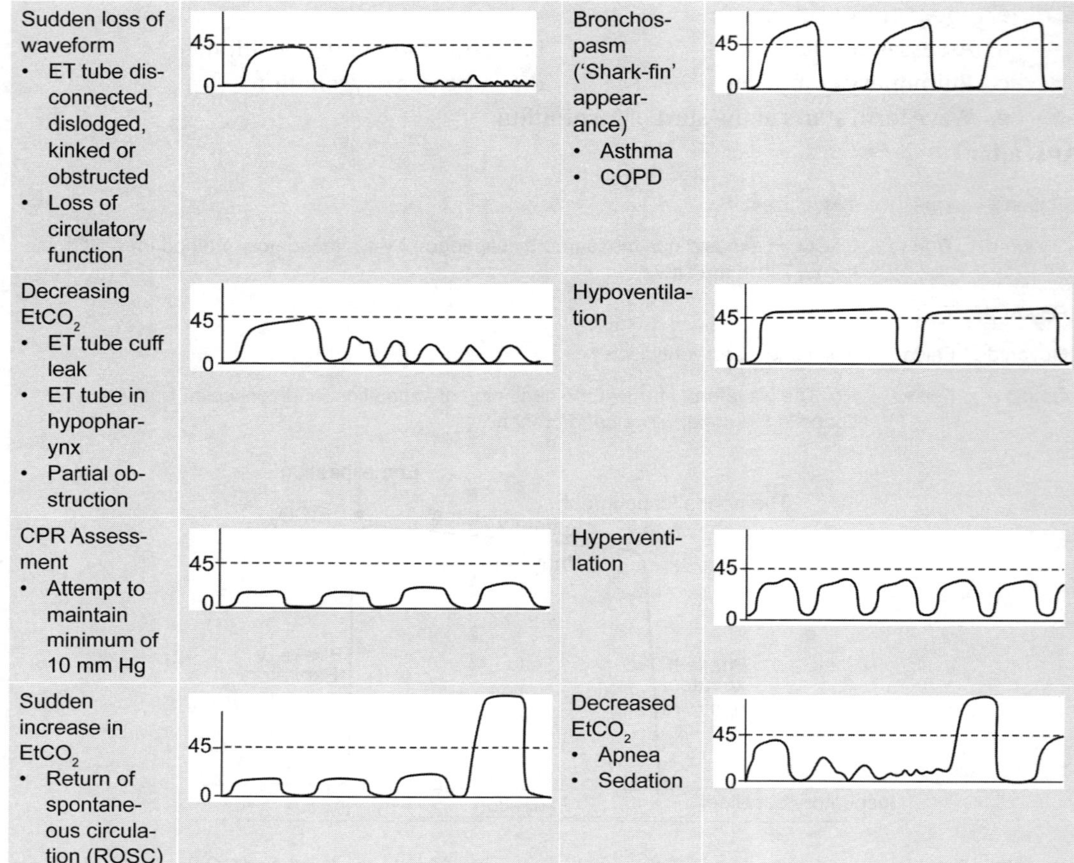

Sudden loss of waveform • ET tube disconnected, dislodged, kinked or obstructed • Loss of circulatory function	Bronchospasm ('Shark-fin' appearance) • Asthma • COPD
Decreasing $EtCO_2$ • ET tube cuff leak • ET tube in hypopharynx • Partial obstruction	Hypoventilation
CPR Assessment • Attempt to maintain minimum of 10 mm Hg	Hyperventilation
Sudden increase in $EtCO_2$ • Return of spontaneous circulation (ROSC)	Decreased $EtCO_2$ • Apnea • Sedation

16. Polyuria of Solute diuresis is seen in:

a. Primary psychogenic polydipsia
b. Diabetes mellitus
c. Diabetes insipidus
d. SIADH
e. Salt wasting nephropathy

Ans. b,e *Ref: Bhavna bhasin. Evaluation of Polyuria: The Roles of Solute Loading and Water Diuresis. Am J Kidney Dis. 2016;67(3):507-511; Textbook of critical care. 7th/ed, Chap 11.*

Option a	False	No, there will be water diuresis, due to excess drinking of water, excess diuresis with low urinary sodium
Option b	True	Yes, correct
Option c	False	No, vasopressin deficiency will lead to water diuresis
Option d	False	No polyuria in SIADH
Option e	True	Yes, correct

Polyuria is an important clinical condition characterized by urine output in excess of 3.0 to 3.5 L/d and low urine osmolality of, 300 mOsm/kg.

Basics

	Water diuresis	Solute diuresis
Etiopathogenesis	Water diuresis can be produced by drinking large amounts of hypotonic fluid	Osmotic diuresis is produced by 1. The administration of compounds such as mannitol and related polysaccharides that are filtered out but not reabsorbed. 2. Naturally occurring substances when they are present in amounts exceeding the capacity of the tubules to reabsorb them.
Pathology	The amount of water reabsorbed in the proximal tubules is normal, and the maximal urine flow that can be produced is about 16 mL/min	Increased urine flow is due to decreased water reabsorption in the proximal tubules and loops and very large urine flows can be produced
Mechanism	Result of a reduced osmotic reabsorption of water, leading to increased solute-free water clearance and a hypoosmotic urine.	Result of reduced solute reabsorption, leading to the presence of large quantities of unreabsorbed solutes in the renal tubules, causing an increase in urine volume

The differential diagnosis of polyuria includes central diabetes insipidus, congenital or acquired nephrogenic diabetes insipidus, psychogenic polydipsia, high protein or hyperglycaemic osmotic diuresis, salt wasting nephropathies, mixed polyuria due to excess solute and water intake, and post-obstructive diuresis following recovery from urinary obstruction.

Causes of Polyuria

1. Polyuria secondary to water diuresis
   a. Excessive intake of water
      i. Psychogenic polydipsia
      ii. Drugs—anticholinergic drugs, thioridazine
      iii. Hypothalamic disease—trauma, sarcoidosis
   b. Defective water reabsorption by the kidney
      i. Central diabetes insipidus (vasopressin deficiency)
      ii. Renal tubular resistance to AVP
2. Congenital nephrogenic diabetes insipidus
3. Acquired nephrogenic diabetes insipidus
   a. Hypercalcemia
   b. Hypokalemia
   c. Drugs—lithium, demeclocycline
   d. Chronic renal diseases—postobstructive diuresis, polyuric phase of ATN
   e. Other systemic diseases—amyloidosis, sickle cell anemia
4. Polyuria secondary to solute diuresis
   a. Electrolyte-induced solute diuresis
      i. Iatrogenic—excessive sodium chloride load, loop diuretic use
      ii. Salt-wasting nephropathy (rarely causes polyuria)

b. Nonelectrolyte solute-induced diuresis
   i. Glucosuria—diabetic ketoacidosis, hyperosmolar coma
   ii. Urea diuresis—high-protein diet, ATN
   iii. Iatrogenic—mannitol

Good to Remember Points

- Polyuria is defined as urinary volume in excess of 3.0–3.5 L/d
- Polyuria can be due to water diuresis or solute diuresis
- Solute load is an important determinant of urinary volume
- Solute diuresis may be seen in hospitalized patients who are given high protein feeds and following relief of urinary obstruction
- High dietary solute intake can cause polyuria in the outpatient setting, particularly with unusually large ingestion of protein and fruits
- Mixed polyuria due to solute loading and habitual excessive water intake can be seen in athletic individuals
- Calculation of urinary osmoles and the nature of the osmoles is helpful in the diagnosis of solute diuresis
- Estimation of daily osmole excretion should be included as a part of the routine workup for polyuria
- Most common cause of nephrogenic diabetes insipidus is chronic lithium ingestion.

Approach to Polyuria

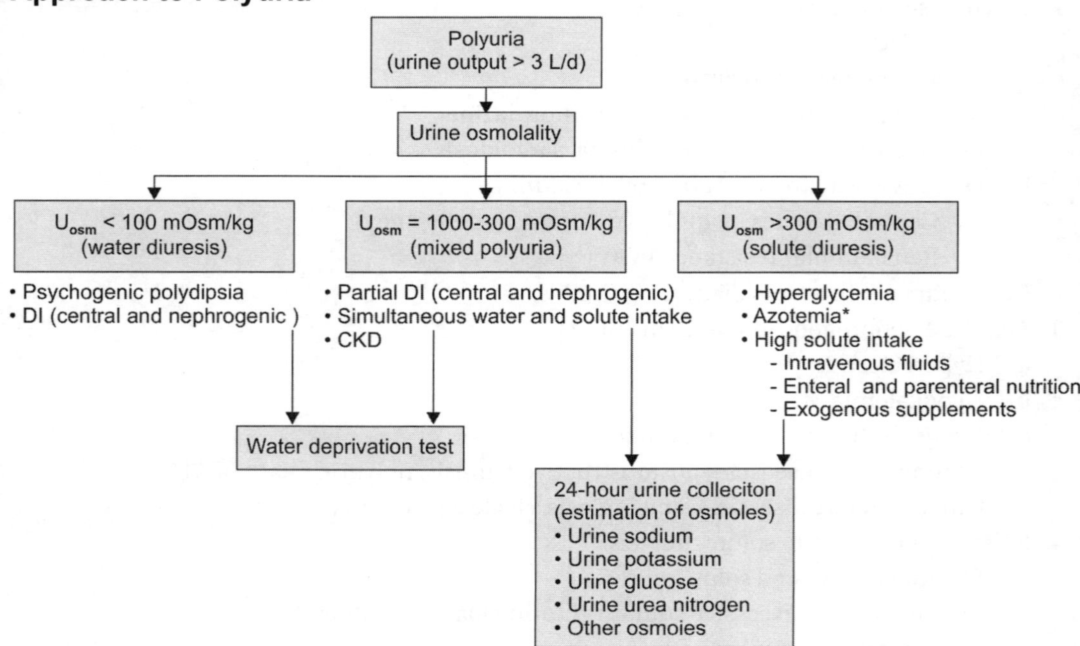

Basic clinical approach:

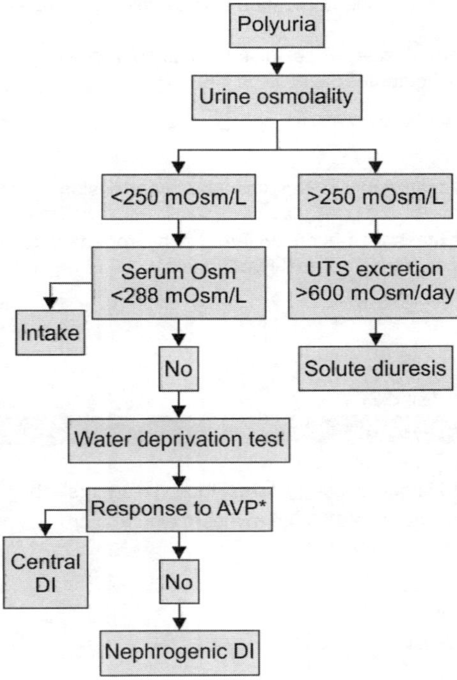

17. A 2-year-old male presents with low potassium, high urinary calcium, high urea, metabolic alkalosis, nephrocalcinosis and shock. The probable differential diagnosis will be:

a. Barter syndrome
b. Renal tubular acidosis
c. Gittleman syndrome
d. Chronic diuretic use
e. Chronic vomiting

Ans. a,b *Ref: Arvind bagga. Approach to Renal Tubular Disorders. [Indian J Pediatr 2005;72(9):771-776*

Option a	True	Yes correct
Option b	True	Yes, correct in distal RTA, these features could be seen
Option c	False	No, Not correct. There is no hypercalcemia but characteristic presence of hypermagnesemia
Option d	False	No, Not correct. There is no calcinosis and no hypercalcuria
Option e	False	No, Not correct. There is no calcinosis and no hypercalcuria

Causes of HypokalAemia

Increased excretion
Nonrenal losses (urine K^+ <20 mmol/L) • Diarrhea, laxative abuse • Vomiting

Contd...

Renal losses (urine K^+ >20mmol mmol/L) • Loop diuretics (furosemide, bumetanide, torsemide): Block chloride-coupled sodium reabsorption in the loop of Henle • Thiazide diuretics (hydrochlorothiazide): Block distal tubule chloride-coupled sodium reabsorption • Osmotic diuresis (uncontrolled diabetes)
Hypokalemia with hypertension • Mineralocorticoid excess • Primary hyperaldosteronism • Glucocorticoid-remediable aldosteronism: Renovascular hypertension, renin-secreting tumor, Liddle syndrome • Apparent mineralocorticoid excess: 11b-hydroxysteroid dehydrogenase deficiency [genetic, durg induced (chewing tobacco, licorice), congenital adrenal hyperplasia]
• Hypokalemia with normal blood pressure • Bartter's syndrome • Gitelman's syndrome • Magnesium depletion (cis-platinum, alcoholism) • Renal tubular acidosis (types 1 and 2)
Transcellular shifts
Drugs-insulin administration
β-Adrenergic agonists (bronchodilators, decongestants, tocolytic agents)- theophyline, caffeine
Acute catecholamine surge from stress (e.g. acute myocardial infarction)
Delirium tremens
Thyrotoxic hypokalemic paralysis
Familial hypokalemic periodic paralysis
Barium poisoning-metabolic alkalosis

Causes of Hyperkalemia

Spurious • Thrombocytosis (>1,000,000/mm³) • Leukocytosis (>50,000/mm³) • Hemolysis • Repeated first clenching with tourniquet in place
Impaired potassium excretion • Renal insufficiency or failure • Mineralocorticoid deficiency • Addison's disease • Hyporenin hypoaldosteronism (type 4 renal tubular acidosis) • Hereditary enzyme deficiencies
Pseudohypoaldosteronism
Drugs • Block sodium channel in distal nephron—trimethoprim, pentamidine, potassium-sparing diuretics (amiloride, triamterene) • Block aldosterone production: ACE inhibitors, angiotensin receptor blockers, NSAIDs, and COX-2 inhibitors, heparin, tacrolimus • Block aldosterone receptors: Spironolactone, eplerenone • Block Na^+, K^+ -ATPase activity in the distal nephron: cyclosporine
Impaired transcelular shift-insuline deficiency
Hypertonicity (uncontrolled diabetes): Familial hyperkalemic periodic paralysis Drugs–beta blockers, digoxin (at toxic levels), succinylcholine, arginine, lysine
Excessive potassium load
Massive tissue breakdown (rhabdomyolysis, burns, trauma)
ACE, angiotensin-converting enzyme; COX-2, Cyclooxygenase-2; NSAID, nonsteroidal anti-inflammatory drug

Common disorders of tubular functions:

Segment	Function	Disorder
Proximal tubule*	Phosphate transport Glucose transport Aminoacid transport	Hypophosphatemic rickets Renal glucosuria Isolated, generalized aminoaciduria
Ascending limb of Henle	Sodium, postassium, chloride transport	Bartter syndrome
Distal tubule	Proton (H+) secretion Sodium, chloride transport	Distal RTA Gitelman syndrome
Collecting duct	Sodium, potassium transport Water transport	Pseudohypoaldosteronism Liddle syndrome Nephrogenic DI

*Generalized dysfunction of the proximal tubule (Fanconi syndrome) may be primary or secondary to various disorders (e.g., galactosemia, Lowe syndrome)

RTA renal tubular acidosis: DI diabetes insipidus

Features of Renal Tubular Acidosis

Clinical

- ❑ Growth retardation, failure to thrive
- ❑ Polyuria, polydipsia: Preferrence for savory foods
- ❑ Refractory rickets
- ❑ Renal calculi, nephrocalcinosis
- ❑ Unexplained hypertension*

Laboratory

- ❑ Hyperchloremic metabolic acidosis
- ❑ Metabolic alkalosis with or without hypokalemia
- ❑ Hyponatremia with hyperkalemia
- ❑ Hypercalciuria with normal serum calcium

*As in Liddle's syndrome, syndrome of apparent mineralocorticoid excess

Evaluation of child with hypokalaemia and metabolic acidosis:

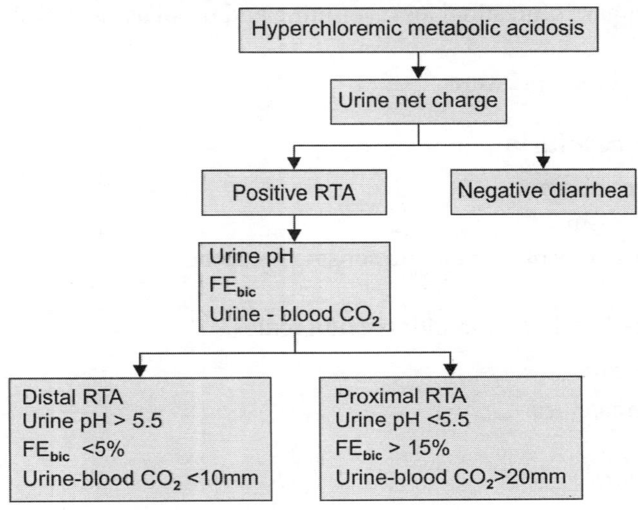

Note: Urine net charge (urinary $Na^+ + K^+ - Cl^-$) provides an estimate of renal ammonium production, differentiating between renal and extrarenal causes of hyperchloremic acidosis.

Evaluation of patient with metabolic alkalosis and hypokalaemia

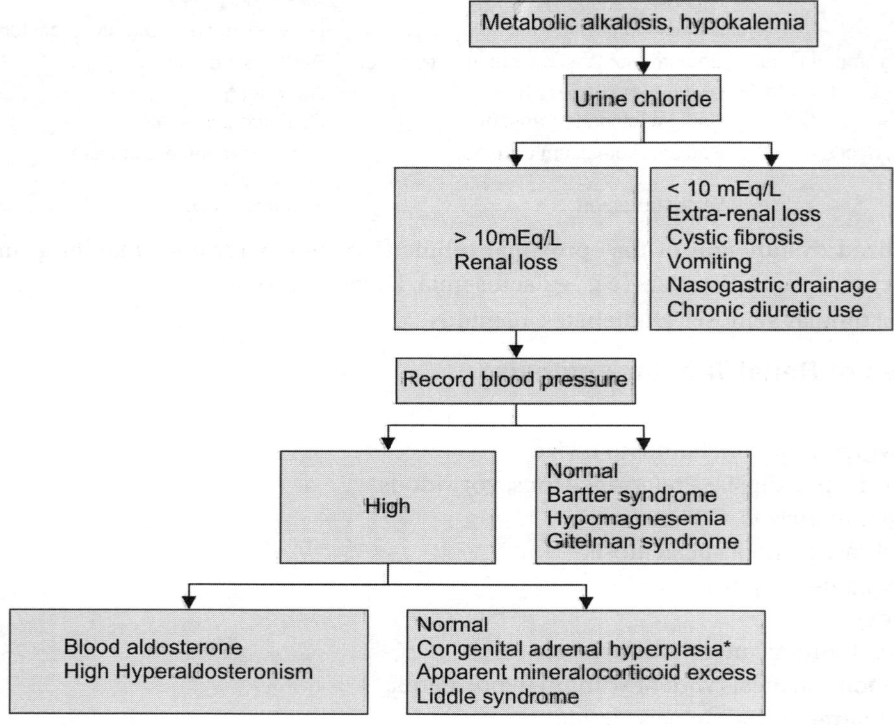

Evaluation of Hypokalemia with Metabolic Alkalosis

Initial evaluation should include

- History of upper gastrointestinal loss (vomiting and nasogastric drainage)
- Diuretic use
- Measurement of blood pressure.

Causes of Hypercalciuria

Secondary to hypercalcemia

- Hyperparathyroidism
- Inactivating mutations of the calcium sensing receptor
- Vitamin D excess
- Granulomatous disorders – sarcoidosis, tuberculosis

Without hypercalcemia

- Idiopathic hypercalciuria
- Distal RTA
- Bartter syndrome

- ❑ Therapy with loop diuretics, corticosteroids
- ❑ Familial hypomagnesemia

Pearls:

1. Normal anion gap in the presence of acidosis (hyperchloremic metabolic acidosis) suggests increased urinary (proximal RTA) or gastrointestinal loss (diarrhea) of bicarbonate or impaired excretion of H^+ ions (distal RTA).
2. Patients with RTA typically show impaired renal $NH4^+$ excretion and a positive urine anion gap
3. The occurrence of metabolic acidosis and hypokalemia suggests RTA or gastrointestinal loss of bicarbonate (diarrhea, ureterosigmoidostomy).
4. The primary defect in proximal RTA is the reduced renal threshold for bicarbonate, resulting in bicarbonaturia.
5. Distal RTA is characterized by decreased proton excretion due to a proton pump defect or back diffusion of protons.
6. Fanconi syndrome is characterized by bicarbonaturia, phosphaturia, sodium and potassium wasting, glycosuria and aminoaciduria.
7. Urine chloride helps in differentiating non-renal (< 10 mEq/L) from renal causes (> 20 mEq/L) of hypokalemic alkalosis.
8. The presence of elevated blood pressure suggests true (hyperaldosteronism, glucocorticoid remediable aldosteronism, congenital adrenal hyperplasia) or apparent mineralocorticoid excess (Liddle syndrome, syndrome of apparent mineralocorticoid excess)
9. Low blood levels of aldosterone and lack of response to glucocorticoid and spironolactone is suggestive of Liddle syndrome.
10. Barter Syndrome: Hypercalciuria (due to dysfunction of the TALH chloride transporters preventing chloride reabsorption)
11. In Gitelman syndrome, dysfunction of the sodium chloride cotransporter (NCCT) leads to hypocalciuria and hypomagnesemia (pathognomonic)

Hence in this MCQ, we get:

- ❑ Hypokalemia
- ❑ Hypercalciuria
- ❑ Hyper-urecemia
- ❑ Metabolic alkalosis
- ❑ Nephrocalcinosis
- ❑ Shock

All features point towards: severe Barter syndrome or distal type RTA

Note: The shock could be secondary to metabolic alkalosis and nephrocalcinosis

18. First line investigation for assessing pituitary tumor is:

a. MRI
b. CT
c. PET
d. IGF-1
e. S. Prolactin levels

Ans. a,d,e

Option a	True	Yes, MRI has been found to be highly specific and sensitive
Option b	False	No, MRI is considered superior for diagnosing the pituitary mass lesions
Option c	False	No, not correct
Option d	True	Yes, it may the first investigation done for growth hormone abnormalities
Option e	True	Yes, it may be the first investigation for prolactinomas

Assessment of pituitary tumour:

1. Pituitary mass – non localised
   a. Visual field evaluation
   b. Neuroimaging
2. Prolactinomas
   a. S. Prolactin levels
3. Growth hormone level
   a. GH levels
   b. IGF-1 levels
   c. GH suppression test
4. Cushing's
   a. 24 hr free cortisol
   b. Dexamethasone suppression test
   c. Metyrapone test
   d. Serum ACTH

Imaging:

1. MRI brain plain
2. MRI brain pre and post gadolinium
3. CT
4. Cerebral angiography
5. Indium-111-DTPA scan (^{111}In-DTPA-octreotide single photon emission CT-SPECT) – for hormone secreting pituitary tumours.

19. Fever during a blood transfusion could be probably due to:

a. TRALI
b. Citrate acidity
c. Haemolytic transfusion reactions
d. Contamination
e. Massive blood transfusion

Ans. b,c,d

Option a	False	No, TRALI is unlikely to present as febrile reaction only in blood transfusion. TRALI may present as shortness of breath, disorientation, tachycardia or other features related to cardiac decompensation
Option b	True	Yes, citrate toxicity, may present as transient rise in temperature (but only a few proportions of cases may present with fever. It is not characteristic of citrate toxicity)
Option c	True	Yes, it may present as fever

Option d	True	Yes, spiking, high grade fever is characteristic
Option e	False	No, massive transfusion rarely would present as fever. However, massive transfusion will present as predominantly with hypothermia and electrolyte abnormalities

Causes of transfusion related reactions:

1. Acute hemolytic reactions
   a. Misidentification of the patient or the receipt/donor blood group
2. Nonhemolytic febrile reactions
   a. Reaction of the normal constituents of blood during transfusion
   b. Fever is characteristic ± chills, rigors
3. Allergic reactions
   a. Rash, fever
4. Anaphylaxis
   a. Dyspnea
   b. Bronchospasm, wheeze
   c. Hypotension
5. Circulatory overload
   a. Cardiac overload features
   b. Tachycardia
6. TRALI
   a. Features of cardiac decompensation
   b. Acute onset dyspnea
   c. Orthopnea
   d. Tachycardia
7. Bacterial contamination
   a. High grade fever
   b. Shock, weak pulse
   c. Orthopnea
   d. Tachypnea
   e. Tachycardia
   f. Distended JVP

Medicine

1. True about factitious fever is:

a. Temperature > 41°C
b. Pulse rate > Temperature
c. Lack of sweating in effervescence
d. CRP is raised
e. Diurnal variation

Ans. a, c

Option a	True	
Option b	False	Pulse rate is not related to increase in temperature
Option c	True	
Option d	False	CRP is normal
Option e	False	No diurnal variation

Factitious fever (fever artificially induced by the patient—for example, by IV injection of contaminated water) should be considered in all patients but is more common among young women in health care professions.

Clues to the diagnosis of factitious fever

- Patient looks well
- Bizarre temperature chart with absence of diurnal variation or temperature related pulse rate
- Temperature > 41 °C
- Normal ESR and CRP despite high fever
- Evidence of self injection or self harm
- Normal temperature during supervised measurements.

2. True diads:

a. Hypophosphatemic rickets–AR
b. DMD–AD
c. Sickle cell anemia–AD
d. Achondroplasia–AD
e. Tuberous sclerosis–AD

Ans. d, e *Ref: Harrison and Robbins*

Option a	False	X linked or autosomal dominant
Option b	False	X linked recessive
Option c	False	Autosomal recessive
Option d	True	
Option e	True	

Hypophosphatemic rickets is either X-linked or autosomal dominant.
DMD–X-linked recessive

Sickle cell anemia–AR

Achondroplasia–AD

Tuberous sclerosis–AD

Genetic disorders and possible interventions

Genetic disorder	*Inheritance*	*Genes*	*Interventions*
Oncologic			
Lynch syndrome (HNPCC)	AD	MLH1, MSH2, MSH6, PMS2	Early endoscopic screening; risk-reducing surgery
Familial adenomatous polyposis	AD	APC	Early and frequent endoscopy; prophylactic colectomy
Hereditary breast and ovarian cancer	AD	BRCA1, BRCA2	Risk reducing salpingo-oophorectomy; intensified breast surveillance including breast MRI; risk-reducing mastectomy
Hereditary diffuse gastric cancer	AD	CDH1	Prophylactic gastrectomy; enhanced breast cancer surveillance
Hematologic			
Factor V Leiden	AD	F5	Avoidance of thrombogenic risk factors
Hemophilia A	XL	F8	Factor VIII replacement
Hemophilia B	XL	F9	Factor IX replacement
Glucose 6-phosphate dehydrogenase deficiency	XL	G6PD	Avoidance of oxidant drugs and certain foods
Cardiovascular			
Hypertrophic cardiomyopathy	AD	> 10 genes including MYBPC3, MYH7, TNNT2, TPM1	Echocardiographic screening; pharmacologic intervention; myomectomy
Long QT syndrome	AD, AR	> 10 genes including KCNQ1, SCNSA, KCNE1 KCNE2	Electrocardiographic screening; pharmacologic intervention; implantable cardiac defibrillator devices
Marfan's syndrome	AD	FBN1	Echocardiographic screening; prophylactic beta blockers; aortic valve replacement as indicated
Gastrointestinal			
Familial Mediterranean fever	AR	MEFV	Colchicine
Hemochromatosis	AR	HFE	Phlebotomy
Pulmonary			
α1 Antitrypsin deficiency	AR	SERPINA1	Avoidance of smoking and occupational and environmental toxins
Cystic fibrosis	AR	CFTR	Chest physiotherapy; agents to promote airways secretion clearance; *CFTR* modulators (G551D mutations); lung transplantation
Endocrine			
Neurohypophyseal diabetes insipidus	AD	AVP	Replace vasopressin
Familial hypocalciuric hypercalcemia	AD	CASR	Avoidance of parathyroidectomy
Multiple endocrine neoplasia type 2	AD	RET	Prophylactic thyroidectomy; screening for pheochromocytoma and hyperparathyroidism
Renal			

Contd…

Contd...

Genetic disorder	*Inheritance*	*Genes*	*Interventions*
Polycystic kidney disease	AD, AR	PKD1, PKD2, PKHD1	Prevention of hypertension; prevention of urinary tract infections; kidney transplantation
Nephrogenic diabetes insipidus	XL, AR	AVPR2, AQP2	Fluid replacement; thiazides with or without amiloride
Neurologic			
Malignant hyperthermia	AD	RYR1, CACNA1S	Avoidance of precipitating anesthetics
Hyperkalemic periodic paralysis	AD	SCN4A	Diet rich in calcium and low in potassium; thiazides or acetazolamide
Duchenne's and Becker's muscular dystrophy	XL	DMD	Corticosteroids; physical therapy
Wilson's disease	AR	ATP7B	Zinc, trientene

Disease	Abnormal protein	Protein type/Function
Autosomal Dominant Inheritance		
Familial hypercholesterolemia	Low-density lipoprotein receptor	Receptor transport
Marfan syndrome	Fibrillin	Structural support: extracellular matrix
Ehlers-Danlos syndrome	Collagen	Structural support: extracellular matrix
Hereditary spherocytosis	Spectrin, ankyrin, or protein 4.1	Structural support: red blood cell membrane
Neurofibromatosis, type I	Neurofibromin-I (NF-I)	Growth regulation
Adult polycystic kidney disease	Polycystic-I (PDK-I)	Cell-cell and cell-matrix interactions
Autosomal Recessive Inheritance		
Cystic fibrosis	Cystic fibrosis transmembrane regulator	Ion channel
Phenylketonuria	Phenylalanine hydroxylase	Enzyme
Tay-Sachs disease	Hexosaminidase	Enzyme
Severe combined immunodeficiency	Adenosine deaminase	Enzyme
α- and β-Thalassemias	Hemoglobin	Oxygen transport
Sickle cell anemia	Hemoglobin	Oxygen transport
X-linked Recessive Inheritance		
Hemophilia A	Factor VIII	Coagulation
Duchenne/Becker muscular dystrophy	Dystrophin	Structural support: cell membrane
Fragile X syndrome	FMRP	RNA translation

3. Which of the following is not useful in diagnosis of DKA?

a. Blood ketones
b. Urinary ketones
c. Serum glucose
d. Acid anion gap
e. Blood pH

Ans. b

Option a	True	Yes, is useful in diagnosis of DKA
Option b	False	No, is not useful in diagnosis of DKA
Option c	True	Yes, is useful in diagnosis of DKA
Option d	True	Yes, is useful in diagnosis of DKA
Option e	True	Yes, is useful in diagnosis of DKA

DKA is characterized by hyperglycemia, ketosis, and metabolic acidosis (increased anion gap) along with a number of secondary metabolic derangements as shown in the following table.

	DKA	HHS
Glucose[a], mmol/L (mg/dL)	13.9 – 33.3 (250 – 600)	33.3 – 66.6 (600 – 1200)
Sodium, mEq/L	125 – 135	135 – 145
Potassium[a,b]	Normal to ↑	Normal
Magnesium[a]	Normal	Normal
Chloride[a]	Normal	Normal
Phosphate[a,b]	Normal	Normal
Creatinine	Slightly ↑	Moderately ↑
Osmolality (mOsm/mL)	300 – 320	330 – 380
Plasma ketones[a]	++++	+/–
Serum bicarbonate[a],mEq/L	< 15	Normal to slightly ↓
Arterial pH	6.8 – 7.3	> 7.3
Arterial pCO_2[a], mm Hg	20 – 30	Normal
Anion gap[a] [Na – (Cl + HCO_3)]	↑	Normal to slightly ↑

In DKA, the ketone body, β-hydroxybutyrate, is synthesized at a threefold greater rate than acetoacetate; however, acetoacetate is preferentially detected by a commonly used ketosis detection reagent (nitroprusside). Serum ketones are present at significant levels (usually positive at serum dilution of ≥ 1:8). **The nitroprusside tablet, or stick, is often used to detect urine ketones; certain medications such as captopril or penicillamine may cause false-positive reactions. Serum or plasma assays for β-hydroxybutyrate are preferred because they more accurately reflect the true ketone body level.** *Harrison's Medicine, 19/e*

Essentials of Diagnosis (CMDT, 2017)

- Hyperglycemia greater than 250 mg/dL
- Acidosis with blood pH < 7.3
- Serum bicarbonate less than 15 mEq/L
- Serum positive for ketones.

Diabetic Ketoacidosis cannot be diagnosed on the basis of large value of ketones in urine, because ordinary fasting can produce such a reading.

Endocrinology and obesity by Gordon c. Weir, 6/e.

4. Which of the following features are seen in hypomagnesemia and not hypermagnesemia?

a. Tremors
b. Muscle weakness
c. Delayed deep tendon reflexes
d. Sinus tachycardia
e. Paradoxical bradycardia

Ans. a, b, d

Option a	True	Seen in only hypomagnesemia
Option b	True	Seen in only hypomagnesemia
Option c	False	
Option d	True	Seen in only hypomagnesemia
Option e	False	

Hypomagnesemia	*Hypermagnesemia*
Generalized alterations in neuromuscular function, including tetany, tremor, seizures, muscle weakness, ataxia, nystagmus, vertigo, apathy, depression, irritability, delirium, and psychosis.	Most prominent clinical manifestations are vasodilation and neuromuscular blockade. Hypotension that is refractory to vasopressors or volume expansion may be an early sign.
Cardiac arrhythmias may occur, including sinus tachycardia, other supraventricular tachycardias, and ventricular arrhythmias. Electrocardiographic abnormalities may include prolonged PR or QT intervals, T-wave flattening or inversion, and ST straightening. Sensitivity to digitalis toxicity may be enhanced.	Nausea, lethargy, and weakness may progress to respiratory failure, paralysis, and coma, with hypoactive tendon reflexes. Other findings may include gastrointestinal hypomotility or ileus; facial flushing; pupillary dilation; paradoxical bradycardia; prolongation of PR, QRS, and QT intervals; heart block; and, at serum magnesium levels approaching 10 mmol/L, asystole.

5. X-ray features of pulmonary TB includes:

a. Presence of cavitation means a stable disease
b. Tuberculoma is present
c. Rasmussen aneurysm is seen
d. Pneumonia is most commonly seen in children
e. No X-ray changes can be seen in about 15% of population

Ans. b, c, d, e *Ref: Harrison's Medicine, 19/e; Clinical TB by PDO Davies, 4/e*

Option a	False	Cavitation gives a likelihood of infectivity
Option b	True	
Option c	True	
Option d	True	
Option e	True	

Primary pulmonary TB occurs soon after the initial infection with tubercle bacilli. It may be asymptomatic or may present with fever and occasionally pleuritic chest pain.

The lesion forming after initial infection (Ghon focus) is usually peripheral and accompanied by transient hilar or paratracheal lymphadenopathy, which may or may not be visible on standard chest radiography.

In the majority of cases, the lesion heals spontaneously and becomes evident only as a small calcified nodule.

- ***TB in young children***:
  - In young children with immature CMI and in persons with impaired immunity (e.g., those with malnutrition or HIV infection), primary pulmonary TB may progress rapidly to clinical illness.

- The initial lesion increases in size and can evolve as pleural effusion or progressive primary Tb.
- Accompanied by hilar or paratracheal lymphadenopathy due to the spread of bacilli from the lung parenchyma through lymphatic vessels.
- Enlarged lymph nodes may compress bronchi, causing total obstruction with distal collapse, partial obstruction with large-airway wheezing, or a ball-valve effect with segmental/lobar hyperinflation.
- Lymph nodes may also rupture into the airway with development of pneumonia, often including areas of necrosis and cavitation, distal to the obstruction.
- Bronchiectasis may develop in any segment/lobe which has been damaged by progressive caseating pneumonia.
- Occult hematogenous dissemination commonly follows primary infection.

❑ ***Postprimary tuberculosis*** is characterised by:
- Fibrosis, and
- Cavitation
- It is usually localized to the apical and posterior segments of the upper lobes, where the substantially higher mean oxygen tension (compared with that in the lower zones) favors mycobacterial growth
- The superior segments of the lower lobes are also more frequently involved
- Cavitation is a common part of tissue destruction. It gives a likelihood of infectivity.

A ***tuberculoma*** is a solid encapsulated mass which may present as a solitary mass on X-ray. The mass has risk of cavitation and spread in 5% of cases. CT scanning shows no enhancement with contrast.

In patients with good immunity, radiologic features typical of post primary TB are seen. As immunity wanes, the host immune response declines resulting in less fibrosis and cavitation. The typical diagnostic features are lost, and in 15% of cases of sputum smear positive pulmonary TB, the chest X-ray is normal.

Hemoptysis develops in 20–30% of cases, and massive hemoptysis may ensue as a consequence of the erosion of a blood vessel in the wall of a cavity. Hemoptysis, however, may also result from rupture of a dilated vessel in a cavity (Rasmussen's aneurysm) or from aspergilloma formation in an old cavity.

6. True about autosomal recessive polycystic kidney disease is/are:

a. Can not be diagnosed in utero
b. Develops in utero
c. End-stage renal disease is never seen in school going children
d. Features like nephromegaly can be seen
e. Biliary dysgenesis

Ans. b, d, e

Option a	False	Diagnosed in utero
Option b	True	
Option c	False	One third of the affected neonates will have end stage renal disease
Option d	True	
Option e	True	

Autosomal recessive polycystic kidney disease:

- ❑ Diagnosed in utero with enlarged (nephromegaly) echogenic kidneys, oligohydramnios and pulmonary hypoplasia.
- ❑ On ultrasonography, kidneys appear large with loss of corticomedullary differentiation.
- ❑ In severe cases the diagnosis may be made in utero as early as 24 weeks of gestation.
- ❑ 30% die shortly after birth.
- ❑ Total 60% mortality occurs in the first month of life.
- ❑ 80% of those who survive neonatal period are still alive after 10 years of age, but one third will have developed end stage renal disease.
- ❑ Clinical features – severe hypertension, progressive renal disease, liver manifestations.
- ❑ Liver manifestations – biliary dysgenesis due to primary ductal plate malformations with associates periportal fibrosis namely congenital hepatic fibrosis (CHF) and dilatation of intrahepatic bile ducts (Caroli disease).

7. True about Dubin-Johnson syndrome is/are:

a. Glucuronyl Uridyl transferase deficiency
b. Autosomal dominant
c. Conjugated hyperbilirubinemia
d. Sulfobromophthalein is not secreted in bile
e. Rise in serum transaminases is usually seen

Ans. c, d

Option a	False	Defect occurs in hepatic excretory function or intrahepatic biliary canalicular dysfunction
Option b	False	Autosomal recessive
Option c	True	
Option d	True	
Option e	False	Not seen

- ❑ Dubin-Johnson syndrome is a familial disease that results from defects in hepatic excretory function or intrahepatic biliary canalicular dysfunction (and not enzyme deficiency).
- ❑ Autosomal recessive, caused by mutations in ABCC2 gene.
- ❑ Benign, relatively rare disorder, characterized by low-grade, predominantly conjugated hyperbilirubinemia.
- ❑ Total bilirubin concentrations are typically between 2 and 5 mg/dL but on occasion can be in the normal range or as high as 20–25 mg/dL and can fluctuate widely in any given patient.
- ❑ The degree of hyperbilirubinemia may be increased by intercurrent illness, oral contraceptive use, and pregnancy.
- ❑ Because the hyperbilirubinemia is due to a pre-dominant rise in conjugated bilirubin, bilirubinuria is characteristically present.
- ❑ Aside from elevated serum bilirubin levels, other routine laboratory tests are normal.
- ❑ Physical examination is usually normal except for jaundice, although an occasional patient may have hepatosplenomegaly.

- Patients with DJS are usually asymptomatic, although some may have vague constitutional symptoms.
- In women, the condition may be subclinical until the patient becomes pregnant or receives oral contraceptives, when chemical hyperbilirubinemia becomes frank jaundice. Even in these situations, other routine liver function tests, including serum alkaline phosphatase and transaminase activities, are normal.
- A cardinal feature of DJS is the *accumulation in the lysosomes of centrilobular hepatocytes* of dark, coarsely granular pigment. As a result, the liver may be grossly *black* in appearance. This pigment is thought to be derived from epinephrine metabolites that are not excreted normally. The pigment may disappear during bouts of viral hepatitis, only to reaccumulate slowly after recovery.

  Bile acid disposition, including hepatocellular uptake and biliary excretion is normal in DJS. Patients have normal serum and biliary bile acid concentrations and do not have pruritus.
- Biliary excretion of a number of anionic compounds is compromised in DJS. These include various cholecystographic agents, as well as sulfobromophthalein (Bromsulphalein, BSP), a synthetic dye formerly used in a test of liver function. In this test, the rate of disappearance of BSP from plasma is determined following bolus IV administration. BSP is conjugated with glutathione in the hepatocyte; the resulting conjugate is normally excreted rapidly into the bile canaliculus. Patients with DJS exhibit characteristic rises in plasma concentrations at 90 minutes after injection, due to reflux of conjugated BSP into the circulation from the hepatocyte. Dyes such as ICG that are taken up by hepatocytes but are not further metabolized prior to biliary excretion do not show this reflux phenomenon. Continuous BSP infusion studies suggest a reduction in the time to maximum plasma concentration (tmax) for biliary excretion.

8. True about congenital adrenal hyperplasia:

a. Deficiency of 5 alpha hydroxylase
b. Deficiency of 21 hydroxylase
c. Deficiency of 17 alpha hydroxylase
d. Deficiency of 11 beta hydroxysteroid dehydrogenase
e. Deficiency of 21 beta hydroxysteroid dehydrogenase

Ans. b, c

Option a	False	
Option b	True	
Option c	True	
Option d	False	
Option e	False	

Congenital adrenal hyperplasia (CAH) is caused by mutations in genes encoding steroidogenic enzymes involved in glucocorticoid synthesis (CYP21A2, CYP17A1, HSD3B2, CYP11B1) or in the cofactor enzyme P450 oxidoreductase.

Variants of congenital adrenal hyperplasia			
Variant	***Gene***	***Impact on steroid synthesis***	***Diagnostic marker steroids in serum (and urine)***
21-Hydroxylase deficiency (21OHD)	CYP21A2	Glucocorticoid deficiency, mineralocorticoid deficiency, adrenal androgen excess	17-Hydroxyprogesterone, 21-deoxycortisol (pregnanetriol, 17-hydroxypregnanolone, pregnanetriolone)
11β-Hydroxylase deficiency (11OHD)	CYP11B1	Glucocorticoid deficiency, mineralocorticoid excess, adrenal androgen excess	11-Deoxycortisol, 11-deoxycorticosterone (tetrahydro-11-deoxycortisol, tetrahydro-11-deoxycorticosterone)
17α-Hydroxylase deficiency (17OHD)	CYP17A1	(Glucocorticoid deficiency), (mineralocorticoid excess androgen deficiency	11-Deoxycorticosterone, corticosterone, pregnenolone, progesterone (tetrahydro-11-deoxycorticosterone, tetrahydrocorticosterone, pregnenediol, pregnanediol)
3β-Hydroxysteroid dehydrogenase deficiency (3bHSDD)	HSD3B2	Glucocorticoid deficiency, (mineralocorticoid deficiency), adrenal androgen excess	17-Hydroxypregnanolone (pregnanetriol)
P450 oxidoreductase deficiency (ORD)	POR	Glucocorticoid deficiency, (mineralocorticoid excess), androgen deficiency, skeletal malformations	Pregnenolone, progesterone, 17-hydroxyprogesterone (pregnanediol, pregnanetriol)

9. Features of MPGN–1 are:

a. C4 normal
b. C3 increased
c. Thick ribbon shaped deposits
d. Gap in basal membrane layers
e. Linear deposits

Ans. a, c *Ref: Robbins and Harrison*

Option a	True	
Option b	False	Consistently decreased serum C3
Option c	True	
Option d	False	Not true
Option e	False	Globular deposits within the mesangium

MPGN or mesangiocapillary glomerulonephritis or lobar glomerulonephritis.

- Is an immune-mediated glomerulonephritis characterized by thickening of the GBM with mesangioproliferative changes;
- Subdivided pathologically into type I, type II, and type III disease:
  - *Type I Disease (Most Common)*
    - Idiopathic
    - Subacute bacterial endocarditis
    - Systemic lupus erythematosus
    - Hepatitis C ± cryoglobulinemia
    - Mixed cryoglobulinemia

- Hepatitis B
- Cancer: Lung, breast, and ovary (germinal)

■ *Type II Disease (Dense Deposit Disease)*
- Idiopathic
- C3 nephritic factor-associated
- Partial lipodystrophy

■ *Type III Disease*
- Idiopathic
- Complement receptor deficiency.

Most patients with dense deposit disease have abnormalities resulting in excessive activation of alternative complement pathway. These patients have consistently decreased serum C3 but normal C1 and C4.

Morphology:

- ***Mostly*** mesangial proliferative pattern of injury.
- May also have an inflammatory and focal crescentic appearance.
- In some cases, dense deposits of cellular material can be seen permeating the glomerular basement membrane (GBM).
- The defining feature is (seen on electron microscopy) ***permeation of lamina densa of GBM*** by ribbon like homogeneous, extremely electron dense material of unknown composition. There is a dense transformation of the glomerular basement membrane with round, globular deposits within the mesangium (and not linear deposits).
- By immunofluorescence, C3 is present in irregular chunky and segmental linear foci in the basement membranes and in the mesangium.
- IgG and the early components of the classical complement pathway (C1q and C4) are usually absent.
- Classically, the glomerular tuft has a lobular appearance; intra mesangial deposits are rarely present and subendothelial deposits are generally absent.

10. True regarding the features of Crohn's disease is/are:

a. Linear ulcer
b. Cobblestone appearance
c. Loss of haustrations
d. Lead stem pipe
e. String sign

Ans. a, b, e *Ref: Harrison's Medicine 19/e; Schwartz Principle of surgery, 9/e*

Option a	True	
Option b	True	
Option c	False	Seen in ulcerative colitis and not Crohn's
Option d	False	Seen in ulcerative colitis and not Cohn's
Option e	True	

- CD can affect any part of the gastrointestinal (GI) tract from the mouth to the anus.
- The most common sites involved by Crohn disease at presentation are the terminal ileum, ileocecal valve, and cecum.
- Some 30–40% of patients have small bowel disease alone, 40–55% have disease involving both the small and large intestines, and 15–25% have colitis alone.

- CD is segmental with skip areas in the midst of diseased intestine.
- Perirectal fistulas, fissures, abscesses, and anal stenosis are present in one-third of patients with CD, particularly those with colonic involvement.
- Rarely, CD may also involve the liver and the pancreas.
- Unlike UC, CD is a transmural process.

Pathology:

- The presence of multiple, separate, sharply delineated areas of disease, resulting in ***skip lesions***, is characteristic of Crohn's disease and may help in differentiation from ulcerative colitis.
- Strictures are common.
- The earliest lesion, the aphthous ulcer, may progress, and multiple lesions often coalesce into elongated, linear or serpentine ulcers oriented along the axis of the bowel.
- Edema and loss of normal mucosal folds are common.
- Sparing of interspersed mucosa results in a coarsely textured, ***cobblestone appearance*** in which diseased tissue is depressed below the level of normal mucosa.
- Crohn's disease generally occurs as a transmural process, affecting all layers of the bowel wall.
- The intestinal wall is thickened as a consequence of transmural edema, inflammation, submucosal fibrosis, and hypertrophy of the muscularis propria, all of which contribute to stricture formation. In cases with extensive transmural disease, mesenteric fat frequently extends around the serosal surface (creeping fat).
- Long lengths of narrowed terminal ileum ***(Kantor string sign)*** may be present in long-standing disease.

Barium enema in ulcerative colitis

Barium enema has been used to diagnose ulcerative colitis and to determine the extent of disease. However, this modality is less sensitive than colonoscopy and may not detect early disease. In long-standing ulcerative colitis, the colon is foreshortened and lacks haustral markings ***("lead pipe" colon)***. Because the inflammation in ulcerative colitis is purely mucosal, *strictures are highly uncommon.*

Thus lead pipe colon and loss of haustrations are features of UC and not Cd.

11. The only monosomy with aneuploidy which survives:

a. Turner's
b. Down's
c. Klinefelter
d. Edward
e. Patau

Ans. a

Option a	True	
Option b	False	
Option c	False	
Option d	False	
Option e	False	

Syndrome	Chromosomal anomaly, karyotype
Turner	X monosomy, 45XO
Klinefelter	XXY Aneuploidy, 47XXY
Down	Trisomy 21
Edward	Trisomy 18
Patau	Trisomy 13

Autosomal monosomies end in abortions.

The only chromosomal monosomy to survive till birth and beyond, is monosomy X or Turner syndrome.

12. Regarding renal manifestations in multiple myeloma, true is:

a. Amyloidosis
b. Nephrocalcinosis
c. Cryoglobulinemia nephritis
d. Interstitial nephritis
e. Bence Jones proteinuria

Ans. a, d, e

Option a	True	
Option b	False	
Option c	False	Cryoglobulinemia is found in as many as 50% of patients with hepatitis C and may be associated with MPGN type I
Option d	True	
Option e	True	

Light chain cast nephropathy or myeloma kidney

Overt renal insufficiency occurs in half of those with multiple myeloma. Several factors contribute to renal damage:

- Bence Jones proteinuria and cast nephropathy: The main cause of renal dysfunction is related to Bence Jones (light chain) proteinuria.
- Amyloidosis of AL type
- Light chain deposition disease
- Hypercalcemia or hyperuricemia.

Renal failure occurs in nearly 25% of myeloma patients, and some renal pathology is noted in more than 50%.

Hypercalcemia is the most common cause of renal failure.

Infections
Acute bacterial pylonephritis Chronic pyelonephritis (including reflux nephropathy) Other infections (e.g., viruses, parasites)
Toxins
Drugs Acute-hypersensitivity interstitial nephritis Analgesics Heavy metals Lead, cadmium

Metabolic diseases
Urate nephropathy
Nephrocalcinosis (hypercalcemic nephropathy)
Acute phosphate nephropathy
Hypokalemic nephropathy
Oxalate nephropathy
Physical factors
Chronic urinary tract obstruction
Neoplasms
Multiple myeloma (light-chain cast nephropathy)
Immunologic reactions
Transplant rejection Sjögren syndrome Sarcoidosis
Vascular diseases
Miscellaneous
Balkan nephropathy Nephronophthisis-medullary cystic disease complex "Idiopathic" interstitial nephritis

Cryoglobulinemia is found in as many as 50% of patients with hepatitis C and may be associated with MPGN type I.

13. Risk of pulmonary embolism is seen in:

a. OCP users
b. Pregnancy
c. Unaccustomed exercise
d. Mitral regurgitation
e. Antiphospholipid antibody syndrome

Ans. a, b, e

Option a	True	
Option b	True	
Option c	False	
Option d	False	
Option e	True	

Acquired causes of venous thrombosis:

- Surgery
  - Neurosurgery
  - Major abdominal surgery
  - Cancer surgery
- Malignancy
- Antiphospholipid syndrome
- Other
  - Trauma
  - Pregnancy

- Long-haul travel
- Obesity
- Oral contraceptives/hormone replacement
- Myeloproliferative disorders
- Polycythemia vera

When deep venous thrombi detach from their site of formation, they embolize to the vena cava, right atrium, and right ventricle, and lodge in the pulmonary arterial circulation, thereby causing acute pulmonary embolism (PE). Thus risk factors for PE are same as that for DVT.

14. True about ankylosing spondylitis includes:

a. B27 association
b. Low backache relieved with rest
c. 40% chance of posterior uveitis
d. Enthesitis
e. Chance of primary heart block is >30%

Ans. a, c, d

Option a	True	
Option b	False	Improves with activity and returns following inactivity
Option c	True	
Option d	True	
Option e	False	

B27 is among the most negatively charged of HLA class I heavy chains, and the overall preference is for positively charged peptides.

HLA-B27:05 subtype is very highly associated with ankylosing spondylitis (AS), both in its idiopathic form and in association with chronic inflammatory bowel disease or psoriasis vulgaris.

Ankylosing Spondylitis

Is an inflammatory disorder of unknown cause that primarily affects the axial skeleton; peripheral joints and extra-articular structures are also frequently involved.

The disease usually begins in the second or third decade; male-to-female prevalence is between 2:1 and 3:1.

The symptoms of the disease are usually first noticed in late adolescence or early adulthood. In 5% of patients, symptoms begin after age 40.

- The initial symptom is usually dull pain, insidious in onset, felt deep in the lower lumbar or gluteal region, accompanied by low-back morning stiffness of up to a few hours' duration that improves with activity and returns following inactivity. Within a few months, the pain has usually become persistent and bilateral.
- Nocturnal exacerbation of pain often forces the patient to rise and move around.
- In some patients, bony tenderness (presumably reflecting enthesitis or osteitis) may accompany back pain or stiffness, whereas in others it may be the predominant complaint.
- The most common extra-articular manifestation is acute **anterior uveitis, which occurs in up to 40% of patients** and can antedate the spondylitis. Attacks are typically unilateral,

causing pain, photophobia, and increased lacrimation. These tend to recur, often in the opposite eye.

- Cataracts and secondary glaucoma are not uncommon sequelae.
- Up to 60% of patients with AS have inflammation in the colon or ileum. This is usually asymptomatic, but frank IBD occurs in 5–10% of patients with AS.
- About 10% of patients meeting criteria for AS have psoriasis.
- Aortic insufficiency, sometimes leading to congestive heart failure, occurs in a **small percentage** of patients, occasionally early. **Third-degree heart block** may occur alone or together with aortic insufficiency.
- Subclinical pulmonary lesions and cardiac dysfunction may be relatively common.
- Cauda equina syndrome and upper pulmonary lobe fibrosis are rare late complications.
- Retroperitoneal fibrosis is a rare associated condition.
- Prostatitis has been reported to have an increased prevalence.
- Amyloidosis is rare.

15. True about silicosis:

a. Lower zone is affected
b. Nodular opacities
c. Progressive massive fibrosis may be seen
d. Increased susceptibility to infections
e. Calcification of hilar lymph nodes

Ans. b, c, d, e

Option a	False	Seen in upper zone
Option b	True	
Option c	True	
Option d	True	
Option e	True	

- Silicosis is one of the oldest known occupational pulmonary hazards,
- Most often, pulmonary fibrosis due to silica exposure (silicosis) occurs in a dose-response fashion after many years of exposure.
- The clinical and pathologic features of acute silicosis are similar to those of pulmonary alveolar proteinosis.
- The chest radiograph may show profuse miliary infiltration or consolidation, and there is a characteristic HRCT pattern known as “crazy paving”.
- The disease may be quite severe and progressive despite the discontinuation of exposure.
- Whole-lung lavage may provide symptomatic relief and slow the progression.
- Simple Silicosis—With long-term, less intense exposure, small rounded opacities in the upper lobes may appear on the chest radiograph after 15–20 years of exposure, usually without associated impairment of lung function.
- Calcification of hilar nodes may occur in as many as 20% of cases and produces a characteristic “eggshell” pattern. Silicotic nodules may be identified more readily by HRCT.
- Complicated silicosis—The nodular fibrosis may be progressive in the absence of further exposure, with coalescence and formation of nonsegmental conglomerates of irregular masses >1 cm in diameter. These masses can become quite large, and when this occurs,

the term progressive massive fibrosis (PMF) is applied. Significant functional impairment with both restrictive and obstructive components may be associated with PMF.

- Because silica is cytotoxic to alveolar macrophages, patients with silicosis are at greater risk of acquiring lung infections that involve these cells as a primary defense (Mycobacterium tuberculosis, atypical mycobacteria and fungi).
- Another potential clinical complication of silicosis is autoimmune connective tissue disorders such as rheumatoid arthritis and scleroderma.
- Also, International Agency for Research on Cancer lists silica as a probable lung carcinogen.

16. All are true about asbestosis except:

a. Pleural effusion
b. Lobar pneumonia
c. Mediastinal lymphadenopathy
d. Mesothelioma
e. Interstitial fibrosis

Ans. b, c

Option a	True	
Option b	False	No, not seen
Option c	False	No, not seen. Asbestosis is associated with basal lobe interstitial fibrosis and peribronchial inflammation
Option d	True	Mesothelioma is the most specific cancer in asbestosis whereas most common cancer is Bronchial cancer (and not mesothelioma)
Option e	True	

- Asbestos is a generic term for several different mineral silicates, including chrysolite, amosite, anthophyllite, and crocidolite.
- The major health effects from exposure to asbestos are pleural and pulmonary fibrosis, cancers of the respiratory tract, and pleural and peritoneal mesothelioma.
- Asbestosis is a diffuse interstitial fibrosing disease of the lung that is directly related to the intensity and duration of exposure. The disease resembles other forms of diffuse interstitial fibrosis. Usually, exposure has taken place for at least 10 years before the disease becomes manifest.
- Past exposure to asbestos is specifically indicated by pleural plaques on chest radiographs, which are characterized by either thickening or calcification along the parietal pleura, particularly along the lower lung fields, the diaphragm, and the cardiac border. Without additional manifestations, pleural plaques imply only exposure, not pulmonary impairment.
- Benign pleural effusions also may occur. The fluid is typically a serous or bloody exudate. The effusion may be slowly progressive or may resolve spontaneously.
- Irregular or linear opacities that usually are first noted in the lower lung fields are the chest radiographic hallmark of asbestosis.
- An indistinct heart border or a "ground-glass" appearance in the lung fields may be seen. HRCT may show distinct changes of subpleural curvilinear lines 5–10 mm in length that appear to be parallel to the pleural surface.
- Pulmonary function testing in asbestosis reveals a restrictive pattern with a decrease in both lung volumes and diffusing capacity. There may also be evidence of mild airflow obstruction (due to peribronchiolar fibrosis).

- Lung cancer is the most common cancer associated with asbestos exposure. The excess frequency of lung cancer (all histologic types) in asbestos workers is associated with a minimum latency of 15–19 years between first exposure and development of the disease.
- In addition, there is a significant interactive effect of smoking and asbestos exposure that results in greater risk than what would be expected from the additive effect of each factor.
- Mesotheliomas, both pleural and peritoneal, are also associated with asbestos exposure. In contrast to lung cancers, these tumors do not appear to be associated with smoking. Relatively short-term asbestos exposures of ≤1–2 years, occurring up to 40 years in the past, have been associated with the development of mesotheliomas (an observation that emphasizes the importance of obtaining a complete environmental exposure history). The risk of mesothelioma is much less than that of lung cancer among asbestos-exposed workers.
- Because epidemiologic studies have shown that >80% of mesotheliomas may be associated with asbestos exposure, documented mesothelioma in a patient with occupational or environmental exposure to asbestos may be compensable.

17. Dyspnea in COPD is due to:

a. Hypoxemia
b. Hypercapnia
c. Increase in respiratory drive
d. Activation of pulmonary receptors
e. Activation of vascular receptors

Ans. a, b, c, d

Option a	True	
Option b	True	
Option c	True	
Option d	True	
Option e	False	

Dyspnea in COPD

Asthma and COPD, the most common obstructive lung diseases, are characterized by expiratory airflow obstruction, which typically leads to dynamic hyperinflation of the lungs and chest wall.

Patients with moderate to severe disease have both increased resistive and elastic loads on the ventilatory muscles and experience increased work of breathing.

Patients with acute bronchoconstriction may also have a sense of tightness, which can exist even when lung function is still within the normal range. These patients are commonly tachypneic; this condition leads to hyperinflation and reduced respiratory system compliance and also limits tidal volume.

Both the chest tightness and the tachypnea are probably due to stimulation of **pulmonary receptors**.

Both asthma and COPD may lead to **hypoxemia** and **hypercapnia** from ventilation-perfusion (V/Q) mismatch (and diffusion limitation during exercise with emphysema); hypoxemia is much more common than hypercapnia as a consequence of the different ways in which oxygen and carbon dioxide bind to hemoglobin.

Mechanism of dyspnea in various disease conditions		
Descriptor	***Clinical examples***	***Pathophysiology***
Chest tightness or constriction	Asthma, CHF	Bronchoconstriction, interstitial edema
Increased work or effort of breathing	COPD, asthma, neuromuscular disease, chest wall restriction	Airway obstruction, neuromuscular disease
"Air hunger", need to breathe, urge to breathe	CHF, PE, COPD, asthma, pulmonary fibrosis	Increased drive to breathe
Inability to get a deep breath, unsatisfying breath	Moderate to severe asthma and COPD, pulmonary fibrosis, chest wall disease	Hyperinflation and restricted tidal volume
Heavy breathing, rapid breathing, breathing more	Sedentary status in healthy individual or patient with cardiopulmonary disease	Deconditioning

18. In cystic fibrosis, organism causing infection is/are:

a. Burkholderia cepacia
b. Staph. aureus
c. P. aeruginosa
d. Burkholderia pseudomallei
e. Strep. pyogenes

Ans. a, b, c

Option	Answer
Option a	True
Option b	True
Option c	True
Option d	False
Option e	False

The major morbidity and mortality associated with CF is attributable to respiratory compromise, characterized by copious hyperviscous and adherent pulmonary secretions that obstruct small and medium-sized airways. CF airway secretions are exceedingly difficult to clear, and a complex bacterial flora that includes Staphylococcus aureus, Haemophilus influenzae, and Pseudomonas aeruginosa, Burkholderia cepacia (among other pathogens) is routinely cultured from CF sputum.

Hypersensitivity to Aspergillus (allergic bronchopulmonary aspergillosis) occurs in approximately 5% of individuals with the disease.

19. QT is prolonged by:

a. Amiodarone
b. Lignocaine
c. Ketoconazole
d. Cisapride
e. Calcium gluconate

Ans. a, c, d *Ref: Echocardiography by OP Yadava; Harrison's Medicine 19/e*

Option	Answer
Option a	True
Option b	False
Option c	True
Option d	True
Option e	False

Long QT syndrome:

- May be familial or sporadic

Familial:

- Autosomal recessive: Jervell and Lange-Nielsen syndrome (with deafness)
- Autosomal dominant: Romano-Ward syndrome (without deafness)

Acquired:

- Electrolyte imbalance: hypokalemia, hypomagnesemia, hypocalcemia
- Antiarrhythmic drugs with class IA and III actions: quinidine, procainamide, disopyramide
- Psychotropic drugs: phenothiazine, tricyclic antidepressants
- Myocarditis
- Myocardial ischemia
- Sinus node disease
- CNS disease: subarachnoid or cerebral hemorrhage
- Liquid protein diets

1. Congenital long QT syndromes (see text for details) Long QT syndrome type 1: Reduced repolarizing current I_{Ks} due to mutation in KCNQ1 gene Long QT syndrome type 2: Reduced repolarizing current I_{Kr} due to mutation in KCNH2 gene Long QT syndrome type 3: Delayed inactivation of the I_{Na} due to mutations in SCN5A gene Others: Several other types of long QT syndromes have been described; long QT types 1, 2, and 3 account for 80–90% of cases 2. Acquired prolongation of QT interval Electrolyte abnormalities Hypokalemia Hypomagnesemia Hypocalcemia	Antihistamines (histamine 1-receptor antagonists) Terfenadine, astemizole, diphenhydramine, hydroxyzine Cholinergic antagonists: Cisapride, organophosphates Citrate (massive blood transfusions) Cocaine Methadone Fluoxetine (in conjunction with other drugs that prolong QT) Cardiac conditions Myocardial ischemia and infarction Myocarditis Marked bradycardia Stress cardiomyopathy
Drugs Antiarrhythmic drugs Class IA: Quinidine, disopyramide, procainamide Class III: Sotalol, amiodarone (QT prolongation common but torsade ventricular tachycardia is rare), ibutilide, dofetilide, almokalant Antibiotics Macrolides: Erythromycin, clarithromycin, azithromycin Fluoroquinolones: Levofloxacin, moxifloxacin, gatifloxacin Trimethoprim-sulfamethoxazole Clindamycin Pentamidine Chloroquine Antifungals: Ketoconazole, itraconazole Antivirals: Amantadine Antipsychotics Haloperidol, phenothiazines, thioridazine, trifluoperazine, sertindole, zimelidine, ziprasidone Tricyclic and tetracyclic antidepressants	Endocrine disorders Hypothyroidism Hyperparathyroidism Pheochromocytoma Hyperaldosteronism Intracranial disorders Subarachnoid hemorrhage Thalamic hematoma Cerebrovascular accident Encephalitis Head injury Nutritional disorders Anorexia nervosa Starvation Liquid protein diets Gastroplasty and ileojejunal bypass Celiac disease

20. Causes of exudative pleural effusion are:

a. Congestive heart failure
b. Hypoproteinemia
c. Inflammation of diaphragm
d. Cancer
e. Tuberculosis

Ans. c, d, e

Option a	False	
Option b	False	
Option c	True	Leading cause of exudative pleural effusion
Option d	True	Leading cause of exudative pleural effusion
Option e	True	Leading cause of exudative pleural effusion

Transudative pleural effusion occurs when systemic factors that influence the formation and absorption of pleural fluid are altered.

An exudative pleural effusion occurs when **local factors** that influence the formation and absorption of pleural fluid are altered.

The leading causes of exudative pleural effusions are **bacterial pneumonia, malignancy, viral infection, and pulmonary embolism.**

Transudative and exudative pleural effusions are distinguished by measuring the lactate dehydrogenase (LDH) and protein levels in the pleural fluid.

Exudative pleural effusions meet at least one of the following criteria, whereas transudative pleural effusions meet none:

1. Pleural fluid protein/serum protein > 0.5
2. Pleural fluid LDH/serum LDH > 0.6
3. Pleural fluid LDH more than two-thirds the normal upper limit for serum.

Options c, d, e affect local factors, while a and b affect systemic factors that influence the formation and absorption of pleural fluid.

21. True about Posterior mediastinal mass is/are:

a. Thymoma
b. Lymphoma
c. Enteric cyst
d. Neurogenic cyst
e. Extramedullary hematopoiesis

Ans. c, d, e *Ref: Harrison's medicine 19/e*

Option a	False	Anterior compartment mass
Option b	False	Anterior compartment mass
Option c	True	
Option d	True	
Option e	True	

	Anterior compartment	*Middle compartment*	*Posterior compartment*
Anatomical boundaries	Manubrium and sternum anteriorly, pericardium, aorta, and brachiocephalic vessels posteriorly	Anterior mediastinum anteriorly, posterior mediastinum posteriorly	Pericardium and trachea anteriorly; vertebral column posteriorly

Contd...

Contd...

Contents	Thymus gland, anterior mediastinal lymph nodes, internal mammary arteries and veins	Pericardium, heart, ascending and transverse arch of aorta, superior and inferior vena cava, brachiocephalic arteries and veins, phrenic nerves, trachea, and main bronchi and their contiguous lymph nodes, pulmonary arteries, and veins	Descending thoracic aorta, esophagus, thoracic duct, azygos and hemiazygos veins, sympathetic chains, and the posterior group of mediastinal lymph nodes
Common abnormalities	Thymoma, lymphomas, teratomatous neoplasms, thyroid masses, parathyroid masses, mesenchymal tumors, giant lymph node hyperplasia, hernia through foramen of Morgagni	Metastatic lymph node enlargement, granulomatous lymph node enlargement, pleuropericardial cysts, bronchogenic cysts, masses of vascular origin	Neurogenic tumors, meningocele, meningomyelocele, gastroenteric cysts, esophageal diverticula, hernia through foramen of Bochdalek, extramedullary hematopoiesis.

22. True about Wilms' tumor is/are:

a. Contralateral kidney is to be explored during surgery
b. Bilateral presentation
c. Presents as asymptomatic abdominal mass in children
d. Histopathological and grading staging is important for prognosis
e. Patency of IVC should be confirmed prior to tumor resection

Ans. a, c, d, e *Ref: Nelson textbook of Pediatrics, 18/e*

Option a	True	
Option b	False	Usually a large solitary, well circumscribed mass
Option c	True	
Option d	True	
Option e	True	

Clinical presentation of Wilms' tumor

- An abdominal mass discovered fortuitously.
- Usually a large solitary, well circumscribed mass.
- Only 10% are either bilateral or multicentric.
- Staging correlates with prognosis.
- Anaplastic histology is a critical determinant of poor prognosis (option D).

Management

Surgical extirpation of the tumor must be done. The patency of inferior vena cava should be established prior to resection, if it is not patent preoperative chemotherapy should be administered.

During operation, contralateral kidney should be examined to exclude bilateral Wilms' tumor.

Liver and retroperitoneal lymph nodes should be examined. Suspicious nodes should be biopsies.

Every attempt should be made to avoid spillage of tumor.

23. True about multiple sclerosis is/are:
  a. Oligoclonal bands may be present in CSF
  b. Autoimmune etiology
  c. Intrathecal IgM production
  d. Callososeptal lesions
  e. Spinal cord involvement may occur

Ans. a, b, d, e *Ref: Harrison's, 19/e; Mathew's, 5/e*

Option a	True	
Option b	True	Acquired immune-mediated
Option c	False	Intrathecal IgG production
Option d	True	Callososeptal interface may have multiple small hypointense lesions (venus necklace)
Option e	True	Partial acute transverse myelitis

Multiple sclerosis (MS) is an acquired immune-mediated, chronic, relapsing inflammatory disease that attacks myelinated axons in the central nervous system, destroying the myelin and the axon in variable degrees and producing significant physical disability within 20–25 years.

It is the second most common cause of neurological impairment in young adults, after trauma.

The hallmark of MS is symptomatic episodes that occur months or years apart and affect different anatomic locations.

Clinical features of multiple sclerosis	
• Fatigue • Motor - Weakness - Spasticity • Altered sensation - Numbness - Pins and needles • Pain - Trigeminal neuralgia - Dysesthesia • Bladder - Frequency, urgency, incontinence	• Bowel (constipation) • Sexual dysfunction (impotence) • Swallowing disorders • Eyes: visual defects on exercise or ↑T° (this is Uhthoff's sign) - Optic neuritis - Diplopia - Nystagmus • Cerebellum: ataxia; intention tremor • Cognition ↓; memory ↓; dementia • Vertigo • Depression* (or, rarely, euphoria) • Rarely: aphasia, epilepsy
*Depression is common, severe, and treatable: fluoxetine may be better than desipramine as anticholinergic effects limit dose. Avoid electroconvulsive therapy if MRI shows contrast-enhancing lesions.	

Diagnosis

Multiple sclerosis is diagnosed on the basis of clinical findings and supporting evidence from ancillary tests. Tests include the following:

- **Magnetic resonance imaging:** The imaging procedure of choice for confirming MS and monitoring disease progression in the CNS.
- **Evoked potentials:** Used to identify subclinical lesions; results are not specific for MS.
- **Lumbar puncture:** May be useful if MRI is unavailable or MRI findings are nondiagnostic; CSF is evaluated for *oligoclonal bands* and *intrathecal immunoglobulin G (IgG) production.*

24. All are true about Sjogren's syndrome *except*:

a. Bilateral parotid gland enlargement
b. Parotid gland enlargement may be painful
c. Xerostomia is present
d. Progression to lymphoma
e. Recurrent infection

Ans. b, e *Ref: Harrison's, 19/e; Mathew's, 5/e*

Option a	True	True for Sjogren's syndrome
Option b	False	Not painful
Option c	True	True for Sjogren's syndrome
Option d	True	True for Sjogren's syndrome
Option e	False	Progressive destruction of exocrine glands

Sjogren's syndrome is an immunologic disorder characterized by progressive destruction of exocrine glands leading to mucosal and conjunctival dryness. Diagnosis is made when there is a triad of—*keratoconjunctivitis sicca, xerostomia and mononuclear cell infiltration of salivary gland.*

Classification and types	
• Primary (sicca syndrome)	The disease occurs by itself, in the absence of any connective tissue disorder
• Secondary	The disease is accompanied by a variety of autoimmune disorders. These include rheumatoid arthritis, SLE, progressive systemic sclerosis, primary biliary cirrhosis, chronic active hepatitis, myasthenia gravis, polymyositis and thyroiditis
• Glandular type	The only clinical manifestations are within the exocrine system
• Extraglandular type	Other tissues are also involved

Incidence:

- ❑ The disease occurs in third to fourth decades and predominantly affects women.
- ❑ The two main mechanisms of tissue destruction in Sjogren's syndrome are lymphocytic infiltration and immune complex deposition.

Clinical features:

- ❑ **Keratoconjunctivitis sicca** is dryness of eyes resulting from lack of lacrimal secretion. This results in grittiness, burning or itching, associated with sticky mucous threads.
- ❑ **Xerostomia** is dryness of mouth resulting from lack of salivary secretion.
- ❑ Renal involvement in the form of interstitial nephritis or glomerulonephritis.
- ❑ Cutaneous and systemic vasculitis.
- ❑ Pulmonary involvement with interstitial pneumonitis.
- ❑ Polyneuropathies or mononeuritis multiplex.
- ❑ Pseudolymphoma is common in Sjogren's syndrome. Approximately 10% of these patients develop a lymphoproliferative process which may go on to develop a non-Hodgkin's lymphoma.
- ❑ Hashimoto's thyroiditis is a common accompaniment of Sjogren's syndrome.
- ❑ Common **laboratory abnormalities** are raised ESR, leucopenia, thrombocytosis, elevated levels of circulating immune complexes, and autoantibodies.

Among patients with Sjögren syndrome, the incidence of non-Hodgkin lymphoma is 4.3% (18.9 times higher than in the general population).

Treatment:

- ❑ Ocular and mucosal lubricants as artificial tears, ophthalmologic lubricating ointments, nasal sprays of normal saline and moisturizing skin lotions.
- ❑ Corticosteroids for management of glomerulonephritis and pneumonitis.
- ❑ Immunosuppressive therapy for systemic vasculitis.

25. Feature(s) of Felty syndrome is/are:

a. Neutrophilia
b. Seropositive for rheumatoid factor
c. Long standing rheumatoid arthritis
d. Splenomegaly
e. Keratoconjunctivitis sicca

Ans. a, b, c, d, e *Ref: Harrison's, 19/e; Mathew's, 5/e*

Option a	True	
Option b	True	
Option c	True	
Option d	True	
Option e	True	

Felty syndrome:

- ❑ Associated with seropositive [rheumatoid factor (RF)-positive] rheumatoid arthritis (RA).
- ❑ Long standing aggressive destructive rheumatoid arthritis (RA) precede the onset of Felty syndrome (FS).
- ❑ Characterized by the triad of RA, splenomegaly, and granulocytopenia.

Physical findings in FS include the following:

- ❑ Splenomegaly, possibly nonpalpable
- ❑ Left upper quadrant pain, initiated by splenic infarcts or capsular distension.
- ❑ Hepatomegaly, usually mild
- ❑ Lymphadenopathy
- ❑ Weight loss
- ❑ Rheumatoid nodules
- ❑ Sjögren syndrome
- ❑ Articular findings of long-standing RA: Joint deformities typical of RA, as well as synovitis (joint swelling and tenderness), which may be mild at presentation
- ❑ Small-vessel inflammation (vasculitis): Lower-extremity ulcers, palpable purpura and brownish pigmentary changes of the lower extremities, and periungual infarcts
- ❑ Signs of systemic vasculitis: Mononeuritis multiplex and extremity ischemia
- ❑ Other findings: Pleuritis, peripheral neuropathy, episcleritis, and signs of portal hypertension.
- ❑ Anemia and thrombocytopenia
- ❑ Antinuclear antibodies (ANAs), antihistone antibodies, and antineutrophil cytoplasmic antibodies (perinuclear pattern; p-ANCA) can be found.
- ❑ Almost all the patients have high titers of *rheumatoid factor (RF).*

Complications:

- ❑ Splenic rupture
- ❑ Life-threatening infection
- ❑ Toxicity due to immunosuppressive regimens

- Portal hypertension and gastrointestinal bleeding due to nodular regenerative hyperplasia of the liver.

Treatment:

- The best way of treating Felty syndrome is to control the underlying rheumatoid arthritis.
- Immunosuppressive therapy for RA often improves granulocytopenia and splenomegaly.
- Splenectomy may be required in certain cases.

26. True about Paterson Brown-Kelly syndrome is/are:

a. Increased TIBC
b. Glossitis
c. Dysphagia
d. Posterior cricoid web
e. Increased risk of Ca esophagus

Ans. a, b, c, d, e *Ref: Harrison's, 19/e; Mathew's, 5/e*

Option a	True	Low serum iron, high TIBC
Option b	True	
Option c	True	Dysphagia to solids initially
Option d	True	Thin web in posterior cricoid area
Option e	True	Post-cricoid carcinoma or carcinoma of the esophagus

- Also known as Plummer-Vinson syndrome.
- Triad of microcytic hypochromic anemia (iron deficiency), atrophic glossitis, and esophageal webs or strictures.
- Most often affects middle-aged women.
- The web (containing mucosa and submucosa) occurs at the anterior post-cricoid area of the upper oesophagus.
- The improvement in dysphagia after iron therapy provides evidence for an association between iron deficiency and postcricoid dysphagia.
- Dysphagia is due to a thin web in the postcricoid area. The web is formed of degenerated epithelial cells.
- Usually seen in post-menopausal women.
- Investigations:
    - Hemoglobin and PCV low.
    - Peripheral smear shows microcytic hypochromic anemia.
    - Serum iron is low and iron binding capacity is increased.
    - Bone marrow iron stores are depleted.
    - Barium swallow may show the web.
- Treatment:
    - Endoscopic dilatation.
    - Treatment of iron deficiency anemia with iron.
- Complication:
    - Post-cricoid carcinoma or carcinoma of the esophagus may develop.

27. Respiratory failure type II is/are seen in:

a. Myasthenia gravis
b. Acute exacerbation in COPD
c. Acute severe asthma
d. Pulmonary edema
e. Pulmonary embolism

Ans. a, b, c *Ref: Harrison's, 19/e; Mathew's, 5/e*

Option a	True	
Option b	True	
Option c	True	
Option d	False	Type-I respiratory failure
Option e	False	Type-I respiratory failure

- Respiratory failure may result from disorders of lungs, chest wall, diaphragm or neuromuscular apparatus.
- Respiratory failure may develop **rapidly** or **slowly** and may be **transient** or **persistent**.
- Consider respiratory failure in a patient with following features, and measure arterial blood-gases in all such patients.

• Breathlessness at rest	• Raised respiratory rate
• Central cyanosis	• Drowsiness, confusion or unconsciousness

Definition:

- Respiratory failure is present when PaO_2 is < 60 mmHg (8.0 kPa) and/or $PaCO_2$ is > 50 mmHg (6.5 kPa).
  - Type I respiratory failure is characterised by low PaO_2 and low or normal $PaCO_2$.
  - Type II respiratory failure is characterized by low PaO_2 and raised $PaCO_2$.

Types of Respiratory Failure:

- Acute hypoxemia without hypercapnia (acute Type I respiratory failure)
- Chronic hypoxemia without hypercapnia (chronic Type I respiratory failure)
- Acute hypoxemia with hypercapnia (acute Type II respiratory failure)
- Chronic hypoxemia with hypercapnia (chronic Type II respiratory failure)
  - Note that hypoxemia is invariable in respiratory failure, but hypercapnia may or may not be present.

Acute Type II Respiratory Failure

Causes:

- Respiratory depressant drugs like diazepam, opiates and alcohol.
- Brain-stem damage from stroke and trauma.
- Disorders of nerves and neuromuscular transmission like acute GB syndrome, paraplegia, poliomyelitis and myasthenia gravis.
- Disorders of muscle affecting respiratory muscles like acute polymyositis.
- Severe airflow obstruction like severe acute asthma, laryngeal and tracheal obstruction.
- Chest injuries resulting in tension pneumothorax, massive hemothorax and flail chest.

Management:

- Treatment of the underlying condition.
- Oxygen therapy to be started with 24% oxygen, and adjusted further based on serial measurements of arterial blood-gas levels.
- Removal of secretions by coughing or emergency bronchoscopic aspiration.
- Bronchodilators in severe airflow obstruction.
- Assisted ventilation must be considered in selected cases.

28. True statement about polymyositis is:

a. F > M
b. MRI monitors disease activity
c. Staphylococcus aureus is the cause
d. Characteristic skin rash
e. Distal muscles are spared

Ans. a, b, e *Ref: Harrison's, 19/e; Mathew's, 5/e*

Option a	True	Polymyositis and dermatomyositis are more common in women than in men (2:1 ratio), while inclusion body myositis is twice as common in men
Option b	True	MRI scans may also be used to guide muscle biopsy and to monitor disease activity
Option c	False	Immune-mediated syndrome secondary to defective cellular immunity
Option d	False	Seen in dermatomyositis
Option e	True	

Polymyositis is an idiopathic inflammatory myopathy characterized by the following:

- Symmetrical, proximal muscle weakness
- Elevated skeletal muscle enzyme levels
- Characteristic electromyography (EMG) and muscle biopsy findings

Clinically similar to polymyositis, dermatomyositis is an idiopathic inflammatory myopathy associated with characteristic dermatologic manifestations.

Classification of polymyositis-dermatomyositis:

- *Group I—Primary idiopathic polymyositis*
- *Group II—Primary idiopathic dermatomyositis*
- *Group III—Polymyositis or dermatomyositis associated with malignancy*
- *Group IV—Childhood polymyositis or dermatomyositis*
- *Group V—Polymyositis or dermatomyositis associated with another connective-tissue disease*
- *Group VI—Inclusion body myositis*
- *Group VII—Miscellaneous (e.g., eosinophilic myositis, myositis ossificans, focal myositis, giant cell myositis).*

Clinical manifestations

- **Primary idiopathic polymyositis**
  - Weakness of the proximal muscles of the lower limbs (hips and thighs) results in difficulty in arising from the squatting or kneeling position and in climbing or descending stairs.
  - Weakness of the proximal muscles of the upper limbs (shoulder girdle muscles) results in difficulty in placing an object on a high shelf or combing hair.
  - Weakness of the trunk muscles and flexor muscles of the neck may be present.
  - Pain and tenderness of the involved muscles of buttocks, thighs and calves may be present.
  - The distal muscles are spared in most of the patients.
  - Others features are dysphagia, respiratory impairment, and myocarditis resulting in ECG abnormalities, heart failure and arrhythmias.
- **Primary idiopathic dermatomyositis**
  - This term is used when polymyositis is associated with characteristic skin changes.
  - The skin changes may precede or follow the muscle syndrome and include a localized or diffused erythema, maculopapular eruption or scaling eczematoid dermatitis.

- The classic lilac-colored (heliotrope) rash is seen on the upper eyelids. In addition, the rashes may be seen on the bridge of the nose, cheeks (butterfly distribution), forehead, chest, elbows, knees and knuckles. Periorbital edema is frequent.
- Most patients over the age of 60 years with dermatomyositis have an underlying malignancy.

Diagnosis:

- ❑ Erythrocyte sedimentation rate (ESR) is usually raised.
- ❑ Elevated serum levels of the muscle enzymes, such as creatine kinase (CK), aldolase, serum glutamic oxaloacetic transaminase (SGOT), lactic dehydrogenase (LDH), and serum glutamic pyruvate transaminase (SGPT).
- ❑ Characteristic EMG findings may be present.
- ❑ Muscle biopsy shows the typical pathologic changes of myositis.

Management:

- ❑ Prednisolone is initially given at a dose of 40–60 mg/day, to induce remission. Maintenance of remission usually requires 10–15 mg/day.
- ❑ Immunosuppressive therapy may be tried when there is no response to prednisolone.

29. Which of the following is/are feature of aortic stenosis?

a. Usually asymptomatic
b. Angina occurs mainly because of fixed coronary blood flows
c. No increase in cardiac output despite exercise
d. Ejection systolic murmur radiating to neck may present
e. Left ventricular hypertrophy

Ans. a, c, d, e *Ref: Harrison's, 19/e; Mathew's, 5/e*

Option a	True	Symptoms develop gradually after an asymptomatic latent period of 10–20 years
Option b	False	Angina results from a concomitant increased oxygen requirement by the hypertrophic myocardium
Option c	True	
Option d	True	
Option e	True	

- ❑ ***Aortic stenosis*** is the obstruction of blood flow across the aortic valve.
- ❑ Symptoms of aortic stenosis usually develop gradually after an asymptomatic latent period of 10–20 years.
- ❑ When the aortic valve becomes stenotic, resistance to systolic ejection occurs and a systolic pressure gradient develops between the left ventricle and the aorta. So, there is increase in left ventricular (LV) systolic pressure. As a compensatory mechanism to normalize LV wall stress, LV undergoes *concentric hypertrophy*.
- ❑ In most patients with aortic stenosis, LV systolic function is preserved and cardiac output is maintained for many years despite an elevated LV systolic pressure. Although cardiac output is normal at rest, it often *fails to increase* appropriately during exercise, which may result in exercise-induced symptoms.
- ❑ Angina results from a concomitant *increased oxygen requirement* by the hypertrophic myocardium and *diminished oxygen delivery* secondary to diminished coronary flow reserve, decreased diastolic perfusion pressure, and relative subendocardial myocardial ischemia.

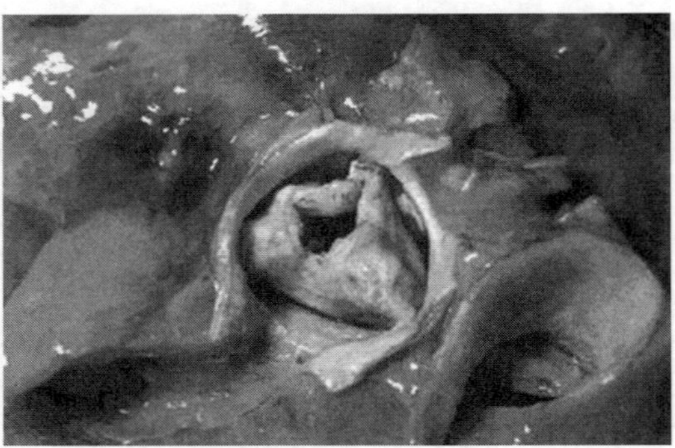

Fig. 12.1: Stenotic aortic valve.

Symptoms of Aortic Stenosis:

- Syncope, angina and dizziness in compensated phase.
- Exertional breathlessness, orthopnea, paroxysmal nocturnal dyspnea, angina and cough in decompensated phase.
- Hematemesis and malena from AV malformations of right colon, small intestine and stomach.

Signs:

- *Pulsus tardus* due to prolongation of ejection phase.
- Low systolic blood pressure.
- Systolic thrill in carotids.
- Systolic thrill at aortic area radiating to carotids, lower left sternal border and mitral area.
- Heaving apical impulse.
- No cardiomegaly in initial stages of concentric hypertrophy. Cardiomegaly develops later with left ventricular dilatation and failure.

On auscultation:

- Aortic component of second heart sound delayed.
- Ejection click of valvular origin.
- Left ventricular third heart sound in left ventricular failure.
- Fourth heart sound
- Ejection systolic murmur best heard at aortic area, conducting to carotids. It is best heard when the patient is sitting up, leaning forward and breath held in expiration.

Investigations:

- Chest radiography shows concentric hypertrophy of left ventricle, post-stenotic dilatation of aorta, and calcification of aortic valve.
- ECG shows left ventricular hypertrophy, first degree AV block or bundle branch block.
- Two-dimensional transthoracic echocardiography can confirm the clinical diagnosis of aortic stenosis and provide specific data on LV function.
- Cardiac catheterization
- Doppler USG

30. True about atrial flutter:

a. Narrow-complex tachycardia of > 150 beats/min
b. P wave absent on ECG

c. Associated with 2 : 1, 3:1, or 4:1 AV block
d. Best therapy is catheter ablation
e. Occur due to macro re-entry circuit within the right atrium

Ans. a, c, e *Ref: Harrison's, 19/e; Mathew's, 5/e*

Option a	True	Atrial rates of 240–400 beats/min
Option b	False	Seen in atrial fibrillation
Option c	True	
Option d	False	Catheter ablation is a minimally invasive procedure to treat atrial fibrillation
Option e	True	Typical atrial flutter, facilitated by the anatomical structure of the right atrium is the most frequent atrial macroreentrant tachycardia

- Definition
  - Atrial flutter is characterized by a regular, rapid atrial rate of 250–350 per minute, where ventricles respond to every second, third or fourth beat (2:1, 3:1 or 4:1 atrioventricular block).
- Common causes
  - Organic heart diseases (ischemic, rheumatic, congenital).
  - Pericarditis.
  - Acute respiratory failure.
  - First week following open heart surgery.
- Electrocardiographic feature
  - Characteristic flutter waves are seen as regular saw-toothed waves.
- Management
  - Immediate conversion to sinus rhythm can be accomplished by direct current cardioversion or atrial pacing.
  - Initial reduction of ventricular rate using digoxin, beta-blockers or verapamil followed by conversion to sinus rhythm using quinidine, amiodarone, disopyramide or flecainide.

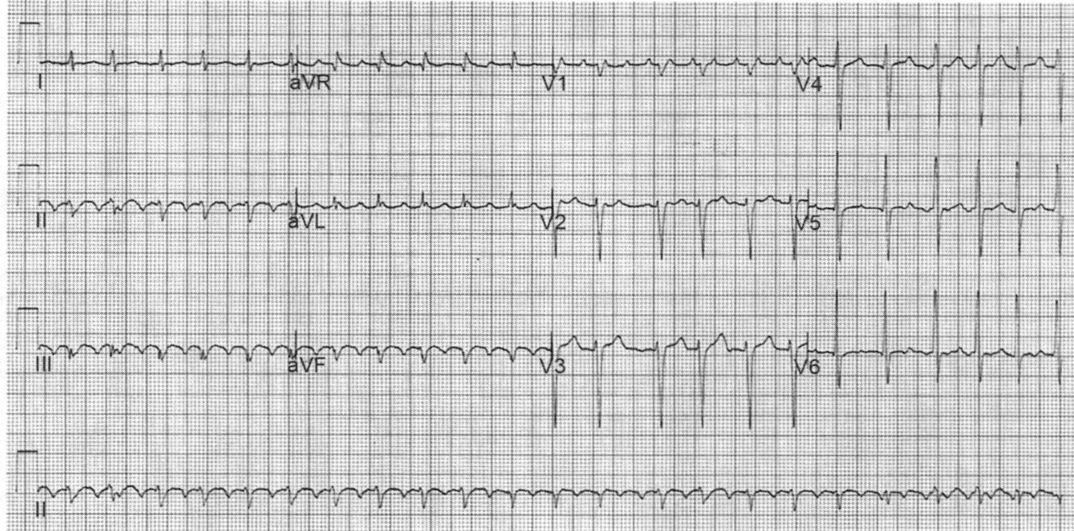

Fig. 12.2: Atrial flutter with 2:1 block.

31. Proximal renal tubular acidosis (RTA) is/are associated with:

a. Fanconi anemia
b. Multiple myeloma
c. Lead poisoning
d. Sjogren's syndrome
e. SLE

Ans. a, b, c, d *Ref: Harrison's, 19/e; Mathew's, 5/e*

Option a	True	
Option b	True	
Option c	True	
Option d	True	
Option e	False	

- **Proximal renal tubular acidosis (Type II RTA)** occurs when bicarbonate is not properly reabsorbed by the kidney's filtering system.
- Type II RTA is less common than Type I RTA. Type I is also called *distal renal tubular acidosis.*
- Type II most often occurs during infancy and may go away by itself.
- Hyperaldosteronism with consequent renal K^+ wasting occurs.
- The hypokalemia may be severe in some cases but as hypokalemia inhibits adrenal aldosterone secretion, this often limits the severity of the hypokalemia.
- Hypercalciuria does not occur and this type of RTA is *not associated with renal stones.* During the NH_4Cl loading test, urine pH will drop below 5.5.
- *Note that the acidosis in proximal RTA is usually not as severe as in distal RTA and the plasma [HCO_3] is typically greater than 15 mmol/L.*

Causes of type II RTA include

- Cystinosis (body is unable to break down cysteine)
- Drugs such as ifosfamide (a chemotherapy drug), certain antibiotics that are no longer used much (tetracycline), or acetazolamide
- Fanconi syndrome
- Inherited fructose intolerance
- Multiple myeloma
- Primary hyperparathyroidism
- Sjögren syndrome
- Wilson disease
- Vitamin D deficiency
- Lead nephropathy
- Amyloidosis.

Comparison of major types of RTA

	Type 1	*Type 2*	*Type 4*
Hyperchloremic acidosis	Yes	Yes	Yes
Minimum urine pH	> 5.5	< 5.5 (but usually > 5.5 before the acidosis becomes established)	< 5.5
Plasma potassium	Low-normal	Low-normal	High
Renal stones	Yes	No	No
Defect	Reduced H^+ excretion in distal tubule	Impaired HCO_3 reabsorption in proximal tubule	Impaired cation exchange in distal tubule

32. Features of stage III sarcoidosis are:

a. Mediastinal node enlargement
b. Pleural effusion
c. Pericardial effusion
d. Hilar lymphadenopathy
e. Parenchymal disease

Ans. e *Ref: Harrison's, 19/e; Mathew's, 5/e*

Option a	False	Stage-I
Option b	False	
Option c	False	
Option d	False	Stage-I
Option e	True	

Pulmonary sarcoidosis may be classified on a chest radiograph into 5 stages:

- *Stage 0: Normal chest radiograph*
  - 5–10% of patients at presentation
- *Stage I: Hilar or mediastinal nodal enlargement only*
  - 45–65% of patients at presentation
  - 60% go onto complete resolution
- *Stage II: Nodal enlargement and parenchymal disease*
  - 25–30% of patients at presentation
- *Stage III: Parenchymal disease only*
  - 15% of patients at presentation
- *Stage IV: End-stage lung (pulmonary fibrosis)*

33. Transudative pleural effusion occurs in:

a. Urinothorax
b. Dressler syndrome
c. Nephrotic syndrome
d. Myxedema
e. Congestive heart failure

Ans. a, c, d, e *Ref: Harrison's, 19/e; Mathew's, 5/e*

Option a	True	Rare case of transudative pleural effusion
Option b	False	Exudative pleural effusion
Option c	True	
Option d	True	
Option e	True	Most common cause

Definition

- Accumulation of serous fluid between parietal pleura and visceral pleura is called pleural effusion. Accumulation of purulent fluid is called empyema.
- The term hydrothorax denotes passive transudation of fluid into pleural cavity. This occurs in congestive heart failure, nephrotic syndrome, cirrhosis of live, severe malnutrition, etc.
- A minimum of 500 mL of fluid is necessary for clinical detection of pleural effusion.
- **Transudate** is an ultrafiltrate of plasma, resulting from increased hydrostatic pressure or decreased serum oncotic pressure. This is essentially an effusion with normal pleura.
- Exudate resembles plasma, and is rich in proteins. This results from increased capillary permeability. This is essentially an effusion with diseased pleura.

Classification and causes of pleural effusion

Transudates	CHF, cirrhosis of liver, nephrotic syndrome, severe malnutrition
Exudates	Tuberculosis, malignancy, pneumonia, pulmonary infarction, rheumatoid arthritis, pancreatitis, systemic lupus erythematosus, drug induced effusion, benign asbestos related effusion, Dressler's syndrome, intra-abdominal abscess, Meigs syndrome, chylous pleural effusion

- *Urinothorax*—Pleural effusion can occur when there is retroperitoneal leakage of urine. Urinothorax can be divided into two categories:
  - Obstructive urinothorax due to bilateral obstructive uropathy, and
  - Traumatic urinothorax due to unilateral traumatic injury of the urinary system, mostly iatrogenic.
- It is a rare cause of transudative pleural effusion secondary to obstructive uropathy.
- Myxedema causes transudative type of pleural effusion.

Difference between transudate and exudates

Test	*Transudate*	*Exudate*
• Appearance	Clear	Clear, cloudy, or hemorrhagic
• Protein - Absolute value - Pleural fluid/serum ratio	 < 3.0 g/dL < 0.5	 > 3.0 g/dL > 0.5
• Lactic dehydrogenase - Absolute value - Pleural fluid/serum ratio	 < 200 IU/L < 0.6	 > 200 IU/L > 0.6
• Glucose	> 60 mg/dL (usually same as in blood)	> 60 mg/dL (variable)
• Leucocytes - Total leucocytes - Differential leucocytes	 < 1000/mm^3 > 50% lymphocytes or mononuclear cells	 > 1000/mm^3 > 50% lymphocytes (tuberculosis, malignancy) > 50% polymorphs (acute inflammation)
• Erythrocytes	< 5000/mm^3	Variable

34. True about severe combined immunodeficiency:

a. Adenosine deaminase replacement may be given for treatment
b. Hematopoietic stem cell transplant (HSCT) is curative
c. Most common inheritance is X-linked and autosomal recessive
d. Lymphocytosis is present in most cases
e. Increased risk of infection by Pneumocystis jirovecii

Ans. a, b, c, e *Ref: Harrison's, 19/e; Mathew's, 5/e*

Option a	True	The primary treatment for adenosine deaminase (ADA) deficiency is ongoing polyethylene glycol–conjugated ADA (PEG-ADA) replacement therapy
Option b	True	
Option c	True	
Option d	False	There is deficiency of both B and T cells in SCID
Option e	True	Bacterial infection

Severe combined immunodeficiency (SCID) is a life-threatening syndrome of recurrent infections, diarrhea, dermatitis, and failure to thrive. It is the prototype of the primary immunodeficiency diseases and is caused by numerous molecular defects that lead to severe compromise in the number and function of T cells, B cells, and occasionally natural killer (NK) cells.

The genetic mutations leading to SCID can be *X-linked, autosomal recessive,* or *sporadic,* depending on the location of the gene affected.

Apart from other causes, d*eficiency of Adenosine deaminase* enzyme has been linked with the pathophysiology of SCID. This is the enzyme that breaks down purines. When it is absent, deoxyadenosine triphosphate (dATP) builds up and inhibits the enzymes necessary for lymphocyte proliferation. It causes B-, T-, and NK-cell deficiency.

Severe *thymic dysgenesis* results in lack of T cells, causing a T– B+ NK+ SCID.

Clinically, most patients present before age 3 months. Without intervention, SCID usually results in severe infection and death in children by age 2 years.

The following are the more common opportunistic infections in SCID:

- **Viral infections**
  - Cytomegalovirus (CMV) (pneumonia, hepatitis)
  - Parainfluenza virus 3, respiratory syncytial virus (RSV), and adenovirus (pneumonia)
  - Enterovirus and rotavirus (diarrhea)
  - Varicella zoster virus (VZV), herpes simplex virus (HSV), and human herpesvirus 6 (extensive cutaneous disease, meningitis)
- **Candida albicans infections**
  - Thrush
  - Diaper dermatitis progressing to diffuse skin involvement
  - Renal and biliary candidiasis
- **Cutaneous fungal infections**
- **Cryptosporidium infections**
- **Aspergillus infections (pneumonia)**
- **Bacterial infections**
  - Staphylococcus aureus, streptococci, and enterococci: (pyodermas, recurrent furunculosis, impetigo)
  - Pseudomonas aeruginosa (ecthyma gangrenosum)
  - Pneumocystis jirovecii (pneumonia)
  - Atypical mycobacteria
  - Pneumococcus and other common bacteria
  - Haemophilus influenzae and Listeria, Legionella, and Moraxella species
- **Protozoan infections (diarrhea)**

Treatment

Hematopoietic stem cell transplantation (HSCT) is the only curative option for most children with SCID.

The primary treatment for adenosine deaminase (ADA) deficiency is ongoing *polyethylene glycol-conjugated ADA (PEG-ADA) replacement therapy.*

35. Risk factors associated with health care associated pneumonia (HCAP):

a. Acute care hospitalization for at least 2 days in the preceding 90 days
b. Nursing home infusion therapy
c. Immunosuppressive disease or immunosuppressive therapy
d. Oral antibiotic therapy in the preceding 90 days
e. Hospitalization for < 48 hours

Ans. a, b, c *Ref: Harrison's, 19/e; Mathew's, 5/e*

Option a	True	
Option b	True	
Option c	True	
Option d	False	Undergone IV therapy (including chemotherapy) or wound care within the previous 30 days
Option e	False	Hospitalized in an acute care hospital for ≥ 2 days within the previous 90 days

Healthcare-associated pneumonia (HCAP) occurs in:

- Non-hospitalized patients who reside in a nursing home or other long-term care facility
- Have undergone IV therapy (including chemotherapy) or wound care within the previous 30 days.
- Have been hospitalized in an acute care hospital for ≥ 2 days within the previous 90 days, or
- Have attended a hospital or hemodialysis center within the previous 30 days.
- In addition to the usual community-acquired pathogens, HCAP pathogens include gram-negative bacilli (including Pseudomonas aeruginosa) and Staphylococcus aureus (including methicillin-resistant S. aureus) and various antibiotic-resistant pathogens.

36. In comparison to Child-Pugh scoring, MELD score have:

a. Bedside assessment easy
b. Prothrombin time expressed as international normalized ratio (INR)
c. Serum creatinine estimation
d. Four component is used in scoring
e. Albumin level estimation

Ans. b, c, d *Ref: Harrison's, 19/e; Mathew's, 5/e*

Option a	False	Used to grade liver dysfunction in preparation for liver transplantation
Option b	True	
Option c	True	
Option d	True	
Option e	False	

- The MELD score (Model for end-stage liver disease) is a classification used to grade liver dysfunction in preparation for liver transplantation.
- It is an estimate of 3 month mortality.
- The range is from 6 (less ill) to 40 (gravely ill).
- The individual score determines how urgently a patient needs a liver transplant within the next three months.

- The number is calculated using the most recent laboratory tests. Lab values used in the MELD calculation:
  - Bilirubin, which measures how effectively the liver excretes bile
  - INR (formally known as the prothrombin time), measures the liver's ability to make blood clotting factors
  - Creatinine, which measures kidney function. Impaired kidney function is often associated with severe liver disease.
- Within the MELD continuous disease severity scale, there are four levels. These are:
  - Score greater than or equal to 25
  - 24–19
  - 18–11
  - Less than or equal to 10
- There are four special case exceptions that will be assigned a higher MELD score than that assigned by the patient's laboratory test results:
  - Hepatocellular carcinoma
  - Hepatopulmonary syndrome (results in severe shortness of breath because of the extremely low level of oxygen. Patient usually needs oxygen therapy).
  - Familial amyloidosis [rare, chronic disease resulting in accumulation of an abnormal fibrillar scleroprotein (amyloid), which infiltrates body organs and can cause life threatening organ damage].
  - Primary oxaluria (metabolic disorder seen in pediatric patients only).

37. True about fourth heart sound:

a. Seen in early diastole
b. Low pitch
c. Due to forceful atrial contraction
d. Produced due to abrupt ending of ventricular filling phase
e. Absent in atrial fibrillation

Ans. b, c, e *Ref: Harrison's, 19/e; Mathew's, 5/e*

Option a	False	Seen in late diastole
Option b	True	
Option c	True	
Option d	False	Produced due to forceful atrial contraction
Option e	True	

- Fourth heart sound (S_4) occurs as a result of forceful atrial contraction ('atrial kick'). It is a low pitched sound heard in pre-systole (late diastole; before first heart sound).
- A fourth heart sound arising from the left side is known as 'left-sided fourth heart sound' and the one arising from right side as 'right-sided fourth heart sound'.

Causes of fourth heart sound

Left-sided S_4	Right-sided S_4
• Systemic hypertension • Hypertrophic cardiomyopathy • Ischemic heart disease (especially acute myocardial infarction) • Acute mitral regurgitation • Anemia, thyrotoxicosis and AV fistulae	Right ventricular hypertrophy due to: • Pulmonary hypertension • Pulmonary stenosis

A S_4 heart sound is often a sign of diastolic heart failure, and it is rarely a normal finding.

A fourth heart sound is never heard with atrial fibrillation because the contraction of the atria is ineffective in this condition.

38. True about Celiac disease is/are:

a. Antiendomysial antibody is present
b. Wheat, rye and barley can be safely given
c. Associated with dermatitis herpetiformis
d. Associated with gliadin
e. No risk for development of cancer

Ans. a, c, d, e *Ref: Harrison's, 19/e; Mathew's, 5/e*

Option a	True	
Option b	False	Gluten is abundantly present in wheat, rye and barley
Option c	True	
Option d	True	An inability to tolerate gliadin
Option e	True	

- ❑ Celiac disease, also known as celiac sprue or gluten-sensitive enteropathy, is a chronic disorder of the digestive tract that results in an inability to tolerate gliadin, the alcohol-soluble fraction of gluten. Gluten is a protein commonly found in wheat, rye, and barley.
- ❑ When patients with celiac disease ingest gliadin, an immunologically mediated inflammatory response occurs that damages the mucosa of their intestines, resulting in maldigestion and malabsorption of food nutrients.
- ❑ Gastrointestinal symptoms may include the following:
  - Diarrhea
  - Flatulence
  - Borborygmus
  - Weight loss—in infants and young children with untreated celiac disease, failure to thrive and growth retardation are common
  - Weakness and fatigue—usually related to general poor nutrition
  - Severe abdominal pain
- ❑ Extraintestinal symptoms may include the following:
  - Anemia
  - Osteopenia and osteoporosis
  - Neurologic symptoms—include motor weakness, paresthesias with sensory loss, and ataxia; seizures may develop
  - Skin disorders—including dermatitis herpetiformis, a condition with pruritic, papulovesicular skin lesions involving the extensor surfaces of the extremities, trunk, buttocks, scalp, and neck
  - Hormonal disorders—Including amenorrhea, delayed menarche, and infertility in women and impotence and infertility in men
- ❑ Investigations:
  - Immunoglobulin A anti-tissue transglutaminase antibody ***(IgA tTG),*** is the best first test for suspected celiac disease.
  - Biopsy is needed for confirmation.

- Other laboratory tests include the following:
  - Electrolytes and chemistries—Electrolyte imbalances; evidence of malnutrition
  - Hematologic tests—Anemia, low serum iron level, prolonged prothrombin time (PT)
  - Stool examination—Fat malabsorption
  - Oral tolerance tests—Lactose intolerance
  - Serology—Immunoglobulin A (IgA) antibodies
- Radiographic evaluation of the small bowel after barium ingestion is helpful in making a diagnosis of untreated celiac disease.

Treatment

The primary treatment of celiac disease is dietary. Removal of gluten from the diet is essential.

39. Which of the following is/are included in management of acute ischemic stroke?

a. Unfractionated heparin
b. LMWH
c. Streptokinase
d. Aspirin
e. Recombinant tissue plasminogen activator (rt-PA)

Ans. d, e *Ref: Harrison's, 19/e; Mathew's, 5/e*

Option a	False	May be given post-operatively to reduce the chance of deep vein thrombosis in stroke immobilized patient
Option b	False	Can be given in embolic stroke after assessing the chances of potential hemorrhage
Option c	False	Used in Myocardial infarction
Option d	True	325 mg orally, within 24–48 hours of ischemic stroke onset
Option e	True	Alteplase given intravenously

The only fibrinolytic agent that has been shown to benefit selected patients with acute ischemic stroke is alteplase (rt-PA). While streptokinase may benefit patients with acute MI, in patients with acute ischemic stroke it has been shown to increase the risk of intracranial hemorrhage and death.

AHA/ASA guidelines recommend giving aspirin, 325 mg orally, within 24–48 hours of ischemic stroke onset. The benefit of aspirin is modest but statistically significant and appears principally to involve the reduction of recurrent stroke.

40. True regarding acromegaly:

a. GH hypersecretion before puberty
b. Thinning of skin
c. Transsphenoidal surgery
d. Somatostatin analogue can be used
e. Pituitary tumor is commonest cause

Ans. c, d, e *Ref: Harrison's, 19/e; Mathew's, 5/e*

Option a	False	GH hypersecretion in adult life
Option b	False	Thickening of skin
Option c	True	
Option d	True	
Option e	True	

Acromegaly:

- Growth hormone hypersecretion occurring in adult life after epiphyseal closure results in acromegaly.
- Pituitary tumor is the commonest cause.

Clinical features:

• Soft tissue changes	Thickening of skin, increased skin tags, acanthosis nigricans, increased sweat and sebum resulting in moist and oily skin, enlargement of lips, nose and tongue, increased heel pad thickness, visceral enlargement, e.g. thyroid, heart and liver, carpal tunnel syndrome, myopathy
• Bone changes	Large spade-like hands, large feet, prognathism, prominent supraorbital ridges, large frontal sinuses, wide-spacing of the teeth, arthropathy
• Metabolic effects	Glucose intolerance or clinical diabetes mellitus, hypertension
• Pressure effects	Refer pituitary tumor

Investigations:

- Investigations of pituitary tumor (refer pituitary tumor).
- GH levels are measured during an oral glucose tolerance test. A failure of suppression or a paradoxical rise of GH indicates acromegaly.
- Demonstration of GH rise after TRH administration.

Treatment:

- Medical therapy with bromocriptine or octreotide (a somatostatin analogue).
- Transsphenoidal surgical removal of adenoma.
- External radiotherapy, or implantation of yttrium into the gland.

Surgery

1. The salivary gland tumor associated with poor survival is/are:

a. Mucin producing mucoepidermoid carcinoma
b. Squamous cell carcinoma
c. Adenoid cystic cancer
d. Adenocarcinoma
e. Acinic cell carcinoma

Ans. b, d

Option a	False	No, it is low malignant
Option b	True	Yes, correct
Option c	False	No, it is low malignant
Option d	True	Yes, it is high grade malignancy
Option e	False	No, it is low malignant

The parotid gland is the most common site for salivary tumors. Most tumors arise in the superficial lobe and present as slow growing, painless swellings below the ear in front of the ear or in the upper aspect of the neck.

Some 80–90% of tumors of the parotid gland are benign, the most common being pleomorphic adenoma. Malignant salivary gland tumors are divided into two distinct sub-groups:

1. *Low-grade malignant tumors,* e.g. acinic cell carcinoma are indistinguishable on clinical examination from benign neoplasms.
2. *High-grade malignant tumors* usually present as rapidly growing, often painless swellings in and around the parotid gland. The tumor presents as either a discrete mass with infiltration into the overlying skin or a diffuse but hard swelling of the gland with no discrete mass. Presentation with advanced disease is common, and cervical lymph node metastases may be present.

	Type	Sub-group	Common examples
I	Adenoma	Pleomorphic	Pleomorphic adenoma
		Monomorphic	Adenolymphomama (Warthin's tumor)
II	Carcinoma	Low grade	Acinic cell carcinoma
			Adenoid cystic carcinoma
			Low-grade mucoepidermoid carcinoma
		High grade	Adenocarcinoma

Contd...

Contd...

	Type	Sub-group	Common examples
			Squamous cell carcinoma
			High-grade mucoepidermoid carcinoma
III	Nonepithelial tumors		Hemangioma, lymphangioma
IV	Lymphomas	Primary lymphomas	Non-Hodgkin's lymphomas
		Secondary lymphomas	Lymphomas in Sjogren's syndrome
V	Secondary tumors	Local	Tumors of the head and neck especially
		Distant	Skin and bronchus
VI	Unclassified tumors		
VII	Tumor-like lesions	Solid lesions	Benign lymphoepithelial lesion
			Adenomatoid hyperplasia
		Cystic lesions	Salivary gland cysts

Malignant Salivary Tumors

- Adenoid cystic carcinoma (cylindroma)
  - Mc cancer of minor salivary gland
  - Tendency to invade perineural tissue
  - TOC – radical parotidectomy]
  - It is radiosensitive (note: Usually all parotid tumors are radioresistant)
- Mucoepidermoid tumor
  - MC malignant tumor (in children and adults)
  - MC radiation induced neoplasm
  - Low grade type
    - Mucin producing
    - More common (especially in children)
  - High grade type
    - Squamous cells predominate
    - Less common
- Acinic cell carcinoma
  - Rare, low grade malignancy
  - TOC- radical excision
- Papillary adenocarcinoma
  - Rare tumor
  - Grow in large sizes
  - Hemorrhage and necrosis may happen
- Squamous cell carcinoma
  - Mc in submandibular gland
- Carcinoma expleomorphic adenoma
  - Carcinoma from pleomorphic adenoma
  - Sudden rapid growth in previously stable parotid mass
  - Tendency for nodal involvement
  - TOC: Radical surgical resection with postoperative radiotherapy.

2. Risk factors for Carcinoma stomach include:

a. Chronic gastritis
b. Smoking
c. Male sex
d. Type A blood group
e. High socioeconomic status

Ans. a,b,c,d *Ref: Sabiston, 20th/ed p1214*

Option a	True	Yes, correct
Option b	True	Yes, correct
Option c	True	Yes, correct
Option d	True	Yes, correct
Option e	False	No, it is not a documented risk factor

Risk Factors

Acquired factors	Genetic factors	Precursor lesion
Nutritional	Type A blood group	Adonomalous gastric polyps
High salt consumption	Pernicious anemia	Chronic atrophic gastritis
High nitrate consumption	Family history	Dysplasia
Low dietary vitamin A and C	Hereditary nonpolyposis colon cancer	Intestinal metaplasia
Poor food preparation (smoked, salt cured)	Li-fraumeni syndrome	Menetrier's disease
Poor drinking water (well water)		Stomach remnant
Occupational		
Rubber workers		
Coal workers		
Cigarette smoking		
Halicobacler pylori infection		
Epstein-Barr virus		
Radiation exposure		
Poor gastric surgery for benign gastric ulcer disease		

Site

- ❑ Mc proximal third >pylorus and antrum > fundus and body
- ❑ Lesser curvature > greater curvature

Lauren Classification

- ❑ Intestinal type (55%)
  - Resemble colon carcinoma
  - Better prognosis

- Diffuse type (30%)
    - Associated with loss of e-codherin
    - Poorer prognosis

Spread

- Mc spread liver > lung > bone
- Tumor at Gastroesophageal (GE) junction have maximum chances of nodal metastases
- Spread along intrathoracic lymphatic channel leads to metastases in;
    - Left supraclavicular node – Virchow nodes – troisir's sign
    - Left axillary node – Irish node
- Spread along lymphatics falciform ligament transperitoneally leads to periumbilical tumor deposits – sister marry joseph nodes.

Investigations

- CEA is the tumor marker
- IOC – endoscopy and biopsy
- CT scan for staging of cancer

Management: Radical subtotal gastrectomy

Signs of Inoperability

- Growth fixed to pancreas
- Transperitoneal spread or distant metastases
- Rectovesical deposits
- Enlarged supraclavicular nodes

* Most important prognostic indicator is: LN involvement and depth of tumor invasion.

3. True about ACUTE Pancreatitis is/are:

a. Necrosis happens
b. Conservative management
c. Most common cause is biliary calculi
d. Ransons scoring system is used
e. ERCP is not indicated for severe pancreatitis with dilated CBD

Ans. a,b,c,d *Ref: Bailey, 27th/ed p1139*

Option a	True	Yes, correct
Option b	True	Yes, correct
Option c	True	Yes, correct
Option d	True	Yes, correct
Option e	False	No, urgent ERCP is recommended for gallstones or severe pancreatitis with dilated bile duct

Acute Pancreatitis

Most common cause is biliary calculi Ranson score, APACHE 2 score is used to assess the severity complication include necrosis, abscess and pseudocyst.

Possible Causes of Acute Pancreatitis

- Gallstones
- Alcoholism
- Post ERCP
- Abdominal trauma
- Following biliary, upper gastrointestinal or cardiothoracic surgery
- Ampullary tumor
- Drugs (corticosteroids, azathioprine, asparaginase, valproic acid, thiazides, oestrogens)
- Hyperparathyroidism
- Hypercalcemia
- Pancreas divisum
- Autoimmune pancreatitis
- Hereditary pancreatitis
- Viral infections (mumps, coxsackie B virus)
- Malnutrition
- Scorpion bite
- Idiopathic

Presentation

- Pain is characteristic
- Nausea, vomiting, retching, hiccoughs maybe associated
- Grey turner's sign - bluish discoloration of the flanks
- Cullen's sign - bluish discoloration of the umbilicus

Scoring Systems for Acute Pancreatitis

Ranson score	Glasgow come scale
On admission	***On admission***
Age > 55 years	Age > 55 years
White blood cell count > 16 × 10^9 l^{-1}	White blood cell count > 15 × 10^9 l^{-1}
Blood glucose > 10 mmol l^{-1}	Blood glucose > 10 mmol l^{-1} (no history of diabetes)
LDH > 700 units l^{-1}	Serum urea > 16 mmol l^{-1} (no response to intravenous fluids)
AST > 250 sigma frankel units percent	Arterial oxygen saturation (PaO_2) < 8 kPa (60 mm Hg)
Within 48 hours	***Within 48 hours***
Blood urea nitrogen rise > 5 mg%	Serum calcium < 2.0 mmol l^{-1}
Arterial oxygen saturation (PaO_2) < 8 kPa (60 mm Hg)	Serum albumin < 32 g l^{-1}
Serum calcium < 2.0 mmol l^{-1}	LDH > 600 units l^{-1}
Base deficit > 4 mmol l^{-1}	AST/ALT > 600 units l^{-1}
Fluid sequestration > 6 liters	
AST, aspartate aminotransferase; ALT, Alanine aminotranferase, LDH, Lactate dehydrogenase; PaO_2, Arterial oxygen tension.	

Table 1: Early management of severe acute pancreatitis

• Admission to HDU/ICU
• Analgesia
• Aggressive fluid rehydration
• Oxygenation
• Invasive monitoring of vital signs, central venous pressure, urine output, blood gases
• Frequent monitoring of hematological and biochemical parameters (including liver and renal function, clotting, serum calcium, blood glucose)
• Nasogastric drainage
• Antibiotic prophylaxis can be considered (imipenem, cefuroxime)
• CT scan essential if organ failure, clincal deterioration or sings of sepsis develop
• ERCP within 72 hours for severe gallstone pancreatitis or signs of cholangitis
• Supportive therapy for organ failure if it develops (inotropes, ventilatory support, hemofiltration, etc.)
• If nutritional support is required, consider enteral (nasogastric) feeding
CT, computerised tomography; ERCP, endoscopic retrograde cholangiopancreatography; HDU, high-dependency unit; ICU, intensive care unit

Note: If gallstones are the cause of an attack of predicted or proven severe pancreatitis, or if the patient has jaundice, cholangitis or a dilated common bile duct, urgent ERCP should be carried out within 72 hours of the onset of symptoms.

4. True about AV fistula is/are:

a. Acquired is mostly due to trauma
b. Surgery is the treatment of choice for congenital rather than acquired
c. Increase in heart rate
d. Osler-Weber-Rendu disease is recessive trait
e. Photodynamic therapy may be done for selected AV fistulas

Ans. a,c,e

Ref:1. Bailey 25th/ed p923
2. Patel AM, Chou EL, Findeiss L, Kelly KM. The Horizon for Treating Cutaneous Vascular Lesions. Seminars in cutaneous medicine and surgery. 2012;31(2):98-104. doi:10.1016/j.sder.2012.02.001.

Option	Answer	Explanation
Option a	True	Yes, correct
Option b	False	No, treatment is by embolization
Option c	True	Yes, correct
Option d	False	No, OWR is autosomal dominant disease
Option e	True	Yes, correct

Arteriovenous fistula (AVF), by definition, describes an abnormal communication between an artery and a vein. These communications are congenital; can occur at any point in the vascular system; and vary in size, length, location and number.

Structural effects on veins

- ❑ Veins become arterialized – dilated, torturous, and thick walled.

Physiological effects of fistula

- ❑ Increased pulse pressure (increased systolic and decreased diastolic)
- ❑ Enhanced venous return result in increased HR and increased CO
- ❑ Left ventricular enlargement and later cardiac failure may occur
- ❑ A congenital fistula in the young may cause overgrowth of limb
- ❑ In the leg, indolent ulcers may result from relative ischemia below the short circuit

Clinical signs

- ❑ A pulsatile swelling
- ❑ A thrill on palpation
- ❑ Continuous bruit on auscultation
- ❑ Nicoladoni-Branham sign pressure on the artery proximal to fistula causes the swelling diminish in size, a thrill or bruit to cease, the pulse rate to fall and pulse pressure return to normal.

Management

Treatment is by embolization. Excisional surgery can be advocated only rarely, perhaps for severe deformity or recurrent hemorrhage.

Osler-Weber-Rendu Disease (OWRD)

Also known as hereditary hemorrhagic telangiectasia [HHT] is a:

- ❑ Rare autosomal dominant disorder that affects blood vessels throughout the body (causing vascular dysplasia) and tendency to bleed.

The four clinical diagnostic criteria are as follows:

1. Epistaxis
2. Telangiectasias
3. Visceral lesions
4. Family history (a first-degree relative with HHT)

Genetic testing of OWRD patients and their family members can confirm the presence of mutations within implicated genes.

Gene involved:

- ❑ Endoglin gene (*ENG*) in chromosome 9 – more common association.
- ❑ Activin receptor-like kinase-I (ALK-1) gene (*ALK1*) in chromosome 12 (involved in HHT type 1 and type 2, respectively).

Photodynamic therapy: PDT involves light activation of a photosensitizer which reacts with local oxygen to generate cytotoxic reactive oxygen species and subsequent tissue injury which may include blood vessel wall damage or destruction. PDT is currently used to treat a wide range of benign, premalignant, and malignant conditions and has promising potential for treatment of PWS, AVMs, VMs, KSs, and angiosarcomas.

5. True about pilonodal sinus:

a. More common in females
b. Due to friction in gluteal area folds
c. Can present as acute or chronic discharges
d. Bascom flap used
e. Chronic repeat abscess predispose to this condition

Ans. c,d,e *Ref: Sabiston, 20th/ed p1408-09, Bailey, 25th/ed p1247*

Option a	False	No, more common in males
Option b	False	No, probably it is due to the friction of the hair in the gluteal cleft which redispose to this condition
Option c	True	Yes, correct
Option d	True	Yes, correct
Option e	True	Yes, correct

- The term pilonidal sinus describes a condition found in the natal cleft overlying the coccyx, consisting of one or more usually noninfected, midline openings which communicate with a fibrous track lined by granulation tissue and containing hair lying loosely within the lumen.
- Pilonidal sinus is more common in men.
- Presence of hair in the gluteal cleft seems to play a central role in the pathogenesis.
- Bascom flap, karydakis flap is used in recurrent disease.
- Bascom's procedure involves an incision lateral to the midline to gain access to the sinus cavity, which is rid of hair and granulation tissue.

6. True about Budd-Chiari syndrome:

a. Can be caused by pericardial disease
b. Primary cause is thrombosis or thickening of veins (hepatic)
c. Anticoagulant therapy is useful
d. Post veno-occlusive
e. Right atrial pressure is normal

Ans. b, d, e *Ref: Bailey 25th/ed p1092*

Option a	False	No, not correct
Option b	True	Yes, correct
Option c	False	No, warfarin anticoagulants are life long management drugs
Option d	True	Yes, correct
Option e	True	Yes, correct

Table 2: Important chronic liver conditions

Condition	Common presentations
Budd-Chiari syndrome	Ascites
Primary sclerosing cholangitis (PSC)	Abnormal LFTs or jaundice
Primary biliary cholangitis (PBC)	Malaise, lethargy, itching, abnormal LFTs
Caroli's disease	Abdominal pain, sepsis
Simple liver cysts	Coincidental finding, pain
Polycystic liver disease	Hepatomegaly, pain

- ❑ Mostly in females
- ❑ Pathophysiology – hepatic venous occlusion due to thrombosis
- ❑ Liver becomes acutely congested with the development of impaired liver function and, subsequently, portal hypertension, ascites and esophageal varices
- ❑ IVC compression or occlusion from the segment I hypertrophy is also a common feature, as is thrombosis of the portal vein
- ❑ Most common presentation is: Hepatomegaly, ascites, and abdominal pain
- ❑ Patient continues on lifelong anticoagulation with warfarin

7. Patent vaginal processes is related to which kind of hydrocele?

a. Juvenile hydrocele
b. Infantile hydrocele
c. Congenital hydrocele
d. Vaginal hydrocele
e. Funicular hydrocele

Ans. c *Ref: Bailey 25th/ed p1381*

Option a	False	No, patent processus vaginalis is congenital hydrocele
Option b	False	No, patent processus vaginalis is congenital hydrocele
Option c	True	Yes, correct
Option d	False	No, patent processus vaginalis is congenital hydrocele
Option e	False	No, patent processus vaginalis is congenital hydrocele

- ❑ A hydrocele is an abnormal collection of serous fluid in a part of the processus vaginalis, usually the tunica. Acquired hydroceles are primary or idiopathic, or secondary to testicular disease
- ❑ Hydrocele can be produced in four different ways:
  1. By excessive production of fluid within the sac, e.g. secondary hydrocele.
  2. By defective absorption of fluid; this appears to be the explanation for most primary hydroceles although the reason why the fluid is not absorbed is obscure.
  3. By interference with lymphatic drainage of scrotal structures.
  4. By connection with the peritoneal cavity via a patent processus vaginalis (congenital).

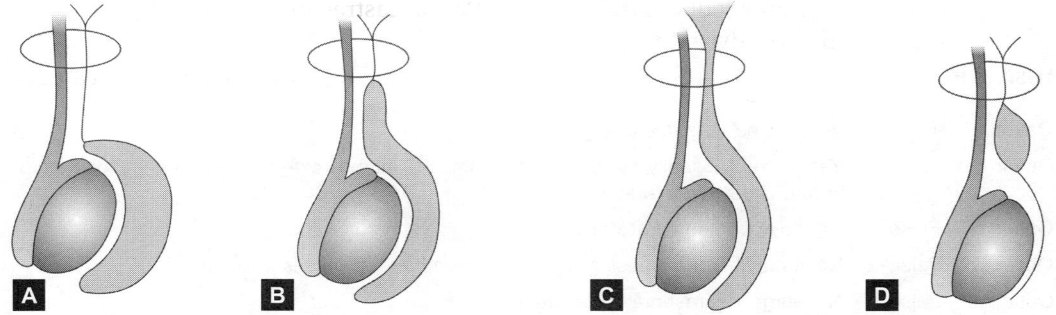

Figure 1: (A) Vaginal hydrocele (Very common). (B) 'Infantile' hydrocele. (C) Congenital hydrocele. (D) Hydrocele of the cord

- ❑ In congenital hydrocele, the processus vaginalis is patent and connects with the peritoneal cavity. The communication is usually too small to allow herniation of intra-abdominal contents. Pressure on the hydrocele does not always empty it but the hydrocele fluid may drain into the peritoneal cavity when the child is lying down; thus, the hydrocele is often intermittent.

Communicating Hydrocele

- *Communicating spermatic cord hydrocele* refers to a fluid collection originating from the pelvis and extending to the scrotum through the deep inguinal ring. This type is virtually the same as a completely patent processus vaginalis.
- Funicular hydrocele results from failure of the processus vaginalis to obliterate at the level of the deep inguinal ring. There is also patency of the proximal funicular process which extends toward the testis where it is closed by a constriction. It resembles a peritoneal diverticulum and is usually found in premature neonates and children.
- Abdominoscrotal hydrocele: Rare

Non-Communicating Hydrocele

- Scrotal hydrocele:
  - Presence of a fluid collection inside the tunica vaginalis.
  - The processus vaginalis is normally obliterated from the internal inguinal ring to the upper extent of the tunica vaginalis. As a result, a scrotal hydrocele does not communicate with the peritoneal cavity through the inguinal canal and can be thus categorized as non-communicating type.
- Encysted hydrocele:
  - Fluid collection that is enclosed between proximal and distal constrictions anywhere along the spermatic cord and does not communicate with the peritoneal cavity.

Management

- Lord's operation
- Jaboulay's operation

8. True about Gastric bezoar:

a. Most common due to fruit fibers
b. Rapunzel syndrome can be upto ileum
c. Gastric antrectomy reduces risk
d. Partial gastrectomy is advantageous
e. Surgery is always advised

Ans. a, b *Ref: Bailey, 25th/ed p1190*

Option a	True	Yes, correct, it is due to organic fibres
Option b	True	Yes, correct. Usually its stays in the stomach, but may extend to duodenum, jejunum or in rare cases even further
Option c	False	No, no documented evidence
Option d	False	No, it may be predisposing to bezoar, but more evidence is awaited
Option e	False	No, surgery is reserved procedure

- Phytobezoars (vegetable—most common)
- Diospyrobezoars, a subset of phytobezoars (excessive intake of persimmon; occur most often in regions where the fruit is grown)
- Trichobezoars (hair; rapunzep syndrome).
- Pharmacobezoars (drugs; particularly common with sucralfate and aluminum hydroxide gel).

- Other (variety of other substances including tissue paper and polystyrene foam products such as cups).

Phytobezoar

They often occur in adult patients as a postoperative complication after gastric bypass or partial gastrectomy especially when partial gastrectomy is accompanied by vagotomy.

Other Risk Factors

- Weight loss surgery: Gastric banding or gastric bypass.
- Hypochloridia.
- Delayed gastric emptying typically due to diabetes, autoimmune disorders, or mixed connective tissue disease.
- Incomplete mastication usually due to absence of teeth or poorly fitting dentures.
- Excessive intake of fibers.

Investigation

CT is best to identify type, location and size.

Management

- Cellulase dosage is 3 to 5 g dissolved in 300 to 500 mL of water; this is taken over the course of a day for 2 to 5 days. Metoclopramide 10 mg PO is often given as an adjunct to promote gastric motility.
- Endoscopic removal for large bezoars or failure to dissolve on primary measures.
- Surgery is final and reserved procedure.

9. Correct statement about Transurethral prostatectomy is/are:

a. Retrograde ejaculation is most common complaint
b. Scissor is used to cut/dissect tissue
c. Laser is used to cut/dissect tissue
d. Can be done in same setting as in cystoscopy
e. Hyponatremia is an avoidable complication

Ans. a, d *Ref: Bailey, 25th/ed p1350*

Option a	True	Yes, correct
Option b	False	No, diathermy with evacuator is used
Option c	False	No, diathermy with evacuator is used
Option d	True	Yes, correct
Option e	False	No, Hyponatermia may occur for which hypotonic glycine is used for irrigation

Most common reason for TURP is a combination of severe symptoms and a low flow rate < 12 mL/ s.

Complications following TURP

- *Retrograde ejaculation:* This occurs in about 65% of men after prostatectomy.
- *Erectile impotence*: This occurs in about 5% of men, usually those whose potency is waning.
- *Risk of re*-operation

Methods of performing prostatectomy

- ❑ Transurethral - TURP
- ❑ Retropubically - RPP
- ❑ Transvesical –TVP

TURP Procedure

Uremic patients with chronic retention are often dehydrated at the time of admission. Owing to the chronic back pressure on the distal tubules within the kidney, there is a loss of the ability to reabsorb salts and water. The result following release of this pressure may be an enormous outflow of salts and water which is known as postobstructive diuresis. It is for this reason that a careful fluid chart, daily measurements of the patient's weight and serial estimations of creatinine and electrolytes are essential.

- ❑ Strips of tissue are cut from the bladder neck down to the level of the verumontanum. Cutting is performed by a high-frequency diathermy current which is applied across a loop mounted on the hand-held trigger of the resectoscope.
- ❑ The 'chips' of prostate are then removed from the bladder using an Ellik evacuator.
- ❑ 1.5% isotonic glycine is used for irrigation to reduce the risk of hyponatremia.
- ❑ Later a three way catheter is inserted into the bladder to prevent further bleeding. The catheter is placed and irrigation continued till the outflow is pale pink. The catheter maybe removed by 2–3 postoperative day.

10. Liver transplant is contraindicated in:

a. Active alcohol drinking b. MELD > 10
c. HIV+ve on HAART d. Metastatic lesions of liver
e. Lack of psycho-social support

Ans. a,d,e *Ref: Bailey 25th/ed p1426; Vibha Varma, Naimish Mehta, Vinay Kumaran, and Samiran Nundy, "Indications and Contraindications for Liver Transplantation," International Journal of Hepatology, vol. 2011, Article ID 121862, Sabiston 20th/ed p640-644*

Option a	True	Yes, it is an absolute contraindication
Option b	False	No, MELD > 10 is an indication for liver transplant
Option c	False	No, it is not absolute contraindication
Option d	True	Yes, it is an absolute contraindication
Option e	True	Yes, it is an absolute contraindication

The indications for liver transplantation fall into four groups:

1. Cirrhosis
2. Acute fulminant liver failure
3. Metabolic liver disease
4. Primary hepatic malignancy

- ❑ Child's score ≥ 7, MELD > 10

Table 3: Contraindications to liver transplantation

• Absolute contraindications
• Severe cardiopulmonary disease
• Extrahepatic malignancy (oncologic criteria for cure not met)
• Active alcohol/substance abuse
• Acute alcoholic hepatitis
• Active infection/uncontrolled sepsis
• Lack of psychosocial support/inability to comply with medical treatment
• Brain death
• Relative contraindications
• Advanced age
• Acquired immune deficiency syndrome
• Cholangiocarcinoma
• Diffuse portal vein thrombosis
• Absolute contraindications
• Age > 60 years
• BMI > 40
• MELD score > 40
• Mean pulmonary artery pressure (PAP) > 50 mm Hg

Good to remember:

- ❑ First liver transplantation done by Starzl
- ❑ Most common indication in children is biliary atresia
- ❑ Most common indication in adults is chronic hepatitis C virus infection
- ❑ Milan criteria for liver transplantation for hepatocellular carcinoma.

11. Abdominal compartment syndrome:

a. Intra-abdominal pressure 1-2 mm Hg
b. Reverse Trendelenburg is harmful
c. Earliest sign is kidney failure
d. Laparotomy is treatment of choice
e. Reperfusion syndrome may occur after evacuation

Ans. c,d,e *Ref: Baily 25th/ed p349*

Option a	False	No, sustained IAP > 20 mmHg with organ dysfunction is known as ACS
Option b	False	No, in few cases reverse Trendelenburg may be used to monitor IAPs
Option c	True	Yes, correct
Option d	True	Yes, correct
Option e	True	Yes, correct

- ❑ Intra-abdominal pressure (IAP) is approximately 5-7 mm Hg in critically ill adults.
- ❑ Intra-abdominal hypertension is defined by a sustained or repeated pathological elevation in IAP of ≥12 mm Hg.

- ACS is defined as a sustained IAP >20 mm Hg associated with organ dysfunction/failure.
- IAH is graded as follows: Grade I: IAP 12-15 mm Hg; Grade II: IAP 16-20 mm Hg; Grade III: IAP 21-25 mm Hg; Grade IV: IAP >25 mm Hg.
- Recommend measuring intra-abdominal pressure when any known risk factor for IAH/ACS is present in critically ill or injured patients.
- Recommend that studies of IAH or ACS adopt the trans-bladder technique as a standard IAP measurement technique.
- Recommend decompressive laparotomy to decrease IAP in cases of overt ACS.
- Suggest brief trials of neuromuscular blockade as temporizing measure in treatment of IAH.

Abdominal compartment syndrome can be divided into the following 3 categories:

- Primary or acute abdominal compartment syndrome occurs when intra-abdominal pathology is directly and proximally responsible for the compartment syndrome
- Secondary abdominal compartment syndrome occurs when no visible intra-abdominal injury is present but injuries outside the abdomen cause fluid accumulation
- Chronic abdominal compartment syndrome occurs in the presence of cirrhosis and ascites or related disease states often in the later stages of the disease.

Causes of primary (i.e. acute) abdominal compartment syndrome include the followings.

- Penetrating trauma
- Intraperitoneal hemorrhage
- Pancreatitis
- External compressing forces such as debris from a motor vehicle collision or after a large structure explosion
- Pelvic fracture
- Rupture of abdominal aortic aneurysm
- Perforated peptic ulcer

Secondary abdominal compartment syndrome may occur in patients without an intra-abdominal injury when fluid accumulates in volumes sufficient to cause IAH. Causes include the following:

- **Large-volume resuscitation:** The literature shows significantly increased risk with infusions greater than 3 L
- **Large areas of full-thickness burns:** Abdominal compartment syndrome may occur within 24 hours in burn patients who had received an average of 237 mL/kg over a 12-hour period.
- Penetrating or blunt trauma without identifiable injury
- Postoperative
- Packing and primary fascial closure which increases incidence
- Sepsis

Therapy should include fluid resuscitation and transfusion if needed. Pharmacologic therapy is less effective than mechanical drainage. Paracentesis may be a superior alternative to decompressive laparotomy in these cases.

Treatments

- ❑ Titrate therapies for IAP ≤ 15 mm Hg
- ❑ Optimize fluid status
- ❑ Optimize systemic perfusion
  - Goal abdominal perfusion pressure (APP) of ≥ 60 mm Hg
    - APP = MAP - IAP
- ❑ Evacuate intraintestinal contents
- ❑ Evacuate intra-abdominal lesions
- ❑ Improve abdominal wall compliance
- ❑ Consider emergent abdominal decompression

Table 4: Effect of raised intra-abdominal pressure on individual organ function

Organ	Effect
Renal	Increase in renal vascular resistance leading to a reduction in glomerular filtration rate and impaired renal function
Cardiovascular	Decrease in venous return resulting in decreased cardiac output because of both a reduction in preload and an increase in afterload
Respiratory	Increased ventilation pressures because of splinting of the diaphragm, decreased lung compliance and increased airway pressures
Visceral perfusion	Reduction in visceral perfusion
Intracranial effects	Severe rises in intracranial pressures

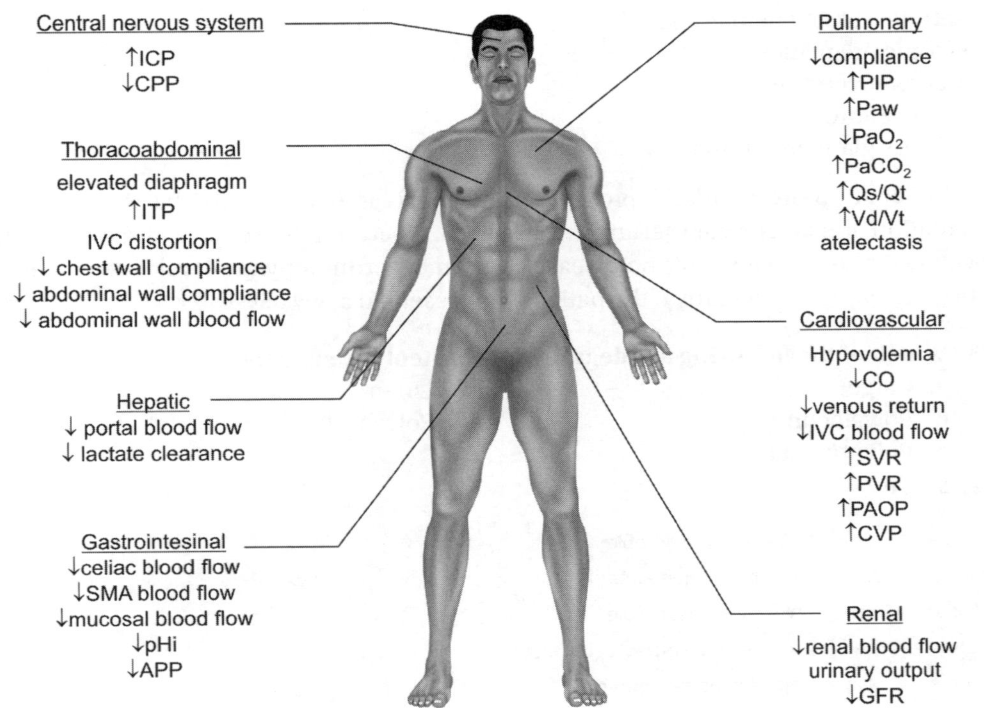

12. Serum amylase is increased in all except:

a. Esophageal rupture
b. Alcohol addicts
c. Burns
d. Ectopic
e. Hemolytic anemia

Ans. b

Option a	True	Yes, it is increased
Option b	False	No, not increased, until liver or pancreas pathology is associated
Option c	True	Yes, it is increased
Option d	True	Yes, it is increased
Option e	True	Yes, it is increased

Serum amylase is increased in:

- ❑ Burns
- ❑ Pregnancy
- ❑ Esophageal rupture
- ❑ Ruptured ectopic
- ❑ Diabetic ketoacidosis
- ❑ Chronic liver disease

Causes of raised serum amylase level other than acute pancreatitis:

- ❑ Upper gastrointestinal tract perforation
- ❑ Mesenteric infarction
- ❑ Torsion of an intra-abdominal viscus
- ❑ Retroperitoneal hematoma
- ❑ Ectopic pregnancy
- ❑ Macroamylasemia
- ❑ Renal failure
- ❑ Salivary gland inflammation

Note for acute pancreatitis: Typically, the diagnosis is made on the basis of the clinical presentation and an elevated serum amylase level. A serum amylase level three to four times above normal is indicative of the disease. A normal serum amylase level does not exclude acute pancreatitis particularly if the patient has presented a few days later.

13. Which of the following are degraded by proteolytic enzymes?

a. Catgut
b. Linen
c. Polyglactin
d. Polyamide
e. Polypropylene

Ans. a ,c, d *Ref: Bailey, 26th/ed p238*

Option a	True	Yes, it is absorbable
Option b	False	No, it is nonabsorbable
Option c	True	Yes, it is absorbable
Option d	True	Yes, it is absorbable (but slow)
Option e	False	No, it is nonabsorbable

Sutures

Silk	Slow absorb over 1-2 years
Linen	Nonabsorbable
Nylon	Slow degradation (15-20% per year)
Polyester	Nonabsorbable
Polybutester	Nonabsorbable
Polypropylene	Nonabsorbable
Catgut	Degrade within 10-60 days
Polyglactin	Complete absorption in 2-3 months
Polyglyconate	Complete absorption by 6 months
Polydioxazone	Complete absorption by 6 months
Polyglycaprone	Absorption by 3-4 months

Absorbable suture are catgut, polyglactin, polyglyconate, polyglycolic acid, polydiaxonone.

14. Correct statement(s) about Esophageal perforation is/are:

a. Middle esophagus
b. Increase in amylase level
c. After 24 hours, modality of treatment is primary repair
d. More common in iatrogenic perforation
e. Conservative management for spontaneous perforation

Ans. b, d *Ref: Sabiston, 20th/ed p1025-26*

Option a	False	No, usually upper or lower esophagus is prone for procedural perforations
Option b	True	Yes, correct
Option c	False	No, delayed presentation is best managed by conservative management
Option d	True	Yes, correct
Option e	False	No, for large spontaneous perforations immediate surgery is advised

Most common cause of perforation is iatrogenic

Barotrauma (spontaneous perforation/Boerhaave syndrome)

- Classically because of vomit against a closed glottis
- Chemical inflammation of the mediastinum
- Acute severe pain in chest
- CXR is confirmatory

Pathological perforation

- Rare
- Aerodigestive fistula is most common

Penetrating injury

- Rare
- In wars or fights or disasters.

Instrumental perforation
- Related to upper GI endoscopy - pharynx, upper (cervical) esophagus.
- Intrathoracic and intra-abdominal perforations are more common.
- May present with chest pain, hemodynamic instability, oxygen desaturation or visual evidence of perforation.

Diagnosis
- CXR
- Water soluble contrast swallow/Dilute barium swallow
- CT is done for all cases of uncertainty.

Treatment:

Conservative management for:
- Pain that is readily controlled with opiates
- Absence of crepitus, diffuse mediastinal gas, hydropneumothorax or pneumoperitoneum
- Mediastinal containment of the perforation with no evidence of widespread extravasation of contrast material
- No evidence of ongoing luminal obstruction or a retained foreign body.

Surgical management for:
- Unstable patient with sepsis
- Large perforation with heavily contaminated mediastinum, pleural space or peritoneum.

Table 5: Management options in perforation of the esophagus

Factors that favor non-operative management	Factors that favour operative repair
Small septic load	Large septic load
Minimal cardiovascular upset	Septic shock
Perforation confined to mediastinum	Pleura breached
Perforation by flexible endoscope	Boerhaave syndrome
Perforation of cervical esophagus	Perforation of abdominal esophagus

In case of delay in presentation with contamination in the mediastinum or pleura.

15. All of the following are true about mesenteric ischemia except:
  a. Abdominal guarding and rigidity develops early
  b. Intestinal atresia
  c. Most common caused by superior mesenteric artery embolism
  d. AMAE has pain which is out of proportion to physical finding
  e. Mesenteric venous thrombosis is usually in young individuals

Ans. a,b *Ref: Bailey, 26th/ed p1173-74)*

Option a	False	No, abdominal guarding develops as late feature (associated with perotinitis)
Option b	False	No, not correct
Option c	True	Yes, correct
Option d	True	Yes, correct
Option e	True	Yes, correct

Types

- NOMI (non-occlusive mesenteric ischemia)
- AMAE (acute mesenteric artery embolism)
- AMAT (Acute mesenteric artery thrombosis - thrombotic AMI)
- MVT (Mesentric venous thrombosis).

AMAE – Acute Mesenteric Artery Embolism

- Mc by embolus of cardiac origin
- Because the vascular occlusion is sudden, patients have not been able to develop a compensatory increase in collateral flow. As a result, they experience worse ischemia than patients with AMAT. Because of its small take-off angle from the aorta and higher flow, the SMA is most susceptible to emboli and the IMA is less commonly affected.

AMAT (Acute Mesenteric Artery Thrombosis - Thrombotic AMI)

- Late complication of preexisting visceral atherosclerosis.
- Causes:
  - Atherosclerotic vascular disease (most common)
  - Aortic aneurysm
  - Aortic dissection
  - Arteritis
  - Decreased cardiac output from MI or CHF (thrombotic AMI may cause acute decompensation)
  - Dehydration from any cause
- Symptoms typically do not develop until two of the three arteries (usually the celiac artery and the SMA) are stenosed or completely blocked.
- Bloody stools develop as the more sensitive mucosa dies first. The bowel gradually becomes necrotic, bacterial overgrowth develops and the resulting bowel perforation causes sepsis and finally death.

NOMI (Non-Occlusive Mesenteric Ischemia)

- Precipitated by a severe reduction in mesenteric perfusion with secondary arterial spasm from such causes as cardiac failure, septic shock, hypovolemia, or the use of potent vasopressors in critically ill patients
- Failure of autoregulation
- Causes:
  - Hypotension from CHF, MI, sepsis, aortic insufficiency, severe liver or renal disease, or recent major cardiac or abdominal surgery
  - Due to drugs – digitalis, cocaine, diuretics, vasopressin

MVT (Mesentric Venous Thrombosis)

- Younger age group
- Primary MVT – non-identifiable factor

- Secondary MVT – more commoner type of MVT
  - Iatrogenic:
    - Ligation of the splenic vein for a splenectomy
    - Ligation of the portal vein for damage control surgery
    - Ligation of the superior mesenteric vein as part of damage control surgery for severe penetrating abdominal injuries
- Causes:
  - Hypercoagulability from protein C and S deficiency, antithrombin III deficiency, dysfibrinogenemia, abnormal plasminogen, polycythemia vera (most common), thrombocytosis, sickle cell disease, factor V Leiden mutation, pregnancy, and oral contraceptive use
  - Tumor causing venous compression or hypercoagulability (paraneoplastic syndrome)
  - Infection, usually intra-abdominal (e.g. appendicitis, diverticulitis, or abscess)
  - Venous congestion from cirrhosis (portal hypertension)
  - Venous trauma from accidents or surgery especially portacaval surgery
  - Increased intra-abdominal pressure from pneumoperitoneum during laparoscopic surgery
  - Pancreatitis
  - Decompression sickness
- **Pathology:** Massive influx of fluid into the bowel wall and lumen which results in systemic hypovolemia and hemoconcentration. The consequent bowel edema and decreased outflow of blood secondary to venous thrombosis impede the inflow of arterial blood, and this leads to bowel ischemia.

Clinical presentation of AMI

- Vomiting, diarrhea
- Pain abdomen – bowel attack
- AMAT – postprandial pain
- AMAE – severe pain abdomen, bowel attack
- NOMI – vague abdominal pain
- MVT – insidious onset abdominal discomfort for weeks.

16. B/L mastectomy is done in:

a. Family history of breast cancer with no mutation
b. BRCA I and II positive
c. Upper torso radiation therapy
d. MEN 2 gene
e. Tumor size greater than 5 cm

Ans. b, c *Ref: 1. Thankamma V Ajithkumar, Oxford desk reference series. Oxford publications 2011. Pg 39, 2. Angelos P, Bedrosian I, Euhus DM, Herrmann VM, Katz SJ, Pusic A. Prophylactic Mastectomy: Challenging Considerations for the Surgeon. Annals of surgical oncology. 2015;22(10):3208-3212*

Surgery		Indication
Option a	False	No, not an indication
Option b	True	Yes, correct
Option c	True	Yes, correct
Option d	False	No, not an indication
Option e	False	No, not an indication

Table 5: Potential indications for risk reducing surgery

Bilateral mastactomy	BRCA1/2 mutations
	Familial breast cancer
	Unilateral breast cancer in < 40 years
Bilateral oophorectomy	BRCA1/2 mutations
	Familial ovarian cancer
Total proctocolectomy	FAP or APC mutations
	HNPCC—germline mutations
Thyroidectomy	RET oncogene mutation
	MEN2

Good to Remember

Indications for mastectomy (contraindications for conservative therapy):

- ❑ Prior radiation therapy to the breast or chest wall
- ❑ Radiation therapy contraindicated by pregnancy (except patients in the third trimester who can receive radiation postpartum)
- ❑ Inflammatory breast cancer
- ❑ Diffuse suspicious or malignant-appearing microcalcifications
- ❑ Widespread disease that is multicentric, located in more than one quadrant, and cannot be removed through a single incision with negative margins
- ❑ A positive pathologic margin after repeat re-excision and suboptimal cosmetic outcome

Relative indications for mastectomy include the following:

- ❑ Active connective tissue disease involving skin (e.g. scleroderma, lupus)
- ❑ Tumors greater that 5 cm in diameter
- ❑ Focally positive margin

17. True about subarachnoid hemorrhage is/are:

a. Most common cause is trauma
b. Tumors are most common cause for nontraumatic hemorrhage
c. Hunt and Hess scale used
d. Hydrocephalus with SAH requires conservative management
e. Rapid control of ICT is the mainstay of management

Ans. a,c *Ref: 1. Bailey 25th/ed p323, 635, 2. https://emedicine.medscape.com/article/2172473-overview, accessed 05th Jan 2018, 3. Welty TE1,Pathophysiology and treatment of subarachnoid haemorrhage; Clin Pharm. 1990;9(1):35-9.*

Option a	True	Yes, correct
Option b	False	No, aneurysm is most common nontraumatic cause for SAH
Option c	True	Yes, correct
Option d	False	No, Surgery is the definitive treatment for the prevention of rebleeding. Hydrocephalus can only be treated surgically most commonly by insertion of a drain
Option e	False	No, the likelihood of rebleeding is increased by measures that rapidly lower intracranial pressure

- Although aneurysms are the most common cause of spontaneous subarachnoid hemorrhage, trauma is by far the most common cause of subarachnoid hemorrhage overall.
- Nontraumatic causes are:
  - Aneurysms (75%)
  - Arteriovenous malformations (AVMs;10%)
  - Idiopathic causes (10%)
  - Tumors (<5%)
- In rare cases, a spontaneous aneurysmal hemorrhage immediately precedes a head injury.
- Traumatic subarachnoid hemorrhage is managed conservatively.
- The most common premonitory symptoms are as follows:
  - Headache (48%)
  - Dizziness (10%)
  - Orbital pain (7%)
  - Diplopia (4%)
  - Visual loss (4%)

The Hunt and Hess scale is used for categorizing severity of SAH:

- Grade 1: Asymptomatic or mild headache
- Grade 2: Cranial nerve palsy or moderate to severe headache/nuchal rigidity
- Grade 3: Mild focal deficit, lethargy, or confusion
- Grade 4: Stupor and/or hemiparesis
- Grade 5: Deep coma, decerebrate posturing, moribund appearance.

18. For French catheter, size used is:

a. Black catheter – 10 f
b. Green – 12 f
c. Orange – 14 f
d. Red – 16 f
e. Yellow – 20 f

Ans. a, e

Option a	True	Yes, correct
Option b	False	No, not correct

Option c	False	No, not correct
Option d	False	No, not correct
Option e	True	Yes, correct

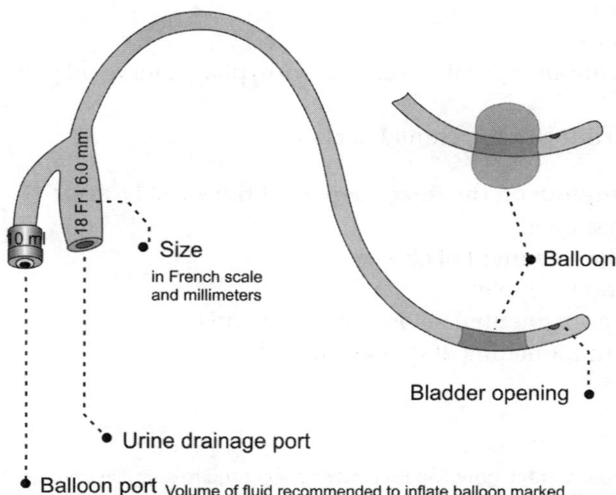

- The french size is a measure of the **outer diameter** of a catheter
- An increasing french size corresponds to a larger external diameter
- To remember, black white GORY
- Black is 10, white is 12, green is 14, orange is 16, red is 18, yellow is 20.

19. Maxillary tumor is staged as T3 from T2 when it involves:

a. Spreads to sphenoid sinus
b. Erosion of pterygoid
c. Middle nasal meatus
d. Hard palate
e. Spreads to frontal sinus

Ans. a, b

Option a	True	Yes, correct
Option b	True	Yes, correct
Option c	False	No, this is T2 stage
Option d	False	No, this is T2 stage
Option e	False	No, this is T4 stage

- Tx – Tumor cannot be assessed
- T0 – No evidence of primary tumor
- Tis – Carcinoma is situ
- T1 – Limited to maxillary sinus mucosa
- T2 – Bone erosion ± may extend to hard palate ± middle nasal meatus

- T3: Tumor invades any of the following:
  - Bone of the posterior wall of the maxillary sinus
  - Subcutaneous tissues
  - Floor or medial wall of the orbit
  - Pterygoid fossa
  - Ethmoid sinuses
- T4 a – Extends to infratemporal fossa, cribriform plate, pterygoid plate, sphenoid or frontal sinuses
- T4 b – Extends to dura, brain, cranial nerves

20. True about ganglion on the flexor aspect of the wrist is/are:

a. It is spindle shaped
b. Surgery is the treatment of choice
c. more common in male
d. Also called as pigmented villonodular synovitis
e. Formed by outpouching of synovial membrane

Ans. a,b,e *Ref: Sabiston, 2008, 10*

Option a	True	Yes, correct
Option b	True	Yes, correct, ganglion on flexor aspect require surgical treatment
Option c	False	No, they are more common in females
Option d	False	Yes, correct
Option e	True	Yes, correct

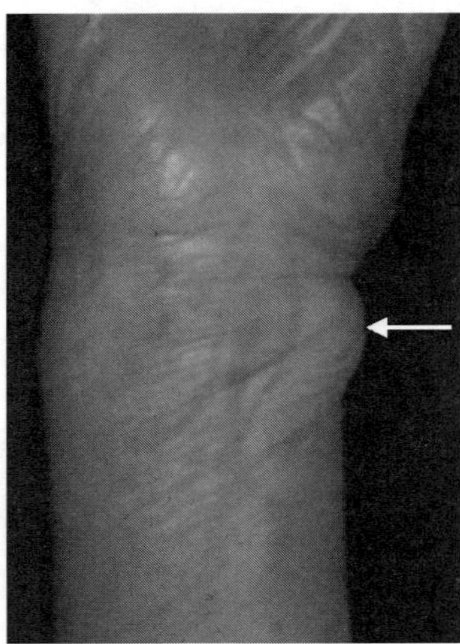

Fig. Volar wrist ganglion

- Ganglion cysts also known as bible cysts are more common in females than males.
- Median age is: 30 years (20–40 years).
- Ganglion cysts most commonly occur on the back of the hand, at the wrist joint, and can also develop on the flexor aspect of the wrist. When found on the dorsum of the wrist, they become more prominent when the wrist is flexed forward.

Management:

- Surgical removal is indicated for pain or for cosmetic reasons.
- High chance of recurrence.

Other cysts: Good to know:

- Ganglion cyst: A cyst around a tendon, most commonly occurring at the wrist
- Baker's cyst: A cyst containing joint fluid that is located in popliteal space behind the knee
- Bartholin's cyst: Cystic enlargement of small glands near the vaginal opening
- Nabothian cyst: A mucus-filled cyst on the surface of the uterine cervix
- Pilonidal cysts: Cysts that arise in the soft tissue at the base of the tailbone (coccyx) of the lower back, just above the natal cleft (the cleavage between the buttocks)
- Dermoid cyst: A type of benign tumor of the ovary that contains multiple cystic spaces and various tissue types
- Ganglion cysts that develop at the end joint of a finger — also known as mucous cysts — are typically associated with arthritis in the finger joint, and are more common in women between the ages of 40 and 70 years.

21. True about primary sclerosing cholangitis is/are:

a. Ulcerative colitis is commonly associated
b. Bile duct scarring
c. Onion skin concentric and periductal fibrosis is characteristic
d. Fever episodes with jaundice is common
e. Affects only extra hepatic biliary tree

Ans. a,b,c *Ref: Sabiston 20th/ed p1508-09; Bailey, 25th/ed p1127; https://emedicine.medscape.com/article/187724-clinical accessed on 5 Jan 2018.*

Option a	True	Yes, correct, 80-90% of PSC cases have ulcerative colitis
Option b	True	Yes, correct
Option c	True	Yes, correct
Option d	False	Yes, correct, Recurrent febrile episodes of bacterial cholangitis (fever with jaundice) occur in 10-15% of patients during the course of PSC
Option e	False	No, it affects both intrahepatic and extrahepatic ducts

- Primary sclerosing cholangitis (PSC) is an idiopathic fibrosing inflammatory condition of the biliary tree that affects both intrahepatic and extrahepatic ducts
- Most common age 30-60 years
- Male > females
- Associated with IBD, especially ulcerative colitis, and Riedel thyroiditis
- Liver biopsy in PSC tends to show onion skin concentric periductal fibrosis

Diagnosis

- Contrast enhanced USG - screening tool
- Percutaneous transhepatic cholangiography (PTC) and endoscopic retrograde cholangio-pancreatography (ERCP) - therapeutic and diagnostic
- Liver biopsy - staging and prognosis of PSC
- The most common characteristic of histologic feature is onion skin fibrosis (concentric periductal fibrosis)

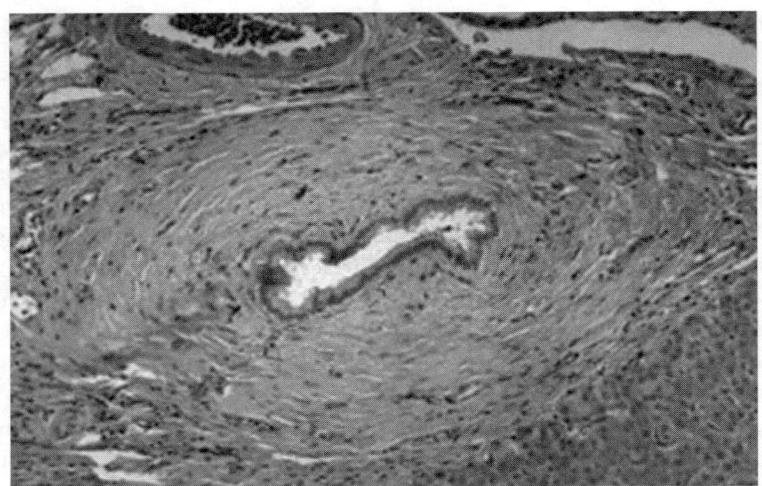

- ❑ LFT is most important for PSC diagnosis
- ❑ Increase in serum alkaline phosphatase
- ❑ Serum gamma-glutamyl transpeptidase levels mirror this rise and can help differentiate cholestasis from bone disease
- ❑ Serum aminotransferase levels are increased in PSC but not very high
- ❑ Serum bilirubin levels with the conjugated component are usually increased, but fluctuations in the level can occur.
- ❑ Serum albumin levels decrease later in the course of the disease, and the presence of hypoalbuminemia earlier in the disease may indicate active inflammatory bowel disease.
- ❑ Antibody markers:
  - P-ANCA (Perinuclear antineutrophil cytoplasmic antibodies)
  - ANA (antinuclear antibodies)
  - aCL (anticardiolipin)
  - ASMA (anti-smooth muscle antibody)

Management: Liver transplant

22. True about Reef knot is/are:

a. Granny's knot is better than reef knot
b. It is standard surgical knot
c. Better than surgeon knot
d. Also called square knot
e. Suture to wound length ratio of 1:2 is optimum

Ans. b,c,d *Ref: Bailey, 25th/ed p241-242*

Option a	False	No, reef knot is better than granny knot. Granny knot must be followed by standard reef knot to ensure security
Option b	True	Yes, correct, standard surgical knot is the reef knot
Option c	True	Yes, correct, reef knot is called square knot and it is better than surgeon knot.
Option d	True	Yes, correct, reef knot is called square knot and it is better than surgeon knot.
Option e	False	No, suture length to wound length ratio of 4:1 indicates the optimum size of tissue bites and of suture spacing.

- Standard surgical knot is the reef knot
- Reef knot is called square knot. It is better than surgeon knot
- Granny knot must be followed by the standard reef knot to ensure security.

Types of Knots used in Surgery

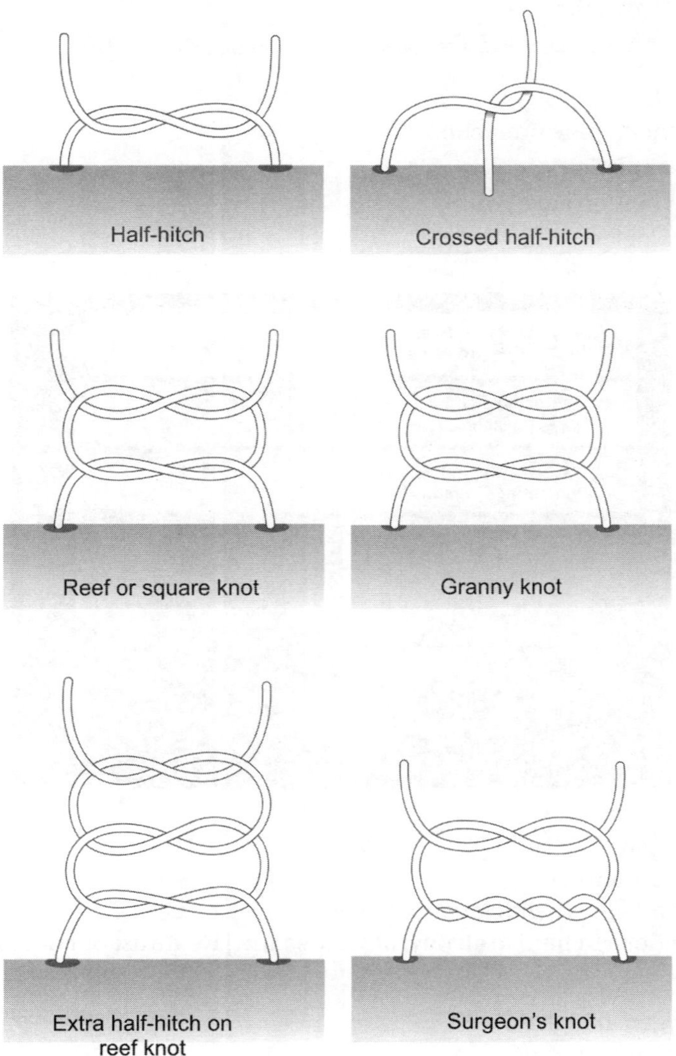

Fig. Types of knot used in surgery

23. Which of the following is/are process for trauma management as per ATLS protocol?

a. FAST
b. Airway
c. Exposure
d. Breathing
e. Cardioversion

Ans. a,b,c,d *Ref: Bailey/25th/290*

Option a	True	Yes, correct
Option b	True	Yes, correct
Option c	True	Yes, correct
Option d	True	Yes, correct
Option e	False	No, cardioversion, if required is part of the ACLS protocol

ABCDE of Trauma

A Airway with cervical spine protection

B Breathing and ventilation

C Circulation with hemorrhage control

D Disability, neurological status

E Exposure

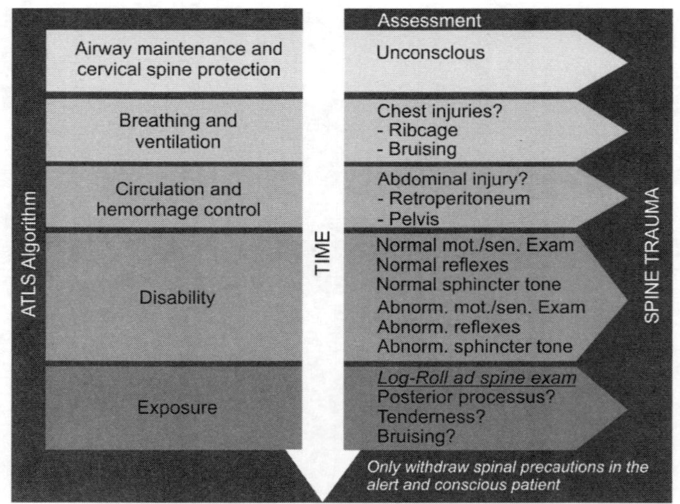

Airway

- ❑ Airway assessment
- ❑ Check verbal response
- ❑ Clear mouth and airway with large-bore sucker
- ❑ If GCS 8, consider a definitive airway; otherwise use jaw thrust or chin lift

Breathing

- ❑ Give 100% oxygen at high flow
- ❑ Check for tension pneumothorax
- ❑ Decompress at once if tension pneumothorax is suspected (needle in the second intercostal space)

Circulation (assessment and warning signs)

- ❑ Deteriorating conscious state
- ❑ Pallor
- ❑ Rapid thready pulse is a more reliable and earlier warning sign than a fall in the blood pressure

Good to remember:

#1 FAST (Focused Assessment with Sonography for Trauma): Identifying the presence of free intraperitoneal or pericardial fluid. In cases of traumatic injury, free fluid is usually due to haemorrhage and contributes to the assessment of the circulation.

FAST examines four areas for free fluid:
1. Perihepatic and hepatorenal space
2. Perisplenic
3. Pelvis
4. Pericardium

FAST assessment is indicated in trauma patients who give a history of abdominal trauma are hypotensive, or are unable to provide a reliable history because of impaired consciousness due to head injury or drugs. FAST is an adjunct to the ATLS primary survey and therefore follows the performance of the ABCs.

#2 Pediatric vitals:

Table 5: Pediatric vital signs

Normal vital signs by age	Pulse (beats per min)	Systolic blood pressure (mmHg)	Respiratory rate (breaths per min)
Infant (< 1 year)	160	80	40
Preschool (<5 years)	140	90	30
Adolescent (> 10 years)	120	100	20

24. True about axillary LN dissection for breast cancer:
   a. Arm kept at 90° abduction
   b. Level I, II, III all are removed
   c. Level III nodes are lateral to the pectoralis minor
   d. Level II lymph nodes are below pectoralis minor
   e. Axillary fat, lymph nodes and long thoracic nerve is dissected enbloc

Ans. a, b, d *Ref: Sabiston, p859*

Arm kept at 90° abduction in axillary lymph node dissection level 1 and 2 group of lymph nodes are removed. Level 2 are located below pectoralis minor.

Option a	True	Yes, correct
Option b	True	Yes, correct
Option c	False	No, level III nodes are medial to the pectoralis minor
Option d	True	Yes, correct
Option e	False	No, long thoracic nerve is preserved

Axillary

Axillary dissection should be reserved for patients with proven axillary disease preoperatively or with a positive sentinel node biopsy.

Axillary dissection is only therapeutic in patients who are node positive. Therefore, performing axillary dissection in all patients would lead to an over treatment of at least 60% of patients who are all node negative.

There are three surgical levels of axillary lymph nodes:

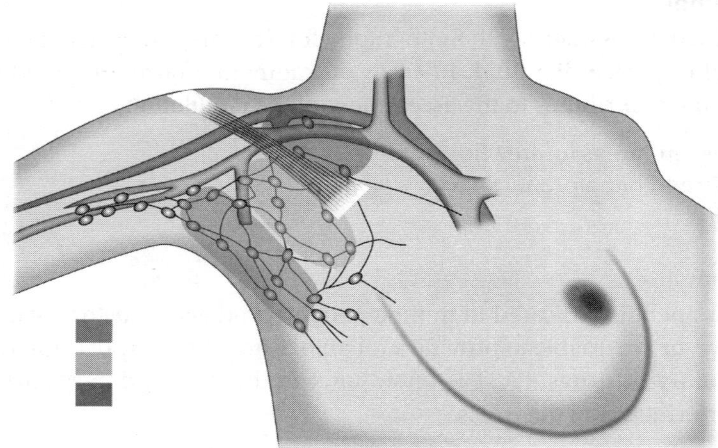

- Level I: Below the lower edge of the pectoralis minor muscle
- Level II: Underneath/posterior to the pectoralis minor muscle
- Level III: Above/medial to the pectoralis minor muscle

Procedure

- Raise head end 30°
- Arm abducted at 90° to chest wall
- Axillary dissection removes all the nodes and fat from this space
- The axillary contents are then separated from the lateral thoracic wall which is the medial boundary of the axilla. This exposes the long thoracic nerve which supplies the serratus anterior muscle (injury to which would lead to winging of the scapula).

25. Features of ischemic colitis:

a. Angiography is diagnostic
b. Caused by small vessel atherosclerosis
c. Griffiths point is most susceptible to ischemia
d. Seen in young atheletes
e. No abdominal tenderness

Ans. b,c *Ref: https://www.ncbi.nlm.nih.gov/pmc/articles/PMC3577613/; Cecil textbook of medicine, volume 24. Elseivers health sciences (2012); Robert D. Odze, John R. Goldblum. Surgical Pathology of the GI Tract, Liver, Biliary Tract, and Pancreas. 2nd/ed p60*

Option a	False	Diagnosis of ischemic colitis is made by CT or colonoscopy Angiography or magnetic resonance angiography is not indicated
Option b	True	Yes correct
Option c	True	Yes correct
Option d	False	Disease of old age >65 years
Option e	False	Abdominal tenderness is seen over the involved area of the abdomen

Bowel ischemia is mainly a disease of old age caused by atheroma of mesenteric vessels. Other causes include embolic disease, vasculitis, fibromuscular hyperplasia, aortic aneurysm, blunt abdominal trauma, disseminated intravascular coagulation, irradiation, and hypovolemic or endotoxic shock.

Areas of the colon most sensitive to decreased blood flow and more likely to suffer from ischemia are the splenic flexure (Griffiths point) and sigmoid colon (Sudek's point). These 'watershed' areas are where the circulation from the superior mesenteric artery and inferior mesenteric artery meet, and where the inferior mesenteric artery and rectal arteries meet.

Patients with ischemic colitis tend to have multiple risk factors for vascular disease such as persons over 65 years of age, persons with cardiac arrhythmia, and thrombophilia. For unclear reasons, patients with irritable bowel syndrome (IBS) have a threefold increased risk for ischemic colitis.

Constipation has also been identified as a risk factor for the development of ischemic colitis. This is believed to be due to increased intraluminal pressures causing compression of the blood vessels and resultant decreased mucosal vessel flow.

Good to Know

Table 3: Drugs associated with ischemic colitis.
Digitalis
Vasopressin
Pseudoephedrine
Amphetamines
Cocaine
Ergot
Sumatriptan
Gold
Danazol
Estrogens
Progestins
Alosetron
Psychotropics
Nonsteroidal anti-inflammatory drugs
Various enemas
Tegaserod
Interferon/ribavirin

Surgery

1. True about prostate-specific antigen:

a. Serum level > 4ng /mL is confirmatory for prostate cancer
b. High probability of prostate cancer if PSA levels are > 10 mg/mL
c. Produced by prostate
d. Useful in prognosis and follow-up
e. Can not be used to monitor recurrence

Ans. b, c, d *Ref: S Das, 9/e; Sabiston, 20/e*

Option a	False	PSA levels between 4 and 10 ng/mL are considered to be suspicious
Option b	True	
Option c	True	Secreted by the epithelial cells of the prostate gland
Option d	True	
Option e	False	PSA levels are periodically monitored after treatment of prostate cancer for recurrence

Prostate-specific antigen (PSA) is a glycoprotein enzyme, belonging to kallikrein-related peptidase family and is secreted by the epithelial cells of the prostate gland. PSA is produced for the ejaculate, where it liquefies semen in the seminal coagulum and allows sperm to swim freely.

PSA is present in small quantities in the serum of men with healthy prostates, but is often elevated in the presence of prostate cancer or other prostate disorders. Hence, the PSA test can be useful for detecting prostate cancer, monitoring its treatment, or assessing its recurrence.

PSA levels between 4 and 10 ng/mL (nanograms per milliliter) are considered to be suspicious and consideration should be given to confirming the abnormal PSA with a repeat test. If indicated, prostate biopsy is performed to obtain tissue sample for histopathological analysis.

For an average man over the age of 50 with a normal digital rectal exam, the average probability of having prostate cancer detectable by prostate biopsy according to his PSA level is as follows:

Probability of prostate cancer detectable by biopsy according to PSA level				
PSA level (ng/mL)	0 to 2.0	2.0 to 4.0	4.0 to 10.0	> 10.0
Prostate cancer on biopsy (%)	10%	25%	17 to 32%	43 to 65%

Since the likelihood of having prostate cancer increases proportionately with PSA level, there is no threshold below which a man can be reassured that prostate cancer is not present.

Most PSA in the blood is bound to serum proteins. A small amount is not protein bound and is called 'free PSA.' In men with prostate cancer the ratio of free (unbound) PSA to total PSA is decreased. The risk of cancer increases if the free to total ratio is less than 25%.

Change in PSA levels over time can be used to assess both cancer risk and aggressiveness of the particular tumor. PSA doubling time is the time it takes the PSA value to increase by 100%, or double. These two measures also have a significant prognostic role in patients that have already been treated for prostate cancer (with either surgery [radical prostatectomy] or radiotherapy [external beam or brachytherapy]).

2. True about insulinoma:

a. Histology similar to normal β-cells.
b. Mostly multiple
c. Encapsulated
d. Enucleation can be done for benign tumor
e. Associated with MEN-I

Ans: a, c, d, e *Ref: S Das, 9/e; Sabiston, 20/e*

Option a	True	
Option b	False	Only 10% have multiple insulinomas
Option c	True	
Option d	True	Insulinomas may be removed by enucleation
Option e	True	

- An insulinoma is a neuroendocrine tumor, deriving mainly from pancreatic islet cells, that secretes insulin.
- Insulinomas are the most common cause of hypoglycemia resulting from endogenous hyperinsulinism.
- The tumor may secrete insulin in short bursts, causing wide fluctuations in blood levels.
- Insulinomas are characterized clinically by the Whipple triad, as follows:
  - Presence of symptoms of hypoglycemia (about 85% of patients)
  - Documented low blood sugar at the time of symptoms
  - Reversal of symptoms by glucose administration
- Approximately 10% of patients have multiple insulinomas; of patients with multiple insulinomas, 50% have multiple endocrine neoplasia type 1 (MEN 1).
- Microscopically, insulinomas are composed of cords and nests of well-differentiated beta cells.
  - **Clinical Features:** Majority of the patients are in the 4th to 7th decades of life. Sex incidence is approximately equal.
  - If the blood sugar falls rapidly, the primary symptoms may be referable to the release of epinephrine caused by hypoglycemia. Sweating, weakness, tachycardia, hunger and trembling result from this. A slower decrease in the blood sugar produces cerebral symptoms such as headache, mental confusion, visual disturbances, convulsions and coma. Symptoms may last for a few weeks or a few years. Bizarre neurologic or psychiatric disorders are not uncommon in this condition.
  - **Treatment:** The only permanent cure of this condition is excision of the tumor or tumors.
- A marked increase in the blood sugar level within 30 minutes of removal of the lesion is confirmatory evidence that the lesion has been removed.

3. Hypercalcemia is seen in which of the following malignancies?

a. Breast cancer
b. Small cell lung cancer
c. Non-small cell lung cancer
d. Prostate cancer
e. Multiple myeloma

Ans. a, c, d, e *Ref: S Das, 9/e; Sabiston, 20/e*

Option a	True	Most common association
Option b	False	
Option c	True	Seen in squamous cell carcinoma variant
Option d	True	Rare phenomenon
Option e	True	

- The main pathogenesis of hypercalcemia in malignancy is increased osteoclastic bone resorption, which can occur with or without bone metastases.
- The enhanced bone resorption is mainly secondary to different humoral factors that alter calcium regulation and are released by tumor cells locally (at the site of metastatic bone lesions) or systemically.
- The main humoral factor associated with cancer-related hypercalcemia is parathyroid hormone-related protein, which is produced by many solid tumors.
- Parathyroid hormone-related protein increases calcium by activating parathyroid hormone receptors in tissue, which results in osteoclastic bone resorption; it also increases renal tubular resorption of calcium.
- Malignancy-associated hypercalcemia occurs in up to 20-30% of patients.
- It is seen in:
  - *Breast cancer:* One of the most common malignancies responsible for hypercalcemia.
  - *Multiple myeloma:* Hypercalcemia is one of the four diagnostic "***CRAB***" criteria (*calcium elevation, renal insufficiency, anemia, or bone disease*) used to distinguish smoldering myeloma from active, symptomatic multiple myeloma.
  - *Non-small cell lung cancer:* Hypercalcemia due to parathyroid-like hormone production occurs most commonly in patients with squamous cell carcinoma.
  - *Prostate cancer:* It is typically associated with metastatic osteoblastic lesions, hypocalcemia and hypophosphatemia. Hypercalcemia is a rarely encountered phenomenon, i.e. 1–2% in prostate cancer.

4. True about gastric adenocarcinoma is:

a. Most common along the lesser curvature
b. Associated with iron deficiency anemia
c. Proliferative type is low grade malignant
d. Linitis plastica causes stomach fibrosis
e. 70% of carcinoid tumors occur in stomach

Ans. c, d *Ref: S Das, 9/e; Sabiston, 20/e*

Option a	False	Most common are pyloric and antral regions of stomach
Option b	False	Associated with pernicious anemia

Option c	True	
Option d	True	
Option e	False	Only 2% of all carcinoid tumors occur in stomach

Gastric cancer is the third most common cause of cancer-related death in the world.
Occurs most commonly between the ages of 50–70 years.

Predisposing factors:

- *Chronic atrophic gastritis:* Decreased or absent normal gastric glands due to which patients are hypo or achlorhydric. Risk of malignancy in such cases increases when associated with intestinal metaplasia.
- Pernicious anemia
- *Helicobacter pylori infection:* Chronic bacterial infection with H pylori is the strongest risk factor for stomach cancer.
- *Chronic gastric ulcer:* A chronic gastric ulcer situated on or within ½ inch of greater curvature should be regarded and treated as malignant.
- *New growths of the stomach:* Adenomatous gastric polyps are considered as premalignant conditions.
- *Menetrier's disease:* Giant hypertrophy of fundic mucosa with cystic changes in the crypts.
- Other factors as smoked food, very hot or iced food, over smoking, alcohol, etc.

Pathology:

- Commonest site of occurrence is pyloric and antral regions followed by lesser curvature.
- Macroscopic types:
  - *Ulcerative type:* Most malignant and commonest variety. Infiltrates widely and rapidly.
  - Proliferative or cauliflower type Bulky, cauliflower-like masses with broad pedicle projecting into the stomach lumen. These are of low grade malignancy. Growths are usually adenocarcinomas composed of columnar epithelial cells. Confined to a limited area.
  - Leather bottle stomach or linitis plastica Local form of disease which starts at pylorus and spreads slowly in the direction of cardia, associated with much fibrosis. This is often called as scirrhous carcinoma of the stomach.

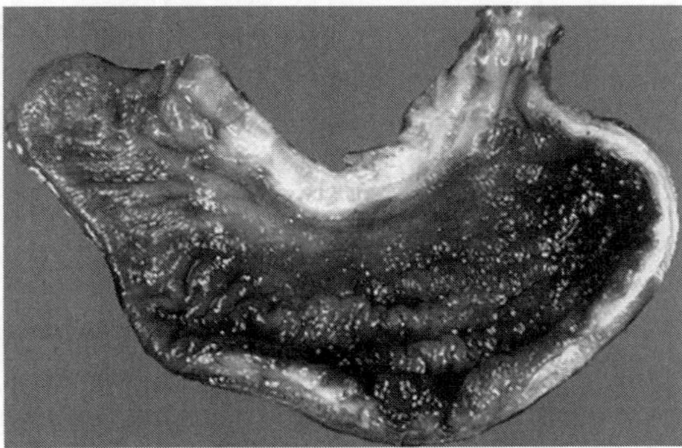

Fig. 13.1: Linitis plastica.

  - Colloid or mucoid carcinoma
  - Carcinoid of the stomach: Only 2% of all carcinoid tumors occur in stomach.

Esophagogastroduodenoscopy has a diagnostic accuracy of 95%.

5. True about spontaneous bacterial peritonitis is/are:

a. Low mortality
b. Antibiotics not required
c. TLC/neutrophils > 500/μL
d. Usually polymicrobial
e. Seen in patients with liver cirrhosis.

Ans. c, e *Ref: S Das, 9/e; Sabiston, 20/e*

Option a	False	Mortality rate is high 40–70%
Option b	False	Since culture is usually positive for microorganisms, antibiotics are definitely indicated
Option c	True	Ascitic fluid neutrophil count of more than 500 cells/μL is the single best predictor of spontaneous bacterial peritonitis
Option d	False	SBP usually results from a single organism
Option e	True	Complication in patients with cirrhosis

- Spontaneous bacterial peritonitis (SBP) is an acute bacterial infection of ascitic fluid. Ominous complication in patients with cirrhosis.
- SBP can occur as a complication of any disease state that produces the clinical syndrome of ascites, such as heart failure and Budd-Chiari syndrome.
- Children with nephrosis or systemic lupus erythematosus who have ascites have a high risk of developing spontaneous bacterial peritonitis.
- Bacterial translocation (viable microorganism passage from the intestinal lumen to mesenteric lymph nodes) plays major role in the development of spontaneous bacterial peritonitis.
- Abdominal tenderness is the most commonly encountered symptom. Findings can range from mild tenderness to overt rebound and guarding.
- Fever, malaise, encephalopathy, worsening hepatic failure, and unexplained clinical deterioration is seen.
- Hypotension or signs of hepatic failure such as jaundice and angiomata may also be seen.
- Diagnosis is made by:
  - Diagnostic paracentesis with culture: An ascitic fluid neutrophil count of more than 500 cells/μL is the single best predictor of spontaneous bacterial peritonitis. Polymorphonuclear neutrophil cell count of > 250 cells/μL is diagnostic of SBP.
  - SBP usually results from a single organism, finding mixed flora on culture suggests a perforated abdominal viscus or contaminated specimen.
  - Blood culture
  - Urine culture
  - Plain radiographs (including abdominal flat plate, abdominal upright, and chest)
  - CT scanning of the abdomen detects small perforations.

The mortality rate in patients with spontaneous bacterial peritonitis ranges from 40–70% in adult patients with cirrhosis.

6. True about Schatzki ring:

a. Contains mucosa and sub-mucosa

b. Web at lower esophagus
c. Occurs above the esophagogastric junction
d. Dysphagia is usually to solid foods
e. Always associated with reflux disease

Ans. b, c, d, e *Ref: S Das, 9/e; Sabiston, 20/e*

Option a	False	
Option b	True	
Option c	True	
Option d	True	Patients typically present with intermittent nonprogressive dysphagia for solids
Option e	True	May rarely be associated with reflux esophagitis

Schatzki Ring

It is an esophageal web in its lower most part. This web contains only mucosa and submucosa. It is covered with squamous epithelium above and columnar epithelium below. So it actually appears at the squamo-columnar junction within 1 to 2 cm above the esophagogastric junction. This condition is in majority of cases asymptomatic. Dysphagia only occurs when the diameter is minimized to less than 15 mm.

Clinical presentation

Most commonly it presents as intermittent dysphagia, especially to solid food. A history of food impaction is also very common. Dysphagia is more common in patients with an associated motility disorder.

Diagnosis: Barium esophagogram is most dependable to diagnose this condition. One thing must be submucosal fibrosis. It may not be associated with gastroesophageal reflux or esophagitis.

Treatment: Intermittent esophageal bougienage is the treatment of choice of this condition. Only when it is associated with reflux esophagitis, an anti-reflux operation is justified.

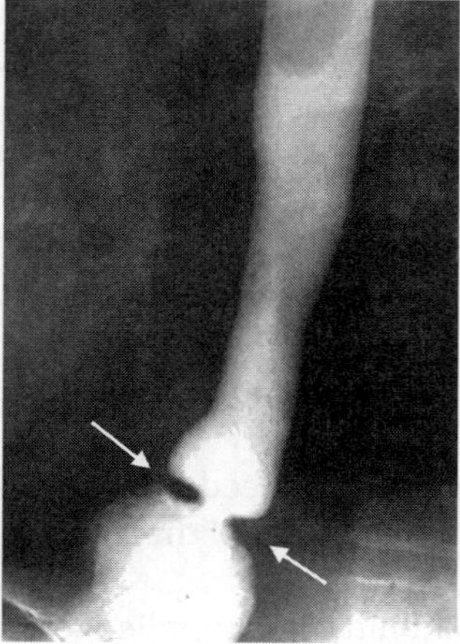

Fig. 13.2: Barium esophagogram showing typical Schatzki ring.

7. **Correct statement(s) about surgical site infection:**
   a. Can occurs due to environment flora in the operation theatre.
   b. Occurs within 2 weeks of surgery

c. Alcohol-based agent is used for skin preparation
d. Shaving helps in preventing SSI
e. Can occur within 1 year in case of implant left in situ

Ans. a, c, e *Ref: S Das, 9/e; Sabiston, 20/e; Centers for Disease Control and Prevention Guideline for the Prevention of Surgical Site Infection, 2017*

Option a	True	
Option b	False	Occurs within 30 days after surgery
Option c	True	
Option d	False	Shaving is not to be done by the patient
Option e	True	

A surgical site infection (SSI) is an infection that occurs after surgery in the part of the body where the surgery took place.

- The most commonly isolated organisms are *Staphylococcus aureus*, coagulase-negative *staphylococci*, *Enterococcus spp.*, *Escherichia coli*, *Streptococcus*, and *Pseudomonas*.
- An SSI typically occurs within 30 days after surgery if no implant is left in place or within one year if implant is in place and the infection appears to be related to the operation itself.
- The CDC describes 3 types of surgical site infections:
  - *Superficial incisional SSI:* This infection occurs just in the area of the skin where the incision was made.
  - *Deep incisional SSI:* This infection occurs beneath the incision area in muscle and the tissues surrounding the muscles.
  - *Organ or space SSI:* This type of infection can be in any area of the body other than skin, muscle, and surrounding tissue that was involved in the surgery. This includes a body organ or a space between organs.

Centers for Disease Control and Prevention: Guideline for the prevention of surgical site infection, 2017:

- Before surgery, patients should *shower or bathe* (full body) with soap (antimicrobial or nonantimicrobial) or an antiseptic agent on at least the night before the operative day.
- *Antimicrobial prophylaxis* should be administered only when indicated based on published clinical practice guidelines and timed such that a bactericidal concentration of the agents is established in the serum and tissues when the incision is made.
- In cesarean section procedures, antimicrobial prophylaxis should be administered before skin incision.
- Skin preparation in the operating room should be performed using an *alcohol-based agent* unless contraindicated.
- For clean and clean-contaminated procedures, additional prophylactic antimicrobial agent doses should not be administered after the surgical incision is closed in the operating room, even in the presence of a drain.
- Topical antimicrobial agents should not be applied to the surgical incision.
- During surgery, glycemic control should be implemented using blood glucose target levels less than 200 mg/dL, and normothermia should be maintained in all patients.
- Increased fraction of inspired oxygen should be administered during surgery and after extubation in the immediate postoperative period for patients with normal pulmonary function undergoing general anesthesia with endotracheal intubation.

- ❑ Transfusion of blood products should not be withheld from surgical patients as a means to prevent SSI.
- ❑ Skin area that the surgeon is planning to operate through should not be shaved by the patient himself.

8. Grade III (contaminated) wound is/are:

a. Surgery over an uninfected site
b. Incision through abscess
c. Wound contaminated with fecal matter
d. Appendicular inflammation
e. Wound in GU tract without unusual contamination

Ans. c, d *Ref: Sabiston, 20/e; http://www.med.umich.edu/surgery/mast/r_surgwoundclass.html*

Option a	False	Grade-I wound
Option b	False	Grade IV wound
Option c	True	Grade III wound
Option d	True	Grade III wound
Option e	False	Grade II wound

Surgical wound classifications

- ❑ *Clean:*
  - Uninfected, no inflammation
  - Respiratory, gastrointestinal, genitourinary tracts not entered
  - Closed primarily

  Examples: Old laparotomy, mastectomy, neck dissection, thyroid, vascular, hernia, splenectomy
- ❑ *Clean-contaminated:*
  - Respiratory, gastrointestinal, genitourinary tracts entered, controlled
  - No unusual contamination

  Examples: Cholecystectomy, Whipple, liver transplantation, gastric surgery, bronchus, colon surgery
- ❑ *Contaminated:*
  - Open, fresh, accidental wounds
  - Major break in sterile technique
  - Gross spillage from GI tract
  - Acute nonpurulent inflammation

  Examples: Inflamed appendix, bile spillage in cholecystectomy, diverticulitis, rectal surgery, penetrating wounds
- ❑ *Dirty:*
  - Old traumatic wounds, devitalized tissue
  - Existing infection or perforation
  - Organisms present BEFORE procedure

  Examples: Abscess I and D, perforated bowel, peritonitis, wound debridement, positive cultures preoperatively.

9. All of the following are Nonabsorbable sutures *except*:

a. Vicryl
b. Silk
c. Linen
d. Polypropylene
e. Catgut

Ans. a, e *Ref: S Das, 9/e; Sabiston, 20/e*

Option a	True	Absorbable
Option b	False	Nonabsorbable
Option c	False	Nonabsorbable
Option d	False	Nonabsorbable
Option e	True	Absorbable

Nonabsorbable sutures	Absorbable sutures
Surgical steel	Surgical gut or catgut
Silk	Polyglycolic acid (Dexon; Syneture)
Linen	Polyglactin 910 (Vicryl; Ethicon)
Nylon	Polydioxanone (PDS; Ethicon)
Polypropylene	Polytrimethylene carbonate (Maxon; Syneture)
Polybutester	Glycomer 631 (caprosyn; Syneture)
Cotton	Polyglytone 6211 (Caprosyn; Syneture) Poliglecaprone (Monocryl; Ethicon)

10. True about Colorectal cancer:

a. Carcinoma of right colon presents with obstructive symptoms
b. Left-sided cancer present with alteration in bowel habit
c. Hepatic flexure is the first one to be involved by cancerous process
d. Left side colon is more commonly involved
e. Associated with familial polyposis coli

Ans. b, d, e *Ref: S Das, 9/e; Sabiston, 20/e*

Option a	False	Obstruction is unusual in right colon
Option b	True	Almost the first symptom
Option c	False	Hepatic and splenic flexures are last to be involved
Option d	True	
Option e	True	

Colorectal cancer:

- Peak incidence is in the 7th decade.
- Rectum is the most affected part followed by sigmoid colon and further followed by cecum.
- Ascending, transverse and descending colons come after cecum.
- Hepatic and splenic flexures are last to be involved.
- Precancerous conditions:
  - Villous adenoma
  - *Familial polyposis coli*

- Gardner's syndrome
- Chronic ulcerative colitis

- Rate of colonic cancer is directly proportional to the amount of animal fat consumed.
- Macroscopically, carcinoma is of following types:
  - Cauliflower or polypoid variety
  - Ulcerative type
  - Tubular or scirrhous type
  - Annular type
- Clinical features:
  - *Carcinoma of right colon:* More broad than left colon and fecal content is fluid, so obstructive symptoms are very unusual. Anemia of varying degree is common. Anorexia, indigestion and weight loss are presenting symptoms. Defined lump can be palpated.
  - *Carcinoma of left colon:* Majority of carcinomas arise in the left region. Due to small lumen and solid fecal content, obstruction of the lumen is more common. Change in the bowel habit is the first symptom. Palpated lump is usually impacted feces. Anemia is uncommon. Sometimes, complete intestinal obstruction may also be seen.
  - *Carcinoma of sigmoid colon:* Tubular variety seen in the recto-sigmoid junction. Tenesmus accompanied by mucus and blood occurs early in the morning. Irritation of bladder can also be noted.
  - *Carcinoma of transverse colon:* Pain and palpable lump are two common modes of presentation. Associated anemia, anorexia are almost always present.

11. True about thyroid cancer:

a. Papillary carcinoma is dependent on TSH stimulation.
b. Hurthle cell carcinoma occurs bilaterally.
c. Follicular cancer is nonresponsive to radioiodine
d. Psammoma bodies can be seen in papillary cancer
e. Medullary carcinoma is associated with MEN-2b

Ans. a, b, d, e *Ref: S Das, 9/e; Sabiston, 20/e*

Option a	True	
Option b	True	
Option c	False	Good response to radioactive iodine
Option d	True	
Option e	True	

Malignant Neoplasms

The *classification* of malignant thyroid tumors should be as follows:

- Follicular cell origin
  - Differentiated:
    - Papillary carcinoma (60%);
    - Follicular carcinoma (15%);
    - Mixed papillary and follicular carcinoma.

- Undifferentiated:
  - Anaplastic carcinoma (13%).
- ❑ Parafollicular cell origin:
  - Medullary carcinoma (6%).
- ❑ Non-thyroid cell origin:
  - Malignant lymphoma (4%);
  - Sarcoma;
  - Metastatic carcinoma

Thyroid carcinoma is rare in children and increases in frequency with increasing age. These tumors also demonstrate a 3 : 1 female predominance.

Papillary carcinoma:

- ❑ Most common form of thyroid carcinoma.
- ❑ Unencapsulated tumors, invade lymphatics and spread to normal surrounding thyroid tissue.
- ❑ Composed of columnar thyroid cells.
- ❑ *Psammoma bodies*: Localized deposits of calcium in connective tissue layers.
- ❑ Multicentricity of primary tumor is the most important feature.
- ❑ Dependent on tumor stimulation.
- ❑ *Most slow growing tumor* among the various malignant tumors of thyroid
- ❑ Three times more common in females than males.
- ❑ Tendency to become malignant with advancing age.

Follicular carcinoma:

- ❑ Encapsulated.
- ❑ Two varieties are:
  - Encapsulated, well-differentiated, low grade malignancy. Capsular invasion and vascular invasion are features. Usually does not metastasize.
  - Early vascular invasion. Primary tumor is most aggressive of all well-differentiated carcinomas.
- ❑ *Hurthle cell carcinomas*: Histologically distinct from follicular type. Prognosis is intermediate between the two types of follicular carcinomas. Occurs bilaterally and metastasize locally with high incidence of recurrence.
- ❑ Good response to *radioactive iodine.*

Anaplastic carcinoma:

- ❑ May develop from a previous *nodular goitre* and pre-existing well-differentiated thyroid carcinoma.
- ❑ Unencapsulated, extends into remaining thyroid tissue, and even outside.
- ❑ Rapid growth, local invasion.
- ❑ *Regional lymph nodes* are frequently enlarged.
- ❑ Distant metastasis to lungs and bones.

Medullary carcinoma:

- ❑ Non follicular, originates from *parafollicular C cells.*
- ❑ Secretes *calcitonin.*

- Associated with *multiple endocrine adenomatosis* and *multiple endocrine neoplasia type-II.*
- *C-cell hyperplasia* is considered as precursor of medullary carcinoma.
- Metastatic lesion in bone is *osteoblastic.*

12. True about gas gangrene:

a. Onset is usually acute
b. Painless condition
c. Wound is swollen initially
d. At first wound is dusky or red, later becomes pale
e. Caused by gram + ve organism

Ans. a, c, d *Ref: S Das, 9/e; Sabiston, 20/e*

Option a	True	
Option b	False	Severe pain in the infected area.
Option c	True	
Option d	True	Initially, the area is swollen and pale but eventually turns red, then bronze, and finally blackish green
Option e	False	

- Gas gangrene is a highly lethal necrotizing soft tissue infection of skeletal muscle caused by toxin- and gas-producing clostridium species.
- Clostridia are gram-positive, anaerobic, spore-forming bacilli commonly found throughout nature.
- Clostridium perfringens, previously known as clostridium welchii, is the most common cause of clostridial gas gangrene (80–90% of cases). Other clostridia species responsible for the condition include Clostridium novyi (40%), Clostridium septicum (20%), Clostridium histolyticum (10%), Clostridium bifermentans (10%), and Clostridium fallax (5%).
- Gas gangrene *develops suddenly*. It usually occurs at the site of trauma or a recent surgical wound.
- In some cases, it occurs without an irritating event. People most at risk of gas gangrene usually have blood vessel disease (atherosclerosis), diabetes, or colon cancer.
- Severe pain in the infected area. Initially, the area is swollen and pale but eventually turns red, then bronze, and finally blackish green. Large blisters often form.
- Gas gangrene can cause myonecrosis, gas production, and sepsis. Progression to toxemia and shock is often very rapid. It can easily be noticed by the large, blackened sores that form, as well as a degree of loud and distinctive crepitus caused by gas escaping the necrotic tissue.
- Treatment is usually debridement and excision, with amputation necessary in many cases.

13. True about postoperative ileus:

a. Right colon recovers earlier than left colon
b. Physiologic ileus usually resolves within 48–72 hour
c. Adhesion is most common cause
d. Succussion splash can be seen
e. Radiographs show diffusely dilated bowel with air in the colon

Ans. a, b, e *Ref: S Das, 9/e; Sabiston, 20/e*

Option a	True	
Option b	True	
Option c	False	Most common reason is intra-abdominal operation
Option d	False	
Option e	True	

- Ileus occurs from hypomotility of the gastrointestinal tract in the absence of mechanical bowel obstruction.
- The postoperative state is the most common setting for the development of ileus.
- Ileus is an expected consequence of abdominal surgery.
- Physiologic ileus spontaneously resolves within 2–3 days, after sigmoid motility returns to normal. The small bowel typically regains function within hours; the stomach regains activity in 1–2 days; and the colon regains activity in 3–5 days.
- The return of propulsive activity to the right colon occurs earlier than to the transverse or left colon.
- Ileus that persists for more than 3 days following surgery is termed postoperative adynamic ileus or paralytic ileus.
- A distinguishing feature from obstruction is absent or hypoactive bowel sounds, in contrast to the high-pitched sound of obstruction. The silent abdomen of ileus shows no peristalsis or succussion splash.
- On plain abdominal radiographs, ileus appears as copious gas dilatation of the small intestine and colon.

14. True about testicular cancer:

a. Seminoma is more common than non-seminoma
b. Teratoma is mostly seen in children
c. Non germinal testicular tumors are always benign
d. Usually presents as painless testicular lump
e. Seminoma always metastasize through blood stream

Ans. a, c, d *Ref: S Das, 9/e; Sabiston, 20/e*

Option a	True	Seminoma is the most common form of testicular tumor in adults
Option b	False	Peak incidence of teratoma is between 25–30 years age
Option c	True	
Option d	True	Painless swelling of testis is common presentation
Option e	False	Seminomas rarely metastasize through blood stream

Classification of testicular tumors:

There are numerous classifications, but the most accepted one is that described by the Testicular Tumor Panel of Great Britain:

- **Germ cell tumors (GCT):**
  - Seminoma—45°
  - Teratoma—38°
    - Teratoma differentiated (TD)
    - Malignant teratoma, intermediate (MTI) (Teratocarcinoma)

- Malignant teratoma, undifferentiated (MTU) (Embryonal carcinoma)
- Malignant teratoma, trophoblastic (MTT) (Choriocarcinoma)

■ Combined tumor consisting of seminoma and teratoma—14%

❑ Non-germ cell tumors:

■ Interstitial tumors—1.5%
■ Lymphoma
■ Other tumors

The **pick incidence** of teratoma is between 25 and 30 years of age and that for seminoma is between 35 and 45 years of age and combined tumors occupy an intermediate are distribution.

Testicular tumors can be broadly classified into 2 main divisions:

❑ *Germinal tumors,* constituting nearly 98% of the total and are presumed to arise from primordial sex or germ cells.

❑ *Non-germinal tumors,* constituting the remaining less than 2% of cases which take origin from the non-germinal elements of testis. *The non-germinal testicular tumors are almost always benign.*

15. Which of the following nipple discharge is most probably physiological:

a. B/l spontaneous discharge
b. B/l milky discharge with squeezing from multiple ducts
c. U/l bloody discharge
d. U/l bloody discharge with squeezing from a single duct
e. U/l spontaneous serous discharge

Ans. b *Ref: S Das, 9/e*

Option a	False	
Option b	True	
Option c	False	
Option d	False	
Option e	False	

According to the nature of nipple discharge the following classification may be made:

Usually seven varieties of nipple discharge may be seen: (i) Milk discharge, (ii) Serous discharge, (iii) Blood discharge, (iv) Greenish discharge, (v) Black discharge, (vi) Pus and (vii) Creamy discharge.

❑ **Milk discharge:** Milk discharge is more commonly seen in very late stages of pregnancy. Lactation may continue for months or years after suckling if the patient continues to express milk because she thinks this should be done. This is called physiological galactorrhea. Drugs including the contraceptive pills may occasionally lead to slight discharge of milk perhaps through pituitary prolactin mechanism.
Milk discharge may be seen in case of milk fistula following chronic subareolar mastitis. Milk discharge may occasionally be seen with *galactocele.*

❑ **Serous discharge:** Physiologically this may be seen, though very rarly and after continuous use of contraceptive pills. Serous discharge may be seen in cases of *fibroadenosis* and *mammary duct ectasis,* though greenish-black discharge is more common in fibroadenosis and thick creamy discharge is more often seen in mammary duct ectasia. *Duct papilloma and non-infiltrating duct carcinoma* may produce serous discharge in the intervals of bloody discharge.

- **Blood discharge:** Though very occasionally blood discharge from the nipple may be seen in bilateral cases in *pregnancy* due to physiological epithelial hyperplasia, yet blood discharge is usually seen in *papilloma* of the duct and in cases of *duct carcinoma*. Benign solitary papilloma is more common in younger women of 15 to 30 years. Multiple papillomas are more often seen in patients nearing menopause. Noneinfiltrating or infiltrating type of duct carcinoma may cause blood stained discharge which are more commonly seen after the age of 50 years.
- **Greenish discharge:** This is typically seen in cases of fibroadenosis. Similar colored fluid can also be obtained from cyst aspiration in similar cases. Serous, brownish or even greenish discharge may also be found it *mammary duct ectasia*.
- **Black discharge:** Old blood looks black and such blackish discharge may occur in *duct papilloma or duct carcinoma* which is notorious for blood discharge. Blackish discharge is also occasionally seen in cases of fibroadenosis.
- **Pus:** Rarely discharge of pus may be seen through nipple in cases of acute mastitis.
- **Creamy discharge:** Thick creamy discharge is seen in *mammary duct ectasia*.

16. True about traumatic fat necrosis in women is/are:

a. Painless lump
b. More common in lactating women
c. Not malignant
d. Biopsy is required for diagnosis
e. Differentiated from malignancy on mammography

Ans. a, c, d *Ref: S Das, 9/e; Sabiston, 20/e*

Option a	True	
Option b	False	Middle aged fatty women
Option c	True	
Option d	True	
Option e	False	

Injury

Traumatic fat necrosis: Some sort of insult to the breast in the form of injury, indirect violence from seat-belt injury and administration of subcutaneous infusion into the breast may produce this condition. Middle aged fatty women are mostly affected. This condition is mostly a chronic one in which the patient presents with a painless lump which simulates in many respects carcinoma of the breast.

Pathology: This is an uncommon lesion. Focal necrosis of fat tissues in the breast followed by inflammatory reaction and subsequent scaring gives rise to a focus of firmer consistency. This is capable of confusing with a new growth. The stages are—that in the beginning there is a focus of hemorrhage, later central liquefactive necrosis of fat surrounded by a zone of inflammation occurs. Later on well-defined nodule of greyish white with firm consistency containing possibly small foci of chalky white debris is formed. The area is converted into a dense fibrous scar. Histologically, the central focus of necrotic fat cells is surrounded by lipid-filled macrophages and intense neutrophilic infiltration. This is followed by progressive fibroblastic proliferation and lymphocytic and histiocytic infiltration to wall off the focus. Still later foreign body giant cells, calcium salts and blood pigments make their appearance and the whole focus is replaced by scarred tissue which is walled off by collagenous tissue.

Clinical features: *This condition is without any clinical significance save for its possible confusion with a tumor*. History of injury, no retraction of the nipple, the feel of the lump which is not very hard and irregular and there is no axillary lymph node enlargement are the features in favour of this condition. Slight skin retraction may be present and the condition cannot be differentiated from carcinoma by mammography. Incision on such a lump will show chalky white area similar to that found in cases of subsiding acute pancreatitis.

Treatment: Whenever in doubt excisional biopsy is the treatment of choice and is usually required for the diagnosis to be certain.

17. True about bronchogenic cyst:

a. May have malignant potential
b. Respiratory distress more common in children
c. Airway compromise rarely occurs
d. Infected cyst may show air fluid levels on chest X-ray
e. Usually multiple

Ans. a, b, d *Ref: S Das, 9/e; Sabiston, 20/e*

Option a	True	
Option b	True	
Option c	False	Airway compromise occurs as a frequent complication with large masses
Option d	True	
Option e	False	Usually single

- Bronchogenic cysts are congenital malformations of the bronchial tree (a type of bronchopulmonary foregut malformation). Although relatively rare, Bronchogenic cysts represent the most common cystic lesion of the mediastinum.
- They can present as a mediastinal mass that may enlarge and cause local compression. It is also considered the commonest of foregut duplication cysts.
- Cysts are believed to result from abnormal development of the ventral foregut and lung budding during the first 4–6 weeks of gestation.
- In many instances, bronchogenic cysts are asymptomatic and are found incidentally when the chest is imaged. When large, mass effect may result in bronchial obstruction leading to air trapping and respiratory distress. An alternative presentation may occur when the cyst becomes infected.
- They are usually single but may be multiple and can be filled with fluid or mucus.
- Cough, wheeze, dyspnea, and respiratory distress are more commonly seen in children.
- Secondary infection of the cyst may occur and may present with fever and respiratory symptoms.
- Complication:
  - Airway compromise
  - Infection
- Chest X-ray typically shows a sharply demarcated spherical mass of variable size, most commonly located in the middle mediastinum around the carina. When the cyst is infected or contains secretions, it may appear as a solid tumor or may demonstrate an air fluid level.
- Surgical resection of all symptomatic bronchogenic cysts is recommended.
- In newborns with asymptomatic bronchogenic cysts, surgical intervention is recommended at age 3–6 months, allowing for compensatory lung growth.

18. True about abdominal aortic aneurysm:

a. Low back pain
b. May presents as pulsatile abdominal mass
c. May be seen in Marfan's syndrome
d. Aneurysms less than 10 cm need no treatment
e. Painful aneurysm treated with NSAIDs

Ans. a, b, c *Ref: S Das, 9/e; Sabiston, 20/e*

Option a	True	Due to tension on retroperitoneal tissues from aneurysm
Option b	True	
Option c	True	
Option d	False	Aneurysms less than 5 cm need no treatment and can be safely observed
Option e	False	Painful aneurysms are an emergency needing immediate surgery

Abdominal aortic aneurysms are most common of all aneurysms.

- Majority are atherosclerotic in origin, occurring below the origin of renal arteries.
- Presents in 6th or 7th decade.
- In minor cases, it can occur in association with Marfan's syndrome, syphilis or trauma.
- If diameter exceeds 10–15 cm, it can be discovered by palpation.
- **Clinical features:**

  Low back pain may be caused by abdominal aneurysms. Sometimes pain may be referred to the groin or thigh due to nerve compression. Virtually any intra-abdominal condition may be simulated by an abdominal aortic aneurysm, e.g. peptic ulcer, cholecystitis, pancreatitis, appendicitis or diverticulitis.

  A few patients only complain of a pulsatile mass in the abdomen.

  With beginning leakage of the aneurysm, it may mimic acute abdominal conditions, e.g. perforated peptic ulcer, hemorrhagic pancreatitis or generalized peritonitis.
- **Physical examination:** A pulsating mass > 1 inch diameter usually establishes the diagnosis of aneurysm.

  During physical examination, peripheral pulses should be carefully palpated for associated occlusive vascular disease. Presence of a bruit over the bifurcation of the carotid artery is particularly significant because an asymptomatic stenosis of the carotid artery may be revealed.

  Leakage may occur either into the peritoneal cavity or into the duodenum or even into the inferior vena cava. Initially bleeding is into the retroperitoneal space, where it may be contained for a while before it proves fatal.
- Straight X-ray abdomen is confirmatory. It shows a thin curved line of calcification in the wall of the sac.
- Other investigations include—ultrasound scanning, and CAT Scan.

Indications for surgery:

- Aneurysms less than 5 cm in diameter can be safely observed till they expand or become symptomatic.
- Asymptomatic aneurysms measuring more than 5 cm require operation unless there are other risk factors.
- When aneurysm becomes painful, an emergency operation needs to be done, as pain denotes impending rupture.

19. Features of congenital esophageal atresia is/are:

a. May be associated with imperforate anus
b. Rubber catheter when passed, feces obstruction
c. Drooling of saliva characteristically absent
d. Abdominal distension
e. Regurgitation of saliva

Ans. a, b, d, e *Ref: S Das, 9/e; Sabiston, 20/e*

Option a	True	In around 12% cases, there is imperforate anus
Option b	True	Rubber catheter encounters obstruction at about 10 cm from lips
Option c	False	Saliva continuously drools from mouth
Option d	True	Seen in type I atresia
Option e	True	

Congenital Esophageal Atresia

Congenital atresia of the esophagus is often associated with tracheoesophageal fistula. Usually 4 types are noticed. In *type I,* which occurs in 90% of cases the upper esophageal segment ends blindly and the lover portion of the esophagus is connected with the trachea through tracheoesophageal fistula. The esophageal fistula usually joins the trachea at or just above the tracheal bifurcation, admitting inspired air into the stomach or in retrograde fashion gastric juice into the lungs, In *type II,* both upper and lower esophageal segment end blindly with a portion of esophagus in between missing. This occurs in about 8% to 10% of cases. In *type III,* the proximal segment of the esophagus are connected with the trachea by tracheoesophageal fistulae. This occurs in only less than 1% of cases.

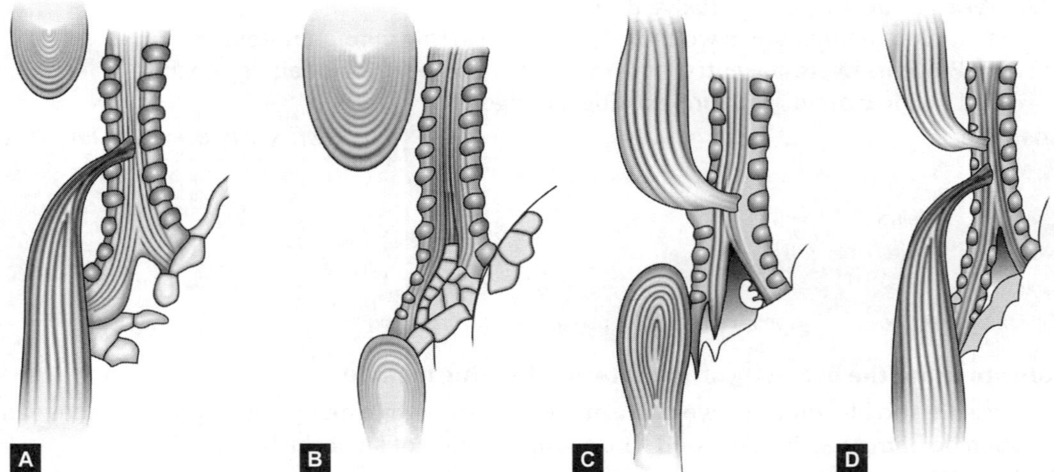

Figs. 13.3A to D: Four types of congenital esophogeal atresia. A is the commonest type (90%); B is type II according to the text and is seen in only 8% to 10% of cases; C is type III of the text and is seen in only 1% to 2% of cases; D is type IV of the text and is extremely rare (less than 1% of cases).

Associated congenital anomalies are quite common and in 20% of babies born with esophageal atresia some variant of congenital heart disease occurs and in 12% of cases there is associated imperforate anus. This condition is often associated with hydramnios (50%), so in all cases of hydramnios such possibility should be considered.

Clinical feature: The earliest and most important clinical feature of esophageal atresia is regurgitation of saliva or feedings. Attempts to feed are met with 'spitting up' or frank vomiting. Saliva pours almost continuously from its mouth. Persistence in feeding may produce aspiration, choking, cyanosis and respiratory distress.

Diagnosis: A soft rubber catheter is introduced into the esophagus through the mouth, which will encounter an obstruction at about 10 cm from the lips. This confirms the diagnosis.

Radiological confirmation may be made by *contrast X-ray* study in which 1 mL of dionosil is used as contrast medium which is instilled down the catheter to demonstrate obstruction. After the radiograph has been taken the dionosil should be aspirated.

In *straight X-ray* air in the stomach confirms the first type of anomaly in which the lower end of the esophagus is connected with the trachea.

Treatment: Surgical intervention should be immediate. The baby should be kept in 30° head-up position. Antibiotic should be started immediately even if aspiration pneumonia is not clinically manifested. Catheter suction of the upper esophageal pouch is started and intravenous infusion is also started.

Gastrostomy is a useful adjunct in the management of many babies before operative repair of the esophagus is undertaken.

Complications:

- Leakage at the anastomosis is not a uncommon complication.
- Mediastinal infection is occasionally seen with esophageal disruption. This may require another operation.
- Gastroesophageal reflux has been sometimes the late complication of this operation.

20. True about surgical occlusive dressing:

a. Maintain moisture in wound
b. No role in pneumothorax
c. Prevents microbial entry
d. Can be used for allergy testing
e. Used in wounds with pre-existing pathogens

Ans. a, c, d *Ref: S Das, 9/e; Sabiston, 20/e*

Option a	True	
Option b	False	
Option c	True	
Option d	True	
Option e	False	Contraindication for use of occlusive dressing

Indications for the necessity of an occlusive dressing include:

- Pressure and bleeding are two of the major concerns when managing any wound, they can often be immediately addressed with the application of an occlusive dressing.
- The dressing allows for ointments to thoroughly penetrate wounds by preventing evaporation.
- Allergy tests sometime require the use of an occlusive dressing as well.
- Sucking chest wounds (open pnuemothorax) are holes in a patient's chest (such as punctures via knife or gun shot) which have created new pathways for air. Occlusive wounds can be utilized to block and treat the puncture.

- Partial evisceration may require the application of an occlusive dressing to contain the bowels until surgery.
- Wound Moisture Maintenance can be achieved by combining an occlusive dressing with a gauze or sponge, which can be soaked in a medicine such as antibiotics, hydrogels and other antibacterial creams utilized for the treatment of the wound.
- Minor wounds and skin conditions can also benefit from an occlusive dressing, which provide protection from contaminants, can help to expedite the healing process and reduce scar tissue.
- New tattoos are sometimes covered with an occlusive dressing to promote healing, prevent infection and preserve the aesthetics of the tattoo.

Contraindications for the application of an occlusive dressing include:

- Pre-existing pathogens in the affected area may create complications when sealed into a wound by an occlusive dressing.
- Occlusive dressings made from polyethylene film have been known to promote the growth of undesirable skin flora in some patients.
- Skin maceration becomes a concern with long-term use of occlusive dressings. With this condition the tissue surrounding the wound is affected by the tape and sealing method utilized in the application of the dressing. When this occurs the skin becomes tender, often feeling moist and looking whiter than usual. In this weakened state, the skin becomes susceptible to bacteria and infections, which could compromise the health of the wound itself.

21. Indications for surgery in tuberculosis is:

a. Streak hemoptysis
b. Empyema TB
c. Bronchiectasis
d. Cough
e. Lobe collapse

Ans. b *Ref: TB: Surgical Protocol LRS Institute of Tuberculosis; S Das, 9/e*

Option a	False	Frank hemoptysis and not streak
Option b	True	
Option c	False	Managed with medical treatment
Option d	False	Managed with medical treatment
Option e	False	Treated by correcting underlying cause

Indications and Protocols for TB Surgery

Indications of surgery in tuberculosis:

- Diagnostic
- Persistent sputum positive state despite therapy
- Complications and sequel:
  - Hemoptysis
  - Destroyed or bronchiectatic lungs
  - Empyema with or without bronchopleural fistula (BPF)

Persistently active disease

The decision about proper case selection is the most important in this situation. There is a justified indication for surgery in only some of the selected cases. These situations are:

- The disease is sufficiently localized

- Adequate trial of anti-tubercular treatment (ATT) has been given
- Drug failure
- Patient is chronic secretor

These are broad indications for surgery in patients of MDR-TB or persistent sputum positive status. There are a few other specific situations where surgery is a good adjuvant in the management plan of persistently positive active disease. These are:

- When sputum smear or culture is positive for AFB, despite 4 to 6 months of appropriate and supervised ATT
- When there have been two or more relapses
- One or more relapse while on therapy
- The organism has been shown to be resistant on culture and sensitivity
- When the patient is likely to relapse in the judgment of the physician
- Anticipated non-compliance in an admitted patient after discharge.

For hemoptysis

- Massive recurrent hemoptysis more than 500 cc on more than two occasions
- Bleeding not controlled on medical measures
- More than two liters in one episode
- Smaller amounts of bleeding continuing for months together
- Significant patient distress.

For destroyed lungs and chest symptomatic

- Three or more episodes of pneumonia like symptoms in a year
- Significant patient distress

For empyema

- The management of empyema tuberculosis depends upon the stage of presentation. Most of the cases are effectively managed with prolonged and expert intercostal tube management.
    - In the sub-acute stage, drainage can be assisted by either video-assisted thoracic debridement or instillation of intrapleural antifibrinolytic agents like streptokinase or urokinase.
    - Decortication is indicated in the presence of persistent pleural infection in late fibrino-purulent stage.
    - Thoracoplasty is partial decostalization of the thoracic cage to obliterate persistent pleural space.
    - Whenever the lung is unlikely to expand because of an extensive disease or multiple bronchopleural fistulae, thoracoplasty is an appropriate intervention and is required quite often in our setting. It is most suitable for management of postoperative empyemas. Results are quite gratifying.
    - It is of vital importance that a patient of pulmonary TB has taken an adequate course of antituberculosis treatment (ATT) before the surgical decision is taken.
    - The patient should be as 'dry' as possible before surgery, meaning thereby that sputum or pus production (in cases of empyema) should be minimized by appropriate measures like antibiotics, postural drainage, respiratory exercises, steam inhalation and nebulized bronchodilators, as appropriate.

22. Increase in serum amylase is seen in:

a. Parotitis
b. Chronic pancreatitis
c. Pseudopancreatic cyst
d. Pelvic inflammatory disease
e. Systemic lupus erythematosus

Ans. a, b, c, e *Ref: S Das, 9/e*

Option a	True	
Option b	True	
Option c	True	
Option d	False	
Option e	True	

Among healthy individuals, the pancreas and the salivary glands account for almost all serum amylase, 40–45% from the pancreas and 55–60% from the salivary glands.

Causes of hyperamylasemia include:

- **Acute or chronic pancreatitis**: Increase in the P-type isoamylase. Other reasons for hyperamylasemia that are associated with pancreatitis are:
  - *Pseudocysts,*
  - *Pancreatic ascites,*
  - *Pancreatic trauma,* and
  - *Choledocholithiasis*
- **Salivary diseases:** Parotitis is associated with increases in the S-type isoamylase. It is usually caused by trauma or surgery of the salivary gland, radiation to the neck area involving the parotid gland followed subsequently by duct obstruction, or calculi of the salivary duct. Chronic alcoholism is another cause which increases salivary amylase levels.
- **Renal failure and liver disease** results in increased S-type and P-type isoamylases.
- **Gut diseases**, including mucosal inflammatory disease of the small intestine, mesenteric infarction, intestinal obstruction, appendicitis, and peritonitis, usually result in increased P-type isoamylase because of increased absorption of amylase from the intestinal lumen.
- **Ruptured ectopic pregnancy**, fallopian or ovarian cysts, and salpingitis.
- **Ectopic amylase production** by lung, ovary, pancreas, and colon malignancies; pheochromocytoma; thymoma; multiple myeloma (increased salivary amylase); and breast cancer (increased pancreatic amylase) are miscellaneous causes of hyperamylasemia.
- **Rare cases** of hyperamylasemia have been reported in association with **systemic lupus erythematosus.**

23. Which of following is true regarding male reproductive system?

a. Sertoli cells produce mullerian inhibition factor
b. Spermatids produce inhibin to inhibit GnRH
c. Cowper's glands are exocrine glands of male reproductive system

d. Testis enters scrotum in the 7th month of gestation
e. Undescended testis is usually fully developed

Ans. a, c *Ref: S Das, 9/e*

Option a	True	Produced by fetal sertoli cells and induces regression of the Müllerian ducts
Option b	False	Small amounts of inhibin are produced by the sertoli cells in the testis
Option c	True	Also known as the bulbourethral glands
Option d	False	Testis enters scrotum in the 9th month
Option e	False	Undescended testis is usually undeveloped

Hormones which control reproduction in males are:

- **Gonadotropin-releasing hormone (GnRH):**
  - The hypothalamus secretes this hormone into the pituitary gland.
  - There are two gonadotropic hormones, FSH and LH.
    - Luteinizing hormone (LH):The pituitary gland secretes this hormone after receiving a GnRH signal from the hypothalamus. LH stimulates Leydig cells, in the testes, telling them to produce testosterone.
    - Follicle-stimulating hormone (FSH): The pituitary gland also secretes this hormone. Testosterone helps FSH run through the bloodstream to make sertoli cells, located in the seminiferous tubules of the testes, to make immature sperm to mature sperm.
- **Testosterone:**
  - Also known as "the male hormone" and "androgen".
  - Testosterone is vital for the production of sperm.

Cells and Glands of Male Reproductive System

Sertoli Cells

- A Sertoli cell (a kind of sustentacular cell) is a 'nurse' cell of the testes which is part of a seminiferous tubule.
- It is activated by follicle-stimulating hormone, and has FSH-receptor on its membranes.
- Its main function is to nurture the developing sperm cells through the stages of spermatogenesis. Because of this, it has also been called the "mother cell." It provides both secretory and structural support.

Cowper's Glands

The Cowper's glands, also known as the ***bulbourethral glands***, are a pair of pea-sized ***exocrine glands*** located inferior to the prostate and anterior to the anus. The Cowper's glands secrete a thin alkaline fluid into the urethra that lubricates the urethra and neutralizes acid from urine remaining in the urethra after urination. This fluid enters the urethra during sexual arousal prior to ejaculation to prepare the urethra for the flow of semen.

Anomalies of Testis

- The testis may be absent on one or both sides.
- The testis may be duplicated.
- The two testes may be fused together.

- *Anomalies of descent (Cryptorchidism)*: Descent of the testis may fail to occur, or may be incomplete, or in the upper part of the scrotum. Some interesting facts about this condition are as follows:
  - The testis may complete its descent after birth.
  - Spermatogenesis often fails to occur in an undescended testis.
  - An undescended testis is more likely to develop a malignant tumor than a normal testis.
  - The condition can be surgically corrected.
- *Abnormal positions (Ectopia)*: The testis may lie
  - Under the skin of the lower part of the abdomen.
  - Under the skin of the front of the thigh.
  - In the femoral canal.
  - Under the skin of the penis.
  - In the perineum behind the scrotum.

Comparison between undescended testis and ectopic testis

Undescended testis	*Ectopic testis*
• The testis is arrested in its normal path of descent.	• The testis deviates from its normal path of descent.
• Undescended testis is usually undeveloped.	• The testis is fully developed.
• Scrotum is not developed on that side and empty.	• Though empty, the scrotum is usually fully developed.
• The length of the spermatic cord may be short.	• The length of the spermatic cord is usually longer.
• Spermatogenesis is poor after 6 years of age.	• Spermatogenesis is perfect.
• Undescended testis may be associated with indirect inguinal hernia.	• This is never associated with indirect inguinal hernia.
• *Treatment*: Mainly operation, though hormone therapy may be tried in selected cases. Operation is not at all successful after puberty.	• *Treatment* is operation and is usually successful.
• *Complications*: List of complications has already been mentioned.	• *Complications*: The main complication is liability to injury.

24. True about blunt trauma abdomen:

a. Liver is most commonly involved
b. RBC > 1000 in peritoneal fluid is indication of diagnostic peritoneal lavage (DPL)
c. There is > 2 liters associated blood loss
d. Grey Turner sign is positive
e. Heimlich maneuver can cause blunt trauma to abdomen

Ans. d, e *Ref: S Das 9/e; Oxford handbook of accident and emergency medicine*

Option a	False	Kidneys are the most common organ involved followed by liver
Option b	False	On DPL, RBC > 100,000/μL is considered positive
Option c	False	Aspiration of > 5 mL free blood is required to produce a microscopically positive DPL result

Option d	True	
Option e	True	Also called abdominal thrusts, first aid procedure used to treat upper airway obstructions by foreign objects

- **Blunt trauma** may involve a direct blow, impact with an object (a fall onto bicycle handlebars), or a sudden decrease in speed (a fall from a height or a motor vehicle crash).
  - The spleen and liver are the two most commonly injured organs. Retroperitoneum, small bowel, kidneys, bladder, colorectum, diaphragm, and pancreas are the other organs to get involved.
  - Hollow organs are less likely to be injured.
  - Blunt abdominal trauma usually results from motor vehicle collisions (MVCs), assaults, recreational accidents, or falls.
  - Ecchymosis involving the flanks (**Grey Turner's sign**) or the umbilicus (**Cullen's sign**): Indicates retroperitoneal hemorrhage, but is usually delayed for several hours to days.
  - In an unstable patient, the abdominal involvement is accomplished by identifying free intra-abdominal fluid with:
    - ***Diagnostic peritoneal lavage (DPL)*** or
    - ***Focused assessment with sonography for trauma (FAST).***
  - DPL results are considered positive in a blunt trauma patient if-
    - 10 mL of grossly bloody aspirate is obtained before infusion of the lavage fluid or
    - If the siphoned lavage fluid contains more than **100,000 red blood cells (RBCs)/μL**, more than **500 white blood cells (WBCs)/μL**, **elevated amylase content**, bile, bacteria, vegetable matter, or urine.
    - Only approximately 30 mL of blood is needed in the peritoneum to produce a microscopically positive DPL result.

Investigations

The need for and choice of investigation depend upon individual circumstances, local policy, facilities, and expertise. Patients who are hemodynamically unstable or who have peritonism require immediate referral for laparotomy.

Perform urinalysis in all patients. Insert a urinary catheter in patients who are present with hemodynamic disturbance or who are critically ill as a result of other injuries (unless there is evidence of urethral injury.

Serum amylase is required on all patients.

Plain abdominal X-ray is rarely useful, unless associated bony injury or bowel perforation is suspected: free intraperitoneal gas may be demonstrated on an erect CXR.

USS is most useful in patients with isolated abdominal injury. Solid organ damage and free fluid may be demonstrated.

CT scan is being increasingly used to evaluate abdominal injuries as well as identifying injuries in other regions (e.g. retroperitoneum, brain, chest).

DPL is helpful in situations where clinical evidence of intra-abdominal injury is equivocal or where CT or USS is not immediately available. It may be employed in other situations (e.g. to search for intra-abdominal hemorrhage in shocked head-injured patients who are unconscious or in patients whose massive pelvic fracture is being externally fixed.

Management of Blunt abdominal trauma:

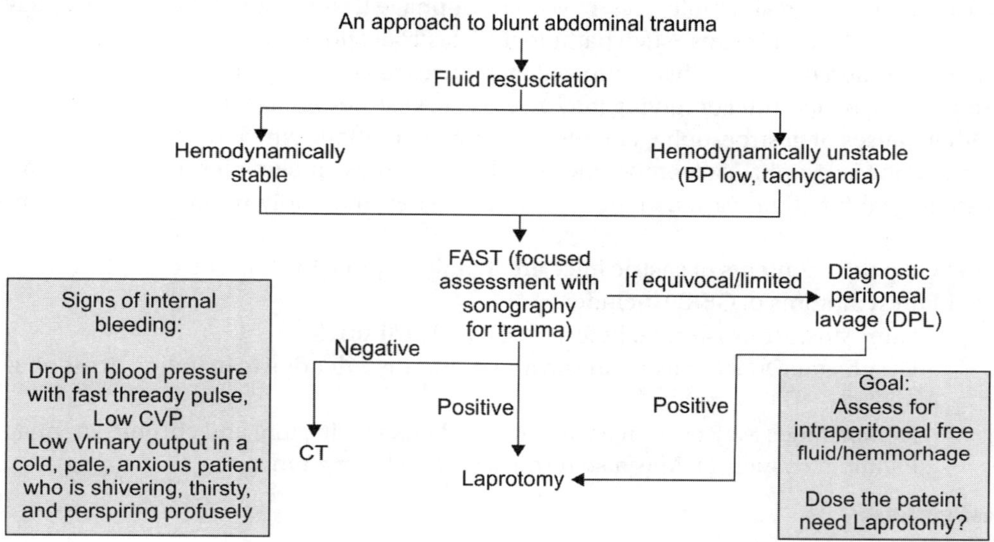

25. Investigation of choice for Gastroesophageal reflux disease (GERD) is:

a. Manometry
b. Endoscopy
c. Multichannel impedance study
d. Histology
e. Barium swallow

Ans. b *Ref: S Das, 9/e*

Option a	False	Manometry measures the strength and muscle coordination of esophagus upon swallowing
Option b	True	
Option c	False	A catheter-based method to detect intraluminal bolus movement within the esophagus
Option d	False	Offers no help in GERD
Option e	False	Not a surefire method of diagnosing GERD

Regurgitation of gastric contents into esophagus is known as gastroesophageal reflux.

- At times, when the stomach is not distended, the gastroesophageal reflux is considered to be pathological. The main reasons are:
  - Reduced intraluminal tension of lower esophageal sphincter.
  - Shorter length of intra-abdominal esophagus than normal.

The lower esophageal sphincter normally works in conjunction with the diaphragm to create a physical barrier against the entry of gastric contents into the esophagus. Transient relaxation of this sphincter may occur more often in patients with GERd.

Aetiology

- The majority of the patients with clinically significant gastroesophageal reflux have associated sliding esophageal hiatal hernia. But the majority of patients with hiatal hernia do not have significant reflux to cause clinical problems.

- Systemic collagen diseases involving esophagus may cause reflux esophagitis. In these cases there is considerable loss of lower esophageal sphincter tone and esophageal peristalsis which may cause such pathological gastroesophageal reflux. Scleroderma is the most common disease in this group which involves the esophagus.
- Impaired gastric-outlet emptying may give rise to gastroesophageal reflux.
- Other causes of gastroesophageal reflux include operations which destroy or by-pass the normal lower esophageal competence mechanism. These include resection of the gastro-esophageal junction, various types of cardioplasties and badly performed myotomy for achalasia.
  - Acid peptic contents of gastric juice are mainly responsible for reflux esophagitis.
  - Main symptoms of GERD include:
    - Pain: Mostly retrosternal. Referred to as "Heartburn".
    - Dysphagia: Due to muscle spasm and motor disorder due to irritation of esophageal mucosa.
    - Hemorrhage: May present as occult blood positive in stool and chronic anemia.
    - Flatulent dyspepsia: May also be an associated symptom.

Investigations

- ***Radiography***: Findings include erosions and ulcerations, strictures, hiatal hernia, thickening of mucosal folds and poor distensibility. Not the test of choice for the diagnosis of GERd.
- ***Endoscopy*** is useful for diagnosing the complications of GERD, such as Barrett's esophagus, esophagitis and strictures.
- ***Ambulatory pH monitoring*** is generally considered as the diagnostic gold standard for use in patients with GERd. In this study, a pH monitor is placed in the esophagus above the lower esophageal sphincter, and the pH is recorded at given moments in time. Over the 24-hour test period, the patient writes down the time and situation in which symptoms occur, in the hope that symptoms can be correlated with the lowering of esophageal pH that occurs with reflux.

Management of GERD

Stage I: Lifestyle modifications

- Head of bed elevated six inches
- Decreased fat intake
- Smoking cessation
- Weight reduction
- Avoidance of recumbency for three hours postprandially
- Avoidance of large meals and certain foods

↓

Stage II: As needed pharmacologic therapy

- Antacid and/or antacid product containing alginic acid
- Over-the-counter histamine H_2-receptor blocker

↓

Stage III: Scheduled pharmacologic therapy

- H_2-receptor blocker or prokinetic agent for 8 to 12 weeks

- For persistent symptoms, high-dose H_2-receptor blocker or proton pump inhibitor for another 8 to 12 weeks (or reconsider diagnosis)
- With documented erosive esophagitis, may use a proton pump inhibitor as first-line therapy

↓

Stage IV: Maintenance therapy

- Appropriate for patient with symptomatic relapse or complicated disease
- Lowest effective dosage of H_2-receptor blocker or proton pump inhibitor

↓

Stage V: Surgery

- May be appropriate in patient with severe symptoms, erosive esophagitis or disease complications
- Laparoscopic Nissen or Toupet fundoplication procedure.

26. Which of following would predispose to malignancy of esophagus?

a. Achalasia cardia
b. Paterson-Kelly
c. Corrosive dye stricture
d. Esophageal ring
e. Schatzki ring

Ans. a, b, c *Ref: S Das, 9/e*

Option a	True	Patients with achalasia cardia have 10 times more chance of developing Ca esophagus
Option b	True	Also called as Plummer-Vinson syndrome
Option c	True	Corrosive esophagitis from dye
Option d	False	Not a premalignant condition
Option e	False	Not a premalignant condition

Schatzki ring

- It is an esophageal web in the lower most part and contains only mucosa and submucosa.
- It appears at squamocolumnar junction within 1–2 cm above the esophagogastric junction.
- In most of the cases, it is asymptomatic.
- Dysphagia occurs only when the diameter is minimized to < 15 mm.
- It is usually associated with sliding hiatus hernia.
- Web is predominantly due to increased submucosal fibrosis.
- Not a pre-malignant condition.

CARCINOMA OF THE ESOPHAGUS

Aetiology

- *Age* and *Sex*: Though esophageal cancer may occur in young individuals, it is *predominantly a disease of the old*. The usual victims are between *45 to 75 years* with *highest incidences between 65 to 75 years. Except the cervical esophagus, where men and women are equally affected, in thoracic and abdominal esophagus men are much more often affected.*

- *Alcohol and tobacco* have been incriminated to increase the incidence of this disease. Native alcohol is more dangerous in this respect.
- *Malnutrition,* vitamin deficiency, anemia, poor oral hygiene also increase the incidence of esophageal carcinoma. This disease is more often *seen in familial keratosis palmaris et plantaris* (dylosis palmaris et plantaris).
- *Plummer Vinson syndrome* is a precancerous condition and increased incidence of carcinoma in cervical esophagus in women is well explained through this.
- *Achalasia*: A direct relation has been seen between achalasia and cancer of esophagus. *Chance is 10 times more in patients with achalasia than normal individuals.* The cancer arising from achalasia is usually of *squamous type* and occurs in *younger age group.* Most unfortunate is that *cancer usually appears in the dilated portion of the esophagus and remains asymptomatic for long time.*

  Various other esophageal lesions are believed to be premalignant. These are:
- *Hiatus hernia and reflux esophagitis,*
- *Barrett's esophagus,*
- *Irradiation esophagitis,*
- *Corrosive esophagitis* from lye, and
- *Esophageal diverticulum.*

Pathology

Highest incidence of esophageal cancer is in its *lower third,* where 50% or more of the esophageal cancers develop. *Histologically, more than 95% of esophageal cancers are squamous cell carcinoma.* Adenocarcinomas, constituting less than 5% of esophageal cancers, usually develop from: (i) the junctional columnar epithelium in the distal esophagus, (ii) Barrett's mucosa, (iii) Glandular epithelium or (iv) Ectopic gastric mucosa.

Modes of Spread

Cancer of esophagus is of equal malignancy to that encountered in growths in other parts of the GI tract. Adenocarcinomas metastasize more rapidly and extensively than squamous growths. *In lower third of the esophagus, the prognosis of adenocarcinoma is much worse.* As other carcinomas in the body esophageal carcinoma also spreads by: (i) *infiltration,* (ii) *lymphatics* and (iii) *blood.*

27. True about undescended testis:

a. Unilateral more common than bilateral
b. During surgery, the other testis should always be explored
c. Non-palpable testis, is most commonly due to testicular agenesis
d. Surgical correction best within 3 months
e. Almost always associated with absent kidney

Ans. a, b *Ref: S Das, 9/e; Bailey and Love, 26/e*

Option a	True	Only about 20% cases are bilateral
Option b	True	
Option c	False	Non palpable testis is commonly due to complete undescended testis
Option d	False	Surgical correction done by 5 years of age
Option e	False	Very very rare combination

Undescended testis

- Is the one which has failed to descend down to scrotum and is retained at any point along the normal path of its descent.
- More common on right side as right testis descends later than the left testis.

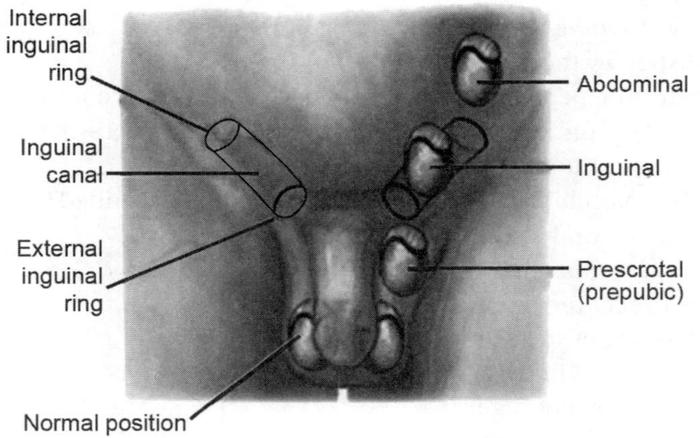

Fig. 13.4: Location of undescended testis.

- According to the position of arrest, the undescended testis are described as:
  - Lumbar testis: Complete failure of descent.
  - Iliac testis: Testis remain deep to deep inguinal ring.
  - Inguinal: Testis is in the inguinal canal.
  - At the superficial inguinal ring: Testis resting just outside the external inguinal ring.
  - Scrotal testis: Testis lies in upper part of scrotum. It is often retractable testis due to contraction of overactive cremaster muscle. Testis and scrotal sac are of normal size and the testis can be brought down to the scrotum.

Complications of incomplete descent

- *Torsion* of the testis.
- *Epididymo-orchitis in an incompletely descended testis* often gives rise to difficulty in diagnosis, but absence of testis in the scrotum of the corresponding side should arouse suspicion.
- *An associated indirect hernia or interstitial hernia* is frequent with incompletely descended testis and it is quoted as high as 80% of cases.
- *Atrophy*: An incompletely descended testis is *smaller than the normally descended testis and it may undergo more atrophy particularly when it is situated in the inguinal canal due to recurrent trauma.*
- *Pain*: A testis situated in the inguinal canal is often *liable to trauma and gives rise to pain in the groin.*
- *Sterility*: *In bilateral cases* this may be seen.
- Malignancy: An incompletely descended testis runs the risk of being malignant 50 times more than a normal descended testis.

Treatment

- Hormone therapy:
  - Not routinely administered.
  - Given ONLY in case of bilateral incomplete descended testis associated with hypo-genitalism and obesity.
- Surgical treatment:
  - **Orchidopexy**: *Treatment of choice:*
    - Accomplished by the age of 5 years.
    - After 6 years, the percentage of successful operation falls considerably.
    - It is absolutely unnecessary to do this operation before the completion of 2nd birthday of the child.
    - In case of cryptorchidism or bilateral incompletely descended testis, one side should be operated 6 months earlier than the other side.
    - During surgery, the other testis should always be explored.
    - Operative procedure involves:
      1. Lengthening of spermatic cord
      2. Retaining testis in the scrotum—done by following operations:
         a. External anchorage
         b. Keetley-Torek operation
         c. Ombredanne operation
         d. Denis Browne's operation
         e. Dartos pouch
  - Orchidectomy: Only done when the other side is normal.
  - Orchidocelioplasty: Abdominal replacement of testis. Indicated when the other testis was removed previously and this testis can't be brought down to scrotum.

28. True about full-thickness grafts in comparison to split-thickness skin grafts is/are:

a. Better for large area
b. Full thickness graft gives better cosmetic result
c. Accumulation of fluid below the graft always indicate rejection
d. Higher risk of hypertrophic scar formation
e. Graft can be expanded by meshing technique

Ans. b, d *Ref: S Das, 9/e; Bailey and Love, 26/e*

Option a	False	Partial-thickness grafts are frequently used as they can cover large areas and the rate of auto-rejection is low
Option b	True	Owing to near same color matching to the recipient site
Option c	False	Significant amount of serous and serosanguineous fluid may drain from the wound during the period of re-epithelialization
Option d	True	Full thickness grafts have higher risk of hypertrophic scar formation
Option e	False	Meshing is used for split thickness skin grafts

Split-thickness skin grafts (STSG):

- Are grafts that include two skin layers of your body: The full epidermal skin layer and part of the dermal skin layer.

- Grafts that are up to four inches wide and 10–12 inches long can be removed from flat body surfaces.
- These surfaces are the abdomen, thigh or back.
- These grafts are sown or stapled into place and covered with compression dressings.
- The dressings are tightly wrapped with elastic bandages in order to offer firm contact.
- Occasionally, the graft sites are left open to air.
- Split-thickness grafts are commonly not performed on hands and feet. These are areas of the body that are subject to abrasion or are a weight-bearing parts your body.
- In general, if there is too little donor skin available STSG is applied as meshed and expanded, in order to maximize graft coverage, or intact sheets.
- Meshing involves cutting tiny holes in the donor skin so it can be stretched to cover more surface area.
- The advantage of STSG includes less tissue use. That offers a higher percentage rate of graft survival and it minimizes the donor site damage.
- The one disadvantage, of STSG, is that it tends to contract more than full-thickness skin grafts.

Full-thickness Grafts:

- Full-thickness skin grafts (FTSG) consists of:
  - Both the epidermal and complete dermal skin layers.
  - This type of graft can offer a better cosmetic outcome than split-thickness grafts.
  - It is also used when skin flap surgery is not available.
  - Advantages of a thicker graft is that if offers less chance for contraction to occur, increased resistance to trauma and less deformation both functionally and cosmetically.

Comparison chart of split, thickness and full-thickness skin grafts

Characteristics	*Split-thickness skin graft (STSG)*	*Full-thickness skin graft (FTSG)*
Structure	100% epidermis and part of the dermis	100% epidermis and dermis. Also a percentage of fat
Graft endurance	High chance of graft survival	Lower chance of graft survival
Confronting to Trauma	Less resistance	More resistance
Cosmetic appearance	Poor cosmetic appearance. Offers poor color and texture match. This also does not prevent contraction	Better-quality cosmetic appearance. Thicker, and prevents contraction or deformation
When performed	Temporarily or permanently performed after excision of a burn injury, as long as there is sufficient blood supply	When aesthetic outcome is important (e.g., facial defects)
Donor site tissue	Abdomen, buttock, inner or outer arm, inner forearm and thigh	Nearby site that offers similar color or texture to the skin surrounding the burned area
Disadvantage	Poor cosmetic appearance, a greater chance of distortion or contraction	A higher risk of graft failure. The donor site requires long-drawn-out healing time and has a greater risk of deformation and hypertrophic scar formation

29. Treatment for increased intracranial pressure includes:

a. IV Mannitol
b. IV Glucose
c. IV Furosemide
d. IV hypotonic saline
e. Barbiturate induced coma

Ans. a, c *Ref: S Das, 9/e; Cerebral Edema and its Management MJAFI, Vol. 59, No. 4, 2003*

Option a	True	
Option b	False	
Option c	True	
Option d	False	IV hypertonic saline is used
Option e	False	May cause systemic hypotension and pulmonary failure, so not used routinely anymore

ICP in adults is normally 5–10 mmHg. Raised ICP can be defined in many ways, but in the acute setting it commonly refers to pressure greater than 20–25 mmHg for more than 5 minutes.

Increased ICP may result from the following:

- **Space-occupying lesions:** Tumor, abscess, intracranial hemorrhage (epidural hematoma, subdural hematoma, intraparenchymal hematoma).
- **CSF flow obstruction (hydrocephalus):** Space-occupying lesion that obstructs normal CSF flow, aqueductal stenosis, Chiari malformation.
- **Cerebral edema:** Due to head injury, ischemic stroke with vasogenic edema, hypoxic or ischemic encephalopathy, postoperative edema.
- **Increase in venous pressure:** Due to cerebral venous sinus thrombosis, heart failure, superior vena cava or jugular vein thrombosis/obstruction.
- **Metabolic disorders:** Hypo-osmolality, hyponatremia, uremic encephalopathy, hepatic encephalopathy.
- **Increased CSF flow production:** Choroid plexus tumors (papilloma or carcinoma).
- **Idiopathic intracranial hypertension**
- **Pseudotumor cerebri**

Raised Intracranial pressure is common presentation of traumatic head injury.

Intractable elevated ICP can lead to death or devastating neurological damage either by reducing cerebral perfusion pressure (CPP) and causing cerebral ischemia or by compressing and causing herniation of the brainstem or other vital structures.

- **Symptoms and signs** that suggest a rise in ICP includes:
  - Headache: The headache is classically a morning headache
  - Vomiting without nausea,
  - Ocular palsies,
  - Altered level of consciousness,
  - Back pain, and
  - Papilledema.

Treatment

- **Mannitol:** Recommended dose is 0.25 to 1 g/kg IV bolus.
  - Establishes an osmotic gradient between plasma and parenchymal tissue, resulting in a net reduction in brain water content.
  - Rapid onset of action and maintains its effect for a period of hours.

- Can be used to decrease ICP and improve cerebral perfusion pressure (CPP) include acute herniation, acute elevation of ICP, and ICP elevation that does not respond to other therapies.
- Possible side-effects:
  - Mannitol administration has the potential side-effects of hyperosmolarity, hypovolemia, electrolyte imbalance, and acute renal failure.
  - More common with chronic or high-dose administration.
  - Serum osmolarity, serum electrolytes, and renal function should be measured at least every six to eight hours.
  - When administered chronically and in high doses, mannitol may cross the injured blood-brain barrier at the site of the cerebral lesion and cause an exacerbation of cerebral edema.

❑ **Furosemide:** The osmotic effect can be prolonged by the use of loop diuretics (furosemide) after the osmotic agent infusion.

❑ **Corticosteroids:** Lower intracranial pressure primarily in vasogenic edema because of their beneficial effect on the blood vessel.
- Not recommended in treatment of edema secondary to stroke or hemorrhage.

❑ **Hyperventilation**
- Can effectively lower ICP via its effect on $PaCO_2$.
- Low $PaCO_2$ causes cerebral vasoconstriction, decreased cerebral blood flow, and consequently, decreased cerebral blood volume and ICP.

In cases of uncontrolled intracranial hypertension, an **intracranial drain** can be placed to remove CSF and monitor ICP.

❑ **Barbiturate coma:** Barbiturates produce a marked decrease in metabolic rate and it seems likely that the fall in cerebral blood flow and ICP is secondary. Complication of barbiturate therapy, in particular systemic hypotension and pulmonary failure, have caused concern. Hence, it is not used routinely.

❑ **Hypertonic saline:** Decreases ICP and increase CPP in patients with elevated ICP that is refractory to conventional therapy.

30. True about liver cirrhosis is/are:

a. Caudate lobe atrophy
b. Nodularity can be seen on USG
c. CT is used for detecting fibrosis
d. Sonoelastography for liver fibrosis
e. Hepatofugal flow by Doppler

Ans. b, c, d, e *Ref: Bailey and Love, 26/e; S Das, 9/e*

Option a	False	Segmental hypertrophy, hepatocellular necrosis
Option b	True	
Option c	True	
Option d	True	
Option e	True	

Investigations for liver cirrhosis:

❑ **Ultrasound**: Major screening tool for cirrhosis and its complications. It is also useful to aid in biopsy. Appearances include:

- Surface nodularity (88% sensitive, 82–95% specific)
- Overall coarse and heterogeneous echotexture
- Segmental hypertrophy/atrophy
  - Caudate width: Right lobe width > 0.65 (43–84% sensitive, 100% specific)
  - Reduction of the transverse diameter (< 30 mm) of the medial segment of the left lobe (segment IV)
- Signs of portal hypertension:
  - Doppler flow changes
    - Portal venous system
    - Enlarged portal vein: > 13 mm (42% sensitive, 95–100% specific)
    - Slow portal venous flow < 15 cm/sec
    - Reversal or to-and-fro portal venous flow
    - Portal venous thrombosis +/– cavernous transformation
    - Enlarged SMV and splenic vein: >10mm
    - Loss of respiratory variation in SMV and splenic vein spectral Doppler waveforms
    - Recanalization and hepatofugal paraumbilical venous flow
    - Portosystemic collaterals
- Hepatic veins
  - Portalization of hepatic vein waveform
- Hepatic arteries
  - "Corkscrew" appearance
  - Increased velocity (compensating for decreased portal vein flow)
- Splenomegaly
- Ascites
- Fatty change (variable)

Sonoelastography may also be useful to assess the amount of liver fibrosis. Suggested values for diagnosis.

- >7 kPa: advanced fibrosis
- 12.5–15 kPa: cirrhosis

❑ **CT**: Is insensitive in early cirrhosis. More established findings include:
- Surface and parenchymal nodularity
- Regenerative nodules (most) are isodense to rest of liver
- Siderotic nodules (minority) are hyperdense due to accumulation of iron
- Fatty change (variable)
- Segmental hypertrophy/atrophy
- Parenchymal heterogeneity both on the pre and post IV contrast scans
- Isodense/hyperdense regenerative nodules
- Predominantly portal venous supply to dysplastic nodules.
- Portal vein enlargement
- Portal venous thrombosis +/– cavernous transformation

❑ **MRI**: Also insensitive in early cirrhosis, but has a significant role in screening cirrhotic livers for small hepatocellular carcinomas. MRI findings include:
- Morphologic changes (same as on CT and ultrasound)
- Regenerative nodules (or cirrhotic nodules)

  MR angiography or a balanced steady state free precession sequence may also be used to assess portal vein patency and portosystemic collaterals.

31. Which of the following is/are cancers of head and neck region?

a. Rhabdomyosarcoma
b. Squamous cell carcinoma
c. Adenocystic carcinoma
d. Ameloblastoma
e. Adenocarcinoma

Ans. a, b, c, d, e

Ref: Curr Opin Otolaryngol Head Neck Surg 12:127-132. (c) 2004 Lippincott Williams and Wilkins.; Atlas of Genetics and Cytogenetics in Oncology and Haematology;

Option a	True	
Option b	True	
Option c	True	
Option d	True	
Option e	True	

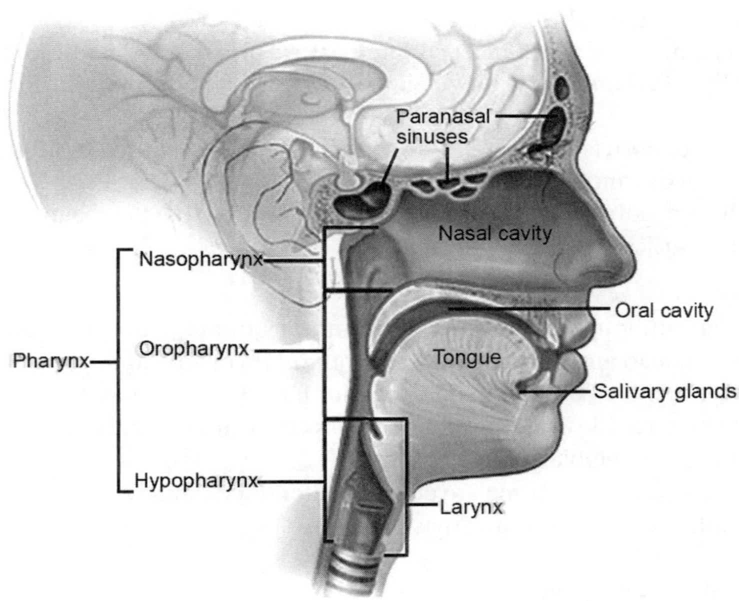

Fig. 13.5: Head and neck cancer regions.

Rhabdomyosarcoma:

- Approximately 40% of rhabdomyosarcoma occur in the head and neck with about 20% in the nasal cavity, nasopharynx, and nasal sinuses.
- Rhabdomyosarcoma is the most common sarcoma in childhood.
- The embryonal subtype predominates in children, while the alveolar subtype predominates in adults.
- The pleomorphic subtype is rare.
- The nasopharynx is more commonly involved than the sinonasal tract.
- In adults, rhabdomyosarcoma is more common in the ethmoid sinuses, followed by the maxillary sinuses and nasopharynx.

- About 40% metastasize to lymph nodes, bones, and lungs, and less commonly bone marrow, soft tissue, liver and brain.
- Adults have a poor prognosis, with 5-year survival of <10%.

Squamous cell carcinoma (SCC):

- Squamous cell cancer of the head and neck is common worldwide.
- Risk factors include chewing betel or areca nuts, smoking bidis, and taking snuff. Epstein-Barr virus has also been implicated in nasopharyngeal carcinoma.
- Most head and neck cancers present with symptoms from the primary site. For example, hoarseness, difficulty in swallowing, or pain in the ear.
- Enlargement of a cervical lymph node as the first presenting feature is common, particularly with certain "silent" sites—the tongue base, supraglottis, and nasopharynx.

Adenoidcystic carcinoma (ACC):

- Adenoid cystic carcinoma is an uncommon salivary gland malignancy that presents insidiously and is generally advanced when diagnosed.
- The parotid gland is the single most common site of origin (25%) in the head and neck.
- Histologically, ACC can be categorized into three growth patterns: cribriform, tubular, and solid.
- A solid growth pattern is associated with a worse prognosis, caused by advanced stage and development of distant metastases.
- The use of fine-needle aspiration biopsy is widely accepted in the diagnostic procedure of head and neck lesions.

Ameloblastoma:

- Ameloblastoma although rare, is the most common odontogenic tumor accounting for 1% of all tumors in head and neck region and around 11% of all odontogenic tumors.
- Arise from remnants of odontogenic epithelium, i.e. from rests of dental lamina. If these rests are situated outside the bone in the soft tissues of gingiva or alveolar mucosa may give rise to peripheral ameloblastoma.
- Four subtypes of ameloblastoma are currently identified namely:
  - Classic/solid/multicystic ameloblastoma
  - Unicystic ameloblastoma
  - Peripheral ameloblastoma
  - Desmoplastic ameloblastoma

Adenocarcinoma:

- Adenocarcinoma is a cancer of epithelial tissue that has glandular characteristics. Several head and neck cancers are adenocarcinomas, can be seen in thyroid.

32. True about thyroid surgery is:

a. In thyroid lobectomy, we divide at isthmus
b. Superior thyroid artery is present inferolateral to superior laryngeal nerve
c. Strap muscles divided in front of anterior jugular vein
d. Horizontal incision with finger below the cricoid cartilage
e. Superior parathyroid gland is normally located in an anterior position

Ans. a, c, d *Ref: Bailey and Love, 26/e; S Das, 9/e*

Option a	True	
Option b	False	Branch of the external carotid artery at the level of the hyoid bone. Origin at the level of the carotid bifurcation (20%) or common carotid artery (10%)
Option c	True	
Option d	True	
Option e	False	Located in posterior position

Anatomical steps of thyroidectomy:

- **Skin incision:** An incision is made in the skin two finger breadths above the sternal notch between the medial borders of the sternocleidomastoid muscles (two muscles make a V shape in front of the neck). The width of the incision may need to be extended for large masses, or for a lateral lymph node removal.
- **Subplatysmal flaps:** Subcutaneous fat and platysma (triangle sheet of muscle at both sides of the neck) are divided, and a subplatysmal dissection is made above the incision up to the level of the thyroid cartilage above, and the sternal notch, but remaining superficial to the anterior jugular veins.
- **Separating the strap muscles and exposing the anterior surface of the thyroid:** The fascia between the sternohyoid, omohyoid and sternothyroid muscles (strap muscles) is divided along the midline and the muscles retracted laterally. This is an avascular plane but care must be taken not to injure small veins crossing between the anterior jugular veins.
- **Identify the middle thyroid vein:** The thyroid gland is rotated medially (using the surgeons fingers). The important vascular structure to identify is the middle thyroid vein (it will be tightly stretched by the medial rotation of the gland), which is then ligated. This permits further mobilization of the gland and moving the bulk of the lobe out the wound.
- **Identify the superior laryngeal artery and the external laryngeal nerve:** Identify the superior laryngeal artery as close to the superior pole of the thyroid parenchyma as possible. Great care should be taken while ligating the superior laryngeal artery so as to avoid injury to the external laryngeal nerve. In some patients the external branch of the superior laryngeal nerve lies on the anterior surface of the thyroid lobe.
- **Identifying superior parathyroid gland:** The superior parathyroid gland is normally located in a posterior position, at the level of the upper two thirds of the thyroid and approximately 1 cm above the crossing point of the recurrent laryngeal nerve and the inferior thyroid artery. It is orange yellow in color, but difficult to identify. The gland must remain in situ with blood supply intact.
- **Identifying the inferior parathyroid gland:** The inferior parathyroid glands are normally located between the lower pole of the thyroid and the isthmus, most commonly on the anterior or the posterolateral surface of the lower pole of the thyroid. Care must be taken to preserve it in situ and to avoid damaging its inferior thyroid artery.
- **Identifying the recurrent laryngeal nerve:** The recurrent laryngeal nerve is located between the common carotid artery laterally, the esophagus medially, and the inferior thyroid artery superiorly.
- **Dividing the thyroid isthmus:** When doing a thyroid lobectomy, the isthmus, which is crossing between the two thyroid lobes, is divided.
- **Removing the thyroid gland.**

33. Change in T stage of maxillary carcinoma can occur due to:

a. Extension to involve the frontal sinus
b. Extension to involve the maxillary sinus
c. Extension to involve the ethmoid sinus
d. Extension to involve the sphenoid sinus
e. Extension to pterygoid plate

Ans. e *Ref: Bailey and Love, 26/e; S Das, 9/e*

Option a	False	
Option b	False	
Option c	False	
Option d	False	
Option e	True	

T categories for maxillary sinus cancer

TX: Primary (main) tumor cannot be assessed.

T0: No evidence of primary tumor.

Tis: Cancer cells are limited to the innermost layer of the mucosa (epithelium). These cancers are known as carcinoma in situ.

T1: Tumor is only in the tissue lining the sinus (the mucosa) and does not invade bone.

T2: Tumor has begun to grow into some of the bones of the sinus, other than into the bone of the back part of the sinus.

T3: Tumor has begun to grow into the bone at the back of the sinus (called the posterior wall) or the tumor has grown into the ethmoid sinus, the tissues under the skin, or the side or bottom of the eye socket.

T4a: Tumor is growing into other structures such as the skin of the cheek, the front part of the eye socket, the bone at the top of the nose ***(cribriform plate),*** the sphenoid sinus, the frontal sinus, or certain parts of the face ***(the pterygoid plates or the infratemporal fossa).*** This is also known as moderately advanced local disease.

T4b: Tumor has grown into the throat behind the nasal cavity ***(nasopharynx),*** the back of the eye socket, the brain, the tissue covering the brain (***the dura***), some parts of the base of the skull (***middle cranial fossa or clivus***), or certain nerves. This is also known as very advanced local disease.

34. Variants of squamous cell carcinoma of lung includes:

a. Papillary
b. Clear cell
c. Large cell carcinoma
d. Merkel's
e. Basaloid

Ans. a, b, e *Ref: Bailey and Love, 26/e; S Das, 9/e*

Option a	True	
Option b	True	
Option c	False	Lacks squamous differentiation
Option d	False	
Option e	True	

Squamous cell carcinoma of lung: A tumor arising from bronchial epithelium showing keratinization or intercellular bridges.

More than 90% of squamous cell carcinomas of lung occur in cigarette smokers.

Variants of squamous cell carcinoma:

- **Papillary:** The papillary variant occurs more frequently as a primarily superficial, endobronchial lesion, with a modestly better prognosis. It shows endobronchial obstructive growth with sometimes limited intraepithelial spread and invasion may be difficult to assess.
- **Small-cell:** Small cell variant of squamous cell carcinoma tends to have coarser chromatin and more prominent nucleoli than does true small cell carcinoma.
- **Clear-cell**
- **Basaloid:** Characterized by a basal bronchial stem cell proliferation shows basaloid pattern predominance and minimal areas of squamous differentiation. Patients with this variant have significantly shorter survival than other variants.
- **Alveolar space-filling peripheral variant:** This subtype appears to have a better prognosis.
- **Transitional cell carcinoma:** Rare.

Of these variants, there is some evidence that the basaloid and poorly differentiated small-cell variants may have worse prognoses than "conventional" squamous-cell carcinomas. Very little data is currently available on the clear-cell variant of squamous-cell carcinoma, and no consensus has been reached on the prognostic implications of clear-cell changes in lung cancer.

35. True about hernias:

a. Direct hernia is more common in children
b. Femoral hernia causes more strangulation
c. Indirect inguinal hernia is due to failure of closure of processus vaginalis
d. Direct hernia presents with more sign and symptoms
e. Direct hernia occurs due to defect in transversalis fascia

Ans. b, c, e *Ref: Bailey and Love, 26/e; S Das, 9/e*

Option a	False
Option b	True
Option c	True
Option d	False
Option e	True

A hernia is a protrusion of any viscus from its proper cavity. A hernia can lead to an incarcerated and often obstructed bowel or a strangulated bowel with a compromised blood supply.

Types of Hernia

- **Indirect inguinal hernia**
  - Follows the tract through the inguinal canal.
  - This results from ***a persistent process vaginalis.***
  - The inguinal canal begins in the intra-abdominal cavity at the internal inguinal ring, located approximately midway between the pubic symphysis and the anterior iliac spine.

- The canal courses down along the inguinal ligament to the external ring, located medial to the inferior epigastric arteries, subcutaneously and slightly above the pubic tubercle.
- Contents of this hernia then follow the tract of the testicle down into the scrotal sac.

❑ **Direct inguinal hernia**
- A direct inguinal hernia usually occurs due to a defect or weakness in the ***transversalis fascia*** area of the Hesselbach triangle.
- The triangle is defined inferiorly by the inguinal ligament, laterally by the inferior epigastric arteries, and medially by the conjoined tendon.

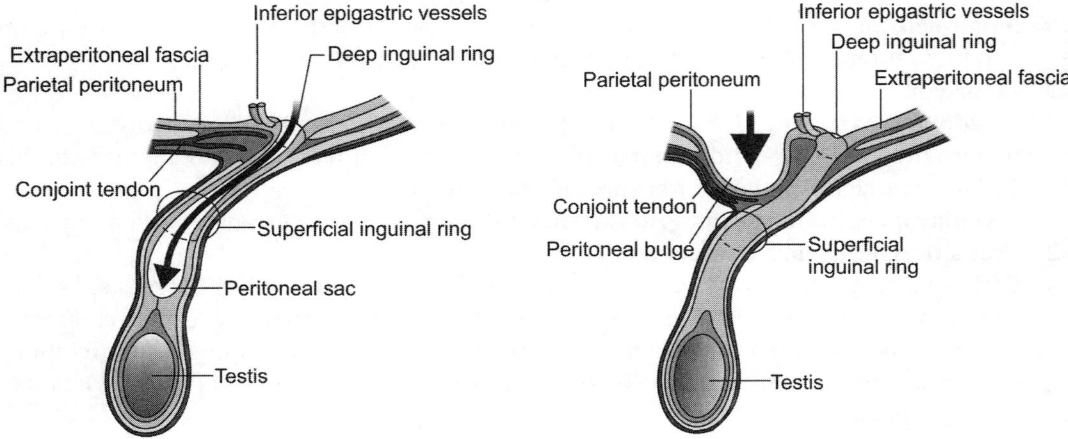

Fig. 13.6: Indirect and direct inguinal hernias.

❑ **Femoral hernia**
- The femoral hernia follows the tract below the inguinal ligament through the femoral canal.
- The canal lies medial to the femoral vein and lateral to the lacunar (Gimbernat) ligament.
- Because femoral hernias protrude through such a small defined space, they frequently become *incarcerated or strangulated.*

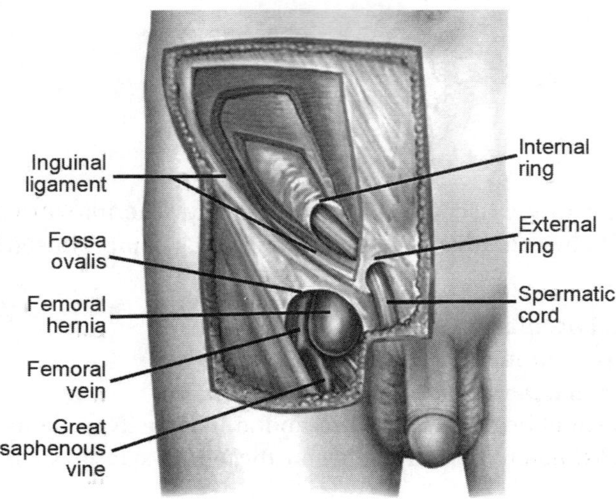

Umbilical hernia

- The umbilical hernia occurs through the umbilical fibromuscular ring, which usually obliterates by 2 years of age.
- They are congenital in origin and are repaired if they persist in children older than age 2–4 years.

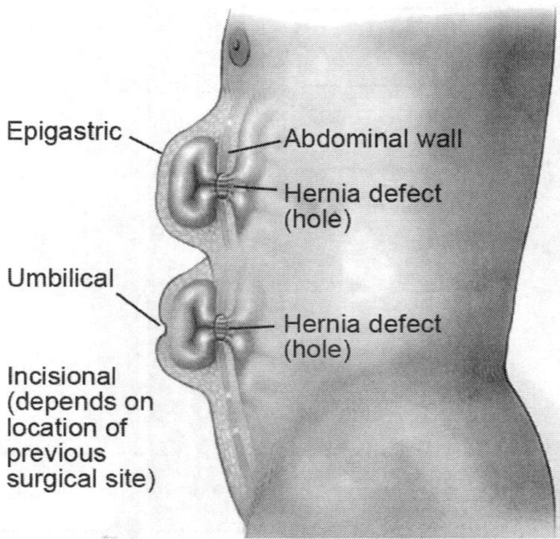

Fig. 13.7: Ventral hernias.

Richter hernia

- The Richter hernia occurs when only the antimesenteric border of the bowel herniates through the fascial defect.
- The Richter hernia involves only a portion of the circumference of the bowel.
- As such, the bowel may not be obstructed, even if the hernia is incarcerated or strangulated, and the patient may not present with vomiting.
- The Richter hernia can occur with any of the various abdominal hernias and is particularly dangerous, as a portion of strangulated bowel may be reduced unknowingly into the abdominal cavity, leading to perforation and peritonitis.

Incisional hernia

- This iatrogenic hernia occurs in 2–10% of all abdominal operations secondary to breakdown of the fascial closure of prior surgery.
- Even after repair, recurrence rates approach 20–45%.

Spigelian hernia

- This rare form of abdominal wall hernia occurs through a defect in the spigelian fascia, which is defined by the lateral edge of the rectus muscle at the semilunar line (costal arch to the pubic tubercle).
- The two subtypes are interstitial and subcutaneous, which are best defined using CT and assist with optimizing the surgical approach when indicated.

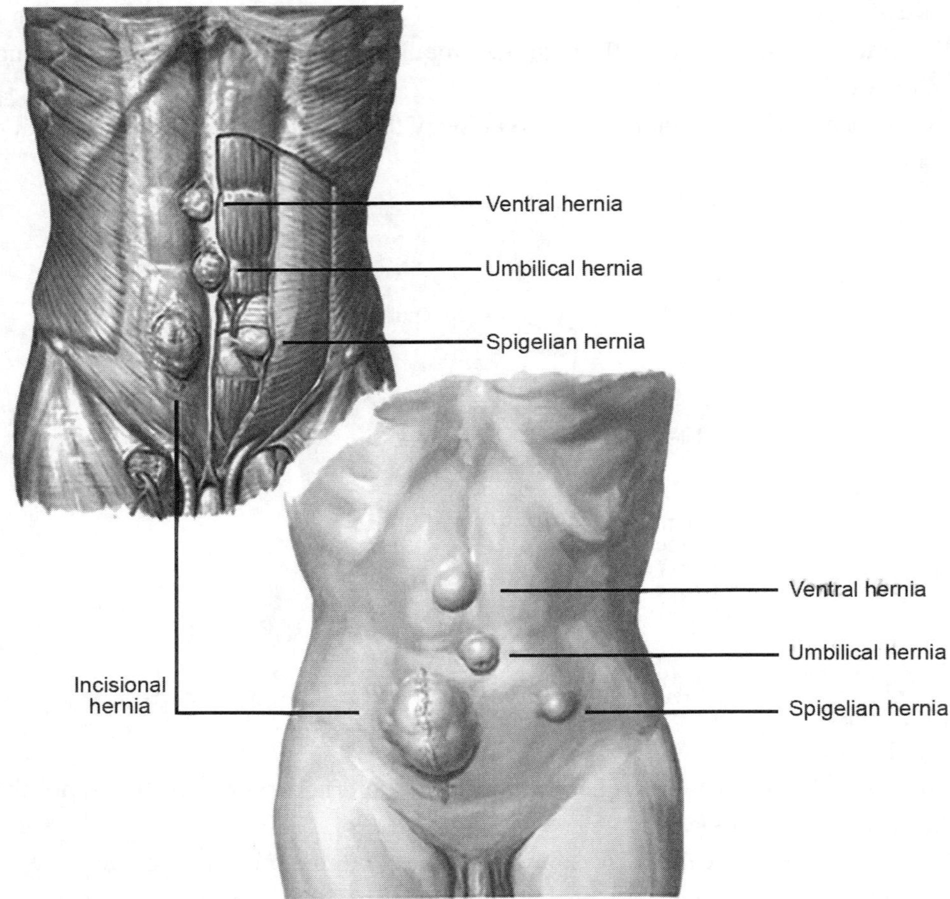

- **Obturator hernia**
  - This hernia passes through the obturator foramen, following the path of the obturator nerves and muscles.
  - Obturator hernias occur with a female-to-male ratio of 6:1, because of a gender-specific larger canal diameter and predominately in the elderly.
  - Because of its anatomic position, this hernia presents more commonly as a bowel obstruction than as a protrusion of bowel contents.

36. Meckel's diverticulum presents with:

a. Hematemesis
b. Volvulus
c. Hemoptysis
d. Hematuria
e. Patent vitelline duct

Ans. a, b, e *Ref: Bailey and Love, 26/e; S Das, 9/e*

Option a	True	Rare clinical manifestation of Meckel's diverticulum
Option b	True	Volvulus of Meckel's diverticulum causing intestinal obstruction is a rare occurrence

Option c	False	
Option d	False	Melena is seen
Option e	True	

- Meckel's diverticulum is present in 2% of cases, 2 feet proximal to ileocecal valve, 2 inches in length and found on antimesenteric border of ileum.
- A Meckel diverticulum is a vestigial remnant of the omphalomesenteric (vitellointestinal) duct.
- As a congenital anomaly, it is a true diverticulum that includes all three coats of the small intestine.
- Clinically important manifestations are found in children, over 60% occurring before the age of 10 years.
- Presence can only be detected if some complication arises in it.

Important complications that may occur in Meckel's diverticulum:

- **Intestinal obstruction**
  - *In adults this is probably the most common complication. Intestinal obstruction* may occur *around a band running from the tip of the diverticulum to the umbilicus.* Intestinal obstruction may result from *volvulus or kinking around this band.*
  - Intestinal obstruction may also be caused by *intussusception due to swollen, inflamed heterotopic epithelium at the mouth of the diverticulum and not due to inversion of the diverticulum.*
- **Bleeding** is also a *common* manifestation. This is *due to peptic ulceration produced by secretion of acid—pepsin by the ectopic gastric mucosa in the diverticulum. Melaena is usual, but frank hemorrhage with passage of dark red clots may occur per rectum. Perforation from such ulceration is rare.* Patient also vomits but *vomitus does not contain blood.* When the abdomen has been explored with the diagnosis of peptic ulceration hemorrhage and no peptic ulcer can be detected in the stomach or duodenum, it is wise to look for Meckel's diverticulum and ulceration there.
- **Meckel's diverticulitis** is the third complication in the adult. *Inflammation in Meckel's diverticulitis* occurs due to lodgement of food residues within it. Symptoms are very much akin to appendicitis. About 50% of cases there may be *perforation and general peritonitis.* It is the usual practice to look for Meckel's diverticulum after performing appendicectomy, as the patient might have been suffering from Meckel's diverticulitis, when the diagnosis of appendicitis was made.
- **Chronic peptic ulceration**: *May occur when there is ectopic gastric mucosa in the diverticulum.* Patient mainly complains of pain around the umbilicus (typical '*hunger pain*'). *Pain relating to Meckel's* diverticulum is always felt around the umbilicus *as it is a part of the midgut.*
- Exceptionally Meckel's diverticulum *may be found in an inguinal or femoral hernia,* when it is called *Littre's hernia.*

37. Surgery safe list includes:

a. Sign in
b. Sign out
c. Time in
d. Timeout
e. Pre-anesthetic checkup

Ans. a, b, d

Ref: WHO Surgical Safety Checklist

Option a	True	
Option b	True	
Option c	False	
Option d	True	
Option e	False	

Surgical safety checklist (First Edition)		
Before induction of anesthesia	***Before skin incision***	***Before patient leaves operating room***
SIGN IN • Patient has confirmed - Identity - Site - Procedure - Consent • Site marked/not applicable • Anesthesia safety check completed • Pulse oximeter on patient and functioning **Does patient have A:** **Known allergy?** • No • Yes **Difficult airway/aspiration risk?** • No • Yes, and equipment/assistance available **Risk of > 500 mL blood loss (7 mL/kg in children)?** • No • Yes, and adequate intravenous access and fluids planned	**TIMEOUT** • Confirm all team members have introduced themselves by name and role • Surgeon, anesthesia professional and nurse verbally confirm - Patient - Site - Procedure **Anticipated critical events** • **Surgeon reviews:** What are the critical or unexpected steps, operative duration, anticipated blood loss? • **Anesthesia team reviews:** Are there any patient-specific concerns? • Nursing team reviews: Has sterility (including indicator results) been confirmed? Are there equipment issues or any concerns? **Has antibiotic prophylaxis been given within the last 60 minutes?** • Yes • Not applicable **Is essential imaging displayed?** • Yes • Not applicable	**SIGN OUT** Nurse verbally confirms with the team: • The name of the procedure recorded • That instrument, sponge and needle counts are correct (or not applicable) • How the specimen is labeled (including patient name) • Whether there are any equipment problems to be addressed • Surgeon, anesthesia professional and nurse review the key concerns for recovery and management of this patient

38. Facial laceration management:

a. Eyebrow should be shaved
b. Clean wounds are repaired with monofilament sutures and removed after few days
c. Both animal and human bites should have delayed closure
d. Eyebrow sutures are removed in 3–5 days
e. Polyfilament suture is associated with lower risk of infection

Ans. b, c, d *Ref: Bailey and Love, 26/e; S Das, 9/e*

Option a	False	It may not regrow
Option b	True	

Option c	True	
Option d	True	
Option e	False	Monofilament suture is associated with a lower risk of infection

- ❑ A systematic approach to facial laceration repair ensures the best chance at an optimum outcome.
- ❑ Cosmetic results are better when minimal tension is placed on the wound edges at the time of repair.
- ❑ All areas should be thoroughly explored, copiously irrigated, cleaned, and debrided of devitalized tissue before closure.
- ❑ Non-contaminated wounds repaired within 6 hours of injury rarely develop infection. Nonabsorbable monofilament suture should be used for skin closure. *Monofilament suture is associated with a lower risk of infection compared with a polyfilament suture.*
- ❑ Deep wounds should be repaired in layers. Unrepaired muscle layers are much more likely to produce noticeable scarring.
- ❑ A simple interrupted technique can be used in areas of low tension or in wounds in which the tension has been reduced with a layer of subcutaneous sutures.
- ❑ All facial wounds should be repaired in less than 24 hours to decrease the risk of infection and achieve the best cosmetic result. If a delay in closure is necessary, wounds should be covered with saline-moistened gauze until the repair can be made.

List of laceration sites and recommendations on suture size and typical time to removal:

- ❑ Scalp: 4–0 suture or staple, with removal in 7–14 days
- ❑ Forehead: 5–0/6–0 sutures, with removal in 5 days
- ❑ Eyebrow: 5–0/6–0 sutures, with removal in 3–5 days
- ❑ Face: 6–0 suture, with removal in 5 days
- ❑ Eyelid: 6–0/7–0 sutures, with removal in 3 days
- ❑ Nose: 5–0 sutures, with removal in 3–5 days
- ❑ Ears: 6–0 sutures, with removal in 10–14 days
- ❑ Lips: 6–0 sutures, with removal in 3–5 days

Incase of human and animal bites, primary closure with sutures is not generally recommended for non-facial bite wounds, especially deep punctures, bites to the hand and clinically infected wounds. Delayed closure is usually more appropriate and should also be considered for wounds more than six hours old.

A laceration that involves the eyebrow should be reapproximated to recreate the natural curve of the eyebrow as well as possible.

Do not shave the eyebrow. The hair may not grow back normally.

39. Acute appendicitis presents as:

a. Nausea and vomiting
b. Constipation
c. Vague pain in periumbilical region in initial stage
d. Passive extension of hip causes pain
e. Passive flexion and internal rotation of hip causes pain

Ans. a, c, d *Ref: Bailey and Love, 26/e; S Das, 9/e*

Option a	True	Murphy's triad—Pain, nausea, temperature
Option b	False	Not present because of appendicitis itself
Option c	True	Pain is present in all cases
Option d	True	Called as obturator test
Option e	False	Passive external rotation of the flexed thigh will elicit pain

Acute appendicitis:

- ❑ Most common acute surgical condition of abdomen.

Aetiology and pathogenesis:

- ❑ OBSTRUCTION OF THE LUMEN seems to be the dominant factor in production of acute appendicitis. This may occur due to obstruction of the lumen, obstruction in the wall or obstruction from outside the wall.
    - In the lumen faecolith and hyperplasia of submucosal lymphoid follicle are the major causes of obstruction. Other causes are intestinal worms, e.g. round worm, thread-worm etc., vegetables, fruit seeds, inspissated feces or barium form previous X-rays.
    - In the wall, stricture (due to fibrosis from earlier inflammation) or neoplasms of which carcinoid is the commonest are the main causes.
    - Outside the wall adhesions and kinks are common in this group.
- ❑ DIET: Rise in incidence of appendicitis is mostly due to diet which is relatively rich with fish and meat and departure from simple diet rich in cellulose and high residue.
  PATHOLOGY: Acute appendicitis may be of obstructive variety or non-obstructive variety.

Clinical features:

- ❑ Pain is present in ALL patients. Initially typical pain is dull and diffuse situated in the umbilical or lower epigastric region. Gradually, it gets localized to right; lower quadrant.
- ❑ Anorexia: Almost always complained by every patient.
- ❑ Nausea: Almost always present. Vomiting is frequently present in children and teenagers, however, adults may not vomit.
- ❑ Typically, Murphy's triad, Pain, Vomiting and temperature.
- ❑ Constipation may be present before the onset of pain, and is not because of appendicitis *per se.* young children may complain of diarrhea.

Examination:

- ❑ Patient looks anxious in pain and the tongue is dry.
- ❑ Maximum tenderness can be found near McBurney's point.
- ❑ Muscle guarding is present on palpation.
- ❑ Rebound tenderness (elicitation of severe pain on pressing at the inflamed area and releasing suddenly) is present.
- ❑ Rovsing's sign (pain in the right lower quadrant on exerting pressure at left lower quadrant) is present.
- ❑ Psoas sign is positive. It is elicited by making the patient lie on his left side. Patient's right thigh is extended which stretches the iliopsoas muscle and produces pain. This sign indicates presence of irritative inflamed appendix in close proximity to the psoas muscle.
- ❑ Obturator test: Passive external rotation of the flexed thigh will elicit pain. This sign is positive in pelvic appendix.

40. True about torsion of testis is/are:

a. Doppler stethoscope with ultrasound is used
b. Differentiated from epididymitis by radionuclide
c. Occurs above processus vaginalis
d. Can never occur during sleep
e. Pain is sudden and agonizing

Ans. a, e *Ref: Bailey and Love, 26/e; S Das, 9/e*

Option	Answer	Explanation
Option a	True	
Option b	False	Doppler ultrasound differentiates it from epididymitis
Option c	False	Testis hangs within processus vaginalis
Option d	False	Can occur during sleep also
Option e	True	

Torsion of testis/torsion of spermatic cord:

- Uncommon condition limited to peripubertal males.
- Causes strangulation of blood to the testis. It can cause testicular atrophy if not treated within 3–4 hours.
- **Predisposing factors:**
  - Inversion of the testis
  - Long mesorchium: In this case the body of the testis only rotates without involving the spermatic cord, that means torsion of the testis occurs without torsion of the spermatic cord.
  - Undescended or ectopic testis.
  - High investment of tunica vaginalis: It causes the testis to hang within the tunica vaginalis which may initiate rotation.
  - A voluminous tunica vaginalis: This also gives adequate space to the testis to rotate.

  It should be borne in mind that the abnormality which causes torsion is usually bilateral.

Clinical features:

- Most commonly seen between 10 and 25 years of age.
- As cause is congenital, second most common incidence seen during infancy.
- Severe, sudden and agonizing pain in one testicle or groin.
- Nausea and vomiting are very common.
- Scrotum is swollen and tender and may mimic epididymo-orchitis. *Elevation of testis normally relieves pain in epididymo-orchitis but increases in torsion of spermatic cord.*
- Torsion can be differentiated from epididymitis by using Doppler stethoscope in combination with ultrasound.
- MRI clearly reveals the twisted stalk of testis and thickened proximal spermatic cord.

Differential diagnosis:

The two most important differential diagnoses are:

- Acute epididymo-orchitis: In case of torsion of completely descended testis. Epididymitis is unusual before the age of 25 years.
- Strangulated inguinal hernia: In case of torsion of incompletely descended testis.

Other important conditions are:
- ❑ Mumps orchitis
- ❑ Trauma.

41. True about lower GI bleeding:
   a. Less common than upper
   b. Aspirin is the cause
   c. Angiography is diagnostic
   d. Patients with moderate bleeding are hemodynamically stable
   e. Hematemesis occurs frequently

Ans. a, b, d *Ref: Bailey and Love, 26/e; S Das, 9/e*

Option a	True	
Option b	True	
Option c	False	Colonoscopy is the initial diagnostic method of choice
Option d	True	
Option e	False	Hematemesis does not occur

Lower gastroIntestinal bleeding (LGIB) is less common than upper GI bleeding (UGIB). **Acute LGIB** is defined as bleeding that is of recent duration, originates beyond the ligament of Treitz, results in instability of vital signs, and is associated with signs of anemia with or without need for blood transfusion.

LGIB presents as
- ❑ Maroon stools, with LGIB from the right side of the colon
- ❑ Bright red blood per rectum with LGIB from the left side of the colon
- ❑ Melena with cecal bleeding

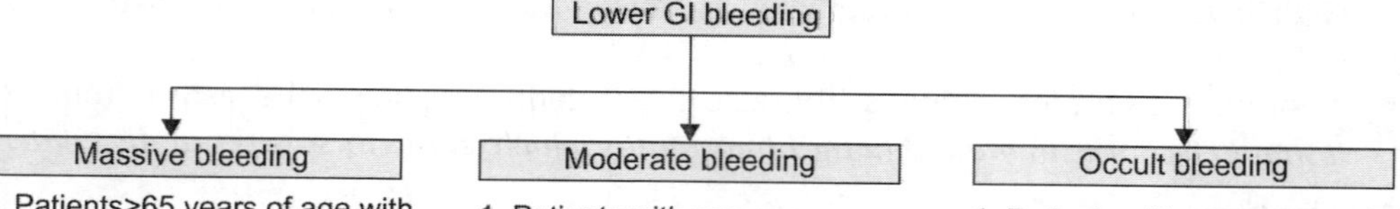

Massive bleeding
1. Patients>65 years of age with multiple medical problems
2. Present as a hematochezia or bright red blood per rectum
3. Hemodynamically unstable
   - SBP=90 mmHg
   - HR> 100/min
   - Low urine output
4. Hemoglobin level=6 g/dL
5. Most commonly due to:
   - Diverticulosis
   - Angiodysplasias
6. Mortality rate may be as high as 21%

Moderate bleeding
1. Patients with any age
2. May present as hematochezia or melena
3. Hemodynamically stable patients
4. Long list of diseases including benign anorectal, congenital, inflammatory, and neoplastic amount of acute or chronic bleeding

Occult bleeding
1. Patients with any age
2. Patients present with microcytic hypochromic anemia due to chronic blood loos
3. Long list of diseases including congenital, inflammatory, and neoplastic diseases may cause chronic occult bleeding

Types of lower GI bleeding.

Massive LGIB is defined as follows:
- ❑ Passage of a large volume of red or maroon blood through the rectum
- ❑ Hemodynamic instability and shock
- ❑ Initial decrease in hematocrit (Hct) level of 6 g/dL or less

- ❑ Transfusion of at least 4 U of packed red blood cells (RBCs)
- ❑ Bleeding that continues for 3 days
- ❑ Significant rebleeding in 1 week

Drug-induced bleeding is caused mainly by NSAID and aspirin use, and it is more common in the elderly.

In most patients with LGIB, colonoscopy is the initial diagnostic method of choice. Emergency angiography as an initial study is indicated ONLY in a highly select group of patients with massive ongoing LGIb.

42. Cancers caused by virus are:

a. Hepatocellular carcinoma
b. Kaposi's sarcoma
c. Nasopharyngeal carcinoma
d. Merkel cell carcinoma
e. Hodgkin lymphoma

Ans. a, b, c, d *Ref: S Das, 9/e; M.e. McLaughlin-Drubin, K. Munger/Biochimica et Biophysica Acta 1782 (2008) 127–150*

Option a	True	Caused by HBV and HCV
Option b	True	Caused by Kaposi sarcoma associated herpes virus, HIV
Option c	True	Caused by Epstein-Barr virus
Option d	True	Merkel cell polyomavirus
Option e	False	Non-hodgkin lymphoma can be caused by Human T-lymphotropic virus-1

Properties of cancer causing viruses of humans

Virus	*Viral taxonomy*	*Genome*	*Cell tropism*	*Human cancers*
EBV	*Herpesviridae*	dsDNA 172 kb ~ 90 ORFs	Oropharyngeal epithelial cells, B-cells	BL, NPC, lymphomas
HBV	*Hepadnaviridae*	dsDNA 3.2 kb 4 ORFs	Hepatocytes, white blood cells	HCC
HCV	*Flaviviridae*	dsRNA 9.4 kb 9 ORFs	Hepatocytes	HCC
HPV	*Papillomaviridae*	dsDNA 8 kb 8–10 ORFs	Squamous epithelial cells	Cervical, oral, and anogenital cancer
HTLV-1	*Retroviridae*	dsRNA 9.0 kb 6 ORFs	T-cells	ATL
KSHV	*Herpesviridae*	dsDNA 165 kb ~ 90 ORFs	B-cells	Kaposi sarcoma, primary effusion lymphoma

ATL, adult T-cell leukemia; BL, Burkitt's lymphoma; EBV, Epstein–Barr virus; HBV, hepatitis B virus; HCC, hepatocellular carcinoma; HCV, hepatitis C virus; HPV, human papillomavirus; HTLV-1, human T-cell leukemia virus; KSHV, Kaposi's sarcoma-associated herpesvirus; and NPC, nasopharyngeal carcinoma.

43. Features of second degree burns include:

a. Dry and leathery skin
b. Severe pain
c. Appearance of blisters
d. Hair can be easily plucked out
e. Charred vessels are seen easily

Ans. b, c *Ref: Bailey and Love, 26/e; S Das, 9/e*

Option a	False	Seen in first degree burns
Option b	True	
Option c	True	
Option d	False	Hair follicles remain intact
Option e	False	Seen in 3rd degree burn

There are many types of burns caused by thermal, radiation, chemical, or electrical contact.

Thermal burns: These burns are due to heat sources which raise the temperature of the skin and tissues and cause tissue cell death or charring. Hot metals, scalding liquids, steam, and flames, when coming into contact with the skin, can cause thermal burns.

Radiation burns: These burns are due to prolonged exposure to ultraviolet rays of the sun, or to other sources of radiation such as X-ray.

Chemical burns: These burns are due to strong acids, alkalies, detergents, or solvents coming into contact with the skin or eyes.

Electrical burns: These burns are from electrical current, either alternating current (AC) or direct current (DC).

Severity of Burn: Burns are classified into 3 grades or degrees according to the depth of necrosis. In *first-degree* burn there is simply hyperaemia of the skin with slight edema of the epidermis. There is only microscopic destruction of the superficial layers of the epidermis, which are desquamated within a few days. It is of little clinical significance as the superficial layers of epithelium are soon replaced from the basal layers, so that there is no scarring. First-degree burns rapidly heal if the patient avoids further exposure to source of heat. First-degree burns are not considered while estimating the magnitude of burn for purposes of planning intravenous fluid replacement. In *second-degree* burns the entire thickness of the epidermis is destroyed. Blebs or vesicles are formed between the separating epidermis and dermis. Vesiculation is the hallmark of the second-degree burn. Second-degree burn is further subdivided into: (a) mild and (b) severe varieties. In mild cases enough epithelium is left in the hair follicles and dermal glands to provide new cells for resurfacing the burned area. In severe cases, there is not enough epithelium left, so that resurfacing of the burned area is not possible and skin grafting becomes necessary. In *third-degree* burn there is complete destruction of the epidermis and dermis with irreversible destruction of dermal appendages and epithelial elements including the sensory nerves. Skin grafting becomes obligatory to cover the area.

The extent of burn is expressed as a percentage of the total surface area displaying either 2nd degree or third degree burn. It is commonly estimated by the rule of nines.

'Rule of nines' for estimating percentage of body surface involved in burns are as follows:

Anatomic area	*Percentage of body surface*
Head, face and neck	9%
Right upper extremity	9%
Left upper extremity	9%
Right lower extremity (thigh–9%, leg and foot–9%)	18%
Left lower extremity	18%
Anterior trunk (chest–9%, abdomen–9%)	18%
Posterior trunk (upper half–9%, lower half–9%)	18%
External genitalia	1%

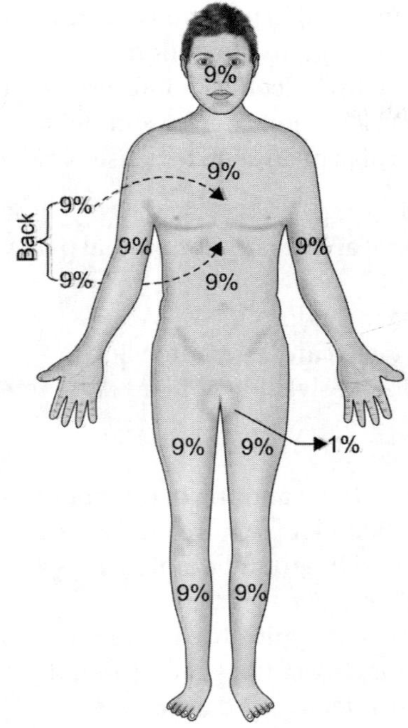

Fig. 13.8: A diagrammatic representation to show how to apply 'Rule of Nines'.

44. True about acute pancreatitis is:

a. Fluid contains activated pancreatic enzyme
b. Fluid mostly contains infectious material
c. Collection of fluid is asymptomatic
d. Pseudocyst may form after 2 weeks
e. Pseudocyst does not contain any wall

Ans. a, c, d *Ref: Bailey and Love, 26/e; S Das, 9/e*

Option a	True	Amylase and lipase
Option b	False	
Option c	True	
Option d	True	
Option e	False	Walled off by granular tissue

Acute pancreatitis is acute inflammation superimposed on a normal gland. When several such episodes occur, it is called as acute relapsing pancreatitis.

- Gallstones, choledocholithiasis and alcohol are two major conditions giving rise to 90% cases of acute pancreatitis.
- Obstruction of the pancreatic duct may lead to stimulation of pancreatic secretion and hence acute pancreatitis.
- Metabolic factors as hyperlipidemia (genetic and diet induced), hypercalcemia (precipitation of calcium phosphate in pancreatic duct) and hemochromatosis (produces pancreatic fibrosis and atrophy) may lead to occurrence of acute pancreatitis.

- Fat emboli may cause obstruction of pancreatic duct and may cause pancreatitis.
- Postoperative causes—due to surgeries on abdomen or biliary tract.
- Certain toxins as alcohol (methyl alcohol), viral diseases (mumps, echovirus, coxsackie virus), drugs (corticosteroids, azathioprine, frusemide) may cause pancreatitis.
- Investigation with ERCP has also been seen to cause pancreatitis.

Physical examination reveals:

- Characteristically dull, boring, and steady abdominal pain with nausea, vomiting and may be anorexia.
- Low grade fever and epigastric tenderness.
- Signs of shock as sweating, tachycardia, hypotension.
- Mild jaundice may occur due to swelling of head of pancreas and excessive hemolysis of red blood cells.
- Hypocalcemia is a known feature.
- Paralytic ileus may be seen in the beginning of duodenum and proximal jejunum.
- *"Sentinel loop"* (solitary gas filled loop of proximal jejunum) may be seen on X-ray.
- *Cullen's sign* (discoloration of skin around umbilicus) is a characteristic finding. When it is seen in loins, it is called as *"Grey Turner's sign"*.
- Acute fluid collections may occur, typically early in the course of acute pancreatitis. These are primarily detected by imaging studies rather than by physical examination. Because they lack a defined wall, non-infective and usually regress spontaneously, most acute fluid collections require no specific therapy.
- Approximately 10 days– 2 weeks after the onset of the disease, a tender palpable mass may appear in the epigastrium, called as, *pseudocyst of the pancreas.* An acute pseudocyst is a collection of pancreatic fluid that is walled off by granulation tissue after an episode of acute pancreatitis. If such mass appears after 3rd week, it is due to the abscess formation.

Investigations:

- **Elevated serum amylase** is an established feature of acute pancreatitis. Higher the serum amylase level, greater is the possibility of having acute pancreatitis.
- **Urinary amylase excretion** is also increased. Urinary amylase levels remain elevated for longer periods of time.
- **Elevated serum lipase along with serum amylase** is diagnostic.
- **Serum lactescence** is a specific indicator of acute pancreatitis. It occurs when circulating triglyceride levels are > 500 mg/100 mL.
- **Hyperglycemia** due to relative hypoinsulinemia is often noticed.
- **Hypocalcemia.**
- **Paracentesis** is sometimes used to confirm the diagnosis. Increased amylase and lipase may be detected in the aspirated fluid when their respective serum levels are normal.

45. True about head injury is:

a. Battle's sign seen around the orbit
b. Subacute subdural hemorrhage occurs 3–5 days later
c. Decompression craniotomy will not produce a better outcome but will decrease ICT
d. Diffuse axonal injury occurs rarely during motion changes
e. Epidural hematoma can occur due to tearing of middle meningeal artery

Ans. b, c, e *Ref: Bailey and Love, 26/e; S Das, 9/e*

Option a	False	Battle's sign is subcutaneous bleed over the mastoid
Option b	True	
Option c	True	
Option d	False	Usually occurs as the result of an acceleration or deceleration motion
Option e	True	

Head injury includes injury to scalp, skull and/or brain.

Skull fracture:

- **Basilar skull fractures** occur because of blunt trauma and describe a break in the bones at the base of the skull. These are often associated with ***bleeding around the eyes (raccoon eyes)*** or ***behind the ears (Battle's sign).*** The fracture line may extend into the sinuses of the face and allow bacteria from the nose and mouth to come into contact with the brain, causing a potential infection.
- In infants and young children, whose skull bones have not yet fused together, a skull fracture may cause a ***diastasis fracture***, in which the suture lines widen.
- Fractures can be ***linear*** (literally a line in the bone) or ***stellate*** (a starburst like pattern) and the pattern of the break is associated with the type of force applied to the skull.
- ***Penetrating skull fractures*** describe injuries caused by an object entering the brain. This includes gunshot and stab wounds, and impaled objects to the head.
- A ***depressed skull fracture*** occurs when a piece of skull is pushed toward the inside of the skull (think of pressing in on a ping pong ball). Depending upon circumstances, *decompression craniotomy* may be required to elevate the depressed fragment and reduce the intracranial tension.

An *open fracture* occurs when the skin is torn or lacerated over the fracture site. This increases the risk of infection, especially with a depressed skull fracture in which brain tissue is exposed.

In a *closed fracture*, the skin is not damaged and continues to protect the underlying fracture from contamination from the outside world.

Bleeding in the skull may or may not be associated with a skull fracture. Epidural, subdural, and subarachnoid bleeding describe bleeding in the spaces between the meninges and the fibrous layered coverings of the brain.

Subdural hemorrhage:

- Significant subdural hemorrhage is caused by rupture of superior cerebral veins.
- It is a common occurrence in elderly.
- Level of consciousness deteriorates very quickly than in extradural hemorrhage.

Epidural hematoma:

- If the head trauma is epidural the blood is trapped in a small area and cause a hematoma to form. Pressure can increase quickly within the epidural space, pushing the clot up against the brain and causing significant damage.
- An epidural hematoma may often occur with trauma to the temporal bone located on the side of the head above the ear *(Battle's sign*). Aside from the fact that the temporal bone is

thinner than the other skull bones (frontal, parietal, occipital), it is also the location of the middle meningeal artery that runs just beneath the bone. Fracture of the temporal bone is associated with tearing of this artery and may lead to an epidural hematoma.

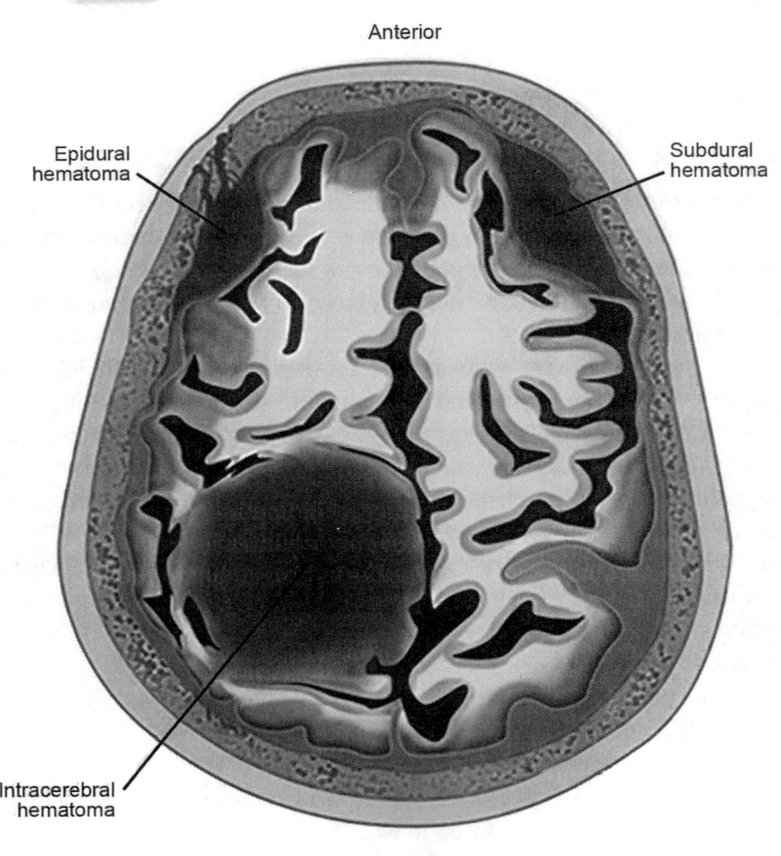

Fig. 13.9: Brain hematoma.

Subarachnoid hemorrhage:

- In a subarachnoid hemorrhage, blood accumulates in the space beneath the inner arachnoid layer of the meninges. The injury is often associated with an intracerebral bleed. This is also the space where cerebral spinal fluid (CSF) flows and affected individuals can develop severe headache, nausea, vomiting, and a stiff neck because the blood causes significant irritation to this meningeal layer.

Diffuse axonal injury:

- Usually occurs as the result of an acceleration or deceleration motion, not necessarily an impact. Axons are stretched and damaged when parts of the brain of differing density slide over one another. Prognoses vary widely depending on the extent of damage.

Symptoms of skull fracture can include:

- ❑ Leaking cerebrospinal fluid (from nose, mouth or ear) may be and is strongly indicative of basilar skull fracture and the tearing of sheaths surrounding the brain, which can lead to secondary brain infection.
- ❑ Visible deformity or depression in the head or face; for example a sunken eye can indicate a maxillary fracture.
- ❑ An eye that cannot move or is deviated to one side can indicate that a broken facial bone is pinching a nerve that innervates eye muscles.
- ❑ Wounds or bruises on the scalp or face.
- ❑ Basilar skull fractures, those that occur at the base of the skull, are associated with *Battle's sign*, a subcutaneous bleed over the mastoid, hemotympanum, and cerebrospinal fluid rhinorrhea and otorrhea.
- ❑ Because brain injuries can be life-threatening, even people with apparently slight injuries, with no noticeable signs or complaints, require close observation; They have a chance for severe symptoms later on. The patient needs to be aroused several times during the next 12 to 24 hours to assess for worsening symptoms.
- ❑ The Glasgow coma scale (GCS) is a tool for measuring degree of unconsciousness and is thus a useful tool for determining severity of injury.

Pediatrics

1. Features of ankyloglossia are:

a. Obstructive sleep apnea
b. More carcinogenic
c. Mandibular prognathism
d. Affects speech
e. Acquired due to trauma

Ans. c,d

Option a	False	No, Not correct
Option b	False	No, it is not cancerous
Option c	True	Yes, correct
Option d	True	Yes, correct
Option e	False	No, it is a Congenital anomaly

Ankyloglossia ('tongue-tie') is a congenital anomaly observed in newborns and children, and is characterized by an abnormally short lingual frenulum. The tight frenulum can cause decreased tongue mobility to varying degrees.

Ankyloglossia varies in degree of severity from mild cases characterized by mucous membrane bands to complete ankyloglossia whereby the tongue is tethered to the floor of the mouth.

Ankyloglossia can affect eating, speech, and oral hygiene as well as have mechanical/social effects. Ankyloglossia can also prevent the tongue from contacting the anterior palate. This can then promote an infantile swallow and hamper the progression to an adult-like swallow which can result in an open bite deformity. It can also result in mandibular prognathism; this happens when the tongue contacts the anterior portion of the mandible with exaggerated anterior thrusts.

Tongue-tie can affect a baby's oral development, as well as the way he or she eats, speaks and swallows.

For example, tongue-tie can lead to:

- **Breast-feeding problems:** Breast-feeding requires a baby to keep his or her tongue over the lower gum while sucking. If unable to move the tongue or keep it in the right position, the baby might chew instead of suck on the nipple. This can cause significant nipple pain and interfere with a baby's ability to get breast milk. Ultimately, poor breast-feeding can lead to inadequate nutrition and failure to thrive.
- **Speech difficulties:** Tongue-tie can interfere with the ability to make certain sounds—such as "t," "d," "z," "s," "th" and "l." It can be especially challenging to roll an "r."
- **Poor oral hygiene:** For an older child or adult, tongue-tie can make it difficult to sweep food debris from the teeth. This can contribute to tooth decay and inflammation of the gums (gingivitis). Tongue-tie can also lead to the formation of a gap or space between the two bottom front teeth.
- **Challenges with other oral activities:** Tongue-tie can interfere with activities such as licking an ice cream cone, licking the lips, kissing or playing a wind instrument.

11. True about tetralogy of fallot:

a. Pulmonary stenosis
b. RV hypertrophy
c. Left to right shunt
d. Single loud S2
e. Most common congenital heart disease in neonates

Ans. a,b,d

Option a	True	Yes, correct
Option b	True	Due to right ventricular outflow tract obstruction (RVOTO)
Option c	False	Right to left shunt
Option d	True	Due to pulmonary stenosis
Option e	False	Transposition of great arteries in the common CHD among infants.

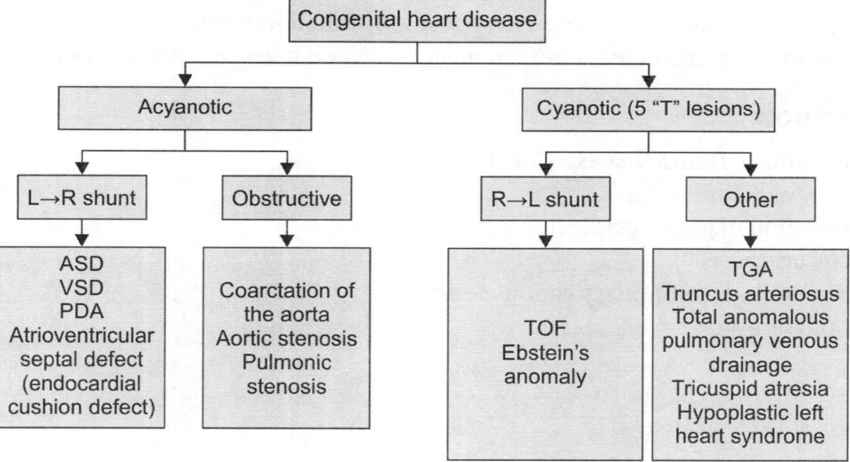

Tetralogy of Fallot

- Epidemiology: 10% of all CHD, most common cyanotic heart defect diagnosed beyond infancy with peak incidence at 2-4 mo of age

Pathophysiology

- Embryological defect due to anterior and superior deviation of the outlet septum leading to:
  1. VSD
  2. Right ventricular outflow tract obstruction (RVOTO) (i.e. pulmonary stenosis ± subpulmonary valve stenosis),
  3. Over-riding aorta
  4. RVH
- Infants may initially have a L → R shunt (therefore no cyanosis); however, RVOTO is progressive, leading to increasing R → L shunting with hypoxemia and cyanosis
- Degree of RVOTO determines the direction and degree of shunt and, therefore, the extent of clinical cyanosis and degree of RVH
  - Clinical presentation

- **History:** Hypoxic spells
  - During exertional states (crying, exercise) the increasing pulmonary vascular resistance and decrease in systemic resistance causes an increase in right-to-left shunting
  - Clinical features include paroxysms of rapid and deep breathing, irritability and crying, increasing cyanosis, decreased intensity of murmur (decreased flow across RVOTO)
    - If severe, can lead to decreased level of consciousness, seizures, death
    - **Physical exam**
    - Single loud S2 due to severe pulmonary stenosis (i.e. RVOTO), SEM at LSB
- Investigations
  - **ECG:** RAD, RVH
  - **CXR:** Boot-shaped heart, decreased pulmonary vasculature, right aortic arch (in 20%)
  - **Echo:** Diagnostic
- **Management of spells:** O_2, knee-chest position, fluid bolus, morphine sulfate, propranolol
- **Treatment:** Surgical repair at 4-6 mo of age; earlier if marked cyanotic spells

Good to Know

Common cyanotic Heart Disease (5 Ts)

- Tetralogy of Fallot
- Transposition of great vessels
- Truncus arteriosis
- Total anomalous pulmonary venous return
- Tricuspid atresia

Pediatrics

1. Neural tube defect in fetus can occur with:

a. Antiepileptic drugs
b. Diabetes mellitus in mothers
c. Hypertension in mothers
d. Methotrexate intake by mother
e. MTHFR mutation

Ans. a, b, d, e *Ref: Ghai, 8/e*

Option a	True	Valproate
Option b	True	Insulin dependent diabetes mellitus
Option c	False	
Option d	True	Causes folate deficiency
Option e	True	

Neural tube defects (NTD) are one of the commonest structural congenital anomalies and occur due to failure of proper closure of neural tube and covering mesoderm and ectoderm. NTDs are birth defects of the brain, spine, or spinal cord. They happen in the first month of pregnancy.

Maternal risk factors for NTD include:

- Alcohol
- Radiation exposure
- Insulin dependent diabetes mellitus
- Valproate and carbamazepine
- Zinc and folate deficiency
- Methotrexate intake which in turn causes folate deficiency
- Maternal malnutrition is another important factor.

The **MTHFR** gene provides instructions for making an enzyme called methylenetetrahydrofolate reductase. Specifically, this enzyme converts 5, 10-methylenetetrahydrofolate to a molecule called 5-methyltetrahydrofolate. Mutation in this gene leads to folate deficiency and hence neural tube defects.

The two most common neural tube defects are spina bifida and anencephaly.

Clinical features

The spectrum includes spina bifida (meningocele, meningomyelocele, spina bifida occuita), anencephaly (absence of brain calvaria, total or partial), encephalocele (herniation of brain and meninges through defect in calvaria), craniorachischisis (anencephaly associated with continuous bony defect of spine and exposure of neural tissue) and iniencephaly (dysraphism of occipital region accompanied by retroflexion of neck and trunk).

Neural tube defects do not occur in isolation but are associated with other congenital anomalies and dysfunction.

Many affected children have:

- Lower body paralysis
- Bladder and bowel dysfunction
- Learning disabilities
- Hydrocephalus due to Arnold-Chiari type II malformation
- Endocrinal abnormality
- Anencephaly is an important cause of fetal and infant mortality.

The spina bifida may be occult in about 5 percent and is asymptomatic. In ***meningocele***, the sac is covered only by skin and generally there is no neurologic deficit. Arnold-Chiari malformation associated meningomyelocele may have a variety of associated CNS anomalies like heterotropias, hypoplasias, and ventricular abnormalities.

In ***meningomyelocele*** the neurologic deficit includes varying degrees of flaccid, areflexic paraparesis and sensory deficit in the trunk and legs correspond to the involved segments of the dysplastic cord. The cord distal to the site of the lesion is severely affected. Involvement of bowel and bladder results in fecal and urinary incontinence. Hydrocephalus is usually present in varying degrees and a shunt is required generally. Arnold-Chiari malformation may cause facial movements may be impaired and there may be laryngeal stridor.

The most common NTD compatible with life is myelomeningocele.

The most common presentation of a **closed NTD** is an obvious *abnormality along the spine* such as:

- A fluid-filled cystic mass,
- Area of hypopigmentation or hyperpigmentation,
- Cutis aplasia,
- Congenital dermal sinus,
- Capillary telangiectasia/hemangioma,
- Hairy patch (hypertrichosis),
- Skin appendages, or
- Asymmetrical gluteal cleft.

2. True about cystic fibrosis is/are:

a. Autosomal recessive
b. CF gene is on chromosome 7
c. Meconium ileus in > 85% cases
d. Poor weight gain even with good appetite
e. CF gene codes for the CFTR protein, which is 1,480 amino acids

Ans. a, b, d, e *Ref: Ghai, 8/e*

Option a	True	
Option b	True	
Option c	False	Meconium ileus is seen in 10–15% cases
Option d	True	
Option e	True	

Cystic fibrosis is an inherited with autosomal recessive transmission. The cystic fibrosis (CF) gene is on the chromosome 7; there are more than 400 mutations at CF locus, of which DF508 (which denotes a single deletion at 508 position of the protein) is the commonest. The mutation affects the gene's protein product, cystic fibrosis transmembrane regulator (CFTR), which acts as a chloride channel and affects other aspects of transmembrane movement of water and ions.

All the exocrine glands in the body especially those in the respiratory and gastrointestinal system are involved and produce abnormal viscid mucus. The inspissated secretions obstruct the pancreatic ducts, and cause distension of acini, which appear like cysts. These are surrounded by fibrosis. Pancreatic secretions do not pass into the duodenum. This leads to impaired digestion and absorption. It has been estimated that 10 percent of patients may not show evidence of pancreatic dysfunction. These patients do not suffer from other gastrointestinal complications.

In the lungs, thick mucus plugs obstruct bronchioles leading to collapse, stasis and infection. Parenchymal and bronchial damage cause chronic pulmonary disease.

In the newborn period, thick meconium plugs which have not been liquefied by the pancreatic juice in the intestinal tract of fetus, may cause intestinal obstruction or meconium ileus.

The patients with malabsorption usually have insufficient or low bicarbonate with low pH in the intestines. Increased secretion of chlorides in the sweat may be an independent associated defect.

Clinical features:

- In 10–15% of newborn infants with CF, the ileum is completely obstructed by meconium (**meconium ileus**).
- Two cardinal symptoms of disease are **Chronic diarrhea with massive steatorrhea** and **recurrent respiratory infections**.
- Failure to thrive is an important feature.
- Rectal prolapsed occurs frequently.

3. True about omphalocele is:

a. Peritoneum covered
b. Amnion covered
c. Not covered
d. Associated heart defects
e. Covered with skin

Ans. a, d *Ref: Ghai, 8/e*

Option a	True	
Option b	False	Sac is covered with peritoneum without overlying skin
Option c	False	
Option d	True	
Option e	False	

- An **omphalocele, also known as exomphalos,** is a herniation or protrusion of the abdominal contents into the base of the umbilical cord.
- In contrast to the more common umbilical hernia, the sac is covered with peritoneum without overlying skin.

- The majority (≈75%) of infants with omphalocele have associated congenital anomalies/syndromes, including Beckwith-Wiedemann syndrome (omphalocele, macrosomia, hypoglycemia), and other chromosomal (29%, including trisomies 13 and 18) and nonchromosomal (45%) multiple and isolated congenital anomalies (musculoskeletal, 24%; urogenital, 20%; cardiovascular, 15%; and central nervous system, 9%).

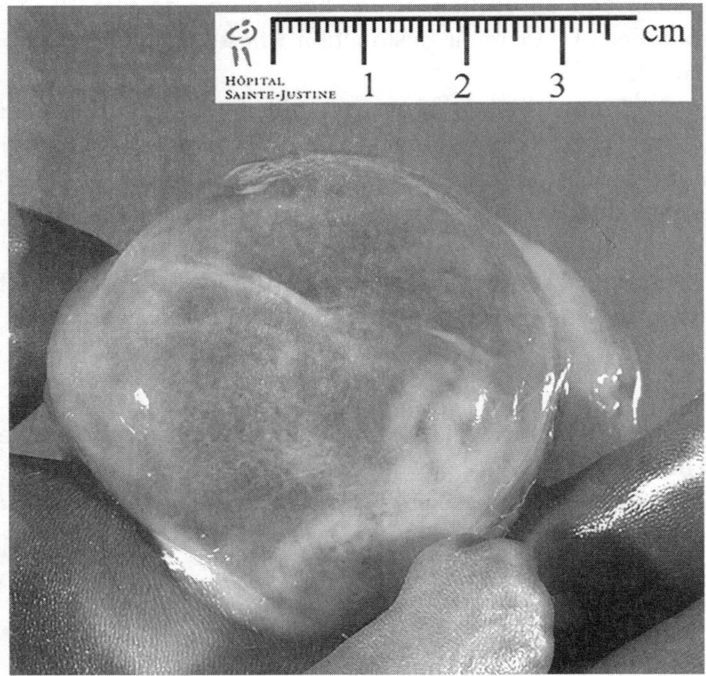

Fig. 14.1: Omphalocele.

4. **True about paracetamol toxicity in children:**
   a. Hypernatremia is a common side effect of N-acetylcysteine
   b. Liver failure may occur after 3–4 days
   c. Renal damage occurs very frequently
   d. N-acetylcysteine is very less effective if given after 24 hours of paracetamol ingestion
   e. N-acetylcysteine be given orally or iv

Ans. b, d, e *Ref: Ghai, 8/e*

Option a	False	Allergic and anaphylactoid reactions may occur
Option b	True	
Option c	False	Hepatotoxicity ensues
Option d	True	
Option e	True	

Paracetamol ingestion flowchart

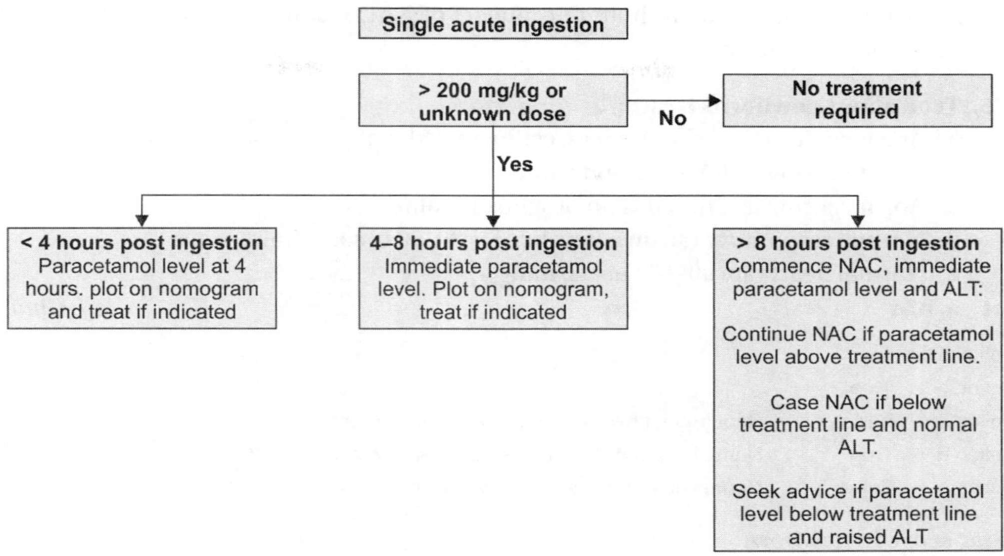

NAC: n-acetylcysteine ; ALT: Alanine transaminase

- The risk of developing toxic reactions to acetaminophen appear to be lower in children than in adults.
- The toxicity of acetaminophen is closely linked to its metabolism. With therapeutic dosing, acetaminophen is predominantly metabolized by conjugation with sulfate and glucuronide.
  Acetaminophen intoxication typically includes 4 phases:
- The first consists of anorexia, nausea, vomiting, malaise, and diaphoresis, which may provoke administration of additional doses of acetaminophen.
- In the second phase, those first-phase signs resolve and are replaced by right upper quadrant pain or tenderness, liver enlargement, and oliguria in some patients. Bilirubin and hepatic enzyme levels become elevated, and the prothrombin time becomes prolonged.
- In the third phase, usually 3 to 5 days into the course, anorexia, nausea, vomiting, and malaise reappear, along with signs of hepatic failure, including jaundice, hypoglycemia, coagulopathy, and encephalopathy. Renal failure and cardiomyopathy may also develop.
- The fourth phase is associated with recovery or progression to death from complete liver failure.
- Acetaminophen poisoning also may present as central nervous system depression, shock, hypothermia, and metabolic acidosis.
- N-acetylcysteine (NAC), is the antidote for acetaminophen.
- Because delays in treatment with NAC are associated with worse outcomes, early treatment is indicated when acetaminophen hepatotoxicity is considered likely. Even delayed therapy may be beneficial. Therefore, treatment should be considered even if 24 hours or more has elapsed since the last dose of acetaminophen was given.
- Most patients' liver enzymes will peak 3 or 4 days after their ingestion.

- ❑ NAC is available in oral and intravenous forms, and both are equally efficacious.
- ❑ Longer infusion periods (48 hours or longer) of NAC result in improved tolerance and reduced adverse effects.

5. True about newborns is/are:

a. Apgar score gives an immediate estimate of the physical condition of the baby
b. Apgar scoring is done at 1 and 5 min
c. Apgar scoring at 5 min has no prognostic value
d. Normal respiratory rate in a new born is 30–60 breaths/min
e. Normal heart rate 90–100 beats/min

Ans. a, b, d *Ref: Ghai, 8/e*

Option a	True	
Option b	True	
Option c	False	Required for hypoxic ischemic encephalopathy
Option d	True	Normal respiratory rate: 30–60 breaths/min
Option e	False	Normal heart rate: 120–160 beats/min

Apgar score in newborn

- ❑ Semi-objective measure of assessing the infant's respiratory, circulatory, and neurological status at birth.
- ❑ Normal babies have an Apgar score of more than 8 at one and five minutes.
- ❑ Apgar score between 4–8 is moderately low, less than 4 is very low.
- ❑ Five minute Apgar scores are more important than one minute scores. Most important cause of cardiopulmonary-neurological depression indicated by low Apgar scores is birth asphyxia. Hence, infants with low Apgar score at 5 minutes should be monitored for hypoxic ischemic encephalopathy.
- ❑ Low Apgar scores can also result from depression due to maternal drugs, fetal/neonatal infection, CNS trauma or malformations, myopathy or motor neuron disease.

Apgar score

Score	*0*	*1*	*2*
Respiratory effort	None	Slow, irregular	Good, crying
Heart rate/min	Absent	< 100	> 100
Color of the body	Blue or pale	Body Pink, extremities blue	Pink
Muscle tone	Flaccid	Some flexion	Actively moving the extremities
Reflex stimulation (catheter in the nose)	No response	Grimace	Cries, coughs or sneeze

6. True about atrial septal defect (ASD):

a. Ostium primum is most common type
b. Surgery usually done before 3 year
c. Surgery done in the first year of life
d. Second heart sound wide and fixed
e. Soft delayed diastolic rumble at the lower left sternal border

Ans. d, e *Ref: Ghai, 8/e*

Option a	False	Ostium secundum is the most common type
Option b	False	Elective closure is usually after the 1st year and before entry into school
Option c	False	
Option d	True	
Option e	True	Due to increased flow through tricuspid valve

Atrial septal defect (ASD):

- Abnormal communication between the two atria.
- Ostium secundum type of defect is 10 times more common than the ostium primum type and located at the *fossa ovalis* (superior or posterior).
- Ostium primum (endocardial cushion defect) type of defect is situated inferior to fossa ovalis.
- ASD leads to leaking of blood from left to right atrium at a minor difference in pressure between the two atria. Thus right to left shunt is *silent* on auscultation.
- The increased volume of right atrium passes through tricuspid valve producing a delayed diastolic murmur at the lower left sterna border.
- Pulmonary ejection murmur is produced.
- Pulmonary valve closes late and P_2 is delayed.
- Second sound is widely split and fixed.
- Lung field appear plethoric due to enlarged pulmonary artery and its branches.
- The timing for elective closure is usually after the 1st year and before entry into school.

Investigations:

The *electrocardiogram* of ostium secundum atrial septal defect is characterized by right axis deviation and right ventricular hypertrophy. The characteristic configuration of the precordial lead V1 is rsR' seen in almost 90 percent patients. Presence of left axis deviation beyond –30° suggests the ostium primum type of atrial septal defect.

The thoracic roentgenogram shows mild to moderate cardiomegaly, right atrial and right ventricular enlargement, prominent main pulmonary artery segment, a relatively small aortic shadow and plethoric lung fields. Echocardiogram shows increased size of the right ventricle with paradoxical ventricular septal motion. 2D echo in subcostal four chambered view identifies the defect.

Assessment of the severity: The size of the left to right shunt is directly proportional to the intensity of the two murmurs and the heart size. The larger to shunt the more the cardiomegaly and the louder the pulmonary and tricuspid murmurs.

Complications: Pulmonary arterial hypertension due to pulmonary vascular obstructive disease is rare in patients of atrial septal defect *below the age of 20 years.* It is recognized by the disappearance of the systolic and diastolic murmurs, appearance of a constant pulmonary ejection click and loud palpable P_2. *The second sound continues to be widely split and fixed.*

Treatment: The medical management consists in treating chest infections. *Infective endocarditis is very rare* in patients of ostium secundum atrial septal defect, unless floppy mitral valve is present.

The risk of operation for closure of atrial septal defect is now so low that asymptomatic patients are sent up for operation.

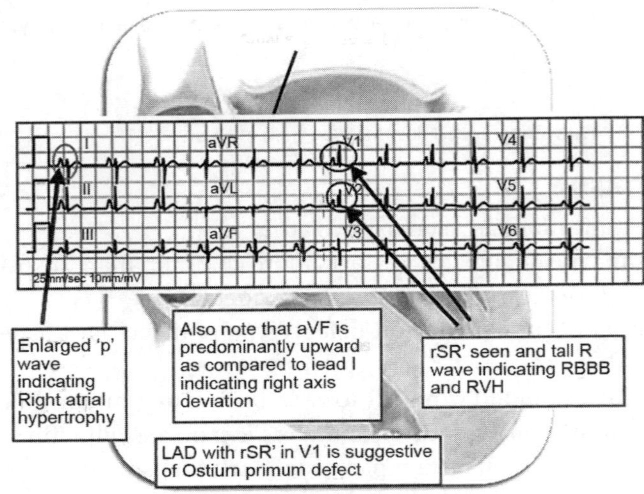

Fig. 14.2: ECG changes in ASD.

7. True about breast milk jaundice is:
- a. Increased bilirubin in urine
- b. Dark urine in diaper
- c. Bilirubin > 10–15 mg/dL
- d. Phototherapy is often required
- e. Usually occurs within first 7 days

Ans. c *Ref: Ghai, 8/e*

Option a	False	Suggests cholestatic jaundice and not breast milk jaundice
Option b	False	
Option c	True	
Option d	False	Not required
Option e	False	Occurs after first 7 days of life

Breast milk jaundice:
- ❑ Exclusive breastfeeding and neonatal jaundice have been seen to have a strong association.
- ❑ It is characterized by indirect hyperbilirubinemia in a breastfed newborn that develops after the first 7 days of life, persists longer than physiologic jaundice, and has no other identifiable cause.
- ❑ A bilirubin level of >20mg/dL may be attained.
- ❑ It is presumed to be due to inhibitory substances in the breast milk that interfere with bilirubin conjugation.
- ❑ Breast milk jaundice is a common cause of indirect hyperbilirubinemia.
- ❑ The prognosis is excellent, although jaundice in breastfed infants may persist for as long as 12 weeks.
- ❑ It should be differentiated from *breastfeeding jaundice*, which manifests in the first 3 days of life and is caused by insufficient production or intake of breast milk.

8. Which of the following is true regarding intussusception in children?

a. Vomiting
b. Most common site is Ileocaecal region
c. Distention
d. Painless in nature
e. Blood in stool

Ans. a, b, c, e *Ref: Ghai, 8/e*

Option a	True	
Option b	True	
Option c	True	
Option d	False	Severe, colicky abdominal pain
Option e	True	

Intussusception is a process in which a segment of intestine invaginates into the adjoining intestinal lumen, causing bowel obstruction.

- A common cause of abdominal pain in children.
- Classic triad of signs and symptoms: vomiting, abdominal pain, and passage of blood per rectum.

Intussusception in infants: Acute intestinal obstruction in infancy may be caused by intussusception. The child around the age of one year presents with severe, colicky abdominal pain manifesting as episodic crying. There is vomiting and stools are blood stained, like *currant jelly*. A sausage shaped mass may be palpable usually in the right quadrant of the abdomen. Right iliac fossa may appear empty Rectal examination may show the tip of the intussusceptum.

Barium enema X-ray film shows cupping, as it is obstructed by the intussusceptum. Ultrasonography may help. Intussusception may reduce under the pressure of barium enema.

Treatment: Intussusception is a surgical emergency. Shock is treated and the patient is rehydrated. In intussusception of short duration, hydrostatic pressure of the barium enema may relieve intussusception. This is not possible in ileoileal intussusception. Surgical management of intussusception carries little risk.

9. Maximum risk to fetus occurs when maternal infection with rubella occurs at which period of gestation (POG)?

a. 6–12 week POG
b. 12–18 week POG
c. 14–20 week POG
d. 20–24 week POG
e. 32–36 week POG

Ans. a *Ref: Ghai, 8/e*

Option a	True	
Option b	False	
Option c	False	
Option d	False	
Option e	False	

Congenital rubella syndrome (CRS) is an illness resulting from rubella virus infection during pregnancy.

- When rubella infection occurs during early pregnancy, serious consequences—such as miscarriages, stillbirths, and a constellation of severe birth defects in infants can result.
- The risk of congenital infection and defects is highest during the ***first 12 weeks of gestation*** and decreases after the 12th week of gestation. The defects are rare after the 20th week of gestation.

- Common congenital defects of CRS include *cataracts, congenital heart disease, hearing impairment, and developmental delay.*
- Infants with CRS usually present with more than one sign or symptom consistent with congenital rubella infection. However, infants may present with a single defect.
- Hearing impairment is the most common single defect.

10. True about constitutional growth delay is:

a. It is a normal variant
b. Delayed puberty
c. Shows after 2–3 months of life
d. Actual height is within normal limits
e. Baseline growth hormone decrease

Ans. a, b, d *Ref: Ghai, 8/e*

Option a	True	
Option b	True	
Option c	False	Growth delay starts between 3–6 months of age
Option d	True	
Option e	False	Growth hormone levels are within normal range

Constitutional growth delay:

- This is a significant cause of short stature in mid-childhood period.
- In this variant of normal growth, linear growth velocity and weight gain slows beginning as young as age 3–6 months but the ultimate height is normal.
- Their birth weight and height are normal.
- Extra years of prepubescent growth make up for the short stature of the earlier years.
- Bone age (epiphyseal development) is slightly less than that expected for the chronological age.
- Ratio between upper and lower segments is normal or slightly immature.
- Human growth hormone and gonadotropin levels after puberty are within normal range.
- No treatment is required.

11. Feature of pallid breath holding spell in comparison to cyanotic breath holding spell:

a. More common than cyanotic breath holding spell
b. Elicited by painful stimulus
c. Bradycardia is prominent
d. Atropine is given in refractory cases
e. Elicited in response to frustration

Ans. b, c, d *Ref: Ghai, 8/e*

Option a	False	Cyanotic spell is the most common type
Option b	True	
Option c	True	
Option d	True	
Option e	False	This is cyanotic spell

Breath holding spells occur only when the child is awake. There are 2 ways in which children with breath holding spells present:

- A **cyanotic spell** is caused by a change in the child's usual breathing pattern, usually in response to feeling angry or frustrated. It's the most common type. The child usually cries or screams loudly and then the cry gradually becomes noiseless as child open the mouth and holds the breath in expiration for about 20–30 sec (apnea). The child turns blue (cyanotic) and then the child may again start breathing or may proceed to lose consciousness. Sometimes, fits or seizure like activity may follow the loss of consciousness.
  The entire episode may last less than one minute and the child generally regains full activity within a few minutes.
- A **pallid spell** is caused by slowing of the child's heart rate, usually in response to pain or a fearful experience. The child becomes pale and often loses consciousness within a single gasp or cry.
  Breath holding spells are seen in 5% of children between 6 months to 6 years of age. They are commonly seen in children between 12 and 18 months and usually disappear by 4–5 years of age.
  Breath holding spells are an involuntary phenomenon (the child does not do it deliberately). They are usually seen in children with temper tantrums and other behavioral disorders.
  A positive family history may be found in about 25% of the cases.
  A breath-holding spell may cause:
- Fainting. It usually lasts for less than a minute.
- Twitching muscles, a stiff body, or a seizure.
- Changes in breathing and heartbeat.
  - In a cyanotic spell: The child may breathe too fast or too hard. When the child breathes out, there may be a long pause before the child takes another breath.
  - In a pallid spell: The heartbeat may slow down.
- Changes in skin color:
  - In a cyanotic spell: The skin may turn red or blue-purple, especially around the lips.
  - In a pallid spell: The skin may be pale and sweaty.
- Crying:
  - In a cyanotic spell: There may be a short burst of intense crying.
  - In a pallid spell: There may be a single cry or no cry at all.

Treatment:

- Behavior modification program may help if a child has frequent tantrums. Parents should be reassured that long term prognosis is very good.
- Pharmacological treatment is usually not required. Anticonvulsants have no role in breath holding spells. Atropine sulphate may be tried in children with frequent pallid spells.

12. High risk infants are:

a. Birth order > 3
b. Artificial feeding
c. Birth weight < 3 kg
d. Failure to gain weight for 3 consecutive months
e. Twinning

Ans. e *Ref: Ghai, 8/e*

Option a	False	Short interpregnancy interval
Option b	False	

Option c	False	Birth weight <2,500 or >4,000 g
Option d	False	Small or large for gestational age
Option e	True	

The term high-risk infant designates an infant who should be under close observation by experienced physicians and nurses.

High risk infants include:

- **Demographic social factors**
  - Maternal age <16 or >40 year
  - Illicit drug, alcohol, cigarette use
  - Poverty
  - Unmarried
  - Emotional or physical stress
- **Past medical history**
  - Genetic disorders
  - Diabetes mellitus
  - Hypertension
  - Asymptomatic bacteriuria
  - Rheumatologic illness (systemic lupus erythematosus)
  - Long-term medication
- **Previous pregnancy**
  - Intrauterine fetal demise
  - Neonatal death
  - Prematurity
  - Intrauterine growth restriction
  - Congenital malformation
  - Incompetent cervix
  - Blood group sensitization, neonatal jaundice
  - Neonatal thrombocytopenia
  - Hydrops
  - Inborn errors of metabolism
- **Present pregnancy**
  - Vaginal bleeding (abruptio placentae, placenta previa)
  - Sexually transmitted infections (colonization: herpes simplex, group B Streptococcus, Chlamydia, syphilis, hepatitis B, HIV)
  - Multiple gestation (Twinning)
  - Preeclampsia
  - Premature rupture of membranes
  - Short interpregnancy time
  - Poly/oligohydramnios
  - Acute medical or surgical illness
  - Inadequate prenatal care
  - Familial or acquired hypercoagulable states
  - Abnormal fetal ultrasonographic findings
  - Treatment of infertility

- **Labor and delivery**
  - Premature labor (<37 weeks)
  - Postdates pregnancy (≥42 weeks)
  - Fetal distress
  - Immature lecithin: Sphingomyelin ratio; absence of phosphatidylglycerol
  - Breech presentation
  - Meconium-stained fluid
  - Nuchal cord
  - Cesarean section
  - Forceps delivery
  - Apgar score <4 at 1 min
- **Neonate**
  - Birth weight < 2,500 or >4 ,000 g
  - Birth <37 or ≥ 42 weeks of gestation
  - Small or large for gestational age
  - Respiratory distress, cyanosis
  - Congenital malformation
  - Pallor, plethora, petechiae

13. Milestones in a 2-year-old child are:

a. Can ride a tricycle
b. Weight increases by 4 times as that of the birth
c. Takes alternate steps in climbing the stairs
d. Upper and lower canines show cusps
e. Knows gender

Ans. b, d *Ref: Ghai, 8/e*

Option a	False	At three years of age
Option b	True	
Option c	False	At 4 years of age, the child can walk upstairs and downstairs on her own with one foot per step
Option d	True	
Option e	False	At 3 years of age

Initially, during the first few months, the weight gain of the child is rapid. Then it slows down. From the second year onwards, till the adolescent period, the child gains just 2 to 2½ kgs every year, i.e. 200 gms a month.

From 2 to 7 years of age, the child's weight in kilograms can be calculated according to the following formula:

(age [years] + 4) × 2

Thus, at 2 years, the child should weigh about 12 kgs. *(Taking average birth weight as 2.9 kg, at the age of 2 years, the weight is almost 4 times that of birth weight).*

DEVELOPMENT AT 2 YEARS OF AGE

Two Years

- A child of 2 years *walks freely* on the ground.
- She can also go up and down the stairs by herself. While going down, *she may stop on each step with both feet before taking another step.*

- She can *stand up on her own* from a supine position. She can now climb onto and come down from furniture without help.
- With her building blocks, she can now *build a tower of 6 cubes* (At 15 months, the child can build a tower of 2 cubes, putting one cube on top of another. At 18 months and 21 months, she can build towers of 3 and 5 cubes, respectively).
- When shown how to, she can *imitate a vertical stroke* with a crayon or a pencil.
- She may now imagine different situations and start playing make-believe games. She can imitate others and wants to be in the company of other children.
- The child can now make simple sentences of 2 to 4 words and may keep chattering all the time.
- The child gives the first signal of bladder control at around 15 months of age when she starts telling that she has wet her pants. After about 18 months, she is mostly dry during the day, but may wet her clothes occasionally.

Tooth eruption times		
Teeth	***Number***	***Age at eruption***
Lower side teeth (lower lateral incisors)	2	12–15 months
First back teeth (first molars)	4	10–16 months
Eye teeth or cuspids (canines)	4	16–20 months
Second back teeth (second molars)	4	20–30 months

14. In which of the following syndrome, CNS malignancy is seen in children?

a. Turner's syndrome
b. Neurofibromatosis-II
c. Fanconi's syndrome
d. Sturge-Weber syndrome
e. Tuberous sclerosis

Ans. b, e *Ref: Ghai, 8/e*

Option a	False	
Option b	True	Auditory neuroma
Option c	False	
Option d	False	
Option e	True	Astrocytomas

Neurocutaneous syndromes in children:

- **Neurofibromatosis**: Inherited as autosomal dominant trait. There are two clinical types:
  - Type NF_1 (von-Recklinghausen's disease or peripheral NF_1)- deletion or inactivation of NF gene on chromosome 17.
  - Type NF_2 (central neuro bromatosis):
    - Gene for NF_2 is probably located on chromosome 22.
    - Presence of *bilateral auditory neuroma*
    - *Unilateral auditory neuroma* along with first degree relative with meningioma, schwannoma or juvenile posterior subcapsular lenticular opacity.
- **Tuberous sclerosis complex (TSC):** Inherited as autosomal dominant trait. Defective organization occurs by 30 weeks of gestation. Findings include:
  - *Neurologic:* result from the location, size, and growth of tubers and the presence of *subependymal nodules (SENs)* and *subependymal giant cell astrocytomas (SEGAs).*
  - *Cutaneous:* The best-known cutaneous manifestation of TSC is *adenoma sebaceum,* which often does not appear until late childhood or early adolescence. Shagreen patches, ungula fibromas.

- *Cardiac:* Cardiac involvement is usually maximal at birth or early in life; it may be the presenting sign of TSC, particularly in early infancy; 50–60% of individuals with TSC have evidence of cardiac disease, mostly *rhabdomyomas.*
- *Ophthalmic:* At least 50% of patients have ocular abnormalities; these lesions are actually *retinal astrocytomas* that tend to become calcified over time.
- *Pulmonary:* cystic pulmonary abnormalities.
- *Renal:* Renal manifestations of TSC are the second most common clinical feature; 4 types of lesions can occur: *autosomal dominant polycystic kidney disease lesions, isolated renal cyst(s), angiomyolipomas (AMLs), and renal cell carcinomas.*
- *Dental: Pitting of the dental enamel* is invariably present in the permanent teeth of patients with TSC ; gingival fibromas occur in 50% of children with mixed dentition (primary and permanent teeth), and in 3% of children with only primary teeth.
- *Gastrointestinal: Hamartomas and polyposis* of the stomach, intestine, and colon may occur.
- *Hepatic: Hepatic cysts.*
- *Skeletal: Sclerotic and hypertrophic lesions of bone* may be found incidentally.

- **Sturge-Weber syndrome:** characterized by:
  - Facial nevus flammeus
  - Contralateral focal seizures
  - Calcification of cortex and subcortical structures
  - Glaucoma on same side as skin lesions.
- **Von-Hippel-Lindau disease:** retinal and cerebellar hemangioblastomas, spinal cord angiomas, cystic tumor of pancreas, kidney and epididymis.
- **Ataxia telangiectasia:** Cerebellar ataxia, oculocutaneous telangiectasia, choreoathetosis, lymphoreticular malignancies, immune deficiency.

15. What can be done in a 2-year-old child with mediastinal mass with stridor and puffy face and enlarged cervical lymph nodes?

a. Oxygen inhalation
b. Tracheostomy
c. Endoscopy and biopsy
d. Aspiration cytology
e. Chemoradiation therapy

Ans. a, e *Ref: Ghai, 8/e*

Option a	True	
Option b	False	Emergency thoracotomy may be done
Option c	False	Not done due to the fear of tumor cell seeding in the biopsy tract
Option d	False	
Option e	True	Done to shrink size of the tumor/mass

A growing tumor in the mediastinum has both respiratory and hemodynamic consequences. Respiratory decompensation is caused by mechanical obstruction of either the trachea or the bronchi. At its most severe this can result in complete ventilation/perfusion mismatch, shunt and consequent hypoxia. Hence, oxygen inhalation support has to be given actively.

Hemodynamic decompensation can occur if the heart or major vessels (pulmonary artery, superior vena cave) are surrounded or infiltrated by the tumor. If impingement of the pulmonary artery occurs, decreased pulmonary perfusion, hypoxemia and acute right ventricular heart failure can occur.

The role of obtaining tissue diagnosis in the evaluation of mediastinal masses remains to be controversial due to the fear of tumor cell seeding in the biopsy tract, especially when thymic neoplasms are likely. As proposed by the National Comprehensive Cancer Network Guidelines on thymic malignancies, surgical biopsy should be avoided if a resectable thymoma is strongly suspected based on clinical and radiologic features. If biopsy is performed, transpleural approaches should be avoided.

Treatment: Chemotherapy/radiotherapy and cystic aspiration is done preoperatively in an attempt to shrink the tumor size and relieve airway compression.

16. Foreign body in children, all are correct *except*:

a. More chances of foreign body in the right bronchus
b. M/c is ingested food
c. Tracheal obstruction causes sudden death
d. Vegetable is not common
e. Treatment of choice is endoscopic removal by rigid bronchoscope

Ans. d *Ref: Ghai, 8/e*

Option a	True	
Option b	True	
Option c	True	
Option d	False	Foreign bodies of vegetable origin are common
Option e	True	

Foreign Body Aspiration

Young children between 1 and 4 years of age are especially prone to aspirate small objects in their air passages. Unless recognized and treated, these children have significant respiratory morbidity, such as recurrent wheezing, cough and pneumonia. Immediate response to foreign body aspiration is a choke, gag, cough or localized wheeze. After the initial episode, symptoms may improve for some time and the whole episode may be forgotten. Subsequently, the course of illness depends on the nature of foreign body, its size, extent and the site of obstruction. Foreign bodies of organic or vegetable source swell up and cause more symptoms.

A ***partial obstruction*** may cause ball valve type effect leading to localized hyperinflation. The overlying chest wall may show hyperresonance, diminished vocal resonance and poor air entry. In small children, it may be difficult to elicit hyperresonance. Thus a localized area of poor air entry in a child with chronic respiratory illness should arouse suspicion of a foreign body.

Complete obstruction and surrounding inflammation cause distal atelectasis and suppuration of the surrounding parenchyma of the lungs. The elastic recoil of the bronchi is lost and the bronchi show segmental dilation with eventual development of bronchiectasis. In children incidence of right and left bronchial location of foreign body is nearly equal.

Treatment: These children are treated by removal of foreign body through a bronchoscope. Appropriate antibiotics are given for secondary infection. Bronchoscopy should be undertaken if the clinical and radiological picture suggests the diagnosis even when the history of foreign body aspiration is not forthcoming.

17. Hepatomegaly seen in 5-month-old child, true is:

a. Gaucher's disease
b. Tuberculosis
c. Hepatoblastoma
d. Hemangioendothelioma
e. Biliary atresia

Ans. a, c, d, e *Ref: Ghai, 8/e*

Option a	True	The age of onset for Gaucher disease type 2 is during early infancy
Option b	False	Seen in older children
Option c	True	
Option d	True	
Option e	True	

Palpability of liver does not always indicate hepatomegaly, it only reflects the relation of liver to adjacent structures. In normal children, liver is palpable 1 cm below the costal margin and in infants, it may be felt up to 2 cm below the costal margin.

Causes of hepatomegaly in children	
Infancy	
Infections	Biliary obstruction
Intrauterine (TORCH) infection	EBHA
Septicemia	*Infiltration*
Neonatal hepatitis	Erythroblastosis fetalis
	Histiocytosis
Storage disorders/metabolic	Tumors
Glycogen storage disease	
Galactosemia	*Congestive cardiac failure*
Peroxisomal disorders	
α_1-antitrypsin deficiency	
Mucopolysaccharidosis	
Hemochromatosis	
Older children	
Infections	*Storage/Metabolic disorders*
Acute hepatitis	Glycogen storage disorders
Chronic viral hepatitis	Mucopolysaccharidosis
Pyogenic/amebic liver abscess	Lipidoses
Infectious mononucleosis	α-1 antitrypsin deficiency
Hydatid cyst	Wilson's disease
Fatty infiltration	*Congestion*
Kwashiorkor	Congestive cardiac failure
Tetracycline toxicity	Pericardial diseases
Tuberculosis	Budd-Chiari Syndrome
Cystic fibrosis	Veno-occlusive disease of the liver

Contd...

Contd...

Cellular infiltration	*Other*
Lymphoreticular malignancies	Congenital cyst
Hepatic neoplasms	
Metastasis	
Histiocytosis	

18. True about Wilson's disease in children:

a. Serum ceruloplasmin< 20 mg/dL
b. Urinary copper < 40 μg/day
c. Kayser-Fleischer ring
d. Copper> 250 μg/gm of dry weight of liver
e. Neurologic disturbances

Ans. a, c, d, e *Ref: Ghai, 8/e*

Option a	True	
Option b	False	Increased to > 100 μg/day
Option c	True	
Option d	True	
Option e	True	

- Inborn error of copper metabolism.
- Inherited as autosomal recessive pattern, defective gene is mapped to chromosome 13.
- Copper accumulates in the cytoplasm of liver cells up to a level of 500–2000μg/gm of dry weight of liver.
- Liver cells are damaged, copper released in the serum and then deposited in other tissues and cells.
- Red blood cells are damaged resulting in hemolysis.
- Deposition in the cornea results in Kayser-Fleischer rings.
- Toxic effects of copper on brain cells cause neurologic disturbances.
- Low levels of ceruloplasmin are characteristic.

Clinical features:

- The clinical presentation can be extremely varied, viz., acute or chronic liver disease with or without neurological disease, psychiatric problems, bony deformities, hemolytic anemia and endocrine manifestations.
- *Hepatic dysfunction.* The patients are younger, generally between 6 and 15 years of age. The illness starts acutely with jaundice and hepatomegaly, progressing rapidly to hepatic coma and death. The course of the illness may simulate chronic active hepatitis.
- *Neurological presentation.* These patients are generally older and present with symptoms of basal ganglia involvement, e.g., rigidity, tremors, difficulty in speech, poor handwriting and abnormal posture. There may also be psychiatric disturbances. Performance at the school may deteriorate. The illness appears as a combination of cerebellar ataxia and Parkinsonism. Although the liver may be enlarged, jaundice is usually absent. Kayser-Fleischer (KF) ring appears rusty brown in color usually along with upper and lower borders of cornea. It should be looked for by slit lamp examination. Absence of the ring does not exclude the diagnosis of Wilson disease, especially in the first decade of life.

Diagnosis. Low ceruloplasmin, high 24 h urinary copper and presence of KF rings help in diagnosis. The serum ceruloplasmin level is less than 20 mg/dL and serum copper concentration is below 20 μg/dL. More than 100 μg of copper is excreted in the urine in 24 hours. Urinary copper estimation is usually done with a penicillamine challenge. Liver copper concentration exceeds 250 μg/g of dry weight. Liver function tests are abnormal.

- Low serum copper and ceruloplasmin levels are not characteristic of Wilson disease in infants up to the age of 6 months and in patients with nephrosis, kwashiorkor or severe malabsorption syndrome.

19. True about benign neonatal seizure is/are:

a. Prolonged convulsions
b. Followed by febrile seizures later in life
c. Followed by infantile spasm later in life
d. More common in preterm children
e. Seizure resolve usually by 6 months

Ans. e *Ref: Ghai, 8/e*

Option a	False	Convulsions last for very brief periods
Option b	False	No neurological sequelae later in life
Option c	False	
Option d	False	Occur in full term or near full term infants
Option e	True	

- Benign neonatal convulsions are defined as seizures with onset after birth through day 28 in an otherwise healthy child with no other known medical or neurologic problems.
- They are not classified as epilepsy.
- Psychomotor development is normal for a full-term or near full-term infant with benign convulsions.
- Between seizures, findings on neurologic examination are normal.
- Clinically, the seizures are frequent and brief, occasionally occurring many times within a day.
- The brief seizures are followed by a short or no postictal state.
- The episodes usually resolve within days but may continue for several months and have no neurologic sequelae.
- Majority of them usually resolve by 6 months of age.

20. True about antiphospholipid antibodies (APLA) is/are:

a. Disease of fetus
b. Increased thrombosis
c. Association with neuropsychiatric symptoms
d. Increased bleeding
e. No association with SLE

Ans. a, b, c *Ref: Ghai, 8/e*

Option a	True	
Option b	True	
Option c	True	

Option d	False	Vascular thrombosis
Option e	False	Clear association with SLE

Antiphospholipid antibodies (APLA) are group of antibodies directed against epitopes on plasma proteins that are uncovered by binding of these proteins to anionic phospholipids on plasma membranes.

The most commonly used tests to detect APLA include:

- Lupus anticoagulant (LAC),
- Anticardiolipin (ACL) antibodies, and
- Anti-β2 -glycoprotein I antibodies.

Antiphospholipid antibodies associated with vaso-occlusive events without any underlying disease process is termed the ***primary antiphospholipid antibody syndrome (PAPS).***

Antiphospholipid antibodies are associated with both venous and arterial thrombosis.

Clinical criteria for APLA include the following:

- **Vascular thrombosis:** One or more clinical episodes of arterial, venous, or small vessel thrombosis in any tissue or organ confirmed by imaging studies, Doppler studies, or histopathology (without significant vessel wall inflammation)
- **Pregnancy morbidity** (normal morphology on ultrasonography or direct examination findings)
  - One or more unexplained fetal deaths at more than 10 weeks' gestation
  - One or more premature births at less than 34 weeks' gestation due to severe preeclampsia, eclampsia, or placental insufficiency
  - Three or more unexplained consecutive spontaneous abortions at less than 10 weeks' gestation, excluding maternal anatomic or hormonal abnormalities and paternal and maternal chromosomal causes.

Laboratory criteria include the following:

- **Anticardiolipin (aCL) antibody** of the immunoglobulin G (IgG)/immunoglobulin M (IgM) isotype in medium/high titer [> 40 IgG phospholipid units (GPL), > 40 IgM phospholipid units (MPL), or > 99th percentile] on 2 or more occasions at least 12 weeks apart [measured by a b2-GPI–dependent enzyme-linked immunosorbent assay (ELISA)].
- **Lupus anticoagulant** on 2 or more occasions at least 12 weeks apart, according to the guidelines set forth by the International Society of Thrombosis and Hemostasis Scientific Subcommittee on Lupus Anticoagulants/Phospholipid-dependent antibodies.
  - *Prolonged phospholipid-dependent coagulation* [e.g., aPTT, Kaolin clotting time (KCT), dilute russell viper venom test, dilute PT]
  - Failure to correct the prolonged coagulation time by a mix with platelet poor plasma (PPP)
  - Shortening or correction of the prolonged coagulation time with excess phospholipid
  - Exclusion of other coagulopathies (e.g., factor VIII inhibitor, heparin)

A patient must meet at least one clinical and one laboratory criterion for a diagnosis of antiphospholipid antibody syndrome.

Vasospastic or vaso-occlusive events can occur in any organ system.

High incidence of APLA has been seen in patients with SLE.

Possible consequences of APS	
Cardiovascular	Cerebrovascular accident, sinus thrombosis, cardiac valvulopathy, myocardial infraction
Dermatologic	Livedo reticularis, purpura, infarcts/ulceration
Hematologic	Thrombocytopenia, hemolytic anemia, arterial or venous thromboembolic disease
Musculoskeletal	Avascular necrosis of bone and other infarctions or hemorrhage
Neurologic	Stroke, transient ischemic attacks, cognitive dysfunction
Obstetric	Spontaneous abortion, preterm delivery (before 34 weeks), pre-eclampsia, eclampsia, or placental insufficiency
Ophthalmic	Ocular thrombosis
Pulmonary	Embolism, pulmonary hypertension

APS = Antiphospholipid syndrome

Obstetrics and Gynecology

1. Dual marker for Down syndrome in second trimester:

a. Beta hCG

b. AFP

c. PAPP-A

d. Inhibin A

e. Acetylcholinesterase

Ans. a, c *Ref: Obstetrics by DC Dutta, 7th/ed p493,493,106*

Option a	True	Yes, it is a part of dual screen
Option b	False	No, not correct
Option c	True	Yes, it is a part of dual screen
Option d	False	No, not correct
Option e	False	No, not correct

Screening	Marker	Period of gestation	Detection rate of Down syndrome
First trimester (NT + dual markers)	Nuchal translucency (NT) Dual markers: PAPP–A Beta HCG	10 - 13+6 weeks	82-87%
Triple screen	AFP Beta HCG uE3	15 – 22 weeks	69%
Quadruple screen	AFP Beta HCG uE3 Dimeric inhibin A	15 – 22 weeks	81%
Penta screen	AFP Beta HCG uE3 Dimeric inhibin A + hyperglycosylated hCG (also known as invasive trophoblast antigen)	15 – 22 weeks	Limited data

Second trimester test for Down syndrome is:

1. Triple marker test
   a. AFP (Alpha-fetoprotein)
   b. uE3 (unconjugated Estriol)
   c. hCG (Human Chorionic gonadotrophin)
2. Quadruple Marker Test (Also called Quad scan) - This includes:
   a. AFP (Alpha-fetoprotein)
   b. uE3 (unconjugated Estriol)
   c. hCG (Human Chorionic gonadotrophin)
   d. Inhibin A

AFP levels:

- ❑ Done between 15 and 20 weeks
- ❑ Elevated MSAFP
  - Wrong gestational age
  - Open NTD (with reasonable sensitivity)
  - Multiple pregnancy
  - Intrauterine fetal death
  - Anterior abdominal wall defects
  - Renal anomalies
- ❑ Low MSAFP
  - In Down: MSAFP and U3 are low with high hCG
  - Edward syndrome (trisomy 18)
  - Gestational trophoblastic disease

Acetylcholinesterase:

- ❑ Elevated in open NTD (better diagnostic value than AFP).

Inhibin A

- ❑ Is a dimeric glycoprotein produced by corpus luteum and placenta. It is increased in Down syndrome.

Down syndrome screening

1. First trimester screening: ↑hCCG, ↓MSAFP, ↓PAPP
2. 2nd Trimester screening:
   - Dual screening: ↑hCCG, ↓MSAFP
   - Triple screening: ↑hCCG, ↓MSAFP, ↓U3
   - Quadruple test: ↑hCCG, ↑inhibin, ↓MSAFP, ↓U3
3. Prenatal genetic testing
   a. Amniocentesis: 14-16 weeks
   b. Chorionic villus sampling: transcervical: 10-12 weeks ; transabdominal 10 weeks
   c. Cordocentesis: 18-20 weeks

2. Patient presents with secondary amenorrhea. The progesterone test is negative but the estrogen and progesterone Challenge test is positive. What is the probable diagnosis?

a. Hypo-pituitary failure
b. Ovarian failure
c. Pregnancy
d. Asherman syndrome
e. Anovulation

Ans. a, b

Option a	True	Low estrogen, low to normal FSH
Option b	True	Hypergonadotropic hypogonadism, low estrogen high FSH, LH
Option c	False	Pregnancy has high levels of estrogen and progesterone
Option d	False	Progesterone Challenge test negative; Normal hormone profile
Option e	False	Eugonadotropic hypogonadism

Primary amenorrhea: It is defined as no menses by
- Age 13- in the *absence* of secondary sexual characteristics
- Age 15- in the *presence* of secondary sexual characteristics

Secondary amenorrhea: It is the absence of menses for more than 3 months in a female who menstruates regularly or absence of menses for 6 months in a female who menstruates irregularly.

Causes: Hypothalamus/Pituitary/Ovary/Outflow Tract

1. Hypothalamus (hypogonadotropic hypogonadism: Low estrogen, low to normal FSH) Diagnosis of exclusion: Hypo-hypo in the absence of any pituitary disease.
   a. Kallmann syndrome
   b. Eating disorders: Anorexia, bulimia
   c. Extreme physical, emotional, nutritional stress
   d. Strenuous exercise
   e. Recent significant weight loss
2. Pituitary (hypogonadotropic hypogonadism – low estrogen, low to normal FSH)
   a. Adenoma
      - Lactotroph adenoma or prolactinoma : Constitutes 40% of all clinically recognized pituitary adenomas. Non-functional macroadenoma causes pituitary amenorrhea while functional micro or macroadenomas that cause hyperprolactinemia lead to anovulatory amenorrhea.
      - **Others:** Gonadotroph adenoma, thyrotroph adenoma, somatotroph adenoma, corticotroph adenoma,
   b. **Other tumors:** Craniopharyngioma, chordoma, glioma, meningioma,
   c. **Non neoplastic masses:** TB, sarcoidosis, cysts
   d. **Infiltrative disorders:** Lymphocytic hypophysitis, hemochromatosis, hemosiderosis

e. Empty sella syndrome
   - **Primary:** Congenital defect in sellar diaphragm (rare)
   - **Secondary:** Post surgery for adenoma, post radiation or infarction

f. Sheehan syndrome

3. Ovary
   a. **Primary gonadal failure:** XX, XY, XO (hypergonadotropic hypogonadism, low estrogen high FSH, LH)
      - XO or XX ovarian dysgenesis: Most common cause of primary amenorrhea
      - **XX:** Testicular disorder of sexual development
      - **XY:** Swyer's syndrome
   b. Premature ovarian failure (hypergonadotropic hypogonadism, low estrogen high FSH, LH)
      - Numerical or structural chromosomal abnormalities
      - FMR1 permutations/Fragile X permutations
      - Autoimmune ovarian failure
      - Destruction of ovary by radiation or surgery
      - Savage syndrome
      - Galactosemia
   c. Anovulation (Eugonadotropic hypogonadism)
      - PCOS
      - Hyperprolactinemia
      - Thyroid disorders (both hypo and hyperthyroidism)
      - Obesity
      - Reproductive ageing (perimenopausal anovulation)
      - Reproductive immaturity (perimenarchal anovulation)
4. **Outflow tract abnormality:** (Normal hormone profile)
   a. Imperforate hymen (0.5–1 in 1000)
   b. Transverse vaginal septum (1 in 70,000)
   c. Cervical stenosis (rare)
   d. Mullerian agenesis, other reproductive tract anomalies, androgen insensitivity syndrome
   e. Vaginal agenesis
   f. Ashermans syndrome
   g. TB endometritis

Evaluation of Secondary Amenorrhea

In any female presenting with amenorrhea, the first test to be done is a urine pregnancy test. Those who test negative will be evaluated further for the causes of secondary amenorrhea.

A clinical examination at this stage will give an idea of presence of any signs of hirsutism or reproductive tract anomalies. Pelvic imaging may be advised if any anomalies are suspected.

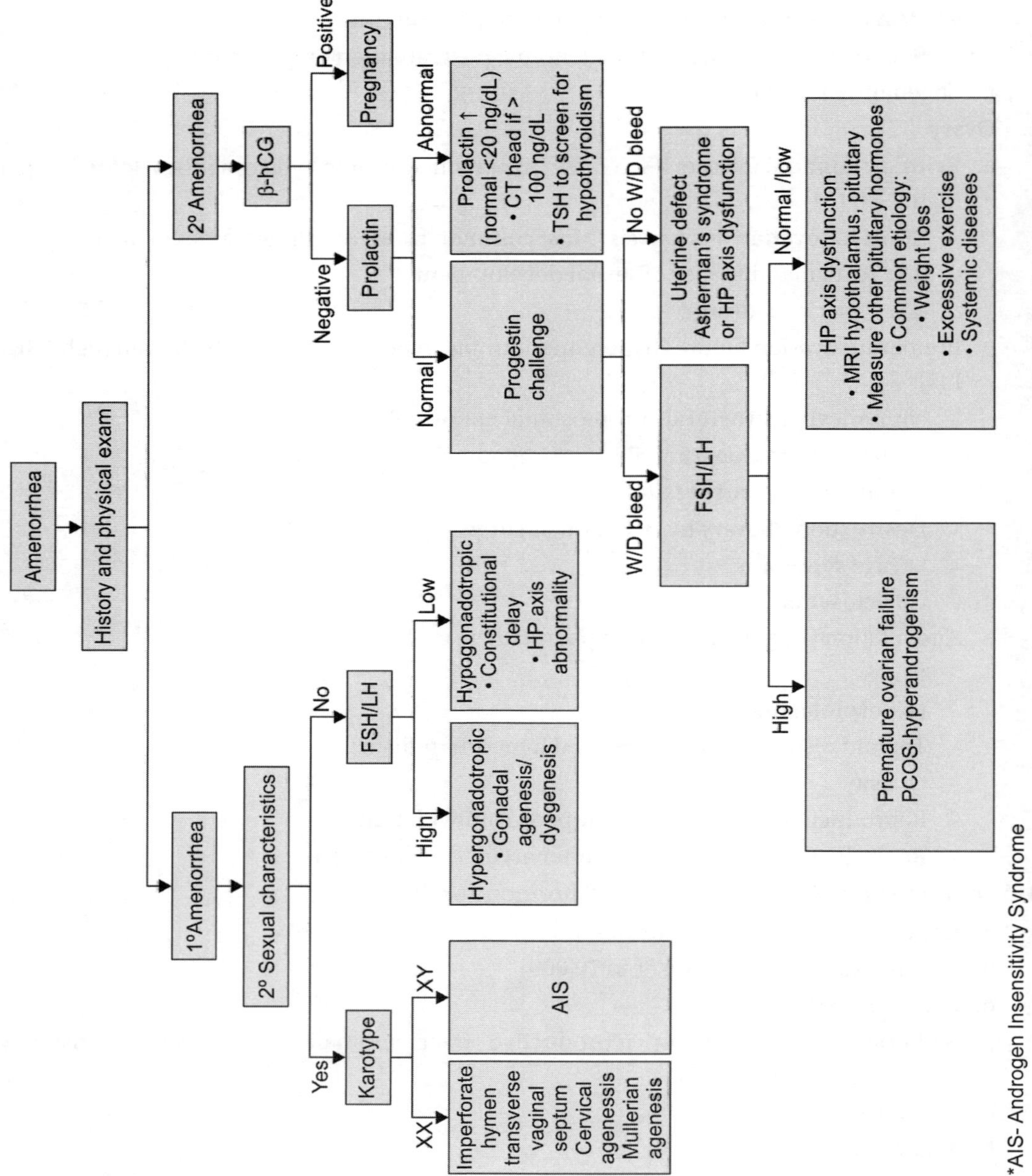

*AIS- Androgen Insensitivity Syndrome

Endocrine disorders (thyroid disorders and hyperprolactinemia) are important causes of amenorrhea and can be easily evaluated and treated. Hence the next tests to be done are serum TSH and prolactin levels. Females with these endocrine disorders will often resume normal menses with correction of the respective hormonal imbalances.

Amenorrheic women with normal TSH and prolactin will need further evaluation for the cause of amenorrhea. These women are subjected to the progesterone challenge test. The progestin challenge test is based on the premise that progestin treatment (e.g., medroxyprogesterone acetate 10 mg daily for 5–7 days) will induce menses only in those having normal circulating estrogen concentrations. A positive test—bleeding within 2–7 days after completion of progestin treatment—implies normal estrogen production and ovarian function, and a negative test—no withdrawal menses—suggests hypogonadism. Scant withdrawal bleeding or spotting suggests marginal levels of endogenous estrogen production.

Those with a negative progesterone challenge test may further be subjected to an Estrogen plus Progesterone challenge. A positive test indicates lack of estrogen production in the body or a state of hypogonadism. Lack of Estrogen can result from two basic mechanisms, 1. Hypothalamo-pituitary dysfunction leading to decreased gonadotropins (hypogonadotropic hypogonadism) or 2. primary gonadal failure with feedback rise in gonadotropins (hypergonadotropic hypogonadism).

In such women serum FSH level will help to differentiate between hypogonadotropic and hypergonadotropic hypogonadism.

A negative estrogen plus progesterone test indicates a need for pelvic evaluation and imaging to rule out reproductive tract and outflow anomalies.

3. A female uses the oral contraceptive pills and accidently misses 3 pills for 3 consecutive days. What is the next management?

a. Barrier method for 10 days and then start new cycle
b. Immediate insertion of an intrauterine device
c. Take missed pills and continue as usual
d. Take levonorgestrel emergency contraception
e. Use Barrier method of contraception for 7 days in the same cycle

Ans. c,d,e

Option a	False	Use barrier method for next 7 days
Option b	False	Take emergency contraception as levonorgestrel
Option c	True	True, Take missed pills as soon as you remember and continue as usual
Option d	True	True, Take levonorgestrel emergency contraception
Option e	True	True, Use barrier method for next 7 days

Missed pills	How to manage
Missed 1 or 2 pills/started new pack 1 or 2 days late	Take one hormonal pill as soon as possible or two pills at scheduled time There is little or no risk of pregnancy
Missed 3 or more pills in the first or second week/started new pack 3 or more days late?	Take one hormonal pill as soon as possible and continue the scheduled pill. Use a backup method for the next 7 days Also can consider taking ECPs, if she had sex in the past 72 hours
Missed 3 or more pills in the third week?	Take one hormonal pill as soon as possible and finish all hormonal pills in the pack as scheduled. Throw away the 7 non-hormonal pills in a 28-pill pack. Start a new pack the next day Use a backup method for the next 7 days Also can consider taking ECPs, if she had sex in the past 72 hours.

Contd...

Contd...

Missed pills	How to manage
Missed any nonhormonal pills? (last 7 pills in 28-pills pack)	Discard the missed non-hormonal pill(s). Keep taking COCs, one each day. Start the new pack as usual.
Severe vomiting or diarrhea	If she vomits within 2 hours after taking a pill, she should take another pill from pack as soon as possible and continue taking the scheduled pills. If she has vomiting or diarrhea for more than 2 days, follow instructions for 1 or 2 missed pills above.

Missed 3 or more pills in the second week – take one pill as soon as possible, also take the scheduled pill (even if it means you have to take two pills on the same day). Use back up contraception for 7 days (most commonly advised – barrier). Use emergency contraception (e.g. Levonorgestrel or LNG) if had sex in the past 72 hours.

4. Cause(s) for secondary postpartum hemorrhage is/are:

a. Retained placenta
b. Uterine atony
c. Trauma
d. Coagulopathy
e. Infection

Ans. a, e

Ref: Babarinsa IA, Hayman RG, Draycott TJ. Secondary post-partum haemorrhage: challenges in evidence-based causes and management. Eur J Obstet Gynecol Reprod Biol. 2011;159:255–60; Mavrides E, Allard S, Chandraharan E, Collins P, Green L, Hunt BJ, Riris S, Thomson AJ on behalf of the Royal College of Obstetricians and Gynaecologists. Prevention and management of postpartum haemorrhage. BJOG. 2016;124:e106–e149.

Option a	True	True, it causes secondary PPH
Option b	False	Cause of early postpartum hemorrhage
Option c	False	Cause of early postpartum hemorrhage
Option d	False	Cause of early postpartum hemorrhage
Option e	True	True, it causes secondary PPH

Causes of secondary postpartum hemorrhage (SPPH)

- ❑ Variant pattern of lochia rubra
- ❑ Idiopathic subinvolution of the uteroplacental vessels
- ❑ Abnormalities of placenta
- ❑ Sub-involution of the placental implantation site
- ❑ Retained placental tissue
- ❑ Placenta accreta, increta or percreta
- ❑ Abnormally adherent isolated lobe of placenta
- ❑ **Infection:** Endometritis, endomyometritis, infection and dehiscence of cesarean section scar
- ❑ Congenital coagulopathies: Von Willebrand's disease/Hemophilia A carrier/Factor XI deficiency/Factor VII deficiency
- ❑ Un-adjusted anticoagulant therapy
- ❑ Pre-existing uterine pathology

- Vascular malformation of the uterus
- Submucous fibroids
- Carcinoma of the cervix
- Trauma
- Rupture of vulval hematoma
- Non-uterine bleeding
- Pseudoaneurysm of the uterine artery
- Gestational trophoblastic disease

The commonest presumed cause of SPPH is 'infection,' specifically endometritis.

Management

In women presenting with secondary PPH, an assessment of vaginal microbiology should be performed (high vaginal and endocervical swabs) and appropriate use of antimicrobial therapy should be initiated when endometritis is suspected.

A pelvic ultrasound may help to exclude the presence of retained products of conception (RPOC).

A color flow Doppler study of the placental bed should be concurrently undertaken. Suspicion of a possible arterio-venous malformation or pseudoaneurysm of the uterus (UAP) may be made from finding an anechoic or hypoechoic pulsatile well defined para-uterine or uterine mass on pelvic scan. Doppler confirms the presence of turbulent flow within the cystic structure.

If the cause of the SPPH is known, then treatment should be specific and focused on the possible underlying pathological process. The specific treatments for SPPH are conservative, pharmacological or surgical; or by interventional radiology.

If the patient is not unwell, not anemic, and no tachycardia and SPPH is not heavy or increasing, it is reasonable to reassure and observe for a few days and make arrangements for regular review, or for her to keep in touch at intervals.

If there are no demonstrable retained products on pelvic scan, no abnormal findings on uterine Dopplers, but the bleeding is persistently heavier than patient's own menstrual blood loss, a course of oral Misoprostol (first week post-partum) or Tranexamic Acid [after the second week] could be considered.

Any patient with SPPH who presents for the first time (or in whom SPPH persists) after 6 weeks, may benefit from a course of antibiotics.

5. Absolute contraindication of medical abortion include-

a. Prostaglandin hypersensitivity
b. Chronic adrenal failure
c. Ectopic pregnancy
d. Anemia
e. Preexisting Heart disease

Ans. a,b,c

Option a	True	True, previous allergic reaction to one of the drugs (mifepristone or misoprostol)
Option b	True	Yes, true

Option c	True	Yes, known or suspected ectopic pregnancy
Option d	False	Caution to be used only in cases of severe anemia, but not an absolute contraindication
Option e	False	Not an absolute contraindication.

Contraindications to medical method of abortion

- Previous allergic reaction to one of the drugs involved (mifepristone or misoprostol)
- Inherited porphyria
- Chronic adrenal failure
- Known or suspected ectopic pregnancy (neither misoprostol nor mifepristone will treat ectopic pregnancy)

Caution and clinical judgement are required in cases of:

- Long-term corticosteroid therapy (including those with severe uncontrolled asthma)
- Hemorrhagic disorder
- Severe anemia
- Pre-existing heart disease or cardiovascular risk factors
- IUD in place (remove before beginning the regimen

Ref: Clinical practice handbook for safe abortion, World Health Organisation, 2014

6. True about benign gestational trophoblastic disease is/are:

a. Placental disorder
b. Snow storm appearance on USG
c. 69XXY
d. 2 spermatozoa fertilize one ovum
e. Some fetal components can be seen

Ans. a,b,c,d

Option a	True	Yes, true
Option b	True	Yes, true
Option c	True	Yes, true
Option d	True	Yes, true
Option e	False	No fetal parts can be seen

Gestational trophoblastic disease (GTD) can be benign or malignant. Histologically, it is classified into:

- Hydatidiform mole,
- Invasive mole (chorioadenoma destruens),
- Choriocarcinoma, and
- Placental site trophoblastic tumor (PSTT).

Those that invade locally or metastasize are collectively known as gestational trophoblastic neoplasia (GTN).

Hydatidiform moles are abnormal pregnancies characterized histologically by aberrant changes within the placenta. Classically, the chorionic villi in these placenta show varying degrees of trophoblast proliferation and edema of the stroma within villi.

Hydatidiform moles are categorized as either *complete hydatidiform moles* or *partial hydatidiform moles.*

Complete Mole

- Most common type of hydatidiform mole
- Diffuse trophoblastic hyperplasia, hydropic, swelling of chorionic villi, no fetal tissues, or membranes present
- 46XX or 46XY, chromosomes completely of paternal origin (90%)
- 2 sperm fertilize empty egg of 1 sperm with reduplication
- 15–20% risk of progression to malignant sequelae
- Risk factors
  - Geographic (South East Asia most common)
  - Others (maternal age >40 yr, β-carotene deficiency, vitamin A deficiency) - not proven
- Clinical features
- Often present during apparent pregnancy with abnormal symptoms/findings
  - Vaginal bleeding (97%)
  - Excessive uterine size for LMP (51%)
  - Theca-lutein cysts >6 cm (50%)
  - Preeclampsia (27%)
  - Hyperemesis gravidarum (26%)
  - Hyperthyroidism (7%)
  - β-hCG > 100,000 IU/L
  - No fetal heart beat detected

Partial (or incomplete) Mole

- Focal trophoblastic hyperplasia and hydropic villi are associated with fetus or fetal parts
- Often triploid (XXY, XYY, XXX) with chromosome complement from both parents
  - Usually related to single ovum fertilized by two sperm
- Low risk of progression to malignant sequelae (<4%)
- Associated with fetus, which may be growth-restricted, and/or have multiple congenital malformations
- Clinical features
  - Typically present similar to threatened/spontaneous/missed abortion
  - Pathological diagnosis often made after D&C.

Investigations

- Quantitative β-hCG levels (tumor marker) abnormally high for gestational age
- U/S findings
  - If complete: No fetus (classic "snow storm" due to swelling of villi)
  - If partial: Molar degeneration of placenta + fetal anomalies, multiple echogenic regions corresponding to hydropic villi, and focal intrauterine hemorrhage
- CXR (may show metastatic lesions)
- Features of molar pregnancies at high risk of developing persistent GTN post-evacuation
  - Local uterine invasion as high as 31%
  - β-hCG > 100,000 IU/L
  - Excessive uterine size
  - Prominent theca-lutein cysts.

Treatment

- ❑ Suction D&C with sharp curettage and oxytocin
- ❑ Rhogam if Rh negative
- ❑ Consider hysterectomy (if patient no longer desires fertility)
- ❑ Prophylactic chemotherapy of no proven benefit
- ❑ Chemotherapy for GTN if develops after evacuation.

Follow-up

- ❑ Contraception required to avoid pregnancy during entire follow-up period
- ❑ Serial β-hCGs (as tumor marker) every week until negative × 3 (usually several weeks), then monthly for 6–12 months prior to trying to conceive again
- ❑ Increase or plateau of β-hCG indicates GTN → patient needs chemotherapy.

7. A 34-year-old female got IUCD inserted a year ago. Now she comes to the clinic with complaints of lower abdominal pain, dyspareunia, abnormal vaginal discharge and dysuria. What is the appropriate management?

a. Start antibiotics immediately and then follow up at 72 hours
b. Remove IUCD first and then start antibiotics
c. First start antibiotics and then remove IUCD
d. No need to remove IUCD
e. Remove IUCD if symptoms do not improve within 72 hours.

Ans. a,d,e

Option a	True	Yes, true
Option b	False	IUCD need not be removed
Option c	False	IUCD need not be removed
Option d	True	Yes, true
Option e	True	Yes, true

According to the latest research, the risk of infection after IUCD insertion, while very low, is highest within the first 20 days after insertion. It is important to note that a pelvic infection does not necessarily develop into pelvic inflammatory disease (PID). PID refers to any infection that ascends into the woman's uterus and fallopian tubes, and that it is caused due to infection with Gonorrhea or Chlamydia, not due to IUCD. However, because PID can lead to infertility and other serious problems, and because diagnosis of PID can be difficult, hence all suspected cases should be treated.

Possible Signs/Symptoms suggesting a pelvic infection:

- ❑ Lower abdominal pain
- ❑ Painful intercourse
- ❑ Postcoital ,intermenstrual or contact bleeding
- ❑ Pain associated with periods (especially if this symptom was absent during the first few months after IUCD insertion but developed later)
- ❑ Abnormal vaginal discharge

- ❑ Painful urination (dysuria)
- ❑ Fever
- ❑ Nausea and vomiting.

Management

Conduct appropriate assessment (including abdominal and pelvic examinations) to identify or rule out other possible causes of the symptoms, such as ectopic pregnancy and appendicitis.

Advise the woman that she should begin treatment immediately to avoid serious potential consequences of the infection, and that the IUCD does not need to be removed during treatment (unless symptoms do not improve within 72 hours).

However, if the woman insists on IUCD removal, arrange to have the IUCD removed under antibiotic coverage for 2 to 3 days.

Treat the woman for gonorrhea, chlamydia, and anaerobic infections according to NACO'sRTI/STI guidelines.

8. Fulminant liver disease in pregnancy is/are:

a. Hep E
b. Hep B
c. HELLP syndrome
d. Acute fatty liver of pregnancy
e. Cholestasis in pregnancy

Ans. a,c,d,e

Option a	True	Yes, correct
Option b	False	No, not a fulminant liver disease in pregnancy
Option c	True	Yes, correct
Option d	True	Yes, correct
Option e	True	Yes, correct

Causes of Acute Liver Failure in Pregnancy

Pregnancy Associated Acute Liver Disease

- ❑ Pre-eclampsia/eclampsia with liver infarction
- ❑ Syndrome of hemolysis, elevated liver enzymes and low platelets (HELLP syndrome)
- ❑ Acute hepatic rupture
- ❑ Acute fatty liver of pregnancy (AFLP).

Exacerbated by Pregnant State

- ❑ Viral hepatitis
- ❑ Budd-Chiari syndrome (BCS) with portal vein thrombosis
- ❑ Gallstone disease.

Unrelated to Pregnant State

- ❑ Drug-induced liver disease
- ❑ Toxins/mushroom poisoning
- ❑ Shock

- Trauma
- Decompensation of pre-existent liver disease.

Ref: Pandey CK, Karna ST, Pandey VK, Tandon M. Acute liver failure in pregnancy: Challenges and management. Indian Journal of Anaesthesia. 2015;59(3):144-149. doi:10.4103/0019-5049.153035

9. True about breech presentations is/are:

a. Frank breech is common in primigravida
b. Incidence of cord prolapse in breech presentation is around 1%
c. Rate of cord prolapse with non frank breech is 5.6%
d. Incidence of breech presentation is 3–4% at term
e. ECV is successful in 50% patients

Ans. a, b, c, d, e *Ref: RCOG Green top guidelines number 20a, 20b, 50; Bedside clinics in Obstetrics, Arup Kumar Majhi*

Option a	True	Yes, correct
Option b	True	Yes, correct
Option c	True	Yes, correct
Option d	True	Yes, correct
Option e	True	Yes, correct

Frank breech is more common in primigravidas and complete breech is more common in multigravidas.

The incidence of breech presentation decreases from about 20% at 28 weeks of gestation to 3–4% at term, as most babies turn spontaneously to the cephalic presentation.

The overall incidence of cord prolapse ranges from 0.1–0.6%. In the case of breech presentation, the incidence is higher at 1%.

A recent observational study of non-frank breech presentations found a high rate of cord prolapse (5.6%) but no increase in abnormal labor nor impaired perinatal outcome.

External cephalic version: Success rates of ECV vary, but in a large series, 47% of women following an ECV attempt had a cephalic presentation at birth. Overall success levels are greater for multiparous women (60%) than for nulliparous women (40%).

Obstetrics and Gynecology

1. During external radiation therapy for cervical cancer which lymph node is/are excluded?

a. External iliac lymph mode
b. Common iliac lymph node
c. Internal iliac lymph node
d. Sacral lymph node
e. Obturator lymph node

Ans. d *Ref: Novak Gynecology, 15/e, NCCN Cervical Cancer Guidelines 2017*

Option a	False	
Option b	False	
Option c	False	
Option d	True	Sacral lymph nodes are not involved in external radiation therapy
Option e	False	

Management options for cervical cancer are:

- ❑ Conization
- ❑ Radical trachelectomy
- ❑ Extrafascial hysterectomy
- ❑ Modified radical hysterectomy
- ❑ Radical hysterectomy
- ❑ Primary radiotherapy—brachytherapy, external beam radiotherapy or EBRT (primary radiation treatment plans usually consist of a combination of EBRT to treat the regional lymph nodes and to decrease the tumor volume, and brachytherapy delivered by intracavitary applicators or interstitial implants to provide a treatment boost to the central tumor)
- ❑ Primary chemoradiation

Principles of radiotherapy for cervical cancer

Stage	***Management***	***NCCN guidelines***
Stage IA1 no LVSI	Conization or simple extrafascial hysterectomy	
LVSI	Radical trachelectomy or modified radical hysterectomy with pelvic lymphadenectomy	
IA2 3–5 mm invasion	Radical trachelectomy or modified radical hysterectomy with pelvic lymphadenectomy	Pelvic radiation with brachytherapy (traditionally 70–80 Gy to total point A dose) is a treatment option for patients who are medically inoperable

Contd…

Contd…

Principles of radiotherapy for cervical cancer		
IB1 < 2 cm	Radical trachelectomy or radical hysterectomy with pelvic lymphadenectomy	Depending on their stage and disease bulk and patients medical condition, patients with stage IB or IIA tumors can be treated with either surgery, or primary radiotherapy, or primary chemoradiation.
> 2 cm	Radical hysterectomy with pelvic lymphadenectomy	
IB2	Radical hysterectomy with pelvic and para-aortic lymphadenectomy or primary chemoradiation	Surgery is the most appropriate option for patients with stage IB1 or IIA1 disease, whereas concurrent chemoradiation is the most appropriate option for those with stage IB2 or IIA2 disease based on randomized trials.
IIA	Radical hysterectomy with pelvic and para-aortic lymphadenectomy or primary chemoradiation	
IIB, III	Primary chemoradiation	
IV A	Primary chemoradiation or pelvic exenteration	
IVB	Primary chemotherapy ± palliative radiation	

2. Drugs for management of PIH include:

a. Methyldopa
b. Nifedipine
c. Labetalol
d. Losartan
e. Clonidine

Ans. a, b, c, e *Ref: KD Tripathi, Essentials of Medical Pharmacology*

Option a	True	
Option b	True	
Option c	True	
Option d	False	Losartan is contraindicated for the management of PIH
Option e	True	

Drugs used in hypertensive disorders in pregnancy (antepartum)		
Drugs used	***Drugs to be avoided***	***Drugs contraindicated***
Alpha methyl dopa	Diuretics (except when indicated, e.g. pulmonary edema)	ACE inhibitors
Labetalol, oxprenolol	Sodium nitroprusside	ARBs or angiotensin antagonists (Candesartan, losartan, etc.)
Nifedipine		Non selective beta blockers, e.g. propranolol
Hydralazine		
Prazosin		
Clonidine		

3. Indications for in-vitro fertilization (IVF):

a. Bilateral tube blockage
b. Normal male factor
c. Hostile cervical factor
d. Proximal tubal block
e. Premature ovarian insufficiency

Ans. a, d, e *Ref: Speroff Gynecology 8/e*

Option	Status	Explanation
Option a	True	
Option b	False	Severe male factor infertility indicates need for IVF
Option c	False	Tubal disease or endometriosis is indication for IVF
Option d	True	
Option e	True	

Explanation

Assisted reproductive technologies (ART) encompass all techniques involving direct manipulation of oocytes outside of the body. The first and still most common form of ART is in vitro fertilization (IVF).

IVF involves a sequence of highly coordinated steps beginning with controlled ovarian hyperstimulation with exogenous gonadotropins, followed by retrieval of oocytes from the ovaries under the guidance of transvaginal ultrasonography, fertilization in the laboratory, and transcervical transfer of embryos into the uterus.

Thus IVF is indicated in conditions when: the female cannot ovulate despite treatment, or cannot get pregnant despite ovulating on treatment, or in vivo fertilization cannot occur due to tubal or pelvic factors, or male partner cannot produce sufficient healthy spermatocytes, etc.

In vitro fertilization indications:

1. Tubal disease
2. Severe male factor infertility
3. Endometriosis associated with infertility
4. Unexplained infertility
5. All other treatments unsuccessful
6. Reproductive ageing (donor oocyte IVF)
7. Fertility preservation before ovarian surgery
8. Müllerian anomalies—surrogacy
9. Preimplantation genetic screening
10. Preimplantation genetic diagnosis

4. All are true about puerperal sepsis *except*:

a. Temperature > 38 °C (100.4 °F)
b. Cesarean section has no increased risk for sepsis
c. Group a beta-hemolytic streptococcus is one of the common causative organism
d. Instrument delivery increases risk
e. Retained placenta is a cause

Ans. b *Ref: RCOG green top guideline number 64b, 2012; Managing puerperal Sepsis, WHO 2008*

Option a	True	
Option b	False	Cesarean section increases risk for sepsis
Option c	True	
Option d	True	
Option e	True	

Puerperal sepsis: Sepsis developing after birth until 6 weeks postnatally.

Sepsis may be defined as local infection plus systemic manifestations of infection;

Severe sepsis may be defined as sepsis plus sepsis-induced organ dysfunction or tissue hypoperfusion.

Septic shock is defined as the persistence of hypoperfusion despite adequate fluid replacement therapy.

Risk factors for maternal puerperal sepsis:

- Obesity
- Impaired glucose tolerance/diabetes
- Impaired immunity/immunosuppressant medication
- Anemia, malnutrition
- Vaginal discharge
- History of pelvic infection
- Amniocentesis and other invasive procedures
- Cervical cerclage
- Prolonged spontaneous rupture of membranes, protracted labor, frequent vaginal examinations
- Vaginal trauma, caesarean section, wound hematoma
- Retained products of conception
- Group A beta hemolytic *Streptococcus* (GAS) infection in close contacts/family members
- Poor socioeconomic status

Major pathogens causing sepsis in the puerperium are:

- GAS, also known as *Streptococcus* pyogenes
- Escherichia coli
- Staphylococcus aureus
- Streptococcus pneumoniae G
- Methicillin-resistant *S. aureus* (MRSA),
- Clostridium tetani, and welchii
- Chlamydia and gonorrhea

The following symptoms and signs occur in puerperal sepsis:

- Fever (temperature of 38 °C or more)
- Chills and general malaise
- Lower abdominal pain
- Tender uterus
- Subinvolution of the uterus
- Purulent, foul-smelling lochia.

Symptoms and signs that may also be present:

- ❑ Light vaginal bleeding
- ❑ Shock.

5. Risk factor for primary dysmenorrhea:

a. Anxiety
b. Low BMI
c. Obesity
d. Smoking
e. Poor socioeconomic status

Ans. b, c, d *Ref: Williams Gynecology 3/e; Novak Gynecology 15/e; American Association of Family Physicians, 1999; Speroff Gynecologic Endocrinology*

Option a	False	Not a risk factor
Option b	True	
Option c	True	
Option d	True	
Option e	False	Not a risk factor

Dysmenorrhea: Pelvic pain during menses

Primary dysmenorrhea: Cyclic menstrual pain without an identifiable associated pathology. It is associated with ovulatory cycles.

Primary dysmenorrhea is by far the most common gynecologic problem in menstruating women.

It usually begins during adolescence, but only after ovulatory cycles are established; 20–45% of teenage girls are ovulatory by 2 years after menarche, and 80% by 4–5 years. The overall prevalence of primary dysmenorrhea among adolescent girls is between 60% and 90% and decreases as age increases.

Secondary dysmenorrhea: Menstrual pain caused by a pelvic pathology like endometriosis, leiomyomas, PID, adenomyosis, endometrial polyps, and menstrual outlet obstruction. For this reason, secondary dysmenorrhea may be associated with other gynecologic symptoms, such as dyspareunia, dysuria, abnormal bleeding, or infertility.

Pathophysiology of primary dysmenorrhea: Prostaglandins play an important role. During endometrial sloughing, endometrial cells release prostaglandins as menstruation begins. Prostaglandins stimulate myometrial contractions with a dysrhythmic pattern, and ischemia. Women with more severe dysmenorrhea have higher levels of prostaglandins in menstrual fluid, and these levels are highest during the first 2 days of menstruation. Uterine hypercontractility, decreased uterine blood flow, and increased peripheral nerve hypersensitivity contribute to pain.

Symptoms

The pain of primary dysmenorrhea usually begins a few hours before or just after the onset of a menstrual period and may last 48 to 72 hours.

The pain is similar to labor, with suprapubic cramping, and may be accompanied by lumbosacral backache, pain radiating down the anterior thigh, nausea, vomiting, diarrhea, and rarely syncopal episodes.

In contrast, women with secondary dysmenorrhea related to pelvic pathology, such as endometriosis, frequently report increasingly severe pain that often occurs at midcycle and during the week preceding menses, in addition to symptoms of deep dyspareunia and dyschezia (painful bowel movements).

Risk factors associated with more severe episodes of dysmenorrhea:

- Earlier age at menarche (before age 12).
- Long menstrual periods, irregular or heavy flow, the severity of dysmenorrhea related directly to the volume and duration of menstrual flow
- Longer intermenstrual intervals
- Premenstrual molimina, body mass index less than 20, obesity
- Smoking, alcohol consumption
- Previous sterilization
- History of sexual assault
- The severity of dysmenorrhea is reduced in women who have delivered a child in the intervening years, but not in those who have had a miscarriage or abortion.
- Some studies have shown, exercise, being married or in a stable relationship, and higher parity decrease the likelihood of dysmenorrhea.

6. In gynecologic surgery:

a. Longitudinal incision is most common
b. Paramedial incision is more common
c. Exposure in transverse incision is less than the longitudinal incision
d. Midline vertical incision is favored when pelvic infection is suspected
e. Transverse incision offers lesser blood loss

Ans. c, d *Ref: Williams Gynecology 3/e*

Option a	False	Midline incision is most common one
Option b	False	
Option c	True	
Option d	True	
Option e	False	

Types of incision in gynecologic surgeries

Vertical incision

Vertical incisions may be midline or paramedian, the midline incision is chosen more often in gynecologic surgeries.

Advantages: This incision offers quick entry, minimal blood loss, superior access to the upper abdomen, generous operating room, and the flexibility or easy wound extension, if greater space or access is needed. No important neurovascular structures traverse this incision. Thus, it may be favored for patients using anticoagulation agents.

Disadvantages: Midline incisions are more frequently associated with greater postoperative pain, poorer cosmetic results, and increased risks of wound dehiscence or incisional hernia compared with low transverse incisions.

Transverse incisions

The Pfannenstiel, Cherney, and Maylard incisions are transverse abdominal incisions used for gynecologic procedures. Of these, the Pfannenstiel incision is the most commonly used incision for laparotomy.

Advantages: Because the transverse incision follows Langer lines of skin tension, excellent cosmetic results can be achieved. Additionally, decreased rates of postoperative pain, fascial wound dehiscence, and incisional hernia are noted.

Disadvantages: Use of the Pfannenstiel incision is discouraged for cases in which greater operating space or upper abdominal access is anticipated. Because o the layers created by incision of the internal and external oblique aponeuroses, purulent fluid can collect between these. Therefore, cases involving abscess or peritonitis favor use o a midline incision, which divides the used linea alba.

7. **Posthysterectomy, vaginal prolapse is due to:**
   a. Level 1 pelvic supports are weakened
   b. Level 2 pelvic supports are weakened
   c. Level 3 pelvic supports are weakened
   d. Ligaments not handled properly
   e. None of the above

Ans. a *Ref: Williams Gynecology 3/e*

Option a	True	
Option b	False	
Option c	False	
Option d	False	
Option e	False	

Supports of vagina

De Lancey's three tier system for vaginal supports

Level 1—parametrium that continues caudally as paracolpium, cardinal and uterosacral ligaments. These attachments are known as level 1 support or suspensory axis and provide connective tissue support to the vaginal apex after hysterectomy. In the standing position, level 1 support fibers are vertically oriented. Clinical manifestations of level 1 support defects include uterine prolapse or posthysterectomy vaginal vault prolapse.

Level 2—or midvaginal support, the lateral walls of the vagina's midportion are attached to the pelvic walls on each side by visceral connective tissue known as endopelvic fascia. These lateral attachments of the vaginal walls blend into the arcus tendineus fascia pelvis and to the medial aspect of the levator animuscles, and in doing so create the anterior and posterior lateral vaginal sulci. These grooves run along the vaginal sidewalls and give the vagina an "H" shape when viewed in cross-section.

Level 3—pelvic floor, suburethral hammock (pubocervical fascia), perineal body. The distal third of the vagina is directly attached to its surrounding structures. Anteriorly, the vagina is fused with the urethra. Laterally it attaches to the pubovaginalis muscle and perineal membrane, and posteriorly to the perineal body. These vaginal attachments are referred to as level III support or the fusion axis and are considered the strongest of the vaginal support components. Clinically, failure of this level of support can result in distal rectoceles or perineal descent. Anal incontinence may also result, if the perineal body is absent.

Level	Supports	Defect results in
I (Upper vagina)	Paracolpium (lower fibers of uterosacral and cardinal ligaments)	Uterine prolapse Post hysterectomy vaginal vault prolapse
II (Mid vagina)	Endopelvic fascia—blends into arcus tendinus fascia pelvis and to the medial aspect of levator ani muscles, thus creating anterior and posterior lateral vaginal sulci	Anterior and posterior vaginal wall prolapse. Stress urinary incontinence
III (Distal vaginal support) also known as the fusion axis	Anteriorly distal vagina is fused with the urethra. Laterally it attaches to pubovaginalis muscles and perineal membrane and posteriorly to the perineal body	Distal rectal or perineal descent Anal incontinence

8. Features of Turner's syndrome is/are:

a. Long stature, wide chest
b. Narrow chest
c. Most common monosomy for survival
d. 20% of first trimester abortions
e. Intelligence normal

Ans. c, d, e *Ref: Speroff Clinical Endocrinology, 8/e*

Option a	False	Short stature
Option b	False	Wide shield chest with widely spaced nipples
Option c	True	
Option d	True	
Option e	True	

Approximately half of first-trimester miscarriages are anembryonic, that is, with no identifiable embryonic elements. The previous term blighted ovum or these pregnancies has fallen out of favor. The remaining pregnancies are embryonic miscarriages, which may be further grouped as either those with chromosomal anomalies (aneuploid abortions) or those with a normal chromosomal complement (euploid abortions).

More than 80 percent of spontaneous abortions occur during the first 12 weeks of gestation

Approximately half of embryonic first trimester miscarriages are aneuploid, an incidence that decreases markedly with advancing gestation at the time of pregnancy loss.

Autosomal trisomy (as a group) is the most frequently identified chromosomal anomaly in early miscarriages (22–32%).

Monosomy X (45, X) is the single most common specific chromosomal abnormality and is also known as Turner syndrome. Most fetuses with monosomy X spontaneously abort, but some are liveborn females. Conversely, autosomal monosomy is rare and incompatible with life.

Chromosomal findings in early abortuses	
Chromosomal studies	*Reported incidence range (Percent)*
Normal (euploid)	
46, XY and 46, XX	45–55
Abnormal (aneuploid)	
Autosomal trisomy	22–32
Monosomy X (45, X)	5–20
Triploidy	6–8
Tetraploidy	2–4
Structural anomaly	2
Double or triple trisomy	0.7–2

Thus most common (or the only) monosomy to survive is Monosomy X. Monosomy X ending in abortions is responsible for 5–20% of first trimester abortions.

Turner syndrome: 45XO or 46XX/45XO mosaic

Incidence 1 in 2000–5000 female live births

Sine qua non - **short stature**

Intelligence—normal (unless small X ring chromosome is present which is associated with severe MR)

Webbed neck, low set ears, low posterior hair line, high palate, wide shield chest with widely spaced nipples, short fourth metacarpals, increased carrying angle, streak gonads.

Associated anomalies:

Renal (30–50% of Turners have renal anomalies): horse shoe kidney, hydronephrosis due to obstruction, etc.

Cardiac: 20–30% patients of Turner have aortic valve disease (Bicuspid aortic valve, aortic root dilatation), Coarctation of aorta in 5–10%. Other anomalies—elongation of transverse aortic arch, persistent superior venal cavalry, QT prolongation.

Predisposition to osteoporosis, ocular anomalies, hearing loss, celiac disease, endocrine disorders.

Mortality increases three fold.

Evaluation on diagnosis: EGG, cardiac 2D echo, renal USG, TFT, CBC, blood sugar, lipid profile, LFT, RFT, antiendomysial antibody (for celiac disease)

Periodic monitoring is to be done with the same investigations

Rx:

- GH—by 2–5 years of age as soon as height falls below fifth percentile for the age

If diagnosed late:

- Start GH + oxandrolone (anabolic steroid) at 9–12 yrs of age.
- Estrogen therapy only after 13–14 years of age to avoid premature epiphyseal fusion.
- Add progesterone after first episode of menses or 12–24 months after starting estrogen (to avoid negative effects of Progestins on breast development)
- Continue COC as source of E + P

Pregnancy is rare and is associated with high risk for sex chromosome aneuploidy and spontaneous abortions.

Pregnancy by oocyte donation carries very high risk due to cardiac anomalies.

9. Abruptio placenta is seen in:

a. HTN
b. Previous fibroids with low placed placenta
c. Higher order multiparity
d. Diabetes mellitus
e. Primigravida

Ans. a, b, c *Ref: Williams Obstetrics, 24/e*

Option a	True	
Option b	True	
Option c	True	
Option d	False	
Option e	False	Increased age and increased parity

Risk factors for abruptio placentae:

1. Previous abruption: Risk of recurrence is 6–16.7%
2. Increased age and parity
3. Race: More common in African-American and Caucasian than Asian
4. First degree relative with abruption
5. Hypertension: Most common condition associated with abruption. There is two to three fold increase in risk
6. Sudden decompression from rupture of membranes especially in polyhydramnios and multiple pregnancy
7. Placental abnormalities especially circumvallate placenta
8. External cephalic version, abdominal trauma
9. Smoking, cocaine abuse
10. Thrombophilias
11. Hyperhomocysteinemia
12. Folic acid deficiency—not confirmed
13. Increased AFP levels
14. Leiomyoma, if located behind the placental implantation site
15. Uterine malformations

10. In case of diabetes with pregnancy:

a. Oxytocin is given with glucose infusion
b. Macrosomia is detected by amniocentesis
c. 10% chances of fetal malformations
d. Higher risk of gestational hypertension
e. Higher risk of hyperemesis gravidarum

Ans. c, d *Ref: Williams Gynecology 3/e*

Option a	False	Oxytocin should not be given in glucose infusion
Option b	False	Macrosomia is detected by clinical examination and USG
Option c	True	
Option d	True	
Option e	False	

Pregnancy outcomes of diabetes

- Increased risk of miscarriages associated with poor glycemic control in pregestational diabetes
- **Congenital malformations:** Seen only with pregestational diabetes or overt diabetes. Not seen in GDM. Rate of malformations in controlled diabetes is 5%. Uncontrolled: 9%. (Williams); 6–10% (James, High risk pregnancy). It is the leading cause of perinatal mortality in infants of diabetic mothers responsible for 40–50% of perinatal deaths. HbA1c >7 before 7 weeks of gestation and periconceptionally is associated with increased risk of malformations.

  Malformations seen are:
  - **Cardiovascular system (most common) 30–40%:** Transposition of the great vessels, ventricular septal defect, atrial septal defect, tetralogy of Fallot, coarctation of aorta, single umbilical artery, hypoplastic left ventricle, cardiomegaly.
  - **Central nervous system (10%):** Open neural tube defects, holoprosencephaly, absent corpus callosum, Arnold-Chiari anomaly, schizencephaly, microcephaly, macrocephaly, agenesis of olfactory tracts, hydrocephaly.
  - **Musculoskeletal system (10%):** Caudal dysgenesis, craniosynostosis, costovertebral anomalies, limb reduction, club foot, contractures, polysyndactyly, sirenomelia
  - **Gastrointestinal system:** Pyloric stenosis, duodenal atresia, microcolon, anorectal atresia, omphaloenteric cyst/fistula, hernias
  - **Urogenital system:** Renal agenesis, renal cysts, hydronephrosis, duplication of ureter, ureterocele, uterine agenesis, hypoplastic vagina, micropenis, hypospadias, cryptorchidism, hypoplastic testes, ambiguous genitalia
  - **Others:** Cleft palate
- **Macrosomia:** Seen in both pregestational and gestational diabetes. Maternal hyperglycemia—fetal hyperglycemia—fetal Hyperinsulinemia. Fetal insulin stimulates excessive fetal growth more fat deposition over shoulder and trunk. Except for fetal brain all tissues are affected. Increased shoulder fat may result in shoulder dystocia and brachial plexus injury. Recurrence of macrosomia in diabetes is seen in 1/3 of all cases. Maternal obesity is an independent and important risk factor for macrosomia.
- **Sudden IUFD:** Unexplained fetal death in last 4–8 weeks of gestation. A/W high fasting glucose > 105. Seen in both pregestational and gestational diabetes
- Polyhydramnios
- **IUGR:** Seen in long standing DM with vascular disease. May also be associated with cong anomalies
- **Preterm delivery:** Spontaneous or indicated

Neonatal effects:

- Hypoglycemia (BG < 35 mg/dl)
- Hypocalcemia
- Polycythemia
- Hyperbilirubinemia
- RDS—Respiratory distress syndrome
- TTN—Transient tachypnea of newborn

Maternal risks:

- Higher risk of gestational hypertension and preeclampsia
- Higher risk of cesarean section
- Higher morbidity associated with cesarean section
- Up to 50% women with GDM will develop diabetes 22–28 years after pregnancy

  Note: For diabetic women in labor glucose and insulin are given by sliding scale. Oxytocin should not be given in glucose infusion as adjusting the infusion rates of glucose and oxytocin will interfere with each other.

  Macrosomia is detected by clinical examination and USG and not by amniocentesis.

11. Blood supply of vagina is:

a. Cervical branch of uterine artery
b. Middle rectal artery
c. Inferior rectal artery
d. Internal pudendal artery
e. Vesical artery

Ans. a, b, d *Ref: Williams Gynecology 3/e*

Option a	True	
Option b	True	
Option c	False	
Option d	True	
Option e	False	

- The main blood supply to the vagina arises from the descending or cervical branch of the uterine artery and from the vaginal artery. Both uterine artery and vaginal artery are branches of the internal iliac artery.
- Additionally, the middle rectal artery from the internal iliac artery contributes to the posterior vaginal wall supply.
- The distal walls of the vagina also receive contributions from the internal pudendal artery.

12. True about anatomy of vagina:

a. Covered by columnar epithelium
b. Covered by nonkeratinized stratified squamous epithelium
c. Vaginal secretion is from transudation of vaginal epithelium
d. Supplied by cervicovaginal branch of the uterine artery
e. Anterior wall is longer than posterior wall

Ans. b, c, d *Ref: Williams Gynecology 3/e*

Option a	False	Nonkeratinized squamous epithelium
Option b	True	
Option c	True	
Option d	True	
Option e	False	Average length of the anterior vaginal wall is 7 cm and that of the posterior wall is 9 cm

Anatomy of vagina

The vagina is a hollow viscus whose shape is determined by the structures that surround it and by the attachments of its lateral walls to the pelvic walls. In the standing or anatomic position, the apex of the vagina is directed posteriorly toward the ischial spines, and the upper two thirds o the vaginal tube lie almost parallel to the plane of the levator plate. Although variable, the average length of the anterior vaginal wall is 7 cm and that of the posterior wall is 9 cm.

The vaginal walls consist of three layers: (1) adjacent to the lumen, a layer of nonkeratinized squamous epithelium with an outer lamina propria; (2) a muscular layer of smooth muscle, collagen, and elastin; and (3) an outer adventitial layer of collagen and elastin. These latter two form the fibromuscular component of the vagina. The vagina lies between the bladder and rectum and, along with its connections to the pelvic walls, provides support to these structures.

13. True about atrophic vaginitis:

a. Low estrogen is a risk factor
b. Low pH
c. Local estrogen therapy gives temporary relief
d. Repeated intercourse decreases chances of atrophic vaginitis
e. None of the above

Ans. a, d *Ref: Novak Gynecology 15/e; Williams Gynecology 3/e*

Option a	True	
Option b	False	pH > 5 in absence of infection, blood, or semen
Option c	False	Estrogen replacement effectively reverses atrophic changes
Option d	True	
Option e	False	

Up to 50% of postmenopausal women have symptoms of atrophic vaginitis.

Symptoms include an external dysuria, pruritus, tenderness, dyspareunia, and bleeding from fissuring or ulcerations.

Clinical findings: A shiny, flat, thin-appearing vaginal mucosa without rugae, Microscopic examination of vaginal secretions reveals an increased number of white blood cells. Treatment with local or systemic estrogens effectively manages the symptoms and restores normal pH levels with ongoing therapy. Systemic absorption does occur with topical estrogen therapy, and rates of absorption differ depending on the degree of atrophy. Topical emollients may be helpful, if estrogens are not desired or are contraindicated. Vaginal lubricants are universally useful in minimizing symptoms of dyspareunia for postmenopausal women.

Etiology: Estrogen deficiency from various causes

- Menopause—Leading cause
- Spontaneous premature ovarian failure
- Radiation therapy/chemotherapy
- Immunologic disorders
- Bilateral oophorectomy
- Postpartum
- Side effects of prolonged treatments with
- Progesterones, Tamoxifen, Danazol, GnRH agonists and antagonists

Management:

- Vaginal moisturisers and lubricants
- *Sexual activity:* Women who participate in regular intercourse have fewer symptoms of vaginal atrophy and less evidence of stenosis and shrinkage on physical exam.These benefits are from improved blood flow and increased androgens, which help to preserve vaginal elasticity and prevent introital stenosis.
- *Vaginal estrogen therapy:*
  Estrogen replacement effectively reverses atrophic changes.
  Vaginal atrophy and diminished vaginal mucosal elasticity, vaginal fluid secretion levels, blood flow, and sensorimotor responses are improved by either topical or systemic estrogen.
  Low doses of estrogen cream (premarin, estrace) (0.5 g) used once or twice a week
  Estradiol vaginal tablet (Vagifem) (10 μg) inserted twice weekly.
  Estrogen-containing vaginal ring (estring) (7.5 μg per day) is placed in the vagina every 3 months
  Studies of the vaginal estrogen therapy of up to 1 years' duration confirmed endometrial safety, but long-term studies on the effects of low-dose vaginal estrogen therapy on the endometrium are not available. Women using vaginal estrogen therapy should be reminded to report any vaginal bleeding, and a thorough evaluation should be performed.

14. Which of the following is/are not fertility awareness based methods?

a. Withdrawal method
b. Rhythm method
c. Cervical mucus method
d. MTP pill
e. Symptothermal method

Ans. a, d *Ref: SK Chaudhuri Practice of Fertility Control*

Option	
Option a	True
Option b	False
Option c	False
Option d	True
Option e	False

Fertility awareness based methods:

The human oocyte has a fertilizable life of 24 hours after ovulation, while spermatocele can fertilize the oocyte for 3 days after deposition in vagina.

For a female with a menstrual cycle length of 28 days, she is most fertile from day 10 to day 18 of her cycle.

The fertile days can be estimated by one of the follow methods

- *Rhythm method:* Shortest cycle length minus 18 to longest cycle length minus 11, e.g., if her shortest and longest cycle lengths are 26 and 30 days respectively, fertile period is from day 8 to day 19.
- *Basal body temperature method:* Progesterone level rises in blood after ovulation and causes a 0.5–0.8 °F or 0.2–0.4 °C rise in basal body temperature. Ovulation occurs 2 days before to 3 days after rise in BBT.

- *Cervical music method or Billings method:* in the ovulation under the influence of high estrogen levels cervical secretion is profuse, transparent, watery and can be drawn out into a thread (spinnbarkeit). This secretion becomes thick and scanty and loses spinnbarkeit in the postovulatory period.
- *Sympto-thermal method:* charting basal body temperature, cervical mucus changes, mid cycle pain, premenstrual breast tenderness all on a sympto-thermal chart, to estimate the fertile period.
- *Standard days method:* A string of color coded beads called 'cyclebeads' may be used by women with cycle lengths of 26 to 32 days to know the days of fertile period in the cycle.

15. Which of the following changes occur during pregnancy?

a. In last trimester blood volume increases by 50%
b. Cardiac output increase by 20% in last trimester
c. Hemodynamic changes can lead to CHF during labor and following delivery in preexisting cardiac lesions
d. Hypercoagulability occurs
e. Hyperreflexia

Ans. a, c, d *Ref: Williams Obstetrics, 24/e*

Option a	True	
Option b	False	Cardiac output increases by 40% during 20–24 weeks. Maximum during second stage of labor and immediately post partum
Option c	True	
Option d	True	
Option e	False	Never seen

Rise in	Starts rising	Maximum value above pre-pregnant level	Maximum at	Later
Blood volume	Early in first trimester	45–50%	32 weeks	Plateaus
RBC volume		30%		
Stroke volume	Early in first trimester	25–30%	12–24 weeks	Plateaus
Heart rate	Progressively rises throughout	At term 15 bpm above baseline		
Cardiac output	Early in first trimester	40%	20–24 weeks	Plateaus
Fall	**Starts falling**	**Minimum value below non-pregnant value**	**Minimum at**	**Later**
BP	I trimester		24–28 weeks	Plateaus
Systemic vascular resistance	I trimester	20–30% below	14–20 weeks	Plateaus
Pulmonary vascular resistance		34% below		

Periods of strain that predispose to heart failure

1. Around 28–32 weeks when pregnancy induced hypervolemia and cardiac output reach their maximum.
2. During delivery.
3. Immediate postpartum – maximum risk.

Coagulation and Fibrinolysis

Both Coagulation and Fibrinolysis are augmented in pregnancy.

Concentration of all clotting factors increases except factor 11 and 13.

Levels of high molecular weight fibrinogen also increases.

Protein C (anticoagulant) is decreased, there is acquired resistance to protein S in pregnancy.

Thus pregnancy is a hypercoagulable state.

16. True about amniocentesis and chorionic villus sampling:

a. In 1st trimester, amniocentesis is a better choice than chorionic villus sampling
b. 2nd trimester amniocentesis has less foetal loss than chorionic villus sampling
c. Amniocentesis may result in oligohydramnios
d. Amniocentesis in 1st trimester has lower risk of foetal loss than 2nd trimester amniocentesis
e. Amniocentesis in 1st trimester has more risk of talipes

Ans. b, c, e *Ref: Williams Obstetrics 24/e*

Option a	False	CVS is generally performed between 10 and 13 weeks' gestation. And amniocentesis usually performed after 15–16 weeks
Option b	True	
Option c	True	
Option d	False	Early amniocentesis is associated with higher rates of procedure-related complications
Option e	True	

Any procedure that involves entering the pregnant uterus logically carries risk to both fetus and the mother.

Amniocentesis: Usually performed after 15–16 weeks. Approximately 20 mL of fluid is then collected for fetal chromosomal analysis.

Maternal risks are quite low:

- Symptomatic amnionitis occurring only rarely (0.1 percent).
- Transient vaginal spotting or minimal amniotic fluid leakage occur in 1 percent or fewer of cases, but almost always these are self-limited in nature.
- Other very rare complications include intra-abdominal viscus injury or hemorrhage.

Fetal risks:

Risk of pregnancy loss secondary to amniocentesis is low.

Other complications of amniocentesis include:

- Amniotic fluid leakage in 1 to 2 percent and
- Chorioamnionitis in less than 0.1 percent. Following leakage of amniotic fluid, which generally occurs within 48 hours of the procedure, fetal survival exceeds 90 percent.
- Needle injuries to the fetus are rare.
- Fetomaternal hemorrhage.

Early amniocentesis

- If performed between 11 and 14 weeks, amniocentesis is termed "early." Also, less fluid is typically withdrawn—approximately 1 mL for each gestational week. Early amniocentesis is associated with significantly higher rates of procedure-related complications than other fetal procedures.

- Rates of amniotic fluid leakage, fetal loss, and talipes equinovarus (clubfoot) are all significantly higher following early amniocentesis than with traditional amniocentesis.
- Compared with chorionic villus sampling, early amniocentesis is associated with a fourfold increased rate of talipes equinovarus.
- Cell culture failure rate is higher, thus necessitating a second procedure. For all these reasons, the American College of Obstetricians and Gynecologists (2012) recommends against the use of early amniocentesis.

Chorionic Villus Sampling (CVS)

Biopsy of chorionic villi is generally performed between 10 and 13 weeks' gestation. The primary advantage of villus biopsy is that results are available earlier in pregnancy, allowing safer pregnancy termination, if desired. A full karyotype is available in 7 to 10 days, and some laboratories provide preliminary results within 48 hours compared to two weeks required to obtain results with amniocentesis.

The overall loss rate following CVS is higher than that following midtrimester amniocentesis because of background spontaneous losses, that is, those that would have occurred between the first and second trimester in the absence of a fetal procedure. The procedure-related fetal loss rate is comparable to that with amniocentesis.

Other complications:

- Vaginal spotting
- Limb deformities and oromandibular dysplasia if performed ≤10 weeks of gestation
- Isolated chromosomal mosaicism
- Fetomaternal hemorrhage

The rate of procedure-related pregnancy loss that is attributable to a prenatal diagnostic procedure currently is estimated to be approximately 0.1–0.3% in procedures performed by experienced healthcare providers.

CVS done before 9 weeks is associated with limb deformities and oromandibular dysplasias.

17. Which of the following is true?

a. Cordocentesis is usually done after 20 weeks gestation
b. Karyotype can be obtained faster with amniocentesis than chorionic villous sampling
c. CVS is done before 10 weeks of gestation
d. Laparoscopic CVS has less fetal injury
e. Cordocentesis can be done to diagnose Fetal inborn errors of metabolism

Ans. a, e *Ref: Williams obstetrics, 24/e*

Option a	True	
Option b	False	Results are obtained faster with CVS
Option c	False	Performed between 10 and 13 weeks' gestation
Option d	False	
Option e	True	

Indications of fetal blood sampling:

- To help clarify chromosome mosaicism detected in cultured amniotic fluid cells or chorionic villi.

- Prenatal evaluation of fetal hematologic abnormalities.
- Fetal blood hematocrit level can be measured directly to assess hemolysis resulting from Rh or other blood antigen isoimmunization states.
- Fetal blood has been used for the diagnosis of blood factor abnormalities like hemophilia A, hemophilia B, or Von Willebrand's disease.
- Assessment of viral, bacterial, or parasitic infections of the fetus.
- Enzyme levels in inborn errors of metabolism
- For Fetal therapy in intrauterine transfusion, introduction of Fetal medication.

Cordocentesis (PUBS) is usually performed from 18 weeks onward, although it can be done as early as 12 weeks.

It is always done under ultrasonography guidance.

Maternal complications are rare, but include amnionitis and transplacental hemorrhage. Fetal risks are more substantive.

Fetal risks:

- Fetal loss 1.4%
- Fetomaternal hemorrhage
- Fetal bradycardia
- Cord thrombosis

Introducing a scope into the uterus of a pregnant female into the amniotic cavity is called fetoscopy.

If chorionic villous sampling is attempted using a scope it should be called fetoscopic CVS and not laparoscopic. Thus, option c is definitely incorrect. (Also refer the previous explanation).

18. True statement(s) regarding investigation in endometrial cancer:

a. MRI is superior to CT in detecting myometrial involvement
b. CT is superior to MRI in detecting omental metastasis
c. USG is initial investigation to be performed
d. USG is the best investigation
e. PET-CT offers no additional use

Ans. a, b, c *Ref: NCCN guidelines for endometrial cancers, 2017*

Option a	True	
Option b	True	
Option c	True	
Option d	False	MRI is used to establish diagnosis
Option e	False	Done in advanced stages and during follow up/surveillance after primary treatment

Imaging in endometrial cancers.

MRI:

- To establish diagnosis (when surgical staging is not planned)
- To assess myoinvasion
- To assess local extent of disease

CT:

- For higher grade carcinoma consider chest/abdominal/pelvic CT to evaluate for metastasis (Note: CT is better than MRI to detect metastatic omentum, pelvic or abdominal lymph nodes, lungs).

Whole body PET CT:

- In advanced stages and during follow up/surveillance after primary treatment if metastasis is suspected.

19. True about delivery of HIV positive woman:

a. Vaginal delivery has lower risk for transmission of HIV to child than Cesarean section
b. Vaginal delivery has higher risk for transmission of HIV to child than Cesarean section
c. Instrumentation has no risk of increased infection
d. Vertical transmission is seen to be more in cases with preterm birth
e. Early cord clamping is of no additional use

Ans. b, d *Ref: Harrison's principle of Internal Medicine, NACO PPTCT guidelines 2013, ACOG committee opinion number 234, 2015.*

Option a	False	Cesarean section offers lesser risk of transmission to the child
Option b	True	
Option c	False	Instrumentation increases the risk of infection through trauma
Option d	True	
Option e	False	Early cord clamping prevents mixing of maternal and fetal blood

HIV in Pregnancy

Vertical transmission

Transplacental HIV transmission can occur early, and the virus has even been identified in specimens from elective abortion.

However, maternal transmission to the fetus occurs most commonly in the perinatal period.

In the absence of prophylactic antiretroviral therapy to the mother during pregnancy, labor, and delivery, and to the fetus following birth, the probability of transmission of HIV from mother to infant/fetus ranges from 15 to 25% in industrialized countries and from 25 to 35% in developing countries.

The relative proportions of mother-to-child transmissions are 23–30% before birth, 50–65% during birth, and 12–20% via breast-feeding.

Vertical transmission is more common with preterm births, especially with prolonged membrane rupture.

Single dose Nevirapine in labor reduces risk of transmission to around 10%.

Multidrug ARV regime started early in pregnancy and continued throughout until cessation of breastfeeding has the potential to reduce vertical transmission rate to less than 5%.

There is increased risk of vertical transmission with HIV-1 and 2 coinfection.

Antenatal PPTCT

Scenario	Recommendations
Newly detected antenatally	Start ARV prophylaxis at 14 weeks and not before. Do CD4 count. Treatment remains same irrespective of CD4 count. CD4 count only determines duration of treatment whether lifelong or up to a week after breastfeeding
Known HIV positive on ART	Evaluate regime. Those who have received Efavirenz or NVP in pregnancy for PPTCT should now receive TDF + 3TC + LPV/r (lopinavir/ritonavir) to overcome NNRTI resistance. Continue modified ART throughout pregnancy. Revaluation and alteration as required after pregnancy
Known HIV positive not on ART	Initiate ARV at 14 weeks. Do CD4
HIV positive detected in labor	SD NVP + AZT (if Hb>9) + 3TC(12 hourly) Confirmation test with confirmatory test Initiate ART/ARV based on CD4 and WHO clinical stage
HIV positive detected after delivery	ART/ARV based on CD4 and WHO clinical staging

ARV prophylaxis is done by—TDF: Tenofovir, EFV : Efavirenz, 3TC : Lamivudine.

Labor and delivery

In theory, the risk of vertical transmission in mothers with high viral loads could be reduced by performing cesarean deliveries before onset of labor and before rupture of membranes.

ACOG Recommendations (American)

Scheduled cesarean section be discussed and recommended at 38 weeks if HIV RNA load exceeds 1000 copies/mL. Though it is unlikely that scheduled CS delivery offers any additional benefits in women already taking ARV regimes.

NACO guidelines (Indian)

Cesarean section is not recommended for prevention of mother to child transmission particularly in women taking ART or ARV prophylaxis as it provides only little additional protection in such women. Moreover Complications of CS are higher in women with HIV. Most common complication is puerperal fever. Thus CS is to be performed only for obstetric indications.

Safe delivery practices:

- No ARM (unless obstetrically indicated)
- Minimal number of PV examinations
- Avoiding shaving parts and enema
- Avoid fetal invasive procedures
- Avoid instrumental delivery. If indicated forceps is preferred over vacuum. As vacuum causes more fetal trauma
- Avoid suctioning unless MSAF
- Early cord clamping.

20. Regarding twin pregnancy correct is:

a. Separation before 72 hours - monochorionic monoamniotic twins
b. Separation after 4–8 days leads to monochorionic diamniotic fetuses

c. Separation after about 8 days most commonly leads to monoamniotic twins
d. Separation after embryonic disc formation leads to conjoined twins
e. Assisted reproductive techniques do not lead to multiple pregnancies

Ans. b, c, e *Ref: Williams Obstetrics, 24/e*

Option a	False	
Option b	True	
Option c	True	
Option d	False	
Option e	True	

Factors affecting dizygotic twinning

- *Race:* Most common in blacks. Intermediate in whites, least common in Asians
- Heredity
- *Maternal age:* Rate of natural twinning peaks at 37. FSH rises as age advances
- Increased parity
- *Nutrition:* Taller, heavier women have higher rates of twinning
- Conception immediately after stopping COC
- Infertility therapy

Infertility treatment	Risk of multiple pregnancy
Clomiphene induction	7–10%
Exogenous gonadotropins	15%
Exogenous GnRH	7–9%
ART	30%

- Previous dizygotic twinning (risk is 10 fold increased).

Types of monozygotic twins

	Period of division	Description
Dichorionic diamniotic	Up to day 3	Division prior to morula stage and differentiation of trophoblast 1/3rd of monozygotic twins
Monochorionic diamniotic	Day 4–8	Division after differentiation of trophoblast but before formation of amnion 2/3rd of monozygotic twins
Monochorionic monoamniotic	Day 8–13	Division after differentiation of amnion. Rare
Conjoined	Day 13–15	Incomplete splitting of embryo after formation of embryonic disc
Incomplete twin	After day 15	For example 2 heads one body - dicephalus

21. True about OCP's:
a. Increased risk of endometrial cancer
b. Increased risk of breast cancer
c. Low risk of venous embolism episode
d. Decreased risk of endometrial cancer
e. Increased hirsutism

Ans. b, d *Ref: Speroff 8/e, WHO Medical eligibility criteria for contraceptive use 5/e, 2015*

Option a	False	Increased risk of breast cancer
Option b	True	
Option c	False	Risk of thromboembolism increases
Option d	True	
Option e	False	Used for treating acne/hirsutism

Metabolic effects of combined OC pills

- **Venous coagulation**
  - With modern combined OC pills (COC) the risk of venous thromboembolism is increased about two fold associated with current use and primarily in the first year of use. Risk declines with increasing duration of use.
  - Risk is mainly influenced by estrogen dose.
  - Risk is slightly more with 3rd gen and drospirenone as compared to second generation Progestins.
  - Risk increases with body weight and age, heavy smoking.
  - Progestin only contraceptives do not increase the risk of venous thrombosis.
- **Arterial thrombosis:** Risk of acute MI and stroke may increase in young women on combined OC pills with 50 μg ethinyl estradiol (high dose) or more. With the use of low dose estrogen contraceptives increased risk occurs only in women who have hypertension or are smoking, not in other young women.
- **Lipoprotein:** Estrogen increases HDL and triglycerides, decreases LDL
  Androgens and androgenic Progestins can antagonize these beneficial effects by reducing HDL and elevating LDL.
  Newer Progestins desogestrel and norgestimate produce potentially beneficial changes by elevating HDL and lowering LDL.
- **Blood pressure:** Small increase in BP can be observed even with 30 μg EE. Rise in BP is because of the estrogen component.
- **Carbohydrate metabolism:** Progesterone exhibits insulin antagonism and increases insulin resistance. The effect is related to its androgenic potential and its dose. Use of POP for postpartum contraception has been associated with development of overt diabetes in Latino women in one study. However larger trials have not confirmed this.
- **Liver:** Active transport of biliary components is impaired by estrogen as well as some Progestins. Cholestatic jaundice and pruritus are occasional complications of high dose COC. Though there is no increased incidence of serious liver disease in COC users.
- **Other metabolic effects:**
  - Increased thyroid binding globulin, sex hormone binding globulin. Thyroid function tests remain normal.
  - The continuous daily use of COC may prevent symptoms of porphyria precipitated by menses.
  - Estrogen increases both free and bound cortisol. But the elevation is slight and cortisol remains in the normal ranges.

Cancers

Increased risk	Carcinoma cervix, breast and liver
Decreased risk	Ca endometrium, ovary, colorectal cancers

- **Cervical cancers:** Increased risk of cervical carcinoma in situ and cervical cancers associated with long term COC use.
  Probable causes:
  - Associated behavior pattern
  - COC may increase the ability of HPV to establish itself in cervix
  - COC may suppress immune response and may increase susceptibility to dysplasia and neoplasia.
- **Breast:** Current or recent use of COC may be associated with about a 20% increased risk of early (under age 35) premenopausal breast cancer, essentially limited to localized disease. Contraindication to COC use : Ca breast (cat IV).
- **Liver:** Oral contraception has been linked to the development of hepatocellular carcinoma.
- **Endometrium:**
  - 12 months of use of COC reduces the risk of Ca endometrium by 50%.
  - Greatest protective effect is obtained after 3 years of use.
  - Protection persists for 20 or more years after discontinuation.
- **Ovary:**
  - Protection seen with use for as little as 3–6 months
  - > 10 years of use—80% protection
  - Protection persists for 20 years after discontinuation
  - Reduced risk of Ca ovary in BRCA mutations
- **Colorectal cancers:** 8 years of use is associated with 40% decrease in risk. Steroid contraception should be offered to women with strong family history of colorectal cancers.

Contraindications to the use of COC:

Absolute contraindications **(WHO category IV)**

1. Postpartum—< 6 weeks + breastfeeding
   < 21 days non breastfeeding but with risk factors of VTE
2. Smoking—> 15 cig/day and age > 35 years
3. Hypertension with vascular disease or BP >160/100
4. Acute DVT/PE, H/O DVT/PE, DVT/PE controlled on Rx, known thrombogenic mutations, i.e. inherited thrombophilias, major surgery with prolonged immobilization
5. Current or past IHD or stroke, complicated valvular heart disease
6. SLE with APLA
7. Current Ca breast
8. DM with vascular disease
9. Acute or chronic cholestatic liver disease, acute flare of hepatitis, severe decompensated cirrhosis, HCC, malignant hepatoma
10. Migraine with aura.

22. True statement about breech delivery:

a. Vasa previa is a complication
b. Fetal congenital malformation increases breech risk
c. Increases fetal and maternal morbidity
d. Oligohydramnios increases breech risk
e. Increases risk of hip joint dislocation of baby

Ans. b, c, d, e *Ref: Williams obstetrics, 24/e*

Option a	False	Not an associated complication
Option b	True	
Option c	True	
Option d	True	
Option e	True	

Breech

Incidence 25% at 28 weeks and 3–4% at term.

Etiology

Maternal	Placental	Fetal
High parity Polyhydramnios Oligohydramnios Uterine anomalies Fibroid uterus Contracted pelvis Preterm delivery Anticonvulsant Substance abuse	Placenta previa Cornual fundal placenta Short umbilical cord	Multiple pregnancy Hydrocephalous Anencephaly Other anomalies Chromosomal anomalies IUGR, IUFD

Maternal morbidity and mortality

Increased rates of maternal and perinatal morbidity can be anticipated with breech presentations.

- Genital tract lacerations—vaginal wall or cervical lacerations, extended episiotomy, deep perineal tears and increased infection risks.
- Increased rate of cesarean delivery.
- Postpartum hemorrhage.
- Slightly increased rate of maternal mortality.

Perinatal morbidity and mortality

- Preterm delivery is a common association.
- There is an increased rate of congenital anomalies.
- Birth trauma:
  - Fractures of the humerus, clavicle, and femur
  - Separation of scapular, humeral, or femoral epiphyses.
  - Neonatal perineal tears have been reported from fetal scalp electrodes.
  - Upper extremity paralysis—Erb or Duchenne— may follow brachial plexus stretching,
  - Spoon-shaped depressions or actual fractures of the skull,
  - The spinal cord may be injured or vertebra fractured if great force is employed,
  - Hematomas of the sternocleidomastoid muscles occasionally develop after delivery, although they usually disappear spontaneously.

- Testicular injury may follow breech delivery
  - Compared with cephalic presentation, umbilical cord prolapse is more frequent with breech.
  - Development of hip dysplasia is more common in breech compared with cephalic presentation and is unaffected by delivery mode.

23. Complications of shoulder dystocia is/are:

a. Humerus fracture
b. Brachial plexus injury
c. Birth asphyxia
d. Sacroiliac joint dislocation of mother
e. Cervical fracture of baby

Ans. a, b, c, d, e *Ref: Williams obstetrics, 24/e; RCOG green top guideline number 42, 2012*

Option a	True	
Option b	True	
Option c	True	
Option d	True	
Option e	True	

Shoulder Dystocia

Risk factors:

- Macrosomic babies of diabetic mothers
- Macrosomia associated with post-term pregnancy
- Maternal obesity and excessive weight gain in pregnancy
- Prolonged labor
- Operative vaginal delivery
- Recurrent shoulder dystocia—10% risk
- Many cases occur in apparently normal labors.

Complications

In general, shoulder dystocia possess greater risk to the fetus than the mother.

Maternal:

- Third and fourth degree perineal tears, vaginal lacerations, cervical tears, bladder rupture, uterine rupture,
- Symphyseal separation, sacroiliac joint dislocation (RCOG, 2012) and lateral femoral cutaneous neuropathy.
- Postpartum hemorrhage from uterine atony or vaginal lacerations.

Fetal and neonatal morbidity and mortality:

- Birth asphyxia, hypoxia and their complications
- Birth injuries:
  - Brachial plexus injury
  - Clavicle, humeral, or rib fracture.
  - Cervical Vertebral dislocation associated with a Zavanelli maneuver. (Williams 24th).

24. Predisposing factor(s) for obstetrical hemorrhage is/are:
   a. Obesity
   b. Placental abruption
   c. Oligohydramnios
   d. Smoking
   e. Instrumental delivery

Ans. a, b, d, e *Ref: RCOG, Green top guideline number 52, 20*

Option a	True	
Option b	True	
Option c	False	Polyhydramnios is an identified complication
Option d	True	
Option e	True	

Causes of PPH can be classified as factors associated with:

- Tone
- Thrombin
- Trauma
- Tissue

80–90% of primary PPH are associated with uterine atony.

Risk factors:

Majority of the cases have no identified risk factors.

Following are the identifiable risk factors that may be present.

	Antepartum	Intrapartum
Tone	Multiple pregnancy Polyhydramnios Big baby Placenta previa Age >40, Obesity Anemia, multiparty	Prolonged labor Uterine inertia Induced labor Chorioamnionitis Prolonged PROM Adherent placenta Uterine inversion
Thrombin	Preeclampsia Liver disease Coagulopathy	Abruptio placentae Pyrexia in labor
Trauma		CS, operative vaginal delivery, episiotomy
Tissue		Retained placenta Adherent placenta

25. All of the following are true about vulvodynia *except*:
   a. Surgery is usually done for localized vulvar lesion
   b. Pain without any significant lesion
   c. May be associated with irritable bowel syndrome
   d. Tricyclic antidepressant is useful
   e. Psychological factor is associated

Ans. a *Ref: Williams gynecology, 3/e*

Option a	True	Behavioral and pharmacological management is done
Option b	False	
Option c	False	
Option d	False	
Option e	False	

Vulvodynia

Definition: "vulvar discomfort, most often described as burning pain, occurring in the absence of relevant visible findings or a specific, clinically identifiable, neurologic disorder".

Limited studies indicate a prevalence of vulvodynia in the general population of 3 to 11 percent. Women from all ethnicities and a wide age range are affected.

Theories propose that some local injury or noxious stimulus results in maladaptive local and/or central nervous system responses leading to a neuropathic pain syndrome added by certain psychological predispositions.

Patients with vulvodynia have an increased prevalence of other chronic pain disorders, including interstitial cystitis, irritable bowel syndrome, fibromyalgia, and temporomandibular pain.

Diagnosis

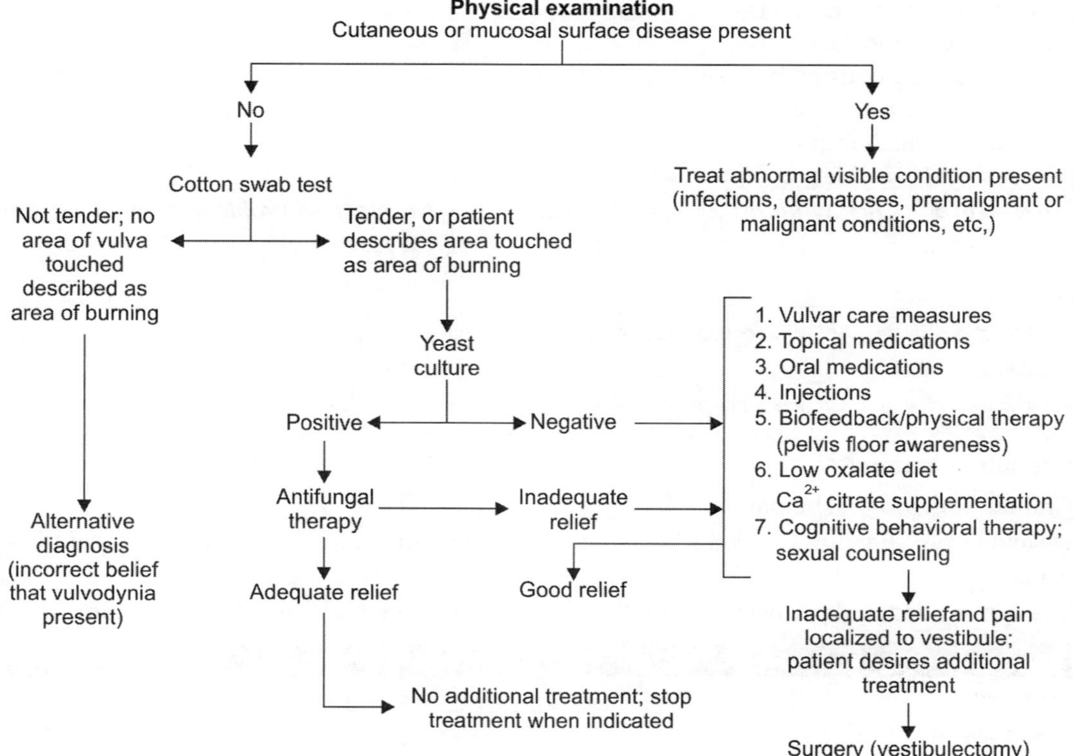

Management

Behavioral therapy:

Biofeedback, physical therapy (pelvic floor awareness). Education regarding foreplay, sexual positions, lubrication, and alternatives to vaginal intercourse is offered if potentially helpful in sexual dysfunction.

Medications:

Topical:

- 5-percent lidocaine ointment applied sparingly to the vestibule 30 minutes prior to sexual intercourse.
- Topical or intravaginal estrogen therapy has yielded mixed results.
- Topical gabapentin cream is well-tolerated, and effective.

Oral medications:

- Antidepressants and anticonvulsants.
- Tricyclic antidepressants (TCAs) have become a first-line agent in the treatment of vulvodynia, and reported response rates may reach 47 percent results.
- Cases resistant to CAs may be treated with the anticonvulsants gabapentin or carbamazepine.
  However, polypharmacy is avoided.

26. Cephalohematoma is:

a. Subperiosteal
b. Self-limiting with in few hours to few days
c. Oedematous fluid
d. Vascular origin
e. 0.01% incidence

Ans. a, b, d *Ref: Williams, 24/e; Gabbe: Obstetrics—Normal and Problem Pregnancies, 4/e*

Option a	True	
Option b	True	
Option c	False	Extracranial bleeding under periosteum
Option d	True	
Option e	False	Incidence is 0.2 to 2.5%

Cephalohematoma

Cranial subperiosteal hematomas.

Develop from shearing forces during labor and delivery that lacerate the emissary or diploic veins.

The densely adhered periosteum impedes rapid enlargement and limits final hematoma size.

Caput succedaneum	Cephalhematoma
Scalp swelling	Extracranial bleeding under periosteum
Very common	Uncommon

Contd...

Contd…

Caput succedaneum	Cephalhematoma
Etiology: Pressure caused by cervical ring obstructs venous return from scalp Seen more often in prolonged labor	Etiology: Prolonged labour Forceps trauma Sudden compression decompression as in precipitate labor
Diffuse swelling, passes suture lines	Sharp borders, confined to individual bones, does not cross suture lines
Largest at birth, grows smaller and disappears in a few hours	Appears few hours after birth, grows larger for a time, disappears after 6–12 weeks
Position of caput varies with position of head	Parietal region is most commonly affected
No treatment required	No treatment required. Vit. K may be given to reduce further bleeding
Large caput in prolonged labor may indicate CPD	

A cephalhematoma occurs in 0.2 to 2.5 percent of live births.

27. All of the following are contraindications to medical method of abortion *except*:

a. Rheumatic heart disease
b. Hypersensitivity to prostaglandins
c. Hemoglobin < 10 gm %
d. Inherited porphyria
e. Adrenal failure

Ans. a, c

Option a	True	Angina, valvular disease, arrhythmia etc. are contraindications but not RHD
Option b	False	
Option c	True	Hb < 8 gm% is a contraindication
Option d	False	
Option e	False	

Medical method of abortion

Drugs used

Commonly used drugs for Medical Methods of Abortion are a combination of Mifepristone and Misoprostol. Drug Controller General of India approved the use of Mifepristone and Misoprostol (in December 2006) for termination of pregnancy up to 49 days gestation period. Also recommended in *Ministry of Health and Family Welfare Government of India, handbook 2016.*

In December 2008, Mifepristone + Misoprostol (1 tab of mifepristone 200 mg and 4 tab of misoprostol 200 mcg each) Combipack was approved by the Central Drugs Standard Control Organization, Directorate General of Health Services for the medical termination of intrauterine pregnancy (MTP) for up to 63 days gestation.

Contraindications *(Ministry of Health and Family Welfare Government of India, handbook, 2016)*

- ❑ Anaemia (haemoglobin < 8 gm %)
- ❑ Confirmed or suspected ectopic pregnancy/undiagnosed adnexal mass

- Uncontrolled hypertension or BP > 160/100 mm Hg
- Known cases of:
  - Heart problems such as angina, valvular disease, arrhythmia which can lead to sudden cardiovascular collapse (note rheumatic heart disease is not included)
  - Renal, liver or respiratory disease (Bronchial asthma is not a contraindication since Misoprostol is a bronchodilator)
  - Current long-term systemic corticosteroid therapy
  - Uncontrolled seizure disorder
  - Chronic adrenal failure
  - Hypersensitivity to Mifepristone/Misoprostol or other prostaglandins
  - Inherited porphyrias.

Contraindications to medical method of abortion *(WHO, Clinical practice handbook for safe abortion, 2014)*

- Previous allergic reaction to one of the drugs involved
- Inherited porphyria
- Chronic adrenal failure
- Known or suspected ectopic pregnancy (neither misoprostol nor mifepristone will treat ectopic pregnancy.

28. True regarding ovarian fibroma is:

a. Fraser syndrome
b. Meigs' syndrome
c. Denys-Drash syndrome
d. 1% chance of malignant transformation
e. Fitz-Hugh-Curtis syndrome

Ans. a, d

Option a	True	
Option b	False	
Option c	False	
Option d	True	
Option e	False	

Fibromas are relatively common, hormonally inactive sex cord stromal tumor variants that usually occur in perimenopausal and menopausal women. These solid, generally benign ovarian neoplasms arise rom the spindled stromal cells that form collagen. Most fibromas are found incidentally during pelvic or sonographic examination.

They are round, oval, or lobulated solid tumors associated with free fluid or less commonly, with frank ascites and possess minimal to moderate vascularization. About 1 percent of women present with Meigs' syndrome, which is a triad of pleural effusion, ascites, and a solid ovarian mass. Pleural effusion is usually right sided, and this, as well as accompanying ascites, is typically transudative and resolve after tumor resection. Despite this association of ascites with benign fibromas, when ascites and a pelvic mass coexist, evaluation is based on an assumption of malignancy.

The prognosis following excision of fibromas is similar to that or any benign tumor of the ovary.

However, 10 percent will demonstrate increased cellularity and varying degrees of pleomorphism and mitotic activity that indicate a tumor better characterized as having low malignant potential. In 1 percent of cases, malignant transformation to fibrosarcoma is found.

Denys-Drash syndrome is characterized by the association of diffuse mesangial sclerosis (DMS), male pseudohermaphroditism with a 46,XY karyotype, and nephroblastoma. Etiology – mutation in WT1gene.

Fraser syndrome is a rare genetic disorder characterized by partial webbing of the fingers and/or toes (partial syndactyly), kidney (renal) abnormalities, genital malformations, and/or, in some cases, complete fusion of the eyelids (cryptophthalmos) that may be associated with malformation of the eyes, causing blindness.

29. $MgSO_4$ is used in eclampsia and preeclampsia for:

a. Treatment of hypertension
b. Therapeutic level is Serum Mg between 4 and 7 mEq/mL
c. Prevents convulsions
d. Loading dose may be given without knowing the renal status
e. Fetal skeletal protection

Ans. b, c, d *Ref: Hypertension in pregnancy by US task force, ACOG, 2013; Williams obstetrics, 24/e; ACOG committee opinion 652, 2016*

Option a	False	Effective anticonvulsant
Option b	True	
Option c	True	
Option d	True	
Option e	False	Possible neuroprotection

$MgSO_4$

Effective anticonvulsant that avoids producing CNS depression of mother or infant. Dose same for both treatment and prevention of convulsions.

Proposed mechanisms of action:

1. Reduced presynaptic release of neurotransmitter glutamate
2. Blockade of NMDA receptors
3. Potentiation of adenosine action
4. Improved calcium buffering by mitochondria
5. Blockade of calcium entry via voltage gated channels.

Indications:

1. Eclampsia
2. Intrapartum magnesium sulphate in severe pre-eclampsia
3. Certain signs and symptoms (headache, altered mental state, blurred vision, scotomata, clonus, and right upper quadrant abdominal pain) have traditionally been considered as premonitory to seizures and should be considered in the choice for initiation of magnesium sulfate therapy.

4. Fetal neuroprotection before anticipated early preterm delivery. (ACOG—32 weeks, NICE—34 weeks).
5. Short-term prolongation of pregnancy (up to 48 hours) to allow for the administration of antenatal corticosteroids in pregnant women who are at risk of preterm delivery within 7 days.

Use of $MgSO_4$ in eclampsia/preeclampsia

Dosage regimes

	Loading dose	Maintenance
Pritchard	4 g iv and 5 g im in each buttock	5 g in each buttock 4 hourly
Zuspan	4 g iv	iv infusion @ 1–2 g/hours
Sibai	6 g iv over 10–15 min	2–3 g in 100 mL infusion every hour
Sardesai (solapur)	4 g iv or im	2 g iv or im every 3 hours

Monitoring required with $MgSO_4$ administration

- Deep tendon reflexes (DTR)
- Respiratory rate (RR)
- Urine output (UOP) >100 mL in 4 hrs
- Some also measure Sr. Mg at 4–6 hours of initial dose to make necessary dose adjustment. $MgSO_4$ is discontinued 24 hours after delivery or 24 hours after last convulsion, whichever is later.

$MgSO_4$ does not treat hypertension

Toxicity:

Therapeutic level	4–7 mEq/L	4.8–8.4 mg/dL
Loss of patellar reflexes	When level reaches 10 mEq/L	12 mg/dL
Respiratory depression	Levels above 10 mEq/L	12 mg/dL
Respiratory paralysis or arrest	≥ 12 mEq/L	
Transient depression of uterine activity	8–10 mEq/L	

Renal dysfunction and $MgSO_4$

The initial 4 gm dose can be given safely regardless of the renal function.

Maintenance dose should be altered in case of decreased GFR indicated by Sr. Creatinine > 1 mg/mL. Infusion rate should be adjusted such that Mg Levels are in the therapeutic range.

With severe renal failure only the loading dose of $MgSO_4$ is required to produce steady state therapeutic level.

Management of Mg toxicity:

Calcium gluconate or calcium chloride 1g IV

Withhold $MgSO_4$

Tracheal intubation, mechanical ventilation if required.

30. Seen in HELLP syndrome:

a. Increase in serum transaminases
b. Low platelet count
c. Increase in conjugate bilirubin
d. Autoimmune hemolysis
e. High platelet count

Ans. a, b *Ref: Hypertension in pregnancy by US task force, ACOG, 2013; Williams obstetrics 24/e*

Option a	True	
Option b	True	
Option c	False	
Option d	False	
Option e	False	

HELLP syndrome

There is no universally accepted strict definition of this syndrome. Some pregnant women present with a specific constellation of laboratory findings—hemolysis, elevated liver enzymes, and low platelet count— that has been labeled as the "HELLP syndrome".

The development of HELLP syndrome may occur antepartum or postpartum. The clinical course of women with HELLP syndrome is often characterized by progressive and sometimes sudden deterioration in maternal and fetal condition.

Laboratory test	Possible result	Cause	Recovery time after postpartum
Haptoglobin	↓	Hemolysis	24–30 hours
LDH	↑	Hemolysis or liver dysfunction	3–5 days
AST or ALT	↑	Liver dysfunction	3–5 days
Bilirubin	↑	Hemolysis	—
Platelets (CBC)	↓	Consumption	6–11 days
Hemoglobin/ Hematocrit (CBC)	↓	Hemolysis	—
PT	Normal		—
PTT	↑	Liver dysfunction	—
D-dimer	↑	Increased coagulation and secondary fibrinolysis	—
Fibrinogen			

Other findings are schizocytosis, spherocytosis, and reticulocytosis in peripheral blood. These derangements result in part from microangiopathic hemolysis (not autoimmune hemolysis) caused by endothelial disruption with platelet adherence and fibrin deposition.

(Rise in Serum bilirubin is not included in the definition or diagnosis of HELLP syndrome. Note that the bilirubin rise in some cases is because of hemolysis and not because of hepatic dysfunction. So if at all there is a rise in bilirubin, it is unconjugated bilirubin that rises primarily).

Management of HELLP syndrome

Period of gestation	Management
Before period of viability (usually < 24 weeks) or after 34 weeks	Delivery should be undertaken soon after initial maternal stabilization.
24 to 33 weeks	Delivery should be delayed for 24–48 hours if maternal and fetal condition remain stable to complete a course of corticosteroids for fetal benefit. There is also evidence of improvement of maternal platelet counts with corticosteroid treatment.

31. Anti-phospholipid syndrome, true is:

a. Recurrent abortions
b. 2nd trimester abortions
c. Accelerated thrombosis
d. Hemoglobinopathy
e. Late onset pre-eclampsia

Ans. a, b, c *Ref: ACOG, Practice bulletin no. 132, 2012; Williams obstetrics, 24/e; Novak gynecology, 15/e*

Option a	True	
Option b	True	
Option c	True	
Option d	False	
Option e	False	

Antiphospholipid antibody syndrome

Phospholipids are the main lipid constituents of cell and organelle membranes. There are proteins in plasma that associate noncovalently with these phospholipids.

Antigenic determinants for antiphospholipid antibodies (like beta 2-glycoprotein I) are ubiquitous, multifunctional plasma proteins with an affinity for negatively charged phospholipids. They have regulatory roles in coagulation, fibrinolysis, and other physiologic systems. Antiphospholipid antibodies are directed against these phospholipids or phospholipid-binding proteins. This antibody group may be of IgG, IgM, and IgA classes, alone or in combination.

The pathophysiology is mediated by one or more of the following:

1. Activation of various procoagulants,
2. Inactivation of natural anticoagulants,
3. Complement activation, and
4. Inhibition of syncytiotrophoblast differentiation.

Antiphospholipid antibodie shave been associated with a variety of medical problems:

- ❑ Arterial thrombosis and venous thrombosis,
- ❑ Autoimmune thrombocytopenia,
- ❑ Obstetrics complications—recurrent pregnancy loss, preeclampsia, intrauterine growth restriction, placental insufficiency, preterm delivery, fetal death.

The antibodies (of diagnostic importance)

Antibody	Diagnosis	Clinical significance
Lupus anticoagulant	Assessed indirectly, and a series of tests are needed for the laboratory • Lupus anticoagulant-sensitive activated partial thromboplastin time • Dilute Russell's viper venom time. Lupus anticoagulant cannot be quantified and is reported only as present or absent. Testing for lupus anticoagulant is ideally performed before the patient is treated with anticoagulants	• More specific, but less sensitive than the other two tests • Associated not with anticoagulation but with thrombosis.
Anti-cardiolipin	Measuring IgG and IgM isotypes of anti-cardiolipin antibody by ELISA Positive anticardiolipin result is greater than 40 GPL or 40 MPL (greater than 99th percentile) GPL and MPL are the new international standard units for quantifying IgG and IgM. However most laboratories still report semi-quantitative results (e.g., negative, low, medium, or high)	
Anti– β2-glycoprotein I	Measuring IgG and IgM isotypes of anti- β2 -glycoprotein 1 by ELISA Reported most commonly in international standard units known as "SGU" or "SMU" for IgG and IgM, respectively. A positive result is greater than the 99th percentile.	**β2-glycoprotein I is the primarily clinically relevant antigen, responsible for the complications.** It has a regulatory role in coagulation, fibrinolysis, and other physiologic systems. Its normal action is to inhibit procoagulant binding and thereby prevent coagulation cascade activation. β2-glycoprotein I is expressed in high concentrations on the syncytiotrophoblastic surface. β2-glycoprotein I may be involved in implantation, and it may result in pregnancy loss via an inflammatory mechanism

32. First trimester aneuploidy screening dual test includes:

a. B-hCG + PAPP-A
b. AFP + hCG
c. PAPP-A + AFP
d. AFP + PAPP-A + B-hCG
e. B-hCG + Estradiol

Ans. a

Option a	True	
Option b	False	
Option c	False	
Option d	False	
Option e	False	

Screening	Marker	Period of gestation	Detection rate of down syndrome
First trimester (NT + dual markers)	NT PAPP –A Beta hCG	11–14 weeks	82–87%
Triple screen	AFP Beta hCG uE3	15–22 weeks	69%
Quadruple screen	AFP Beta hCG uE3 Dimeric inhibin A	15–22 weeks	81%
Penta screen (New)	AFP Beta hCG uE3 Dimeric inhibin A + hyperglycosylated hCG (also known as invasive trophoblast antigen)	15–22 weeks	Limited data

33. PAP smear was done and it shows HSIL. Next step/steps in management would be:

a. Colposcopy
b. Repeat PAP smear
c. Liquid based cytology
d. Hysterectomy
e. HPV DNA estimation

Ans. a

Option a	True	Colposcopy is the acceptable method
Option b	False	
Option c	False	
Option d	False	
Option e	False	

Cervical precancerous lesions and cervical cancers.

Screening methods:

1. Vaginal exfoliative cytology by pap smear
2. Liquid based vaginal exfoliative cytology
3. HPV DNA testing from the vaginal swab
4. Visual inspection with acetic acid
5. Visual inspection with Lugol's iodine

Screening guidelines:

Screening recommendations American society for colposcopy and cervical pathology ASCCP Guidelines 2014

< 21 years	No Screening	
21–29 years	Cytology alone, every 3 years	

30–65 years	HPV and Cytology "Co-testing" every 5 years (Preferred) Cytology alone every 3 years (Acceptable)	Screening by HPV testing alone is not recommended
> 65 years	No Screening following adequate negative prior screening	Women with a history of CIN 2 or a more severe diagnosis should continue routine screening for at least 20 years after spontaneous regression or appropriate management of CIN 2, CIN 3, or adenocarcinoma in situ.
HPV vaccinated	Same as age specific recommendations	
After hysterectomy	No screening	Applies to women without a cervix and without a history of CIN 2, CIN 3, adenocarcinoma in situ, or cancer in the past 20 years.

Management:

Management based on cytology

Cytology	≥ 30 years		21–24 years
Unsatisfactory	HPV (+)	Colposcopy/rpt cytology at 2–4 months	Rpt cytology at 2–4 months
	HPV (–)	Rpt cytology at 2–4 months	
NILM, EC/TZ absent	HV (+)	Genotyping or Rpt cotesting at 1 year	Routine screening
	HPV (–)	Routine screening	
Negative/HPV (+)	©Genotyping		
	HPV 16/18 (+)	Colposcopy	
	16/18 (–)	Rpt cotesting at 1 year	
	©Rpt co-testing at 1 year	Anything (+) do Colposcopy	
ASCUS	€HPV testing		Rpt cytology at 1 year
	HPV (+)	Colposcopy	ASCH, HSIL, AGC – Colposcopy
	HPV (–)	Rpt co-testing at 3 years	
	©Rpt cytology at 1 year	≥ ASC – Colposcopy	ASCUS, LSIL – rpt cytology at 1 year – ASCUS – Colposcopy
LSIL	HPV (+), unknown	Colposcopy	Same as above
	HPV (–)	€rpt co-testing at 1 year	
		©Colposcopy	
LSIL + Pregnant		Colposcopy	Colposcopy
ASCH, HSIL, AGC		Colposcopy	Colposcopy

©Acceptable method

€Preferred method

American Society for Colposcopy and Cervical Pathology (ASCCP) Guidelines 2014

Management of women with high-grade squamous intraepithelial lesions (HSIL)

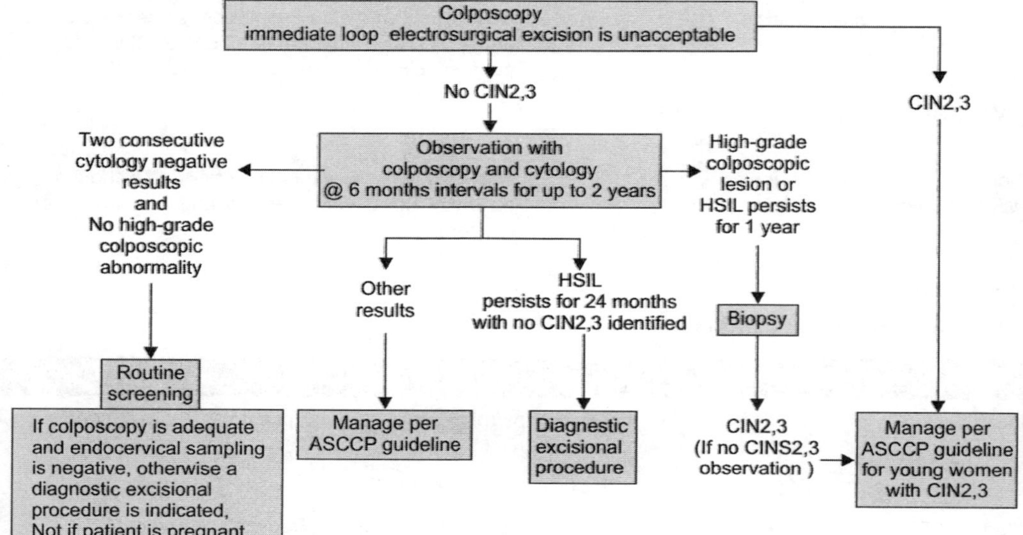

34. True about vacuum extraction is:

a. 5 cm cervical dilatation is required
b. Placed 2 cm anterior to posterior fontanelle
c. Completely dependent on maternal forces
d. Applied at one, extracted after 2 mins
e. Applied to non-engaged head

Ans. b, d *Ref: Williams obstetrics 24/e, ACOG Practice bulletin 154, 2015*

Option a	False	Completely dilated cervix is required
Option b	True	
Option c	False	Maternal forces are not required
Option d	True	
Option e	False	Head has to be engaged

Operative vaginal delivery:

Indications

Maternal	Fetal
Maternal exhaustion and prolonged second stage*	Nonreassuring fetal heart status
Heart disease	Premature separation of placenta
Pulmonary injury or compromise	Cord prolapse

Contd...

Contd…

Maternal	Fetal
Intrapartum infection	
Certain neurologic conditions	

*Prolonged second stage	Without regional analgesia (hrs)	With regional analgesia (hrs)
Primi	2	3
Multi	1	2

	Criteria
Outlet forceps	Scalp visible at the introitus without separating labia Fetal skull has reached pelvic floor Fetal head is at or on perineum Sagittal suture is in AP diameter (OA, LOA, ROA, MA, RMA, LMA, OP, ROP, LOP) Rotation is <45°
Low forceps	Station ≥ +2 but above pelvic floor Rotation is (1) <45° or (2) >45°
Midforceps	Station between 0 and +2

Prerequisites
- Experienced operator
- Engaged head
- Ruptured membranes
- Vertex presentation
- **Completely dilated cervix**
- Precisely assessed fetal head position
- No suspected CPD
- No fetal Coagulopathy
- No fetal bone demineralization disorder
- Bladder emptied

Additional prerequisites for vacuum
- Gestational age > 34 weeks
- Cephalic presentation (face contraindicated)
- No recent fetal scalp blood sampling

Operative vaginal delivery is contraindicated if the above prerequisites are not fulfilled

35. Effects of estrogen are:

a. Cornified vaginal epithelium
b. Growth of mammary ducts
c. Thickened cervical mucus
d. Acidified vaginal pH
e. Tubal motility

Ans. a, b, d, e *Ref: Ganong physiology; Speroff clinical endocrinology, 8/e*

Option a	True	
Option b	True	
Option c	False	Makes cervical mucus thin and elastic
Option d	True	
Option e	True	

Effects of estrogen on the female reproductive system:

Vagina:

- Under the influence of estrogen, the vaginal epithelium becomes cornified.
- Presence of estrogen is required for acidic vaginal pH, which protects against vaginal infections.

Cervix:

- Mid cycle estrogen peak makes cervical mucus thinner and copious. Estrogen is responsible cervical mucus elasticity or spinnbarkeit observed toward the end of follicular phase. In addition getting can be seen on a slide under microscope.

Uterus:

- Endometrial proliferation
- Increased uterine blood flow

Ovaries:

- Synergistic action with FSH on growth of ovarian follicles
- Successful ovulation requires Estrogen milieu in the mature follicle.

Tubes:

- Increased motility of uterine tube

Breasts:

- Duct growth, proliferation of ducts (progesterone has role in development of lobules)
- Pigmentation of areola at puberty and during first pregnancy
- Antagonizes milk producing effect of prolactin on the breasts.

36. True about management of pregnancy with NYHA class 3 or 4 heart disease:

a. Delivery should be done in specialized hospitals
b. Often tolerate major surgical procedures poorly
c. Caesarean delivery is limited to obstetrical indication
d. Mortality is 5–20%
e. Epidural is preferred for delivery and labour pain management

Ans. a, b, c, d, e *Ref: ESC Guidelines on the management of cardiovascular diseases during pregnancy, 2011; Williams obstetrics, 24/e*

Option a	True	
Option b	True	
Option c	True	
Option d	True	
Option e	True	

Conditions in which pregnancy risk is WHO IV (pregnancy contraindicated)

- Pulmonary arterial hypertension of any cause
- Severe systemic ventricular dysfunction (LVEF <30%, NYHA III–IV)
- Previous peripartum cardiomyopathy with any residual impairment of left ventricular function
- Severe mitral stenosis, severe symptomatic aortic stenosis
- Marfan syndrome with aorta dilated >45 mm

- ❑ Aortic dilatation >50 mm in aortic disease associated with bicuspid aortic valve
- ❑ Native severe coarctation

Patients in NYHA class III/IV or with severely reduced function of the systemic ventricle are at high risk during pregnancy, surgical tolerance is poor due to poor cardiac reserve.

Labor and delivery

Vaginal delivery is generally to be preferred, except for obstetric indications for cesarean. The general principle of is to minimize cardiovascular overload. In most cases this is achieved by use of early slow incremental epidural analgesia and assisted vaginal delivery.

Delivery should take place in a multispeciality hospital with obstetrician, cardiologist, anaesthesiologist, pediatrician, trained nursing staff.

CS is the preferred mode of delivery in the following cardiac conditions:

1. Marfan with dilated aortic root > 4 cm or aortic aneurysm
2. Acute severe congestive heart failure
3. Recent MI
4. Severe symptomatic AS
5. Warfarin administration within two weeks of delivery (e.g. in preterm labor) as there is increased risk of neonatal intracranial hemorrhage.
6. Need for emergency valve replacement immediately after delivery.

CS may be considered in:

1. Coarctation of aorta.

37. Most common uterine cause of abortion is/are:

a. Septate uterus
b. Bicornuate uterus
c. Uterus didelphys
d. Unicornuate uterus
e. Arcuate uterus

Ans. a *Ref: Novak gynecology, 9/e*

Option	
Option a	True
Option b	False
Option c	False
Option d	False
Option e	False

Uterus anomalies associated with recurrent pregnancy loss:

- ❑ Congenital uterine malformations
- ❑ Uterine fibroids, polyps
- ❑ Intrauterine adhesions

During development, the uterus forms via the apposition of a portion of bilateral hollow tubes called the müllerian ducts. The dissolution of the walls of these ducts along their site of apposition allows formation of the intrauterine cavity, the intracervical canal, and the upper vagina.

Congenital uterine anomalies may, therefore, include incomplete müllerian duct fusion, incomplete septum resorption, and uterine cervical anomalies.

Additionally prenatal exposure to maternally ingested diethylstilbestrol (DES) results in complex congenital uterine, cervical, and vaginal changes.

All congenital reproductive tract abnormalities have been linked to both isolated spontaneous pregnancy loss and to recurrent pregnancy loss, although the presence of an intrauterine septum and prenatal exposure to DES demonstrate the strongest associations. Women with an intrauterine septum may have as high as a 60% risk for spontaneous abortion. Uterine septum-related losses most frequently occur during the second trimester. However, if an embryo implants into the poorly developed endometrium overlying the uterine septum, abnormal placentation and resultant first trimester losses may occur.

The most common uterine congenital anomaly associated with in utero DES exposure is hypoplasia, which may contribute to first- or second-trimester spontaneous abortions, incompetent cervix, and premature labor.

Acquired anatomic anomalies have likewise been linked to both isolated and recurrent pregnancy losses. These abnormalities include intrauterine adhesions, uterine fibroids, and endometrial polyps.

Endometrium that develops over an intrauterine synechiae or over a fibroid that impinges in the intrauterine cavity (submucous) may be inadequately vascularized. This may promote abnormal placentation for any embryo attempting to implant over such lesions. Although data supporting these concepts are limited, this abnormal placentation may lead to spontaneous pregnancy loss.

The septate uterus is by far the most common uterine developmental anomaly, accounting for 80–90% of all major malformations in both women with recurrent pregnancy loss (3.5% prevalence) and in the general population. It is also the malformation most highly associated with poor pregnancy outcomes. Data from numerous case series indicate that the miscarriage rate associated with septate uteri is approximately 65%.

Bicornuate uterus results from incomplete fusion of the müllerian ducts at the level of the fundus, creating two separate uterine cavities with a common lower segment and a single cervix; externally, the uterus has a midline cleft with a depth that varies with the severity of the fusion anomaly. Data from collected series of women with bicornuate uteri reveal miscarriage and overall fetal loss rates of approximately 30% and 40%, respectively.

Ref: Speroff clinical endocrinology, 8/e

Dermatology

1. Immunotherapy in leprosy is done by using:
   a. Candida albicans
   b. BCG vaccine
   c. Mycobacterium indicus pranii
   d. Human Ig
   e. Polyvalent leprosy vaccine

Ans. b, c *Ref: Katoch K. Immunotherapy of leprosy. Indian J Lepr. 1996;68(4):349-61. https://www.dermnetnz.org/topics/cutaneous-tuberculosis/*

Option a	False	Not correct
Option b	True	Yes, correct
Option c	True	Yes, this is recently launched vaccine
Option d	False	No, there is no availability of passive immunization using immunoglobulins
Option e	False	Not correct

Immunotherapy is a modality which aims to modify the defective cell-mediated immune response in leprosy cases.

Rationale: The addition of immunotherapy to chemotherapy aims at achieving.
- ❑ More efficient killing of viable bacilli including persister organisms
- ❑ Faster clearance of dead bacilli and their components from the body
- ❑ Effectively reduces the duration of treatment and help in greater compliance of patients specially in bacilliferous leprosy cases.

a. Antigenically related mycobacteria sharing antigens with *M. leprae*:
- BCG
- BCG + *M. leprae*
- *Mycobacterium indicus pranii (MIP),* earlier known as Mw is a rapidly growing non-pathogenic mycobacterium. When administered intradermally, it increases cell-mediated immunity in the host.
- Indian Cancer Research Centre (ICRC) bacilli
- *M. vaccae*

b. Immunomodulators:
- Levamisole
- Zinc

c. Other promising immunomodulators:
- Transfer factor
- Interferon gamma
- Interleukin 2
- Acetoacetylated *M. leprae.*
- Detalipified Cell Components of (DCC) *M. leprae*

2. Purpuric contact dermatitis is caused by:
a. Nickel
b. Gold
c. Poison Ivy
d. Para-phenylenediamine
e. Fiber glass

Ans. d, e *Ref: Bonamonte D, Foti C, Vestita M, Angelini G. Noneczematous contact dermatitis. ISRN Allergy. 2013;2013:361746.*

Option a	False	No, it may produce pulmonary symptoms or even Ca lung. Skin manifestations may include allergic contact dermatitis
Option b	False	No, Gold handlers have an increased risk of nephropathy to renal failure
Option c	False	No, not correct. A substance called urushiol found in these plants causes the rash. The rash is 'allergic contact dermatitis' which is delayed hypersensitivity reaction. The most common cause is *rhus dermatitis* or dermatitis from poison ivy or poison oak
Option d	True	Yes, correct
Option e	True	Yes, correct

Purpuric contact dermatitis is a form of non-eczematous contact dermatitis occurring secondary to various textile fabrics, rubber antioxidants or other chemicals and pressure.

Agents producing purpuric contact dermatitis

Rubber compounds	Textile compounds	Plants	Miscellaneous
N-isopropyl-N′-phenyl-paraphenylenediamine Mercaptobenzothiazole	Optical whiteners Azoic dyes Formaldehyde resins	Agave americana Zea mais	Paraphenylenediamine Fiberglass Balsam of Peru Epoxy resin Oxyquinoline Proflavine Cobalt Benzoyl peroxide

3. Sporotrichoid lesions seen in?
a. Sporotrichosis
b. Tuberculosis
c. Blastomycosis
d. Swimming pool granuloma
e. Lichen nitidus

Ans. a, d *Ref: Bolognia Textbook of Dermatology, Page 1416*

Option a	True	Yes, correct
Option b	False	No, TB has other manifestations as lupus vulgaris, verrucosa cutis, scrofulderma (refer explanation)
Option c	False	No, the skin manifestation of blastomycosis include: Purplish-gray verrucous lesions with heaped borders or friable lesions that ulcerate. Munro's Microabscess and subcutaneous nodules can also be seen. The skin is the second most common site of spread after the lungs.
Option d	True	Yes, correct
Option e	False	No, these are reddish brown hypopigmented papules on (usually) a darker skin. These are usually non-pruritic

Linearity is an important feature in the skin lesions as it generally denotes an exogenous influence. The most common clinical presentation of sporotrichosis is the lymphocutaneous or "sporotrichoid" pattern which refers to the primary inoculation site plus spread of the infection along the lymphatics in a nodular pattern.

Differential diagnosis for skin nodules in a sporotrichoid-spread pattern includes:

1. Sporothrix schenckii
2. Mycobacterium marinum (Swimming pool granuloma), other nontuberculous mycobacteria
3. Nocardia
4. Cutaneous Leishmaniasis due to *L. luyanensis*
5. Cat scratch disease, Tularemia.

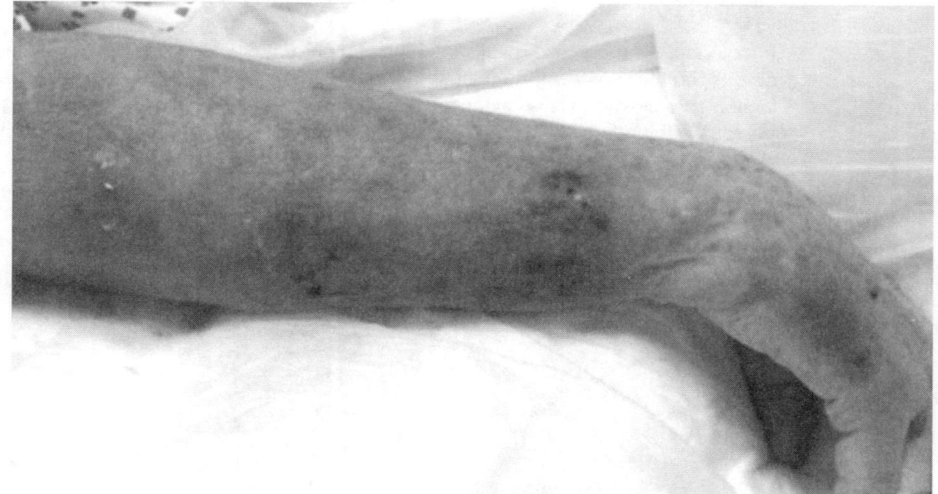

(TB) must remember points for cutaneous manifestations of tuberculosis which are as follows:

Types of cutaneous TB	Features
TB verrucosa cutis	Occurs after direct inoculation of TB into the skin in someone who has been previously infected with mycobacteria Presents as a purplish or brownish-red warty growth Lesions most often occur on the knees, elbows, hands, feet and buttocks Lesions may persist for years but can clear up even without treatment
Lupus vulgaris	Persistent and progressive form of cutaneous TB Small sharply defined reddish-brown lesions with a gelatinous consistency (called apple-jelly nodules) Lesions persist for years leading to disfigurement and sometimes skin cancer
Scrofuloderma	Skin lesions result from direct extension of underlying TB infection of lymph nodes, bone or joints Often associated with TB of the lungs Firm, painless lesions that eventually ulcerate with a granular base May heal even without treatment but this takes years and leaves unsightly scars

Contd...

Contd…

Types of cutaneous TB	Features
Miliary TB	Chronic TB infection that has spread from the primary infection (usually in the lungs) to other organs and tissues via the bloodstream Skin lesions are small (millet-sized) red spots that develop into ulcers and abscesses More likely in immunocompromised patients, e.g. HIV, AIDS, cancer The patient is generally sick Prognosis is poor (many patients die even if diagnosed and treated)
Tuberculid	Generalized exanthem in patients with moderate or high degree of immunity to TB because of previous infection Usually in good health with no identifiable focus of active TB in skin or elsewhere Erythema induratum (Bazin disease) presents as recurring nodules or lumps on the back of the legs (mostly women) that may ulcerate and scar. It is a type of nodular vasculitis. Papulonecrotic tuberculid results in crops of recurrent crusted skin papules on knees, elbows, buttocks or lower trunk that heal with scarring after about 6 weeks. Lichen scrofulosorum is an extending eruption of small follicular papules in young persons with underlying TB

Erythema induratum

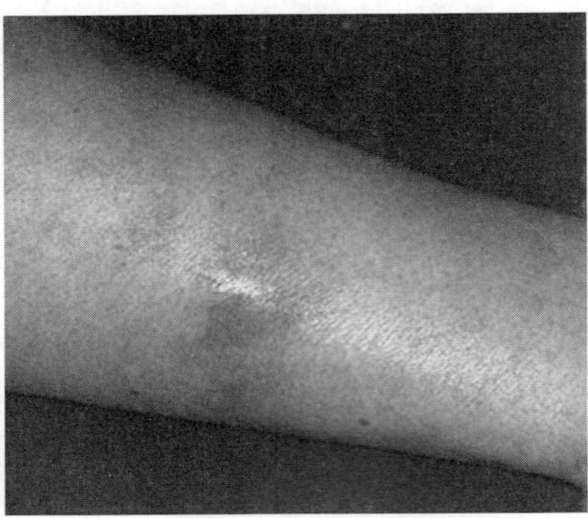

Milliary TB

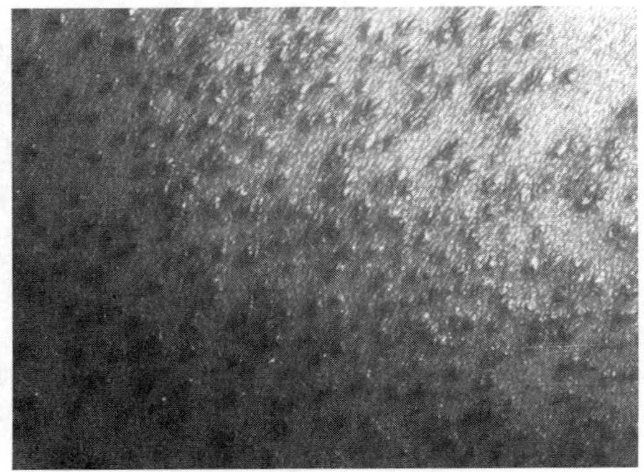

Lupus vulgaris

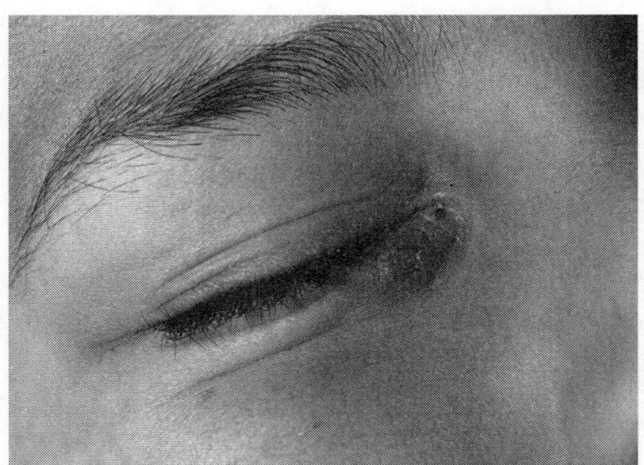

Lupus vulgaris

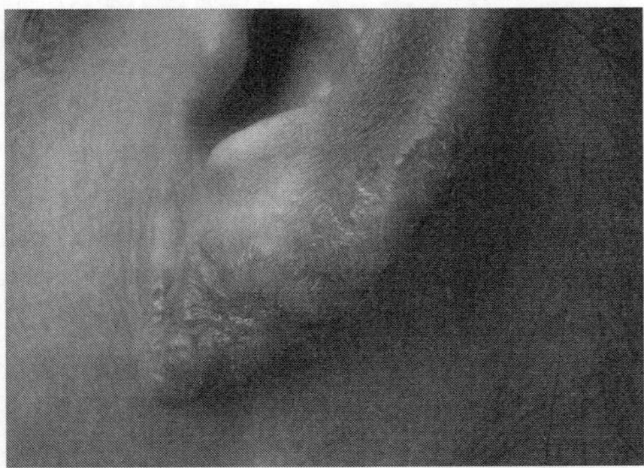

Tuberculosis verrucosa cutis

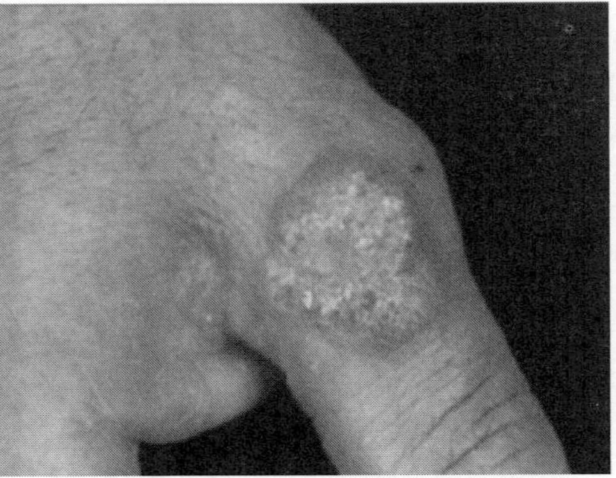

4. **Bacteria involved in rosacea is/are:**
   a. Staphylococcus epidermidis
   b. Propionibacterium acnes
   c. Demodex mite
   d. Malassezia furfur
   e. Bacillus oleronius

Ans. a, c, e *Ref: Bolognia Textbook of Dermatology, page 599*

Option a	True	Yes, correct
Option b	False	No, Propionibacterium acnes also known as Cutibacterium acne is gram positive rod responsible for acne
Option c	True	Yes, correct
Option d	False	No, it is responsible for seborrheic dermatitis
Option e	True	Yes, correct

Rosacea is a chronic inflammatory skin disorder typically involving the nose, forehead, and chin that is characterized especially by flushing, telengiectasia.

Pathogenic hypothesis in Rosacea:

- **Aberrant innate immune system:** In Rosacea, there is upregulation of cathelicidin (Antimicrobial peptides) and its processing serine protease suggesting dysfunction of the innate immune system.
- **Ultraviolet radiation (UVR):** Upregulates of matrix metalloproteinases (MMPs) which inturn result in damage to blood vessels and the dermal matrix.
- **Vascular changes**: An increase in blood flow is seen within affected skin in rosacea especially in response to spicy food, sun light exposure and hot beverages.
- **Epidermal barrier dysfunction**: Increased transepidermal water loss, lowered threshold for skin irritancy has been documented.
- **Neurogenic inflammation**
- **Microbes:**
  - **Demodex mites** (folliculorum and brevis) which are commensal of normal skin, are found in greater numbers in rosacea patients. Demodex infestation is associated with an intense perifollicular infiltrate of predominantly CD4+ helper T cells.
  - **Bacillus oleronius** isolated from a demodex folliculorum mite produces antigens that induces an inflammatory immune response in rosacea.
  - **Staphylococcus epidermidis** is also thought to play a role in rosacea pathogenesis.

5. **Treatment options in Condyloma accuminata include:**
   a. 10–25% Podophyllin
   b. 50–75% Podophyllin
   c. 10– 25% Trichloroacetic acid
   d. 80–90% Trichloroacetic acid
   e. Iodine

Ans. a, d *Ref: IADVL Textbook of Dermatology (2nd Edition): Page 1920*

Option a	True	Yes, correct
Option b	False	No, not correct
Option c	False	No, not correct
Option d	True	Yes, correct
Option e	False	No, not correct

Anogenital warts are referred to as condylomata acuminata.

Treatment is classified into two therapy which are as follows:

1. **Home therapy:**
   - Podophyllotoxin (0.5% solution or 0.15% cream)
   - **Imiquimod:** 3.75% or 5% cream (Toll Like Receptor- 7 agonist)
2. **Office/hospital therapy:**
   - **Podophyllin:** Podophyllin inhibits mitosis at metaphase and causes swelling and necrosis of cells. It is used in a concentration of **10%–25%** dissolved in tincture of benzoin
   - Trichloroacetic acid: 80%–90% solution
   - **Cryotherapy:** Treatment of choice in pregnancy
   - Electrosurgery
   - Laser ablation.

6. Nongonococcal urethritis is produced by the following organism/s:

a. *Calymmatobacter granulomatis*

b. *Mycoplasma genitalium*

c. *Chlamydia trachomatis*

d. *Trichomonas vaginalis*

e. *Adenovirus*

Ans. b,c,d,e

Option a	False	***Klebsiella granulomatis*** is Gram-negative, rod-shaped bacterium of the genus *Klebsiella* known to cause the sexually transmitted disease granuloma inguinale (or donovanosis). It was called *Calymmatobacterium granulomatis.*
Option b	True	Yes, correct
Option c	True	Yes, correct
Option d	True	Yes, correct
Option e	True	Yes, correct

Parameter	Gonococcal urethritis	Nongonococcal urethritis
Etiology	Neisseria gonorrhoeae	Chlamydia trachomatis, ureaplasma urealyticum, mycoplasma genitalium, trichomonas vaginalis, herpes simplex virus (HSV) types 1 and 2, adenovirus
Incubation Period	2-6 days	1-5 weeks with peak at 2-3 weeks
Onset	Abrupt	Gradual
Constitutional symptoms	Fever, malaise	Absent
Discharge	Profuse, purulent and yellowish green	Scanty, mucoid or mucopurulent
Dysuria	Intense burning sensation	'Smarting' feeling in the urethra on passing urine

Syndromic management of urethral discharge: Kit No. 1 (Gray Color)

Cefixime 400 mg + Azithromycin 1g STAT.

7. True about sexually transmitted ulcers include:

a. Syphilis: Painless ulcer with rubbery lymphadenopathy
b. Chancroid: Tender ulcer with suppurative lymphadenopathy
c. Genital herpes: Painful ulcer with tender lymph nodes
d. LGV: Painful ulcer with bubo formation
e. Donovanosis: Beefy red granulation tissue with bubo

Ans. a, b, c

Ref: Sexually transmitted diseases by King K Holmes: Page 448

Option a	True	Yes, correct
Option b	True	Yes, correct
Option c	True	Yes, correct
Option d	False	No, it is painless ulcer
Option e	False	No, the ulcer in donovanosis is with pseudo-bubos

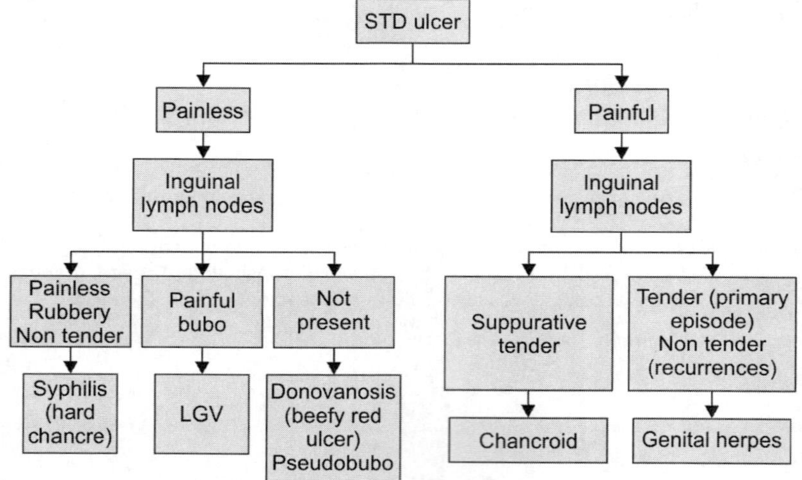

LGV: Lymphogranulorna venereum

Dermatology

1. Nikolsky sign is positive in all of the following *except*:

a. Pemphigus vulgaris
b. Hailey-Hailey disease
c. Transient acantholytic dermatosis
d. Staphylococcal scalded skin syndrome
e. Toxic epidermal necrolysis

Ans: b, c *Ref: Seshadri D, Kumaran M S, Kanwar AJ. Acantholysis revisited: Back to basics. Indian J Dermatol Venereol Leprol 2013; 79:120-6.*

Option a	True	Nikolsky sign is positive
Option b	False	Nikolsky sign is negative
Option c	False	Nikolsky sign is negative
Option d	True	Nikolsky sign is positive
Option e	True	Pseudo-Nikolsky sign is positive

Nikolsky's sign:

- Elicitation: Application of tangential pressure with a finger or thumb to the affected skin, perilesional skin, or normal skin in patients with suspected pemphigus
- Interpretation: Intraepidermal cleavage
- Elicitation on normal looking skin in the vicinity of the blister: Marginal Nikolsky's sign
- Elicitation on normal looking skin away from the blister: Direct Nikolsky's sign.
- The sign also predicts the activity of the disease while on therapy.
- Mechanism: Acantholysis
- Conditions: **Pemphigus vulgaris, Staphylococcal scalded skin syndrome.**

Pseudo Nikolsky sign or Epidermal peeling sign:

- Elicitation: "Involved" erythematous areas
- Mechanism: Necrosis of the cells
- Conditions: Stevens-Johnson syndrome, **toxic epidermal necrolysis**, in some cases of burns and bullous ichthyosiform erythroderma.

2. Photosensitivity is not seen in:

a. Variegate porphyria
b. Erythropoietic porphyria
c. Acute intermittent porphyria
d. Congenital erythropoietic porphyria
e. Porphyria cutanea tarda

Ans. c *Ref: Rook's text book of Dermatology, 9/e, 60.6 (p 1616)*

Option a	True	Yes, Photosensitivity is seen
Option b	True	Yes, Photosensitivity is seen
Option c	False	Acute intermittent porphyria (AIP) belongs to the group "inborn errors of metabolism". Since the porphyrin precursors do not cause light sensitivity and tissue porphyrins are not markedly increased most patients with AIP are not light sensitive
Option d	True	Yes, Photosensitivity is seen
Option e	True	Yes, Photosensitivity is seen

Mechanism of photosensitivity in porphyria: Accumulation of **Tetrapyrrole intermediates.**

First tetrapyrrole structure to be formed during heme synthesis: **Hydroxymethyl- bilane (HMB)**

Enzyme defect **prior to synthesis of Hydroxymethyl bilane**: Accumulation of delta amino levulinate (ALA) and Porphobilinogen (PBG) → Highly reactive oxidants and neurotoxic → Abdominal pain and Neuropsychiatric signs (**No Photosensitivity**)

Enzyme defect	Porphyria
δ-ALA Dehydratase	ALA- Dehydratase deficiency porphyria
PBG Deaminase	Acute intermittent porphyria

3. In a patient with leprosy, 2 nerves are involved. What is the management?

a. MB treatment for 12 months
b. PB treatment for 6 months
c. MB treatment for 6 months
d. ROM Therapy
e. Corticosteroids

Ans. a *Ref: Jopling's Handbook of Leprosy*

Option a	True	This is categorized as multibacillary leprosy
Option b	False	PB includes involvement of no or one nerve only
Option c	False	MB treatment is given for 12 months
Option d	False	
Option e	False	Corticosteroids are given for lepra reactions

	Paucibacillary	Multibacillary
Skin Lesions	1-5	6 and above
Nerves	No nerve/ 1 Nerve	**> 1 Nerve irrespective of skin lesions**
Slit Skin Smear	Negative at all sites	Positive at any site

WHO recommended MDT regimens in leprosy			
	Regimen		*Duration of treatment*
Type of Leprosy	*Monthly supervised*	*Daily Administered*	
Paucibacillary (PB)	Rifampicin 600 mg	Dapsone 100 mg	6 months
Multibacillary (MB)	Rifampicin 600 mg Clofazimine 300 mg	Dapsone 100 mg Clofazimine 50 mg	12 months

Color coded MDT regimes:

Maroon (MB- Adult), Green (PB- Adult), Blue (PB- Child)

ROM therapy:

Single Lesion Paucibacillary (SLPB) Leprosy (1998)

Single supervised dose of combination therapy: Rifampicin (600 mg), ofloxacin (400 mg), and minocycline (100 mg).

Indications of corticosteroids in leprosy:

Type 1 reaction: Neuritis

Type 2 reaction:

a. Neuritis when muscle paralysis is threatened
b. Iritis not responding to steroid eye drops
c. Epididymo-orchitis
d. Erythema necroticans (Vesicular/Bullous erythema nodosum leprosum)

4. True about lepromin test is/are:

a. Prognostic
b. Diagnostic
c. Used for disease classification
d. Used to see the mycobacterial resistance
e. Used to check the drug response

Ans. a, c, e *Ref: Nagar R, Pande S, Khopkar U. Intradermal tests in dermatology-I: tests for infectious diseases. Indian J Dermatol Venereol Leprol. 2006 ;72(6):461-5.*

Option a	True
Option b	False
Option c	True
Option d	False
Option e	True

Lepromin test:

Definition: Intradermal skin test performed using lepromin antigen, which is a suspension of killed M. leprae obtained from infected human/armadillo tissue.

Response: Biphasic (Early Fernandez, Late Mitsuda Reaction)

Lepromin test				
Response	***Timing***	***Reading***	***Inference***	***Remarks***
Early fernandez reaction	48-72 hours	Erythema and induration > 16 mm	Strongly Positive: +++	More prominent with Dharmendra lepromin. Measures existing Delayed type hypersensitivity
Late mitsuda reaction	3-4 weeks	Red nodule > 10 mm or of any size with ulceration	Strongly Positive: +++	More prominent with Mitsuda lepromin. Indicates the ability to mount a cell-mediated immune response

Utility of lepromin test:

- Prognostic test
- Classification of leprosy
- Monitor response to treatment with chemotherapy (Positive: Good prognosis)
- Evaluate host resistance to leprosy.

Disadvantages:

Not diagnostic (Positive: Significant number of normal people, Negative: Lepromatous pole of the disease).

5. **Cutaneous marker(s) of internal malignancy is/are all *except:***
   a. Onychomycosis
   b. Sign of Leser-Trelat
   c. Dermatomyositis
   d. Migratory thrombophlebitis
   e. Seborrheic patch at back

Ans. a, e *Ref: IADVL Textbook of Dermatology 4/e, p 1347*

Option a	False	Not a marker of internal malignancy
Option b	True	GI Adenocarcinoma
Option c	True	Ca Ovary, nasopharyngeal carcinoma
Option d	True	Pancreatic carcinoma
Option e	False	Not a marker of internal malignancy

Cutaneous manifestations of internal malignancy

- **Sign of Leser–Trélat:** Sudden appearance of multiple pruritic seborrheic keratoses, associated with an internal malignancy (Most common: GI Adenocarcinoma)
- **Dermatomyositis:** Women (Ca. ovary), Asian men (Nasopharyngeal carcinoma)
- **Migratory thrombophlebitis (Trousseau's sign)**: Pancreatic carcinoma
- Glucagonoma syndrome: Necrolytic migratory erythema.
- Ca Lung: Erythema gyratum repens "Wood grain-pattern" scales
- Paraneoplastic pemphigus: Non-Hodgkin's Lymphoma, chronic lymphocytic leukemia, Castleman's disease
- Chloromas (granulocytic sarcomas): M1, M2 subtypes of acute myelogenous leukemia
- Malignant Acanthosis nigricans (80%–90%): Intra-abdominal adenocarcinomas and gastric carcinoma
- Most common Malignancy-associated ichthyosis: Hodgkin's lymphoma

Note:

Proximal subungual onychomycosis: Early clinical marker of HIV infection (Not malignancy)

Seborrhoeic keratosis: Common benign tumour of the skin seen in elderly, arising from keratinocytes.

6. **True about acute paronychia:**
   a. Pus under nail bed
   b. Pus may extend to base of nail
   c. Swelling of nail fold
   d. Candida is most common causative organism
   e. Treatment often not required

Ans. c *Ref: Andrews' Diseases of the skin 11/e, p 249*

Option a	False	
Option b	False	
Option c	True	
Option d	False	
Option e	False	

Paronychia: Inflammatory reaction involving the folds of the skin surrounding the fingernail.
Classification: Acute/chronic.

Acute paronychia:

Etiology: Nail biting, finger sucking, aggressive manicuring, a hang nail or penetrating trauma.

Microbiology: Most common infecting organism is **Staphylococcus aureus**, followed by streptococci and pseudomonas organisms.

Most common infecting organism for Chronic paronychia: Candida albicans.

Pathogenesis: Barrier breakdown → Microscopic/macroscopic portal of entry for microbes in the environment, into what is normally an impermeable sealed anatomical apparatus → Acute infection of the soft tissues surrounding the nail and occasionally under the nail plate.

Clinical features: Localized pain, redness and tenderness of the perionychium. The perionychial area usually appears erythematous and inflamed.

Fluctuance and local purulence at the nail margin may occur, and infection may extend beneath the nail margin to involve the nail bed.

Treatment:

Treatment is necessary as if left untreated, a collection of pus may develop as an abscess around the perionychium.

Topical and systemic antibiotics

Surgical drainage (Abscess)

7. **True about electrocautery is/are:**
   a. High voltage - cutting
   b. Low voltage - coagulation
   c. Monopolar
   d. Current goes on one side
   e. None of the above

Ans. d *Ref: Bolognia's textbook of Dermatology: p 2462*

Option a	False
Option b	False
Option c	False
Option d	True
Option e	False

Electrocautery:

- Technique using electrical current to heat a metal wire that is then applied to the target tissue in order to burn or coagulate the specific area of tissue.
- It is not used to pass the current through tissue, but rather is applied directly onto the targeted area of treatment.
- Electrocautery is **not a true form of electrosurgery** as no current flows through the patient.

Electrosurgery:

Application of a high-frequency (radio frequency) alternating polarity, electrical current to biological tissue as a means to cut, coagulate, desiccate, or fulgurate tissue.

Wet field electrosurgery:

Cut mode: High voltage level → Heat vapor pocket generated → Vaporizes and explodes a small section of soft tissue → Incision.

Coagulate mode: Voltage lower than the cut mode → less heat generated → cells and small vessels at the point of contact are destroyed and sealed.

8. Dermatophytes are:

a. Favus
b. Kerion
c. Taenia
d. M. audouinii
e. None

Ans. a, b, d *Ref: IADVL textbook of Dermatology: 2/e, p 256*

Option a	True	
Option b	True	
Option c	False	**Taenia** = Tapeworm infection. Tinea = Dermatophyte infection
Option d	True	
Option e	False	

Dermatophytosis: Superficial fungal infections of keratinized tissue → Skin, hair and nail.

- 3 species of dermatophytes:
  - Trichophyton (Involves skin, hair, nail), Epidermophyton (Skin, Nail), Microsporum (Skin, Hair).
- **"Tinea"** is a term used for dermatophytic infections (**Taenia:** Tapeworm Infestation).
- Various types of Tinea include capitis (scalp), faciei (face), barbae (beard), manuum (palms), glabrous skin with the exclusion of the palms, soles and groins (corporis), groin and buttocks (cruris), pedis (feet).

Tinea capitis:

- Non-inflammatory variants:
  - **Black dot** (T. tonsurans, T. violaceum)
  - **Grey patch** (M. audouinii, M. canis)
- Inflammatory variants:
  - **Favus: Yellow coloured cup shaped crust → Scutula** (T. schoenleinii)
  - **Kerion: Boggy indurated scalp swelling + easily pluckable hair** (T. verrucosum, T. mentagrophytes).

9. Red lesions of tongue include:

a. Erythroplakia
b. Lichen planus
c. Leukoplakia
d. Geographic tongue
e. Osler-Weber-Rendu Disease

Ans. a, b, d, e *Ref: http://www.consultant360.com/article/erythematous-oral-lesions-when-treat-when-leave-alone*

Option a	True	
Option b	True	
Option c	False	Whitish lesion of the tongue
Option d	True	
Option e	True	

Red lesions of the oral cavity

Mucosal alterations	*Reactive lesions*
Erythroplakia Geographic tongue Candidiasis: Atrophic candidiasis a. Acute atrophic candidiasis/ Antibiotic sore mouth b. Chronic atrophic oral candidiasis: - Denture sore mouth - Median rhomboid glossitis Erosive lichen planus Nutritional deficiencies: Vit B12 deficiency (Beefy Red tongue) Vit B2 deficiency (Magenta coloured tongue) Plasma cell gingivostomatitis Granulomatous disorders (Sarcoidosis, Crohn's disease, orofacial granulomatosis)	Pyogenic granuloma Peripheral Giant cell granuloma Vascular lesions Vascular tumours (Hemangioma, Kaposi Sarcoma) Arteriovenous malformations Genodermatoses Osler-Weber-Rendu disease Blue rubber bleb nevus syndrome Fabry's disease

Note:

Leukoplakia: "A white patch or plaque that cannot be characterized clinically or pathologically as any other disease".

Oral leukoplakia: Most common premalignant oral mucosal lesion. Total lifetime risk of malignant transformation is estimated to be 4 to 6%.

Proliferative verrucous leukoplakia: Form of verrucous leukoplakia has a strong potential for malignant transformation and is resistance to treatment.

Erythroplakia: Fiery red patch that cannot be clinically or pathologically distinguished as any other definable disease (Less common than leukoplakia, but higher chance of malignant transformation).

Oral lichen planus: Increased malignant transformation risk occurs greater in **erosive** and **atrophic forms** and in cases of lesions of **lateral border of the tongue.**

10. Subepidermal bullae are seen in:

a. Pemphigus vulgaris
b. Pemphigus vegetans
c. Bullous SLE
d. Bullous pemphigoid
e. Dermatitis herpetiformis

Ans. c, d, e *Ref: Andrews' Diseases of the skin 11/e, p 455*

Option a	False	Intraepidermal bullae
Option b	False	Intraepidermal bullae
Option c	True	
Option d	True	
Option e	True	

Bulla: Fluid filled primary lesions > 0.5 cm

1. **Intra-epidermal autoimmune bullous disorders:** Disruption above the basement membrane results in flaccid bullae (sometimes no bullae are seen and there are mostly erosions).
   - Pemphigus group of diseases
   - Hailey-Hailey disease (benign familial pemphigus)
   - Darier disease
   - **Grover** disease (transient acantholytic dermatosis)

2. **Subepidermal bullae**

Clinical presentation: Tense Bullae

A. **Subepidermal immunobullous diseases**

B. **Subepidermal mechanobullous diseases:**

Junctional epidermolysis bullosa (Laminin Defect: Dermoepidermal Junction)

Dystrophic Epidermolysis bullosa (Type 7 Collagen defect : Dermis)

C. **Porphyria cutanea tarda**

Defective Enzyme: Uroporphyrinogen decarboxylase (UROD)

Subepidermal autoimmune blistering diseases

Subepidermal blistering diseases	Target antigen/ enzyme	Clinical features	Histopathology subepidermal bullae with	Direct immuno-fluorescence
Linear IgA Disease (adults) Chronic Bullous Disease of childhood: CBDC	LAD1 antigen (BP-120) BPAG-2 (BP-180)	Annular arrangement of vesicles (Cluster of Jewel appearance)	Neutrophilic Infiltrate	Linear IgA along BMZ
Bullous Pemphigoid	BPAG-1 BPAG-2	Tense bullae often on urticarial plaques Nikolsky Sign (-)	Eosinophilic Infiltrate	Linear C3 + IgG along BMZ
Bullous SLE	Type 7 Collagen	Tense bullae predominantly on sun exposed areas	Neutrophilic Infiltrate Vacuolar inter-face dermatitis	IgG (with or without IgA and IgM) deposits at BMZ
Cicatricial Pemphigoid	BPAG-2	Predominantly mucosal involved	Mixed inflamma-tory infiltrate with few eosinophils	Linear IgG + C3 along BMZ
Dermatitis Herpetiformis	Epidermal Trans-glutaminase	Intensely pruritic, papulovesicles, grouped excoriations on extensors	Papillary tip microabscess	Granular IgA deposition along BMZ and dermal papilla
Epidermolysis bullosa acquisita	Type VII Collagen	Multiple tense bullae, scarring, milia among elderly at trauma prone sites	Mixed inflammatory infiltrate	Linear IgG + C3 along BMZ
Pemphigoid/ Herpes Gestationis	BPAG-2 (Type XVII collagen)	Extremely pruritic, polymorphic eruption involving periumbilical region	Eosinophils with few neutrophils	Linear C3 along BMZ

Note: Pointer to identify bullous disorder in exams

Pemphigus (Intraepidermal bullae) Pemphigoid (Subepidermal bullae)

11. Skin manifestations of lithium toxicity include:

a. Rash
b. Acne
c. Pemphigus
d. Psoriasis
e. Folliculitis

Ans. a, b, d, e *Ref: IADVL textbook of Dermatology: 2/e, p 1656*

Option a	True	
Option b	True	
Option c	False	Not seen in lithium toxicity
Option d	True	
Option e	True	

Cutaneous manifestations of lithium toxicity:

1. **Papulosquamous lesions:** Psoriasis/Exanthematic type of pustular psoriasis
2. **Drug induced maculopapular rash, erythroderma**
3. **Disorders of appendages**
   a. **Drug induced acne/acneiform eruption:** Most common adverse effect of lithium. Persistent monomorphic pustules on an erythematous base on the limbs and trunk.
   b. **Folliculitis:** Lithium-induced folliculitis presents on the extensor surfaces of the forearms and legs several months after initiating lithium.
   c. **Hair changes:** Alopecia (Telogen effluvium), alteration in hair texture and drying of hair
4. **Vesiculobullous lesions:** Linear IgA dermatosis
5. **Miscellaneous:** Pruritus, nail dystrophy, Lichenoid drug eruption, keratoderma, SLE like syndrome, hidradenitis suppurativa, exacerbates Darier's disease, erythema multiforme.

12. True about hypertrophic scar is/are:

a. Triamcinolone is used for treatment
b. Silicon is used for treatment
c. Negative pressure dressing is done
d. Dark skin is more vulnerable
e. Wound healing is not proper

Ans. a, b, e *Ref: Rook's text book of Dermatology: 9/e, 96.45*

Option a	True	
Option b	True	
Option c	False	Topical negative pressure (vacuum) significantly enhances healing of superinfected chronic leg ulcers with a substantial tissue loss
Option d	False	No racial predilection
Option e	True	

Hypertrophic scars (HTSs): Disorder of **wound healing**

Definition: Visible and elevated scars that do not spread into surrounding tissues and that often regress spontaneously

	Hypertrophic scar	Keloid
History of trauma	Always	Not always, can be spontaneous
Onset	Sudden	Delayed
Predisposing factors	Poor approximation of wound edge, Tension while closure, Poor surgical technique No racial predilection or familial tendency	**Race: Blacks and Asians** Familial Tendency Diseases like Ehlesr-Danlos Syndrome, Osteogenesis imperfecta

Contd...

Contd...

	Hypertrophic scar	Keloid
Symptoms like itching and pain	Present sometimes	Usually present
Anatomic sites	Anywhere on the body	High risk sites: sternal area, upper back, upper arms
Confinement to wound margin	Yes	No
Histopathology	Nodules containing fibrillar collagen of fairly regular thickness arranged parallel to epidermis. bundles, increased myofibroblasts	Pale staining, hypocellular collagen, irregular, abnormally thick, unidirectional arrangement No evidence of nodule/ excess myofibroblast
Spontaneous resolution	Sometimes	Rare
Response to treatment	Good	Poor

Treatment options in hypertrophic scars:

1. **Corticosteroids**
   - Topical: Used for superficial lesions
   - Intralesional steroids: Triamcinolone
   - Mechanism: Decreases fibroblast proliferation, collagen and glycosaminoglycan synthesis
2. **Silicone gel sheet:**
   - Hydration and occlusion affects local keratinocytes to alter growth factor secretion and secondarily influences fibroblast regulation.
   - Increased skin hydration is most likely responsible for decreased capillary activity, reduced hyperemia and reduced collagen deposition.
3. **Pressure therapy:** Reduces scar height and erythema
   - Proposed mechanism: Pressure controls collagen synthesis by limiting the supply of blood, oxygen and nutrients to scar tissue. It encourages realignment of collagen bundles already present.
4. **Onion extract and heparin gel:**
   - Onion extract (Allium cepa) possesses fibroblast inhibiting properties that reduce production of extracellular matrix and increases expression of MMP-1 (Matrix metalloproteinase-1).
   - Heparin strongly interacts with collagen molecules, inducing formation of thicker fibrils typical of mature tissue.
5. **Surgery:** Simple excision + Primary closure due to complicated wounds.
   - Z-plasty for scars not oriented along relaxed skin tension lines.

Note:

Negative pressure wound therapy: Application of controlled suction to the wound bed via a computerized unit attached to an open-cell foam dressing placed in the wound and held in place by an adhesive clear dressing.

Utility: Topical negative pressure (vacuum) significantly enhances healing of superinfected chronic leg ulcers with a substantial tissue loss.

13. True about basal cell carcinoma is:

a. Yellowstone pigmentation
b. Associated with Bowen's disease
c. Arises from non-keratotic basal cells
d. Appears as rodent ulcer
e. Most commonly involved site are extremities

Ans. c, d *Ref: Rook's text book of Dermatology: 9/e, 109.49*

Option a	False	
Option b	False	Bowen's disease is a form of intraepidermal (in situ) squamous cell carcinoma
Option c	True	
Option d	True	
Option e	False	Most common Site is Sun-exposed areas of head and neck region

Basal cell carcinoma:

- Most common skin malignancy
- **Origin:** Non-keratinizing cells forming the basal layer of epidermis
- **Most common clinical type**: Nodular Basal Cell Carcinoma
- **Most common site:** Sun-exposed areas of **head and neck region (80%)**
- Morphology of nodular BCC: Translucent papule/nodule with telangiectasias and rolled border
- Larger lesions with central necrosis **(Rodent ulcer)**
- Most common site of recurrence of BCC: The H-zone (i.e., nasolabial fold, nasal alar, orbital area and auricular area)

Bowen's disease: Form of intraepidermal (in situ) **squamous cell carcinoma (SCC)** characterized by a persistent, non-elevated, red, scaly or crusted plaque with a small potential for invasive malignancy.

14. True about donovanosis is/are:

a. Sodium stibogluconate is given
b. Miltefosine is given
c. Caused by Klebsiella granulomatis
d. Caused by Leishmania donovani
e. Pseudobubos are present

Ans. c, e *Ref: IADVL Textbook of Dermatology, 4/e, p 1884*

Option a	False	Azithromycin is given
Option b	False	This is not correct
Option c	True	
Option d	False	Caused by Klebsiella granulomatis
Option e	True	

Donovanosis (Synonym: Granuloma inguinale)

- **Causative organism:** Klebsiella granulomatis (Previously calymmatobacterium granulomatis)
- Incubation period: 8–80 days
- Primary lesion: Papule/nodule

- Secondary lesion: Genital ulcer: **Beefy red**, exuberant granulation tissue, **Bleeds on touch**
- Inguinal lymph nodes: Normal
- **Pseudobubo** (Not a Lymph node): Subcutaneous nodule/granuloma in the groin region (Granuloma inguinale)
- **Complications: Squamous cell carcinoma (Long standing)**
- **Giemsa stain from crushed tissue smear: Donovan bodies** (Rod-shaped, oval organisms seen in the cytoplasm of mononuclear phagocytes or histiocytes reveal characteristic bipolar staining, giving a **"safety pin"** appearance).
- **Treatment:**
  - **Recommended regimen:** Azithromycin 1 g orally once per week or 500 mg daily for at least **3 weeks** and until all lesions have completely healed.
  - **Alternate regimen drugs:** Doxycycline, Erythromycin, Ciprofloxacin, Trimethoprim-sulfamethoxazole.
  - Addition of an aminoglycoside to these regimens is an option (gentamicin 1 mg/kg IV every 8 hours).

Leishmaniasis:

- **Visceral form (Kala azar):** Causative organism: **Leishmania donovani**, Leishmania infantum
- **Cutaneous form**: Leishmania tropica, Leishmania major
- **Diagnosis: Giemsa stain:** Direct visualization of the amastigotes **(Leishman-Donovan bodies)**: Aflagellate, small, round bodies 2–4 μm in diameter with indistinct cytoplasm, nucleus and a rod-shaped kinetoplast seen within monocytes.
- **Treatment options:**
  - Pentavalent antimonial compounds: **Sodium Stibogluconate**
  - Liposomal amphotericin B
  - **Oral Miltefosine** (FDA approval in March 2014)

15. Which of the following is a small vessel vasculitis?

a. Carcinoma induced vasculitis
b. Takayasu vasculitis
c. Kawasaki vasculitis
d. IgA vasculitis
e. Anti-GBM disease

Ans. d, e *Ref: Chapel hill consensus conference vasculitis 2012*

Option a	False	
Option b	False	Large vessel vasculitis
Option c	False	Medium vessel vasculitis
Option d	True	
Option e	True	

Small vessel vasculitis (SVV):

1. Antineutrophil cytoplasmic antibody (ANCA)-associated vasculitis (AAV)
2. Immune complex SVV

ANCA associated vasculitis (AAV):

Necrotizing vasculitis, with few or no immune deposits, associated with MPO-ANCA or PR3-ANCA

1. Microscopic polyangiitis (MPA)
2. Granulomatosis with polyangiitis (Wegener's/(GPA)
3. Eosinophilic granulomatosis with polyangiitis (Churg-Strauss) (EGPA)

Immune complex SVV:

Moderate to marked vessel wall deposits of immunoglobulin and complement components. Glomerulonephritis is frequent

1. **Anti-glomerular basement membrane (anti-GBM) disease**
2. Cryoglobulinemic vasculitis (CV)
3. **IgA vasculitis (Henoch-Schönlein) (IgAV)**
4. Hypocomplementemic urticarial vasculitis (HUV) (anti-C1q vasculitis).

Note:

- **Large vessel vasculitis:** Takayasu's arteritis, Giant cell arteritis
- **Medium vessel vasculitis:** Kawasaki's disease, Polyarteritis nodosa
- **Cancer associated vasculitis**
- **Categorization in classification: Vasculitis associated with probable etiology**
  - Vasculitis can be associated with certain malignancies, particularly iymphoid or reticuloendothelial neoplasms
  - Most common finding: Leukocytoclastic vasculitis confined to the skin
  - Widespread systemic vasculitis may occur (Association of hairy cell leukemia with polyarteritis nodosa)

16. Syphilis, true is:

a. Tabes dorsalis–hyper reflexia, paresthesia
b. Penicillin is given in both primary and secondary syphilis
c. VDRL is most common investigation
d. Treatment is done for all contacts prior to three months from date of exposure.
e. Jarisch Herxheimer reaction is IgE mediated

Ans. b, c, d *Ref: Manual of Practical Medicine: R Alagappan: 5/e, p 114*

Option a	False	Argyll Robertson pupils, **areflexia** and loss of proprioceptive sense
Option b	True	
Option c	True	
Option d	True	
Option e	False	Not IgE mediated. Does not signify allergy to Penicillin

Late parenchymatous form of neurosyphilis

1. **Tabes dorsalis:**
   - Lightning pains: Most characteristic early symptom (90% of cases)
   - Triad of symptoms (lightning pains, dysuria and ataxia)
   - Triad of signs (Argyll Robertson pupils, **areflexia** and loss of proprioceptive sense)
2. **Generalised paresis of insane**

Treatment of syphilis:

Intramuscular injection of **Benzathine penicillin G** (2.4 million units)

Single dose: Primary, secondary or early latent syphilis.

Three doses at weekly intervals: Late latent syphilis /latent syphilis of unknown duration.

Jarisch-Herxheimer reaction

Aggravation of existing clinical picture of syphilis with fever and constitutional symptoms during treatment.

Mechanism: Treatment with Penicillin → Destruction of spirochetes→ Release of endotoxin-like material from the spirochete + Increased cytokines → Symptoms

Not IgE mediated. Does not signify allergy to Penicillin

Treatment: Resolves spontaneously within 24 hours

Note: Anaphylactic shock secondary to Penicillin is **IgE** mediated reaction

Management of sex partners in syphilis:

Persons who have had sexual contact with a person who receives a diagnosis of primary, secondary, or early latent syphilis should be treated presumptively for early syphilis:

- Within 90 days preceding the diagnosis even if serologic test results are negative.
- > 90 days before the diagnosis if serologic test results are not immediately available and the opportunity for follow-up is uncertain.

17. Premalignant lesions of tongue include:

a. Erythroplakia
b. Lichen planus
c. Behcet's disease
d. Bowen's disease
e. Plummer-Vinson syndrome

Ans. a, b, e *Ref: Yardimci G, Kutlubay Z, Engin B, Tuzun Y. Precancerous lesions of oral mucosa. World Journal of Clinical Cases: WJCC. 2014;2(12):866-872. Bailey and Love's Short Practice of Surgery 26/e, p 707*

Option a	True	
Option b	True	
Option c	False	
Option d	False	
Option e	True	

Conditions associated with malignant transformation		
High-risk lesions	***Medium-risk lesions***	***Low-risk/Equivocal risk lesions***
Leukoplakia	Oral submucous fibrosis	Lichen Planus
Speckled erythroplakia	Sideropenic dysphagia (Plummer Vinson Syndrome)	Discoid lupus erythematosus
Chronic hyperplastic candidiasis	Syphilitic glossitis	Dyskeratosis congenita

18. A 40-year-old female presents with multiple wheals over body. True statement is:

a. Treatment should be targeting against IgE
b. Mast cells are not involved
c. H pylori is associated
d. Anti-H1 antihistamines can be given
e. 25-hydroxycholecalciferol levels can be tested

Ans. c, d *Ref: Rook's text book of Dermatology, 9/e: 42.1 (p 1297)*

Option a	False	
Option b	False	Urticaria is a mast cell driven disease
Option c	True	
Option d	True	
Option e	False	

Urticaria

Definition: Urticaria is a vascular reaction pattern characterized by **wheals** which are intensely pruritic, evanescent, edematous skin lesions.

Urticaria is classified based on the duration

1. Acute urticaria (< 6 weeks)
2. Chronic urticaria (> 6 weeks)

Urticaria is a **mast cell** driven disease.

Investigations of spontaneous urticaria

Acute urticaria	Chronic urticaria
Infection Throat swab if pharyngeal symptoms	• **H1 antihistamine responsive:** • Full blood count, erythrocyte sedimentation rate • Others as indicated by the presentation
Drugs: Withdraw suspected drugs	• H1 antihistamine unresponsive • Thyroid autoantibodies, Thyroid function tests (all patients) • Additional tests dependent on clinical presentation • C4 complement (angio-edema without weals) • Non-organ specific autoantibodies (if associated autoimmune disease possible) • Basophil histamine release assay /Basophil activation tests (if functional autoantibodies suspected) • **Helicobacter pylori (stool antigen or urea breath test)** • Stool for ova, cysts and parasites (Foreign travel) • Chest X-ray (if lymphoma considered)
Foods: Investigate for IgE sensitization (skin prick tests)	• **Optional tests for extensive work-up** • 25-hydroxycholecalciferol (vitamin D) • 3-week trial of a low pseudoallergen diet

H. pylori infection should be included in diagnostic workup of patients with **no response to habitual treatment for chronic urticaria** or **symptomatic gastrointestinal patients.**

Treatment of chronic urticaria:

- **Mainstay of treatment**: Avoidance of triggers, if identified.
- **First-line pharmacotherapy:** Second-generation, non-sedating anti-H1 antihistamines.
- **Other treatment options:** Leukotriene receptor antagonists, Systemic corticosteroids, Cyclosporine, Omalizumab.

Bullous pemphigoid (Subepidermal Bulla)

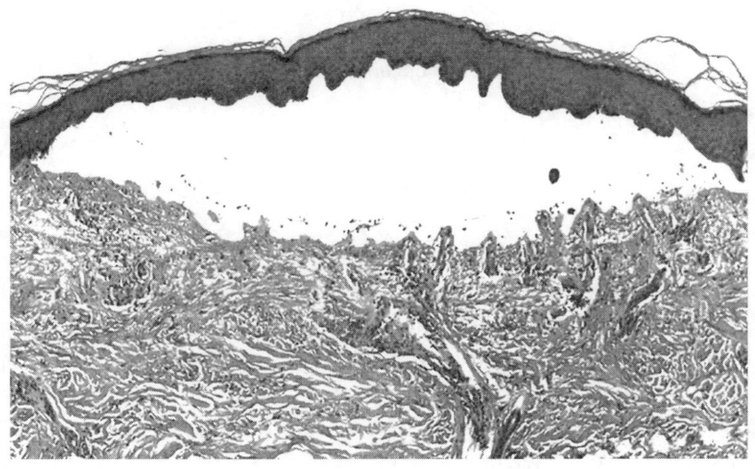

Basal cell carcinoma (Rodent ulcer)

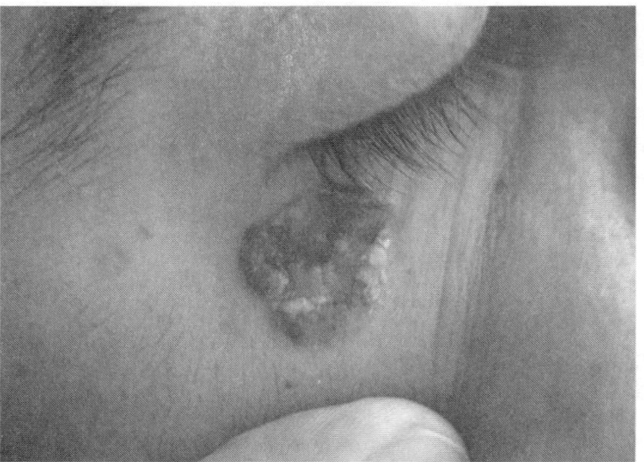

Donovanosis

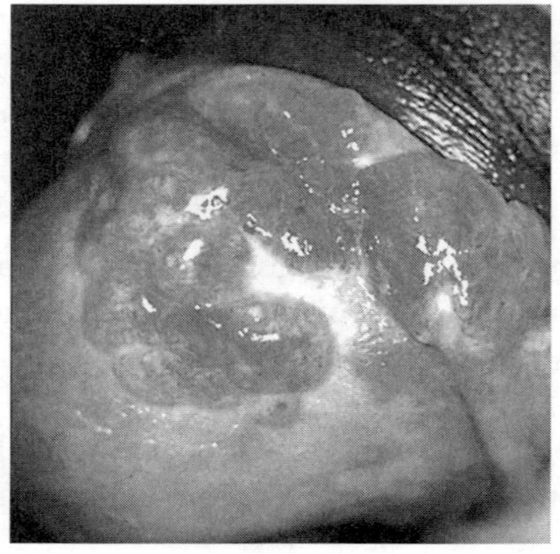

Cutaneous small vessel vasculitis

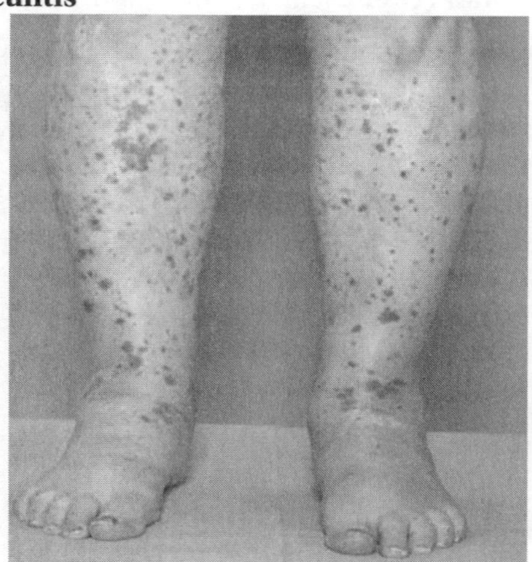

Wheals in urticaria

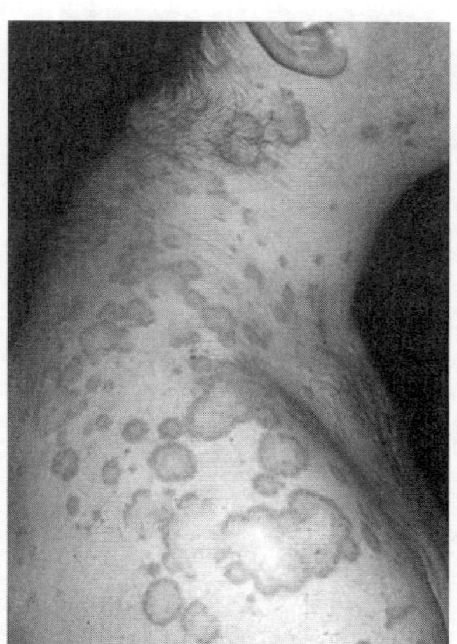

Nikolsky sign

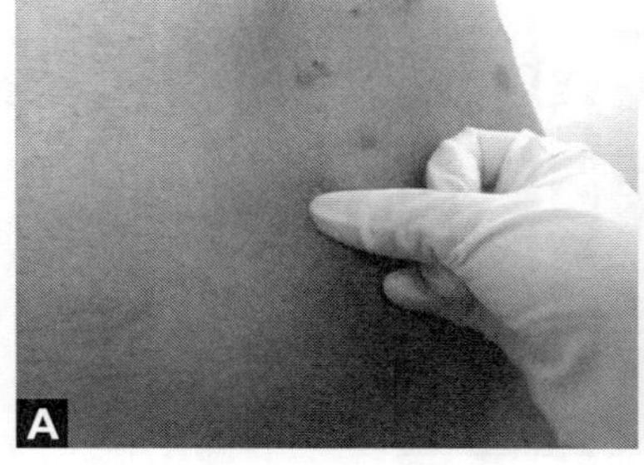

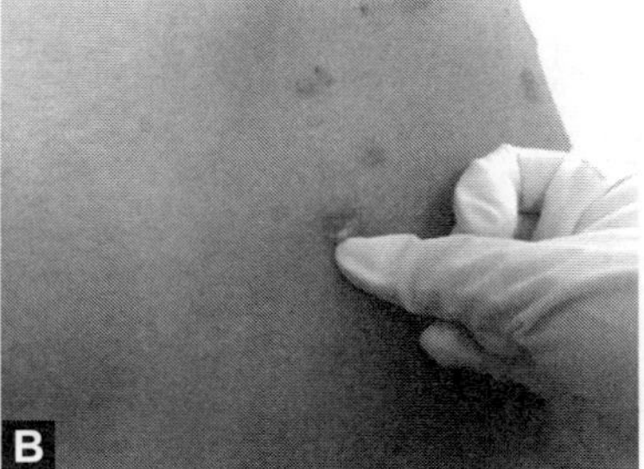

Multi-drug therapy: PB- Adult (Green), MB- Adult (Maroon)

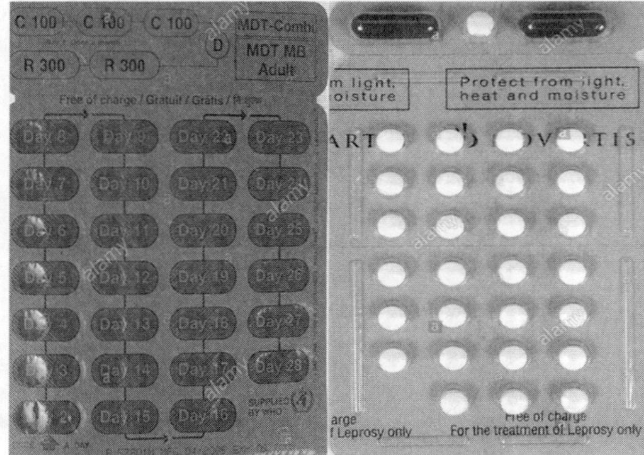

Acute paronychia

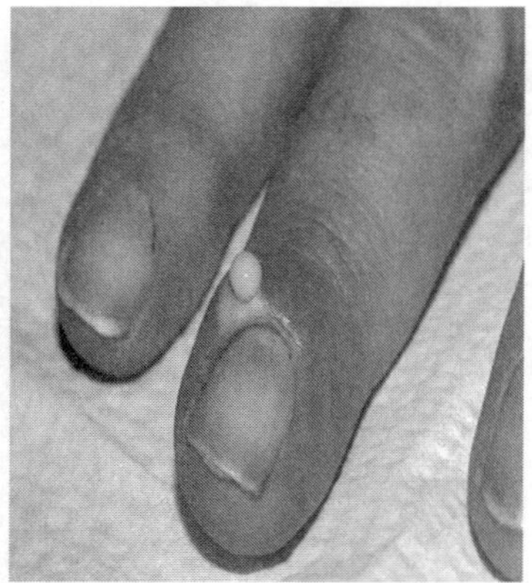

Electrocautery

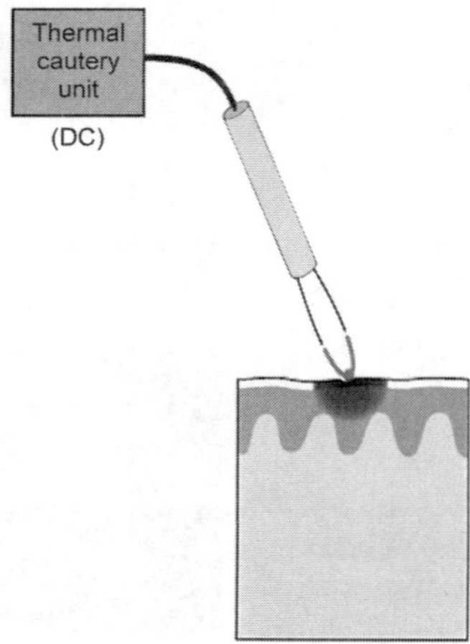

Favus kerion

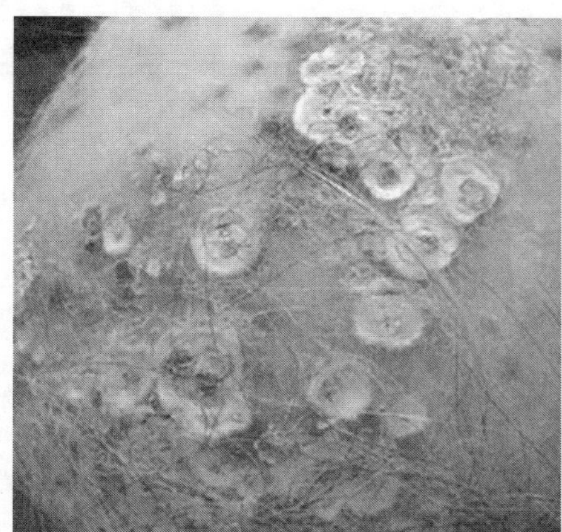

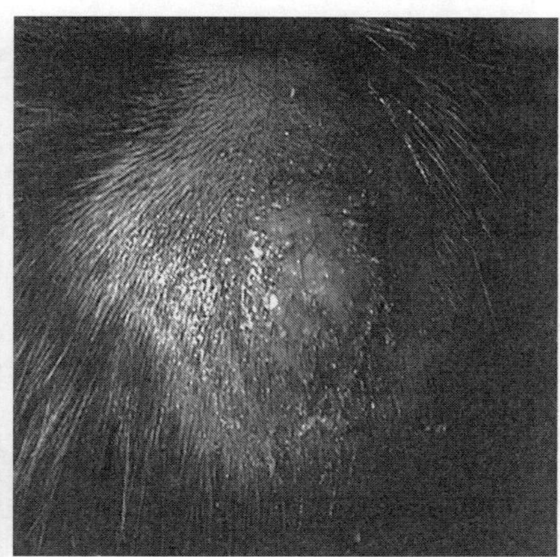

Geographic tongue

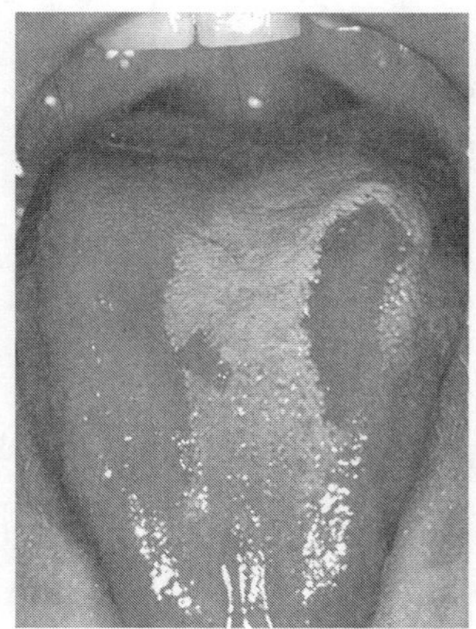

Anesthesia

1. Post-dural-puncture headache is controlled by:

a. Caffeine
b. Blood patch
c. Steroids
d. Hydration
e. Sumatriptan

Ans. a,b,d and e

(Ref: Miller's Anesthesia 8th/ed p1172)

Option a	True	Yes, correct, it does have a transient benefit
Option b	True	Yes, correct, it is the gold standard management
Option c	False	No, it does not have role to manage post-dural headaches
Option d	True	Yes, correct, it is the mainstay for a conservative management of the case
Option e	True	Yes, correct

Management of post-dural-puncture headache

- Analgesics
- Sumatriptan
- Hydration
- Intravenous caffeine
- Autologous blood patch
- Supine positioning

2. Drugs used in monomorphic ventricular tachycardia in hemodynamically stable patient:

a. Amiodarone
b. Propranolol
c. Lignocaine
d. Diltiazem
e. Procainamide

Ans. a,c,e

Ref: Braunwald's Cardiology, Page 801

Option a	True	Yes, correct
Option b	False	No, not used
Option c	True	Yes, correct
Option d	False	No, not used
Option e	True	Yes, correct

- In an acute attack of monomorphic ventricular tachycardia with stable hemodynamics the drugs that can be used are:
  - Amiodarone: Drug of choice
  - Lidocaine
  - Procainamide
- In hemodynamically unstable patients with hypotension, shock, angina or CHF these drugs are not preferred and rather DC cardioversion is preferred.

3. Sugammadex developed for?

a. Induction of anesthesia
b. Intubation
c. Reversal of muscle relaxants
d. Opioid detoxification
e. Cardioprotective anesthesia

Ans. c *Ref: Miller's Anesthesia 8th/ed p1014*

Option a	False	No, not correct
Option b	False	No, not correct
Option c	True	Yes, correct
Option d	False	No, not correct
Option e	False	No, not correct

- Sugammadex is a (gamma)-cyclodextrin which encapsulates the muscle relaxants and removes them from plasma and neuromuscular junction.
- It is used for emergency reversal of muscle relaxants like rocuronium and vecuronium.

Anesthesia

1. Indications of tube thoracostomy:

a. Pneumothorax
b. Coagulopathy
c. Empyema
d. Pleural adhesions
e. Blood in aspirate

Ans. a, c, e *Ref: Miller's 7/e*

Option a	True	
Option b	False	It is a contraindication to tube thoracostomy
Option c	True	
Option d	False	Pulmonary, pleural, or thoracic adhesions are contraindications
Option e	True	

Tube thoracostomy is a flexible plastic tube that is inserted through the chest wall and into the pleural space or mediastinum. Traditionally, this is inserted in the pleural space percutaneously through blunt dissection and connected to a drainage device with an underwater seal. The procedure may be image-directed.

Indications for chest drain insertion:

1. Pneumothorax
   a. In any ventilated patient
   b. Tension pneumothorax after initial needle relief
   c. Persistent or recurrent pneumothorax after simple aspiration
   d. Large secondary spontaneous pneumothorax in patients over 50 years
2. Malignant pleural effusion
3. Empyema and complicated parapneumonic pleural effusion
4. Traumatic or non traumatic (aortic rupture) hemopneumothorax
5. Postoperative—for example, thoracotomy, oesophagectomy, cardiac surgery.

Contraindications:

There are no absolute contraindications to tube thoracostomy, particularly if the patient is in respiratory distress or has a tension pneumothorax.

Relative contraindications include the following:

- Coagulopathy
- Pulmonary bullae
- Pulmonary, pleural, or thoracic adhesions
- Pulmonary abscess
- Skin infection at the chest tube insertion site
- Presence of a diaphragmatic hernia
- Hepatic hydrothorax.

The drain should ideally be inserted in the 'safe triangle', which is delineated by the lateral border of the pectoralis major, the anterior border of the latissimus dorsi and a line horizontal with the nipple.

2. While recovering from general anesthesia, the patient may feel:

a. Muscle aches
b. Sedation
c. Delirium
d. Cognitive dysfunction
e. Hyperthermia

Ans. a, c, d, e *Ref: Miller's 7/e*

Option a	True	
Option b	False	This side effect is not seen
Option c	True	
Option d	True	
Option e	True	

General anesthesia: The side effects of general anesthesia can include:

1. *Nausea and vomiting:* Very common side effect, can occur within the first few days of having surgery and can be triggered by a number of factors such as the medication, motion and type of surgery.
2. *Sore throat:* The tube that is put in the throat to assist in breathing can leave a sore throat after removal.
3. *Confusion:* Confusion when waking up from surgery is common.
4. *Muscle aches:* The medications used to relax the muscles so a breathing tube can be inserted can cause soreness.
5. *Itching:* This is a common side effect of narcotics, sometimes used during general anesthesia.
6. *Chills and shivering (hypothermia):* This is common when patients regain consciousness after surgery. It can occur in up to half of patients.

Rarely, general anesthesia may cause more serious complications, including:

1. Postoperative delirium or cognitive dysfunction: In some cases, confusion and memory loss can last longer than a few hours.
   a. *Delirium:* This can last for a few days after surgery. Occasionally, patients can become confused, disoriented or have problems remembering things. It can come and go, and usually disappears after about a week. This condition can be more common when patients are transferred to intensive care after surgery and remain there for several days.
   b. *Cognitive dysfunction:* People with heart disease, lung disease, Alzheimer's disease and Parkinson's disease, or who have had a stroke, may be at risk for long-term memory loss. Their ability to learn, concentrate and think may be lessened.
2. *Malignant hyperthermia:* Some people inherit this serious, potentially deadly reaction to anesthesia that can occur during surgery, causing a quick fever and muscle contractions.

Regional anesthesia: The potential side effects of regional anesthesia (such as an epidural or spinal block), include:

1. *Headache:* This can occur a few days after the procedure if some of the spinal fluid leaks out.

2. *Minor back pain:* Soreness can happen at the site where the needle was inserted into the back.
3. *Difficulty urinating:* Because the area below the waist is numbed, it may be difficult to urinate.
4. *Hematoma:* Bleeding beneath the skin can occur where the anesthesia was injected.

Serious but rare complications include:

1. *Pneumothorax:* When anesthesia is injected near the lungs, the needle may accidentally enter the lung. This could cause the lung to collapse and require a chest tube to be inserted.
2. *Nerve damage:* Although very rare, nerve damage can occur, causing temporary or permanent pain.

Local anesthesia injection: Side effects are minimal and usually are related to how much anesthesia is injected.

3. Which of the following anaesthetic agents are epileptogenic?

a. Enflurane
b. Atracurium
c. Sevoflurane
d. Halothane
e. Desflurane

Ans. a, b, c *Ref: Miller's 7/e*

Option a	True	Seen at concentrations above 2 MAC
Option b	True	
Option c	True	
Option d	False	Has potent anticonvulsant effect
Option e	False	No evidence that desflurane has epileptiform activity

Seizures are the clinical manifestation of the brain's abnormal electrical activity with enhanced synchrony. They emerge from a hyper excitable focus within the brain where synchronized electrical activity has been formed. Epilepsy can be defined as recurrent seizures unprovoked by acute systemic or neurologic insult.

Anesthetic drugs and epilepsy

Chloral hydrate: This drug is used to promote sedation in preanesthetic medication in children. It has been shown to have some anticonvulsant properties. There is a risk of respiratory depression and hypoxemia, especially in patients at risk for airway obstruction, for example, Down syndrome, or obstructive sleep apnea after tonsillectomy.

Benzodiazepines: They have anticonvulsant activity. However, benzodiazepines can cause short periods of seizure activity, and in EEG, in patients with Lennox-Gastaut syndrome, a form of epilepsy of difficult treatment in children. Benzodiazepines are commonly used to treat acute seizures. Midazolam has potent anticonvulsant activity and is commonly used in the treatment of status epilepticus mainly in children.

Flumazenil may precipitate seizures in patients treated with benzodiazepines or who received this drug as part of premedication due to its competitive antagonism. Given its proconvulsant effects, flumazenil should be used with caution in patients with epilepsy.

Propofol: In spite of the conflicting results in the literature, there is clinical evidence that propofol has anticonvulsant effect and is considered a safe drug for sedation, induction and maintenance of general anesthesia in children and adults. The antiepileptic activity of propofol is probably related to inhibition of pre-and postsynaptic chloride channels mediated by GABA. Propofol can cause abnormal movements, as opisthotonus and myoclonia in both epileptic and healthy patients, but these changes do not seem to relate to epileptogenic activity. Propofol is an effective alternative in the treatment of refractory epileptic seizures to usual antiepileptic drugs and in cases of status epilepticus.

Etomidate: Etomidate appears to have anticonvulsant activity at high doses and pro-convulsant characteristics in usual clinical doses. Therefore, it is recommended to avoid its use in epileptic patients.

Ketamine: Although there are reports of anticonvulsant property of ketamine, especially when associated with drugs with GABAergic activity (benzodiazepines and propofol) for cases refractory to usual therapy, most of the clinical evidence shows that ketamine, at usual doses, has significant epileptogenic potential and should be, therefore, avoided in epileptic patients.

Droperidol: It does not produce neuron excitability nor induce seizures in epileptics; it can be used safely in these patients.

Dexmedetomidine: Sedation with dexmedetomidine observed in the EEG shows a pattern similar to stage II sleep. It presents no pro- or anticonvulsant effects and has been used successfully in children with autism undergoing EEG. This drug has been safely used in adult patients for epilepsy surgery, allowing an adequate mapping of epileptic foci and subsequent resection. Thus, dexmedetomidine can be used safely in the epileptic patient.

Clonidine: The effect of clonidine in epileptic patients is controversial. There are reports that the drug lowers the seizure threshold in epileptic patients (pro-convulsant effect).

There is not enough clinical evidence at present that the use of clonidine is contraindicated in epilepsy patients.

Barbiturates: Barbiturates, except for the methohexital, present a significant anticonvulsant activity in the EEG, and its use is considered safe for induction of anesthesia in epileptic patients, as well as treatment of status epilepticus.

Opioids: Meperidine has neuroexcitatory effect attributed to its metabolite normeperidine. Clinically, it is characterized as tremors, myoclonus and seizures. At the doses commonly used as adjuvant drug in general or regional anesthesia, it appears safe in the epileptic patient.

However, in situations where there may be accumulation of normeperidine, such as prolonged use (patient-controlled analgesia), anticonvulsants (phenytoin and phenobarbital) and phenothiazines (chlorpromazine), patients with renal failure, advanced malignancy and sickle cell disease, the drug can cause seizures; it shall then not be used in epileptic patients.

Morphine has no pro-convulsant effect when used intravenously and can be used safely in epileptic patients. However, tonic-clonic seizures were observed when employing epidural drug in epileptic patients.

Nitrous oxide: Although nitrous oxide has excitatory effects on central nervous system, the epileptogenic potential of the drug is very low and can be used safely in epileptic patients.

Halothane: Halothane has potent anticonvulsant effect, and can be used safely in epileptic patients. However, there are reports of seizures associated with halothane.

Enflurane: It may produce epileptiform EEG activity and seizures, especially at concentrations above 2 MAC and hypocapnia in the presence of stimulation, tactile, visual or hearing impairment; then it should be avoided in epileptic patients.

Isoflurane: Although there are reports of potential epileptogenic with isoflurane, most studies show potent anticonvulsant effect of the drug, that is also used in the treatment of status epilepticus, and certainly in epileptic patients.

Sevoflurane: The epileptiform activity of sevoflurane has been extensively studied. A review of 30 studies evaluated the correlation between the use of sevoflurane and epileptiform EEG changes and/or presence of convulsive movements in patients with or without epilepsy. The incidence of these changes ranged from 0–100%. The depth of anesthesia with sevoflurane and/or the presence of hyperventilation (hypocapnia) were risk factors for the emergence of excitatory activity of the central nervous system.

Desflurane: Although there are few studies, there is no evidence that desflurane has epileptiform activity, even when used in high concentrations or in the presence of hypocapnia, and has even been administered in the treatment of status asthmaticus and safely in epileptic patients.

4. Gas(es) stored as liquid in cylinders is/are:

a. Nitrous oxide
b. Cyclopropane
c. CO_2
d. Helium
e. Nitrogen

Ans: a, b, c

Ref: https://www.ncbi.nlm.nih.gov/pmc/articles/PMC3821266
Drugs and equipment in anaesthetic practice, Arun Kumar, 6/e

Option a	True
Option b	True
Option c	True
Option d	False
Option e	False

The medical gases commonly used for anesthesia and critical care are oxygen, nitrous oxide, medical air, entonox, carbon dioxide and heliox. Medical gases such as oxygen and air can be supplied in bulk and others such as nitrous oxide, medical air and entonox can be supplied from the cylinder manifolds. These gases are then delivered through pipelines to the wall outlets. Medical gases can also be provided directly from the portable cylinders.

The cylinders are made up of molybdenum steel so that they may withstand high pressure. Special cylinders made from aluminum are useful in magnetic resonance imaging (MRI) room. Typical wall thickness of steel cylinders is 3 mm and that of an aluminum alloy cylinder is 6 mm^2.

Size: AA (smallest) to H (biggest). Cylinders are manufactured in different sizes (A-J). Sizes A and H are not used for medical gases. Cylinders attached to the anaesthetic machine are usually of size E.

Agents: O_2, N_2O, Cyclopropane , Entonox , Air etc.

Duration of Gas Flow

- An E cylinder contain 22 cubic feet (cu. ft.) of oxygen when full (2200 psi pressure).
- One cubic foot of oxygen equals 28.3 L.
- Now, Tank Factor: (22×28.3) L/2200 psi = 0.28 L/psi.

- Therefore, the time duration for which the tank would last (in minutes).
  = [Tank factor (gauge pressure – 500)]/L flow.
  = [0.28 L/psi (2000 psi – 500 psi)]/8 L/min.
  = 52.5 min.

Liquid Oxygen

Liquid oxygen is derived by the fractional distillation of liquid air. One volume of liquid oxygen yields 842 times of its volume of oxygen in gaseous form at 15 °C temperature and one atmospheric pressure.

Physical properties of Medical gases in cylinders and their Pin Index				
Agent	***Colour***	***State***	***Pressure***	***Pin Index***
Oxygen	Black with white shoulders	Gas	2000 psi	2.5
Nitrous oxide	Blue	Liquid	750 psi	3.5
CO_2	Grey	Liquid	750 psi	1,6/2,6
Cyclopropane	Orange	Liquid	75 psi	3, 6
Air	Grey with black and white shoulders	Gas	2000 psi	1,5
Entonox (50% O_2 + 50% N_2O)	Blue with black and white shoulders	Gas	2000 psi	7

5. **Advantages of xenon is/are:**
   a. Eco friendly
   b. Inert
   c. Cost effective
   d. Highly stable
   e. High blood solubility

Ans. a, b, d *Ref: Miller's, 7/e*

Option a	True	
Option b	True	
Option c	False	Since it is rare, xenon is expensive
Option d	True	
Option e	False	Low blood solubility

- Xenon is a rarest noble gas, non-flammable and non-explosive.
- It is present in atmospheric air in a concentration of about 0.086 ppm.
- Since it is rare, xenon is expensive. Because xenon is rare and expensive, it can be used as an anesthetic agent only if its waste is reduced to the absolute minimum. It must be applied via rebreathing systems using the lowest possible gas flows. Closed-system anesthesia is the only economically acceptable technique for application of xenon for anesthetic purposes.
- Xenon has many of the properties of an ideal anaesthetic agent.
  - Inhalational induction is smooth and rapid with rapid emergence regardless of duration of anesthesia.
  - So far, it has not been found to have any toxic, allergic, mutagenic, foetotoxic or carcinogenic properties.
  - Xenon appears to be environmentally safe.
  - It has a MAC of 63% in humans and a MAC-awake of 33%.

- Effects of xenon on the cardiovascular system are minimal with left ventricular performance apparently unaffected.
- Xenon does not trigger malignant hyperthermia.

6. True about Advanced Cardiovascular Life Support (ACLS) as per AHA guidelines, includes:
   a. Chest compressions at a rate of 100 to 120/min
   b. The adult sternum should be depressed at least 2 inches (5 cm)
   c. Interrupt compressions for greater than 10 seconds
   d. Vasopressin in combination with epinephrine is drug of choice in cardiac arrest
   e. Ventilate adequately, i.e. 2 breaths after 30 compressions

Ans. a, b, e *Ref: Highlights of the 2015 AHA Guidelines Update for CPR and ECC*

Option a	True	
Option b	True	
Option c	False	Interruption should be for < 10 seconds
Option d	False	Antiarrythmics as Beta blockers are given at first to patients after doing CPR
Option e	True	

Advanced cardiovascular life support (ACLS) refers to a set of clinical interventions for the urgent treatment of cardiac arrest, stroke and other life-threatening medical emergencies, enabling the health care practitioner with knowledge and skills to deploy those interventions. The American Heart Association and the International Liaison Committee on Resuscitation updates and publishes the recommendations and educational material after every five years.

The 2015 Guidelines Update

BLS and CPR Quality: There is a new recommendation to consider use of social media to summon rescuers who are willing and able to perform CPR and are in close proximity to someone with a suspected cardiac arrest, meaning that the rescuers can activate an emergency response (i.e., through use of a mobile telephone) without leaving the victim's side.

Notable changes in BLS include:

- ❑ A single rescuer is to initiate chest compressions before giving rescue breaths (**C-A-B** rather than A-B-C) to reduce delay to first compression. The single rescuer should begin CPR with **30 chest compressions** followed by **2 breaths.**
- ❑ The new upper limit for compression rate is **100–120/min**. The clarified recommendation for chest compression depth for adults is at least **2 inches (5 cm)** but not greater than 2.4 inches **(6 cm)**.
- ❑ Bystander-administered naloxone (IM or Intranasal) may be considered for suspected life-threatening opioid-associated emergencies in patients with known or suspected opioid addiction who are unresponsive with no normal breathing but a pulse.
- ❑ The use of the impedance threshold device (ITD) alone during CPR isn't recommended. However, the use of the ITD combined with active compression-decompression CPR may be considered as an alternative to standard CPR.

Advanced Cardiovascular Life Support (ACLS):

- ❑ There are limited changes in ACLS care during cardiac arrest.
- ❑ Recommendations for defibrillation are unchanged.

- ❑ Review of existing data demonstrated no superiority of bag-valve mask ventilation, supraglottic airways or endotracheal (ET) intubation as strategies for airway management and ventilation during CPR.
- ❑ Although waveform capnography remains the recommended strategy for confirmation of ET tube placement during CPR, ultrasound has been added as an alternative strategy when capnography is not available.
- ❑ On reviewing the use of vasopressors during CPR, vasopressin is removed from the ACLS algorithm based on lack of evidence for additional benefit compared to standard dose epinephrine therapy alone. It is also now recommended that epinephrine, when used, should be administered as soon as possible in patients with non-shockable rhythms.
- ❑ Although there were no new recommendations on the use of physiologic monitoring or ultrasound to guide resuscitation during cardiac arrest, the inability to achieve an end-tidal carbon dioxide value ≥ 10 mm Hg in intubated patients after 20 minutes of CPR has been added a potential component of a multimodal criteria to guide the decision to terminate of resuscitation efforts.
- ❑ The Guidelines restated that the use of extracorporeal cardiopulmonary resuscitation as a rescue therapy for refractory cardiac arrest may be considered when the suspected etiology of the cardiac arrest is potentially reversible during a limited period of mechanical cardiorespiratory support. However, implementation of such a strategy is resource intensive and requires a highly coordinated system of care to be successful.

Summary of high-quality cPR components for BLS providers

Component	*Adults and adolescents*	*Children (Age 1 year to puberty)*	*Infants (Age less than 1 year, Excluding newborns)*
Scene safety	Make sure the environment is safe for rescuers and victim		
Recognition of cardiac arrest	Check for responsiveness No breathing or only gasping (i.e. no normal breathing) No definite pulse felt within 10 seconds (Breathing and pulse check can be performed simultaneously in less than 10 seconds)		

Post-Cardiac Arrest Care:

- ❑ The most important change in post-cardiac arrest care is in targeted temperature management. The target temperature range has been expanded to 32–36 °C, and the use of rapidly infused cold saline in the prehospital setting isn't recommended due to lack of impact on patient outcomes.
- ❑ Emergency coronary angiography is recommended for all patients with ST elevation and for hemodynamically or electrically unstable patients without ST elevation for whom a cardiovascular lesion is suspected.

7. All of the following are true about epidural caudal anesthesia in children *except:*

a. 1 ml/kg of Bupivacaine with epinephrine provides 3–6 hours of anesthesia for all procedures below the umbilicus
b. A dose of 33 mcg/kg of morphine in the caudal epidural solution can provide prolonged analgesia but coupled with risk of delayed respiratory depression
c. An intraosseous injection is equivalent to an intramuscular injection
d. Sacral hiatus is more prominent in children above 8 years of age
e. A caudal catheter should not be left in situ for more than 36–48 hours.

Ans. b, c, d *Ref: Update in Anaesthesia 1998 No. 8*

Option a	True	True for epidural caudal anesthesia in children
Option b	False	Not true, hence the answer
Option c	False	Not true, hence the answer
Option d	False	Not true, hence the answer
Option e	True	True for epidural caudal anesthesia in children

Caudal Block

Pediatric caudal epidural anesthesia is a well-accepted technique commonly used in combination with general anesthesia or occasionally alone in high-risk patients.

Caudal epidural anesthesia is most commonly used in children upto 7 years of age. As the child advances in age the sacral plate tends to flatten out, making the insertion of the needle through the sacrococcygeal ligament more difficult. By far the easiest insertion is in the child below the age of 7 years.

Indications:

- Lower abdominal surgery: (incision below the umbilicus-T10 sensory level) especially perineal, genitourinary or ilioinguinal surgery.
- Lower extremity surgery.
- Newborn and premature infants: If used as the sole anesthetic, caudal epidural anesthesia reduces the risk of respiratory depression from residual neuromuscular blockade (pancuronium) and inhalation anesthetics. Post-operative apnea associated with general anesthesia, is reduced with caudal anesthesia but not abolished.

Monitoring for caudal epidural anesthesia must include monitoring of ventilation, oxygenation, and circulation at least every 3 minutes.

Bupivacaine: provides reliable, long-lasting anesthesia and postoperative analgesia. An easy rule is 1 ml/kg of Bupivacaine 0.25% with epinephrine 1:200,000 provides 3–6 hours of anesthesia for all procedures below the umbilicus.

Opioids: A dose of 50 mcg/kg of preservative free morphine or diamorphine 30 mcg/kg added to the local anesthetic solution will provide 12 to 24 hours of analgesia but can produce urinary retention, nausea, and itching and respiratory depression. However, a dose of 33 mcg/kg of preservative free morphine in the caudal epidural solution can provide prolonged analgesia, with less risk of delayed respiratory depression.

Clonidine: A dose of 0.5–1.0 mcm/kg improves the quality and duration of analgesia with bupivacaine without causing significant bradycardia or respiratory depression, lasting for up to 12 hours. Doses greater than 1 microgram/kg are associated with increased sedation.

Ketamine: Causes significant prolongation of postoperative analgesia.

Complication:

1. Failed or incomplete block.
2. Unilateral block: Although rare, but it can occur if the injection is given too rapidly. Local anesthetics should be injected slowly over 2 minutes after test dose.
3. Local anaesthetic toxicity due to intravascular, intrathecal or intraosseous injection. If accidently, an intraosseous injection is done, it is equivalent to an intravenous injection.
4. Penetration of sacrum: In infants and young babies, the vertebral bodies can be soft due to incomplete calcification and the anesthetist can pass the needle into the body of the

sacrum and through the vertebral body into the pelvis damaging either pelvic viscera or aorta.

5. Bleeding and infection.

8. APACHE- II includes:

a. GCS
b. Age
c. $PaCO_2$
d. FiO_2/PaO_2 ratio
e. FiO_2

Ans. a, b, e *Ref: Miller's, 7/e*

Option a	True	
Option b	True	
Option c	False	
Option d	False	
Option e	True	

- Acute Physiologic Assessment and Chronic Health Evaluation II (APACHE- II) is a type of ICU scoring system that has been developed to grade the severity of illness in critically ill adult patients who have been admitted within 24 hrs in the ICU.
- Point score ranging from 0 to 71 are awarded on the basis of 12 physiologic variables, age, and underlying health of the patient.
- As the score grows higher, the disease severity and risk of death increases.

The point score is calculated from a patient's age and 12 routine physiological measurements

Acute Physiologic Assessment and Chronic Health Evaluation (APACHE-II) scoring system	
$AaDO_2$ or PaO_2 (depending on FiO_2)	
Temperature (rectal)	Mean arterial pressure
pH arterial	Heart rate
Respiratory rate	Sodium (serum)
Potassium (serum)	Creatinine
Hematocrit	White blood cell count
Glasgow Coma Scale	

9. True about ET tube is:

a. Disposable
b. Made of PVC
c. Made of red rubber and the collar is uncuffed in children
d. High volume and low pressure cuff
e. Nasal and oral insertion can not be done

Ans. a, b, c, d *Ref: Miller's, 7/e*

Option a	True	
Option b	True	
Option c	True	
Option d	True	
Option e	False	Nasal and oral insertion can be done

- Endotracheal tube is used to maintain:
  - Airway patency
  - Oxygenation and ventilation
  - Suctioning of secretions
  - Helping in the use of inhalation anesthetics.

Features of ET Tube:

- It is made of transparent polyvinyl chloride (PVC) and is about 33 cm long.
- It has a transparent body, so that blood or vomit can be easily seen .
- ET tubes meant for adults are cuffed. The High volume low pressure (HVLP) cuff is used to seal the trachea.
- The Standard low pressure endotracheal tubes are ideal for short-term intubation while the VentiSeal High Volume Low Pressure cuff is disposable & designed for longer term anesthesia or intensive care where the cuff forms a seal without putting excess pressure on the wall of the trachea.
- The Murphy eye is standard on all Endotracheal tubes to ensure that adequate ventilation is maintained even if the tip of the Tube was fixed to the tracheal wall or occluded by secretions.

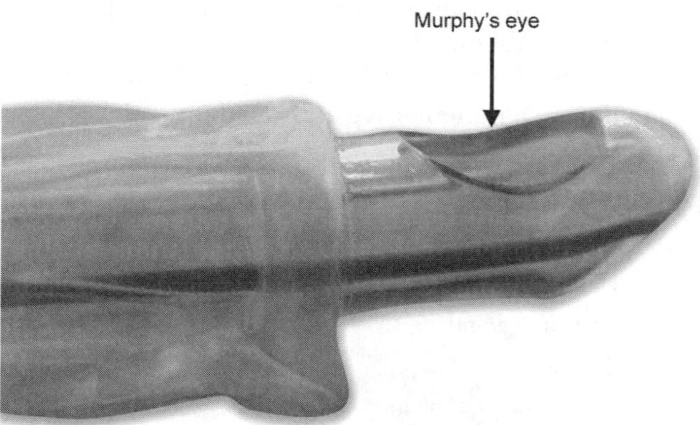

Fig. 17.1: Murphy's eye

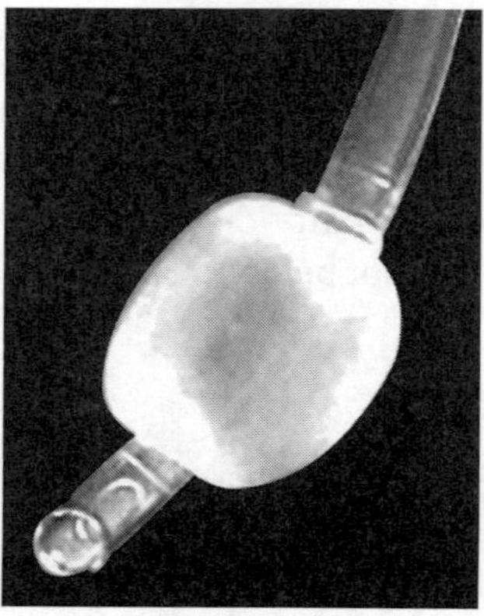

Fig. 17.2: Typical HVLP disposable PVC Cuff

- Uses of cuffed ET tubes:
  - To seal the trachea, so that positive pressure cannot escape from the lower airway.
  - To seal the upper airway, so that material above the glottis cannot enter the trachea.

Complications of excessive cuff pressure seal (> 40 cm H_2O)

Postextubation pain, necrosis, bleeding, stenosis, tracheal rupture and tracheoesophageal fistulae.

Ideal intracuff pressures for adults using traditional PVC cuffed tubes (high volume low pressure ET tube)		
Pressure	***cm H_2O***	***mm Hg***
Ideal	20–30	15–22
High	> 40	30
Low	< 20	15

PVC: Polyvinyl chloride

ET Tube in Children

- The cricoid ring is narrow enough to form a seal all by itself, so the paediatric ET tubes can be uncuffed.
- Nowadays, cuffed ET tubes are considered fairly safe for use in children < 8 years of age.
- Use of cuffed tubes requires smaller internal diameter of the ET tube, hence limiting the suctioning ability.

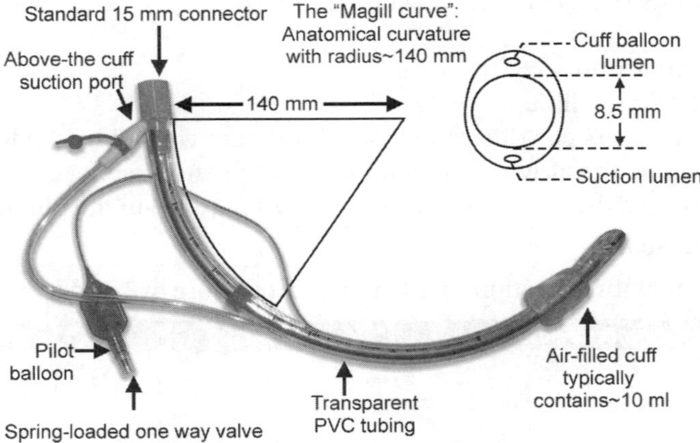

Fig. 17.3: Anatomy of an ET Tube

Difference between High Pressure Low Volume & High Volume Low Pressure ETT Cuffs.

Characteristic	HPLV	HVLP
Material	Non disposable, made of silicone	Disposable, made of PVC
Diameter	Small diameter, low residual volume	1.5–2 times the diameter of trachea when fully inflated
Pressure	Causes ischemic damage to tracheal wall due to high pressure	Intracuff pressure closely correlates with tracheal mucosal pressure
Aspiration	Better protection against aspiration	Microleaks can occur
Visibility	Tube and cuff more easily visible during intubation	
Complications	More	Less

10. The indication of intubation in head injury includes:

a. GCS < 8
b. Non-cooperative patient
c. Full stomach
d. Cervical spine injury
e. Near herniation of brain

Ans. a, b, c, d, e *Ref: Trauma scoring systems and databases. British Journal of Anaesthesia 113 (2): 286–94 (2014)doi:10.1093/bja/aeu242. Accessed on 15 May 2017.*

Option a	True	
Option b	True	
Option c	True	
Option d	True	
Option e	True	

The main aim of assessment and management of head-injured patients is to maintain adequate cerebral blood flow (CBF) and to avoid cerebral ischemia and hypoxia.

As brain injury may be worsened by airway or circulatory compromise, *'ABCDE' approach is used for early identification and treatment of life-threatening injuries.*

Indications for intubation in a patient with head injury include:

- GCS ≤ 8
- Risk of raised ICP due to agitation (i.e. sedation required)
- Inability to control/protect the airway or loss of protective laryngeal reflexes
- A fall of 2 or more points in the motor component of the GCS
- In order to optimise oxygenation and ventilation
- Seizures
- Bleeding into mouth/airway
- Bilateral fractured mandible
- Brain herniation can occur due to increased pressure caused by swelling from the head injury. In such case, the airway is maintained though endotracheal intubation to increase the breathing rate so that the levels of carbon dioxide (CO_2) in the blood may be reduced.

The Glasgow Coma Scale:

The scale is made up of three sections, with a minimum score of 3 and a maximum of 15.

Components of Glasgow coma scale	
• **Eye Opening**	
- Spontaneously	4
- To speech	3
- To pain	2
- None	1
• **Verbal response**	
- Orientated	5
- Confused	4
- Inappropriate	3
- Incomprehensible	2
- None	1
• **Motor response**	
- Obeys commands (for movement)	6
- Purposeful movement to painful stimuli ('localises')	5
- Purposeful movement to painful stimuli ('withdraws')	4
- Abnormal (spastic) flexion, decorticate posture	3
- Extensor (rigid) response, decerebrate posture	2
- None	1

11. Agents used for induction of anesthesia:

a. Thiopentone
b. Ketamine
c. Propofol
d. Morphine
e. Fentanyl

Ans. a, b, c *(Ref: Peck T, Hill S, Williams M. Pharmacology for anesthesia and intensive care. Greenwich medical media, 2003.)*

Option a	True	Acts within 30 seconds of intravenous injection
Option b	True	Produces 'dissociative' anaesthesia.
Option c	True	Short acting general anaesthetic
Option d	False	
Option e	False	

Induction agents provide rapid loss of consciousness, blunt sympathetic responses, and can improve intubating conditions.

Use of induction agents:

- To induce anesthesia prior to other drugs being given to maintain anesthesia.
- As the sole drug for short procedures.
- To maintain anesthesia for longer procedures by intravenous infusion.
- To provide sedation

The commonly used induction agents are:

Barbiturates (Thiopentone): A dose of 4–5 mg/kg of thiopental produces a smooth onset of hypnosis with good definitive endpoints within 30 seconds of intravenous injection. Recovery after a single dose is rapid due to redistribution and there is a low incidence of restlessness and nausea and vomiting.

Advantages of thiopentone:

- Reduces cerebral blood flow, cerebral metabolic rate and oxygen demand
- Lowers cardiac output and blood pressure
- Potent anticonvulsant properties
- In Brain injury, lowers intracranial pressure by producing Barbiturate Coma.

Disadvantages of thiopentone:

- Respiratory Depression
- May precipitate porphyria in susceptible patients due to hepatic enzyme induction

Phenols (Propofol):

- Short acting general anesthetic.
- [Q]**Out of all the induction drugs, it *causes marked fall in blood pressure* due to systemic vasodilatation.**
- Respiratory depression with probable periods of apnoea.
- May cause epileptiform movements.
- Reduces cerebral blood flow, metabolic rate and intra-cranial pressure.
- Can be safely used in patients with porphyrias.
- Contraindicated for infusion in children due to "propofol infusion syndrome".

Imidazoles (Etomidate):

- Induction of anesthesia can be accompanied by involuntary movements.
- Recovery is unpleasant, accompanied by nausea and vomiting.
- **[Q]Out of all the IV anaesthetic drugs,it causes *least cardiovascular depression.***
- Causes transient apnoea.

Phencyclidines (Ketamine):

- Hypnotic, analgesic and local anaesthetic properties.
- Produces 'dissociative' anesthesia.
- A bronchial smooth muscle relaxant.
- Psychic sensations including alterations in mood state, floating sensations, vivid dreams and hallucinations
- **[Q]Ketamine is *unique* amongst induction drugs in that it can be administered *i.v, i.m, orally, nasally, rectally,* and the preservative-free solution *epidurally*.**
- Causes tachycardia, increased blood pressure, and increased cardiac output, hence can be used in a patient with shock.
- Can be safely used in patients with porphyria.

Benzodiazepines (Midazolam):

- Useful premedication drug in children.
- Mild cardiovascular and respiratory depressant effects.
- Effect can be reversed by flumazenil

12. Treatment of bupivacaine toxicity:

a. Intralipid
b. Bretylium
c. Adrenalin
d. Esmolol
e. Calcium chloride

Ans. a, b *Ref: Miller's, 7/e*

Option a	True	20% intralipid especially when unresponsive to standard therapy
Option b	True	Ventricular arrhythmias may be treated with bretylium
Option c	False	
Option d	False	
Option e	False	Increases toxicity

Bupivacaine is most cardiotoxic anaesthetic agent among all the amide local anaesthetics.

Mechanism of cardiotoxicity:

- Blockade of sodium channel: Binds more strongly to resting/inactivated Na channels.
- Bupivacaine dissociates from Na channels during diastole more slowly than lidocaine.
- Calcium channels, release of calcium from sarcoplasmic reticulum, and mitochondrial energy metabolism. Thus cardiotoxic potential is greatly enhanced.

Effects of bupivacaine toxicity:

- Initial CNS excitation followed by a rapid CNS depression.
- Myocardial depression
- Cardiac dysrhythmias

- ❑ Vasoconstriction at low doses, vasodilatation at higher doses
- ❑ Chest pain, shortness of breath, palpitations, lightheadedness, diaphoresis

Treatment:

- ❑ Seizures: GABA agonists
- ❑ Convulsions: Paralytics and airway management as needed
- ❑ Hypotension: Vasopressors
- ❑ Cardiovascular collapse: 20% intralipid especially when unresponsive to standard therapy.
- ❑ Ventricular arrhythmias may be treated with bretylium, but **preferable is Amiodarone.**

13. True about epidural anesthesia in comparison to spinal anesthesia is:

a. Shorter needle required
b. Less post spinal headache
c. Less dose requirement
d. Dense blockade is there
e. Single injection is required

Ans. b

Option a	False	Seen in spinal block
Option b	True	Post spinal headache is profound & common in spinal block
Option c	False	Seen in spinal block
Option d	False	Seen in spinal block
Option e	False	Spinal block is given as single injection.

A spinal block is a single injection of local anaesthetic medications and so there is only one opportunity to deliver the medications. With an epidural, a catheter sits in an epidural space so drugs can be delivered as needed to extend the duration of the block. An epidural block can be made to last longer than a spinal block.

Spinal anesthesia is induced by injecting small amounts of local anaesthetic into the cerebro-spinal fluid (CSF). The injection is usually made in the lumbar spine below the level at which the spinal cord ends (L2).

Complications following spinal anesthesia:

- ❑ Hypotension—common
- ❑ Post dural puncture headache—common
- ❑ Cauda equina injury—rare
- ❑ Cardiac arrest—very rare
- ❑ Epidural abscess—rare

Complications of epidural anesthesia:

- ❑ Pain at the injection site, unintentional dural puncture (21), and vasovagal syncope (minor complications).
- ❑ Major complications include damage to neural structures, epidural hematoma, and epidural abscess.
- ❑ An epidural block interrupts both somatic and sympathetic nerve conduction; thus, cardiovascular changes, including hypotension and tachycardia, may occur.
- ❑ Respiratory compromise or failure can occur if the phrenic nerve or respiratory centers of the brain stem are inadvertently blocked.

Difference between Spinal Block and Epidural Block

Spinal block	*Epidural block*
Smaller needle is required	
Small dose of anaesthetic is required about 1.5–3.5 mL	Larger doses of drug required about 10–20 mL
A spinal anaesthetic delivers drug to the intrathecal space (the CSF), and acts on the spinal cord directly.	An epidural delivers drugs outside the dura (outside CSF), and has its main effect on nerve roots leaving the dura at the level of the epidural, rather than on the spinal cord itself.
Almost always a single injection	Drug delivered through indwelling catheter for longer duration of block
Effect lasts for shorter duration.	Longer duration.
Post spinal headache common	Post spinal headache less common
A spinal gives profound block of all motor and sensory function below the level of injection	Epidural blocks a 'band' of nerve roots around the site of injection, with normal function above, and close-to-normal function below the levels blocked.
	Does not cause as significant a neuromuscular block as a spinal unless specific local anesthetics are also used which block motor fibres as readily as sensory nerve fibres
A spinal must be injected below L2 to avoid piercing the spinal cord	May be given at a cervical, thoracic, or lumbar site

Radiology

1. Radiation absorption units are:

a. Sievert
b. RAD
c. Becquerel
d. REM
e. Gray

Ans. b,e *Ref: Grainger & Allison's Diagnostic Radiology 4th/ed p679*

Parameters	Non-SI Unit	SI Unit
Radioactivity	Curie	Becquerel
Exposed dose	Roentgen	Coulombs/kg
Radiation absorption	Rad (Radiation absorbed dose)	Gray
Equivalent dose	Rem (Roentgen equivalent in man)	Sievert (SV)
Effective dose	milliSievert (mSV)	

2. Advantage of MRI over CT

a. Bone artefact b. IUGR is seen

Ans. a, b *Ref: CT and MRI of the Whole Body, 6th/ed by John R. Haaga, p38*

Beam-Hardening Artefacts (CT Scan)

Beam-hardening artefacts result from the preferential absorption of low-energy photons from the beam as a beam traverses the body, the average beam photon energy is progressively increased. Accordingly, toward the end of the X-ray path the attenuation is less than at the beginning because the attenuation coefficient is smaller for the remaining beam, which has higher average energy. The assigned attenuation coefficients are thus in error, and the densities seen on the image are in error. The effect is most pronounced in regions of strong attenuation, such as bone. The artefact is seen as a shadow beneath the ribs, for example, or increased shadows in the mediastinum or skull. This effect occurs throughout the image, but qualitatively it is not usually perceived except where there is a great deal of hardening (e.g., in the vicinity of bone).

Advantages of MRI over CT Scan

1. No use of ionizing radiation (Preferred in children and those who require multiple imaging)
2. Can be performed in any imaging plane without physically moving the patient
3. Contrast agents used in MRI are less likely to produce a severe lethal reaction
4. Better contrast resolution and lesion characterization than CT
5. Safer modality in pregnancy (if absolutely indicated).

Radiology

1. Chest X-ray features of stage II sarcoidosis include:

a. Enlarged paratracheal nodes
b. Mediastinal adenopathy
c. Bilateral hilar lymphadenopathy
d. Pulmonary infiltrates
e. Pulmonary fibrosis

Ans. b, c, d *Ref: Lippincott's Fundamentals of Diagnostic Radiology, 4/e*

Option a	False	Hilar and mediastinal lymphadenopathy is seen
Option b	True	
Option c	True	
Option d	True	
Option e	False	Stage IV

Sarcoidosis is a non-caseating granulomatous multi-system disease with a wide range of clinical and radiographic manifestations. Majority of patients with sarcoidosis are asymptomatic. The main reason patients seek medical attention is an abnormal imaging study.

- The chest roentgenogram is the most commonly used radiologic imaging technique to evaluate patients with pulmonary sarcoidosis.

Scadding staging system

- In the 1960s, Scadding proposed a staging system of the chest roentgenogram.
- The original staging system has been modified and now includes:
  - Stage 0: No adenopathy or infiltrates;
  - Stage 1: Hilar and mediastinal adenopathy alone
  - Stage 2: Adenopathy and pulmonary infiltrates
  - Stage 3: Pulmonary infiltrates alone
  - Stage 4: Pulmonary fibrosis.

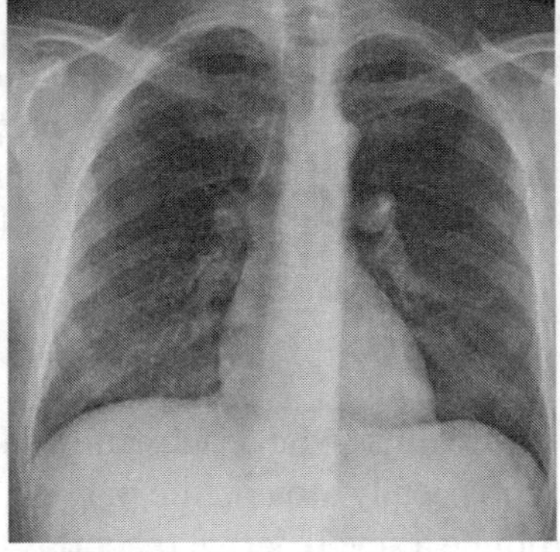

Stage I: Note the bilateral hilar and mediastinal adenopathy.

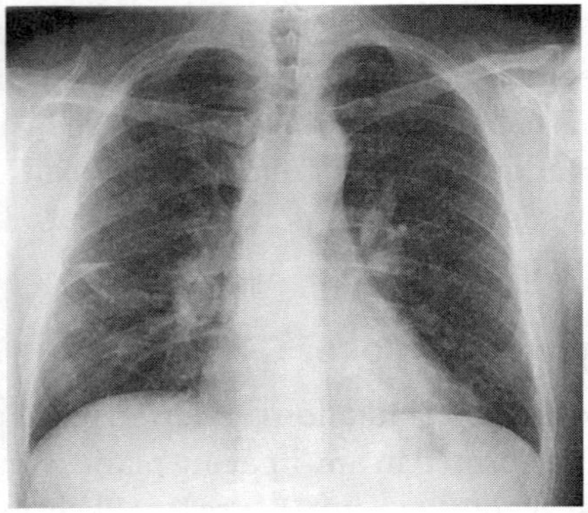

Stage II: Adenopathy and pulmonary infiltrates.

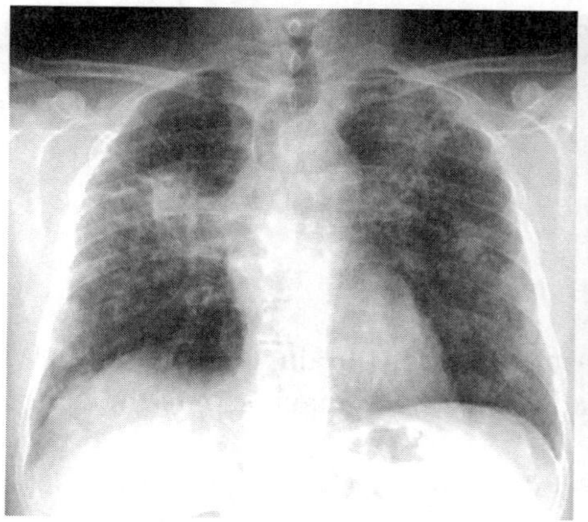

Stage III: Disease associated with a tumefactive type of lung parenchymal involvement: opacities in the right and left midlung zones that mimic neoplasm.

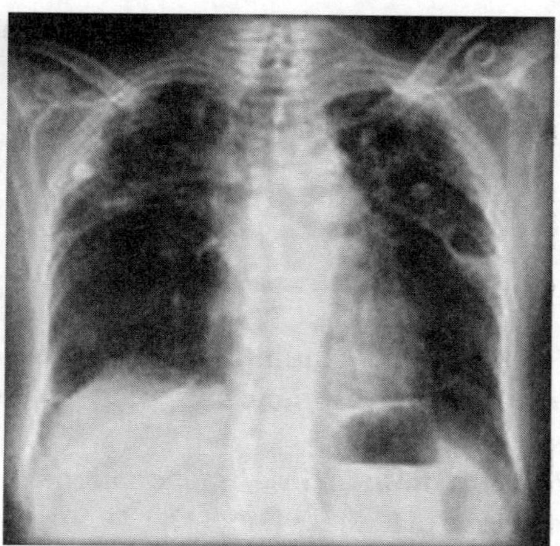

Stage IV: Pulmonary fibrosis.

- The Scadding staging system has important prognostic significance. Scadding noticed that stage I patients have more than 90% resolution of their radiographic findings within 2 years, while those with stage III disease demonstrate resolution in less than 1/3rd of cases.
- However, the chest radiograph does not correlate well with sarcoidosis symptoms (e.g. dyspnea) or functional parameters such as spirometry nor the six-minute walk test.
- The characteristic histology of sarcoidosis is the granuloma formation. Granulomas may be seen along the lymphatics of the bronchovascular bundle, interlobular septa, major fissures and subpleural areas. These are the anatomic areas that deserve attention on regular chest X-rays.
- The majority of patients present with stage I disease in which the differential diagnosis includes lymphoma, infectious diseases (fungal, mycobacterial) or occupational diseases (berylliosis) require biopsy for confirmation.

Mediastinal and hilar lymphadenopathy

- This is the main radiologic feature of sarcoidosis.
- Symmetric hilar adenopathy is the most typical followed by disease in the subcarina and paratracheal lymph nodes stations.
- The hilar nodes are almost always involved.
- It is rare to have middle mediastinal nodal involvement without hilar involvement also.
- Unilateral hilar enlargement without mediastinal involvement is rare, seen only in 1–3% of cases.
- Nodes can be very large but typically do not continue with the cardiac silhouette, in contrast to lymphoma in which the nodes are continuous with the pericardial outline.

Calcification and necrosis are rare features in sarcoidosis.

2. Whole brain radiotherapy for brain metastasis is given as:

a. 30 gray (Gy) in 5 fractions
b. 30 gray (Gy) in 10 fractions
c. 20 gray (Gy) in 10 fractions
d. 15 gray (Gy) in 5 fractions
e. 15 gray (Gy) in 10 fractions

Ans. b *Ref: Lippincott's Fundamentals of Diagnostic Radiology, 4/e*

Option a	False	
Option b	True	
Option c	False	
Option d	False	
Option e	False	

- In patients with multiple cerebral metastases, whole brain radiotherapy (WBRT) is generally the treatment of choice, as it addresses both macroscopic and microscopic disease.
- The most common dose/fractionation schedule used is 30 Gy delivered in 10 fractions over the course of 2 weeks (10×3 Gy).
- In addition to treating patients with known brain metastases, WBRT is also used to treat cancer patients with a high risk of developing brain metastases, termed prophylactic cranial irradiation (PCI). The possible utility of PCI for prevention of *small cell lung cancer (SCLC)-associated intracranial metastases* is one that has been recognized and studied since the 1970s.

3. Which of the following is true about concurrent chemoradiation therapy?

a. Can be given with cytoprotective agent amifostine
b. Uses radiosensitizing property of chemotherapy
c. Risk is more in concurrent than sequential chemotherapy
d. Used for treating solid tumors
e. It is not useful in preventing distant metastases

Ans. a, b, d *(Ref: Huang O, Wu D, Zhu L, Li Y, Chen W, Shen K. Concurrent adjuvant radiochemotherapy versus standard chemotherapy followed by radiotherapy in operable breast cancer after breast conserving therapy: A meta-analysis. J Can Res Ther 2016;12:84-9)*

Option a	True	
Option b	True	
Option c	False	Concurrent chemotherapy is found to have more positive outcome and prevention of distant metastasis
Option d	True	
Option e	False	Concurrent chemoradiation may act systemically and potentially prevent distant metastases

Concurrent chemotherapy: The use of chemotherapy delivered concurrently with radiation. Either chemotherapy can act as a radiosensitizer, improving the probability of local control and potentially the survival, by aiding the destruction of radio-resistant clones, or it can be used with organ-preserving intent, resulting in improved function and/or cosmetic results compared with surgical resection with/without adjuvant treatment. In addition, chemotherapy given as part of concurrent chemoradiation may act systemically and potentially prevent distant metastases.

Chemotherapy can sensitize tumors to radiotherapy by:

- ❑ Inhibiting tumor repopulation,
- ❑ Preferentially killing hypoxic cells,
- ❑ Inhibiting the repair of sublethal radiation damage,
- ❑ Sterilizing micrometastatic disease outside of the radiation fields, and
- ❑ Decreasing the tumor mass, which leads to improved blood supply and reoxygenation. These can be continued for weeks or months, depending on how well the cancer responds to treatment.
- ❑ Radiation actively destroys cancerous cells to break up tumors.
- ❑ Research on concurrent chemotherapy indicates that the medications may make cells more susceptible to radiation.
- ❑ *Taking drugs at the same time as radiation therapy (concurrent) can result in a more positive outcome when compared to patients who take one treatment at a time (sequential).*

Currently, concomitant chemoradiotherapy is widely used in the treatment of solid tumors. In almost all malignancies in which locoregional control is necessary, concurrent chemoradiotherapy is either an established treatment modality or is actively being investigated.

The most recent chemical radioprotector to become available clinically is ***amifostine***. On the basis of efficacy data from a phase III randomized trial in patients with head and neck cancer, which showed reduced acute and chronic xerostomia with preserved antitumor response, some institutions are now adding amifostine to their chemoradiation regimens.

4. Diffuse axonal injury (DAI) is diagnosed by:

a. Single-photon emission CT
b. MR spectroscopy
c. Radiography
d. MR diffusion and susceptibility
e. Doppler USG

Ans. a, b, d, e *Ref: Lippincott's Fundamentals of Diagnostic Radiology, 4/e*

Option a	True	
Option b	True	
Option c	False	Conventional radiography has no role in DAI
Option d	True	
Option e	True	

Diffuse axonal injury (DAI) is a frequent result of traumatic acceleration/deceleration or rotational injuries and a frequent cause of persistent vegetative state in patients. It typically consists of several focal white-matter lesions measuring 1–15 mm in a characteristic distribution.

- ❑ *Magnetic resonance imaging (MRI)* is the preferred examination for DAI (particularly with gradient-echo sequences), although CT scanning may demonstrate findings suggestive of DAI and is more practical and available.
- ❑ The most common MRI finding of DAI is the presence of multifocal areas of abnormal signal (bright on T2-weighted images) at the white matter in the temporal or parietal corticomedullary junction or in the splenium of the corpus callosum.

- ❑ Traumatic microbleeds are considered to be a radiologic marker for DAI. Gradient echo-sequence-based susceptibility-weighted imaging has been found to be sensitive and accurate for microbleed detection.
- ❑ No specific findings related to diffuse axonal injury can be made using conventional radiography, the degree of confidence is low, as conventional radiography cannot demonstrate subtle soft-tissue changes; however, other signs of head trauma can be appreciated, such as facial bone fractures or fluid levels within the paranasal sinuses. Radiographs can also clearly demonstrate skull fractures, but this is not helpful in DAI, as DAI is rarely associated with skull fracture. Thus, many false negatives are possible, because a negative skull radiograph in no way excludes a parenchymal brain injury.
- ❑ *Delayed CT scanning* may be helpful in demonstrating edema or atrophy, which are later findings. Small petechial hemorrhages located at the gray-white matter junction as well as in the corpus callosum and brainstem, are characteristic of CT-scan findings in the acute setting.
- ❑ Transcranial doppler ultrasound is now widely used to detect intracranial hemodynamic phenomena because it is noninvasive and repeatable.
- ❑ Nuclear medicine currently has no role in the routine diagnostic workup of patients with possible diffuse axonal injury; however, studies have suggested that *iodine-123 (123I) single-photon emission CT (SPECT) imaging* demonstrates areas of hypoperfusion in areas of known injury and reveals additional areas of injury not visualized with MRI.
- ❑ *Nuclear magnetic resonance (NMR) spectroscopy*, is a sensitive, accurate and non-invasive method by which changes in brain metabolites can be evaluated after a trauma.

5. True about brachytherapy is:

a. Done by linear accelerators
b. In Ca cervix, more useful than any other treatment
c. Used for esophagus carcinoma
d. Short range isotopes given directly to the tumor
e. Extensive damage to surrounding tissues

Ans. c, d *Ref: Lippincott's Fundamentals of Diagnostic Radiology, 4/e*

Option a	False	External bean radiotherapy is given by linear accelerator
Option b	False	Effective when combined with EBRT
Option c	True	
Option d	True	
Option e	False	The irradiation affects only a very localized area around the radiation sources

Brachytherapy, also called *internal radiation therapy,* uses a higher total dose of radiation to treat a smaller area and in a shorter time than is possible with external beam radiation treatment (EBRT).

- ❑ It is commonly used as an effective treatment for:
  - Cervical cancer—When female does not want to maintain fertility. Used in combination with EBRT, brachytherapy can provide better outcomes than EBRT alone.
  - Prostate—Most often given in the form of a permanent radioactive seed implant.
  - Breast, and
  - Skin cancer.

- Brachytherapy can also be used in the treatment of tumors of the:
  - Brain,
  - Eye,
  - Head and neck region (lip, floor of mouth, tongue, nasopharynx and oropharynx),
  - Respiratory tract (trachea and bronchi),
  - Digestive tract (esophagus, gall bladder, bile-ducts, rectum, anus),
  - Urinary tract (bladder, urethra, penis),
  - Female reproductive tract (uterus, vagina, vulva), and soft tissues.
- Brachytherapy involves the precise placement of *short-range radiation-sources* (radioisotopes) directly at the site of the cancerous tumor.
- These are enclosed in a *protective capsule or wire*, which allows the ionizing radiation to escape to treat and kill surrounding tissue but prevents the charge of radioisotope from moving or dissolving in body fluids.
- The capsule may be removed later, or (with some radioisotopes) it may be allowed to remain in place.
- A feature of brachytherapy is that the irradiation affects only a very localized area around the radiation sources. Exposure to radiation of healthy tissues farther away from the sources is therefore reduced.
- Brachytherapy may be either temporary or permanent:
  - In *temporary brachytherapy*, a highly radioactive material is placed inside a catheter or slender tube for a specific amount of time and then withdrawn. Temporary brachytherapy can be administered at a low-dose rate (LDR) or high-dose rate (HDR).
  - *Permanent brachytherapy*, also called seed implantation, involves placing radioactive seeds or pellets (about the size of a grain of rice) in or near the tumor and leaving them there permanently. After several months, the radioactivity level of the implants eventually diminishes to nothing. The inactive seeds then remain in the body, with no lasting effect on the patient.

Psychiatry

1. Somatic symptom disorder includes all except:

a. Passivity syndrome
b. Illness anxiety disorder
c. Factitious disorder
d. Body dysmorphic disorder
e. General anxiety disorder

Ans. b,c *Ref: DSM 5, Americam Psychiatric Association 2013; Kristy Kultas-Ilinsky, Igor A. Ilinsky. Basal Ganglia and Thalamus in Health and Movement Disorders. Springer Science & Business Media, 2001, p336*

Option a	False	No, it is a neurological disorder with psychopathology, pertaining to frontal cortex damage
Option b	True	Yes, correct
Option c	True	Yes, correct
Option d	False	No, it has been classified under the Obsessive compulsive and related disorders
Option e	False	No, it is an anxiety disorder

This is one expected MCQ and has been in various discussion forums.

There have been significant changes in this group in the recent DSM 5 categorizations.

Specific Somatic Symptom Disorders diagnoses include:

1. Somatic symptom disorder
2. Conversion disorder
3. Psychological factors affecting a medical condition
4. Factitious disorder
5. Other specific and nonspecific somatic symptom disorders

Somatic symptom disorder replaces the *DSM-IV-TR* diagnosis of somatization disorder. Hypochondriasis, pain disorder, and body dysmorphic disorder, conditions listed in the Somatoform Disorders category in *DSM-IV-TR* have been removed.

Somatic symptom disorder replaces somatization disorder with the following criteria:

- At least one somatic symptom that results in significant disruption in everyday life
- Significant actions, thoughts, or feelings about the symptoms
- Somatic symptom actions, thoughts, or feelings are excessively time consuming, out of proportion to the degree of seriousness, or accompanied by a high level of anxiety.

Pain disorder is now clubbed under the broad term of the somatic symptom disorder

Illness anxiety disorder (formerly known as hypochondriasis):

- In patients with/without objective symptoms—with preoccupation for the symptoms (which is clearly in excess or disproportionate to the symptoms)
- Excessive health-related behaviour or concerns or exhibition of clear maladaptive avoidance

Body dysmorphic disorder is now classified under obsessive compulsive and related disorders.

- ❑ Skin, hair, nose, weight are most common organ or features involved

Passivity syndrome (athymhormic syndrome): is essentially a neurological syndrome involving specific pathology of apathy, blunted affect and profound low esteem. There has been evidence of damage to basal ganglia or specifically areas of striatum and globus pallidus

- ❑ Includes abulia, disorders pertaining to frontal cortex
- ❑ May occur after pallidal surgery.

2. True about ADHD is/are:

a. 2/3 develop personality disorder
b. ADHD, combined type is most common
c. Methylphenidate is used
d. Increased chances of learning difficulties
e. Increased chances of schizophreniform illness

Ans. a,b,c,d

Option a	True	Yes, correct
Option b	True	Yes, correct
Option c	True	Yes, correct
Option d	True	Yes, correct
Option e	False	No, it is not commonly associated with ADHD

ADHD is characterised by any or all of the following:

1. Inattention
2. Impulsivity
3. Hyperactivity

Three presentations of ADHD are defined in DSM-5™ based on the predominant symptom pattern for the past 6 months:

- ❑ **Combined presentation**—all three core features are present and ADHD is diagnosed when ≥6 symptoms of hyperactivity/impulsivity and ≥6 symptoms of inattention have been observed for ≥6 months
- ❑ **Predominantly inattentive presentation** - diagnosed if ≥6 symptoms of inattention (but <6 symptoms of hyperactivity/impulsivity) have persisted for ≥6 months
- ❑ **Predominantly hyperactive/impulsive presentation**—diagnosed if ≥6 symptoms of hyperactivity/impulsivity (but <6 symptoms of inattention) have been present for ≥6 months.

Furthermore, the DSM-5™ also states that it must be specified whether the individual with ADHD is in '**partial remission**' (when partial ADHD criteria have been met for the past 6 months with full criteria met previously, and the symptoms still result in impairment in social, academic or occupational functioning) and the current severity of the disease.

Specify current severity:

Mild: Few, if any, symptoms in excess of those required to make the diagnosis are present, and symptoms result in only minor functional impairments.

Moderate: Symptoms or functional impairment between "mild" and "severe" are present.

Severe: Many symptoms in excess of those required to make the diagnosis, or several symptoms that are particularly severe, are present, or the symptoms result in marked impairment in social or occupational functioning.

Behaviors typical of ADHD occur more commonly in children who have experienced violence and emotional abuse.

ADHD is commonly associated with:

1. Depression
2. Anxiety disorders
3. Bipolar disorders
4. Personality disorders
5. Learning disabilities, Tourette syndrome
6. Substance abuse (alcohol most common), sleep disorders may also be associated.

Psychiatry

1. Which of the following is not a defense mechanism in OCD?

a. Reaction formation
b. Projection
c. Isolation
d. Suppression
e. Undoing

Ans. b, d *Ref: Kaplan and Sadock's comprehensive textbook of psychiatry, 9/e*

Option a	False	Is a defense mechanism
Option b	True	Projection is a primitive form of paranoia
Option c	False	Is a defense mechanism
Option d	True	Delay paying attention to an emotion
Option e	False	Is a defense mechanism

Three ego defense mechanisms are common in OCD:

- Isolation,
- Undoing, and
- Reaction formation
- *Isolation*—People unconsciously isolate and disown undesirable thoughts, experiencing them as foreign intrusions.
- *Undoing*—People unconsciously cancel out an unacceptable desire or act by performing another act.
- *Reaction formation*—A person suppresses an unacceptable desire by taking on a lifestyle that expresses the opposite desire.

Projection—It is a psychological defense mechanism in which individuals attribute characteristics they find unacceptable in themselves to another person. For example, a husband who has a hostile nature might attribute this hostility to his wife and say she has an anger management problem.

Suppression—The conscious decision to delay paying attention to an emotion or need in order to cope with the present reality; able to later access the emotion and accept it.

2. Features of delirium tremens include:

a. Seen in methanol withdrawal
b. Visual hallucination
c. Auditory hallucination
d. Not a severe alcohol withdrawal syndrome
e. Predominantly low voltage fast activity on EEG

Ans. b, c, e *Ref: Kaplan Sadock's comprehensive textbook of psychiatry, 9/e*

Option a	False	Most severe form of ethanol withdrawal
Option b	True	
Option c	True	
Option d	False	Most severe form of ethanol withdrawal
Option e	True	

Delirium tremens (withdrawal tremens):

- Most severe form of ethanol withdrawal.

DSM-5 criteria for withdrawal delirium (Delirium tremens).*
Criteria of alcohol withdrawal Cessation of or reduction in heavy and prolonged use of alcohol. At least two of eight possible symptoms after reduced use of alcohol: • Autonomic hyperactivity • Hand tremor • Insomnia • Nausea or vomiting • Transient hallucinations or illusions • Psychomotor agitation • Anxiety • Generalized tonic-clonic seizures. **Criteria for delirium** • Decreased attention and awareness. • Disturbance in attention, awareness, memory, orientation, language, visuospatial ability, perception, or all of these abilities that is a change from the normal level and fluctuates in severity during the day. • Disturbances in memory, orientation, language, visuospatial ability, or perception. • No evidence of coma or other evolving neurocognitive disorders.

*The criteria are based on the *Diagnostic and Statistical Manual of Mental Disorders*, fifth edition (DSM-5). A patient who meets the criteria for both alcohol withdrawal and delirium is considered to have withdrawal delirium.

- Chronic intake of alcohol affects:
  - Increased release of endogenous opiates.
  - Activation of the inhibitory gamma-aminobutyric acid-A (GABA-A) receptor producing increased GABA inhibition, with a resultant influx of chloride ions.
  - Upregulation of the postsynaptic N-methyl-D-aspartate (NMDA) type of glutamate receptor, which mediates the postsynaptic excitatory effects of glutamate.
  - Interactions with serotonin and dopamine receptors.
- During alcohol withdrawal, the loss of GABA-A receptor stimulation causes a reduction in chloride flux and is associated with tremors, diaphoresis, tachycardia, anxiety, and seizures.
- Withdrawal delirium usually begins about 3 days after the appearance of symptoms of alcohol withdrawal and lasts from 1 to 8 days or more.
- Clinical manifestations include:
  - Agitation,
  - Global confusion,
  - Disorientation,
  - Hallucinations (visual, auditory and tactile),
  - Fever,
  - Hypertension,
  - Diaphoresis,
  - Heavy sweating, and
  - Autonomic hyperactivity (tachycardia and hypertension).

Profound global confusion is the hallmark of delirium tremens.

EEG shows low voltage fast activity. *Recovery is slower if the low voltage fast activity is in great amount.*

3. Brain stimulation techniques are all *except*:

a. Electroconvulsive therapy
b. Cognitive therapy
c. Repetitive transcranial magnetic stimulation
d. Deep brain stimulation
e. Transcranial magnetic stimulation

Ans. b *Ref: Kaplan Sadock's comprehensive textbook of psychiatry, 9/e*

Option a	False	Is a brain stimulation technique
Option b	True	Is a psychotherapy
Option c	False	Is a brain stimulation technique
Option d	False	Is a brain stimulation technique
Option e	False	Is a brain stimulation technique

1. **Transcranial magnetic stimulation (TMS)** is a *non-invasive* clinical treatment option, usually reserved for those suffering from severe treatment-resistant depression. Currently TMS is the most commonly practiced brain stimulation technique in the medical field.
2. **Repetitive transcranial magnetic stimulation (rTMS)** is an electromagnetic, *non-invasive* therapy similar to TMS. Due to the increase in strength of electromagnetic induction, rTMS has the potential to solidify longer lasting changes in the brain.
3. **Electroconvulsive therapy** (previously known as electroshock therapy) is also a *non-invasive* brain stimulation technique, utilized in controlled clinical and research settings. ECT is reserved to treat only severe psychiatric illnesses which have proven resistant to other forms of treatment, and is usually considered as a "last resort" treatment option.
4. **Deep brain stimulation** is an invasive stimulation technique. Invasive brain stimulation involves a preliminary procedure to surgically implant parts of the stimulation device into the patient's brain.

Cognitive-behavioral therapy is a relatively short-term, focused psychotherapy for a wide range of psychological problems including depression, anxiety, anger, marital conflict, loneliness, panic, fears, eating disorders, substance abuse, alcohol abuse and dependence and personality problems.

4. Beck's cognitive triad of depression includes:

a. Self
b. Future
c. Past experience
d. World
e. Others

Ans. a, b, d *Ref: An Overview of Beck's Cognitive Theory of Depression in Contemporary Literature. Rochester Institute of Technology*

Option a	True	
Option b	True	
Option c	False	
Option d	True	
Option e	False	

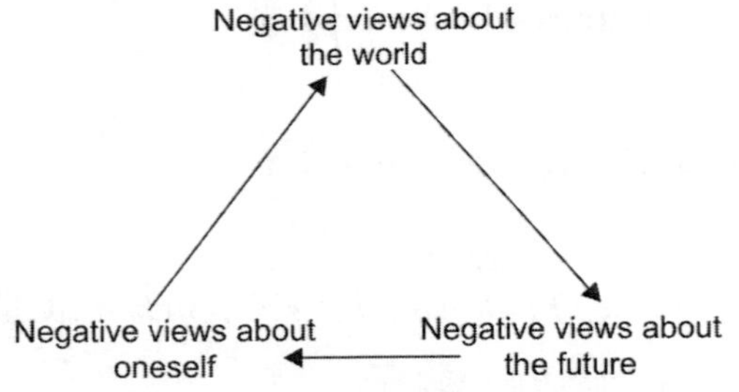

Fig. 19.1: Beck's cognitive triad.

Beck's cognitive triad, also known as the negative triad, is an irrational and pessimistic view of the three key elements of a person's belief system present in depression. It was proposed by Aaron Beck in 1976.

The triad involves "automatic, spontaneous and seemingly uncontrollable negative thoughts" about:

- The *self*
- The *world or environment*
- The *future*

Examples of this negative thinking include:

The self—'Nobody loves me.'
The world—'The world is an unfair place.'
The future—'I will always be a failure.'

5. Personality type associated with coronary artery disease:

a. A
b. B
c. C
d. D
e. E

Ans. a *Ref: Kaplan Sadock's comprehensive textbook of psychiatry, 9/e*

Option a	True	People with personality type A seem to be more prone to heart disease, are typically more driven, impatient, energetic and ambitious
Option b	False	
Option c	False	
Option d	False	
Option e	False	

- Persons with ***Type A personality*** tend to focus on competition. They love to achieve greatness and they don't like it when it takes a lot of time to experience success. When type A behavior was studied in different countries and social groups, it was found not to be a robust predictor of CHD.
- People who have a ***Type B personality*** tend to be more relaxed. They don't take stressful situations personally.
- People who have a ***Type C personality*** like to focus on the fine details of any given situation.
- People who have a ***Type D personality*** tend to see the world in a very negative way. Although there may be situations that most people would find to be optimistic, this personality type will always be pessimistic about any potential outcome.

6. Not included in diagnostic criteria for major depressive disorder:

a. Hypersomnia
b. Insomnia
c. Loss of pleasure in every activity
d. Guilt feeling
e. Sudden mood changes

Ans. e *Ref: Kaplan Sadock's comprehensive textbook of psychiatry, 9/e*

Option a	False	Included in diagnostic criteria for major depressive disorder
Option b	False	
Option c	False	
Option d	False	
Option e	True	Not included in diagnostic criteria for major depressive disorder

Diagnostic criteria for major depressive disorder and depressive episodes

DSM-IV criteria for major depressive disorder (MDD)

- ❑ Depressed mood or a loss of interest or pleasure in daily activities for more than two weeks.
- ❑ Mood represents a change from the person's baseline.
- ❑ Impaired function: Social, occupational, educational.
- ❑ Specific symptoms, at least 5 of these 9, present *nearly every day*:
  1. **Depressed mood or irritable** most of the day, nearly every day, as indicated by either subjective report (e.g., feels sad or empty) or observation made by others (e.g., appears tearful).
  2. **Decreased interest or pleasure** in most activities, most of each day.
  3. **Significant weight change (5%) or change in appetite.**
  4. **Change in sleep:** Insomnia or hypersomnia.
  5. **Change in activity:** Psychomotor agitation or retardation.
  6. **Fatigue or loss of energy.**
  7. **Guilt/worthlessness:** Feelings of worthlessness or excessive or inappropriate guilt.
  8. **Concentration:** Diminished ability to think or concentrate, or more indecisiveness.
  9. **Suicidality:** Thought of death or suicide, or has suicide plan.

7. True about generalized anxiety disorder (GAD) are:

a. Benzodiazepines are drug of choice
b. Duration is for a few days
c. Because of drug abuse
d. SSRIs offer effective treatment
e. Physical activity can improve symptoms of GAD

Ans. d, e *Ref: Kaplan Sadock's comprehensive textbook of psychiatry, 9/e; DSM5 Diagnostic Criteria Generalized Anxiety Disorder*

Option a	False	Use is limited by risk of abuse and adverse effect profiles.
Option b	False	Symptoms occurring for more number of days for at least 6 months
Option c	False	Not attributable to the physiological effects of a substance
Option d	True	Used as first line of therapy
Option e	True	Physical activity is a cost-effective approach in the treatment of GAD

Generalized anxiety disorder (GAD)- DSM-5™ diagnostic criteria

A. Excessive anxiety and worry (apprehensive expectation), occurring more days for at least 6 months, about a number of events or activities (such as work or school performance).
B. The individual finds it difficult to control the worry.
C. The anxiety and worry are associated with three (or more) of the following six symptoms (with at least some symptoms having been present for more days than others for the past 6 months):
(Note: Only one item required in children).
1. Restlessness, feeling keyed up or on edge.
2. Being easily fatigued.
3. Difficulty concentrating or mind going blank.
4. Irritability.
5. Muscle tension.
6. Sleep disturbance (difficulty falling or staying asleep, or restless, unsatisfying sleep).

D. The anxiety, worry, or physical symptoms cause clinically significant distress or impairment in social, occupational, or other important areas of functioning.
E. The disturbance is not attributable to the physiological effects of a substance (e.g., a drug of abuse, a medication) or another medical condition (e.g., hyperthyroidism).
F. The disturbance is not better explained by another medical disorder (e.g., anxiety or worry about having panic attacks in panic disorder, negative evaluation in social anxiety disorder [social phobia],contamination or other obsessions in obsessive-compulsive disorder, separation from attachment figures in separation anxiety disorder, reminders of traumatic events in posttraumatic stress disorder, gaining weight in anorexia nervosa, physical complaints in somatic symptom disorder, perceived appearance flaws in body dysmorphic disorder, having a serious illness in illness anxiety disorder, or the content of delusional beliefs in schizophrenia or delusional disorder).

Treatment:

- Selective serotonin reuptake inhibitors and/or
- Psychotherapy, both of which are highly effective.
- Among psychotherapeutic treatments, cognitive behavior therapy has been studied widely and has an extensive evidence base.
- Benzodiazepines are effective in reducing anxiety symptoms, but their use is limited by risk of abuse and adverse effect profiles.
- Physical activity can reduce symptoms.

8. Maximum score in mini mental state examination (MMSE) include:

a. 5 b. 10
c. 20 d. 30
e. 40

Ans. d

Ref: Folstein M, Folstein SE, McHugh PR "Mini-mental state" A practical method for grading the cognitive state of patients for the clinician. Journal of Psychiatric Research, 12(3); 189-198.

Option a	False	
Option b	False	
Option c	False	
Option d	True	Maximum score is 30
Option e	False	

- **The mini mental state examination (MMSE)** is a tool that can be used to systematically and thoroughly assess mental status.
- Effective as a screening tool for cognitive impairment with older, community dwelling, hospitalized and institutionalized adults.
- It is an 11-question measure that tests five areas of cognitive function:
  - Orientation,
  - Registration,
  - Attention and calculation,
  - Recall, and
  - Language.
- The maximum score is 30.
- A score of 23 or lower is indicative of cognitive impairment.
- When used repeatedly the instrument is able to measure changes in cognitive status that may benefit from intervention.
- However, the tool is not able to diagnose the case for changes in cognitive function and should not replace a complete clinical assessment of mental status.
- In addition, the instrument relies heavily on verbal response and reading and writing. Therefore, patients that are hearing and visually impaired, intubated, have low English literacy, or those with other communication disorders may perform poorly even when cognitively intact.

Section	Questions	Max points	Score
1. Orientation	a. Can you tell me today's (data)/(month)/(year)? Which day is today? Can you tell me which (season) it is?	5	
	b. What town/city are we in? What is the (county)/(country)? What (building) are we in and on what (floor)?	5	
2. Registration	I should like to test your memory. (Name three common objects: "ball, car, man") Can you repeat the words I said? (*1 point per word*) (Repeat up to 6 trials until all three are remembered)	3	
3. Attention and Calculation	a. From 100 keep subtracting 7 and give each answer. Stop after 5 answers. (93–86–79–72–65). Alternatively: b. Spell the word "World" backwards (D_L_R_O_W)	5	
4. Recall	What were the three words I asked you to say earlier? (*Skip this test if all of these objects were not remembered during the registration test*)	3	
5. Language Naming Repeating	Name the following objects (show a watch) and (show a pencil)	2	
	Repeat the following: "No ifs, ands or buts"	1	

Contd...

Contd...

Section	Questions	Max points	Score
6. Reading Writing	(Show card or write: "Close your Eyes") Read this sentence and do what it says	1	
	Now can you write a short sentence for me?	1	
7. Three stage command	(Present paper) Take this paper in your left (or right) hand, fold it in half, and place it on the floor	3	
8. Construction	Will you copy this drawing please?	1	
Total score		**30**	

Image: Mini mental state examination

MMSE Scoring	
24–30	No cognitive impairment
18–23	Mild cognitive impairment
0–17	Severe cognitive impairment